1995
YEAR BOOK OF
SURGERY®

Statement of Purpose

The YEAR BOOK Service

The YEAR BOOK series was devised in 1901 by practicing health professionals who observed that the literature of medicine and related disciplines had become so voluminous that no one individual could read and place in perspective every potential advance in a major specialty. In the final decade of the 20th century, this recognition is more acutely true than it was in 1901.

More than merely a series of books, YEAR BOOK volumes are the tangible results of a unique service designed to accomplish the following:

- to *survey* a wide range of journals of proven value
- to *select* from those journals papers representing significant advances and statements of important clinical principles
- to provide *abstracts* of those articles that are readable, convenient summaries of their key points
- to provide *commentary* about those articles to place them in perspective

These publications grow out of a unique process that calls on the talents of outstanding authorities in clinical and fundamental disciplines, trained literature specialists, and professional writers, all supported by the resources of Mosby, the world's preeminent publisher for the health professions.

The Literature Base

Mosby subscribes to nearly 1,000 journals published worldwide, covering the full range of the health professions. On an annual basis, the publisher examines usage patterns and polls its expert authorities to add new journals to the literature base and to delete journals that are no longer useful as potential YEAR BOOK sources.

The Literature Survey

The publisher's team of literature specialists, all of whom are trained and experienced health professionals, examines every original, peer-reviewed article in each journal issue. More than 250,000 articles per year are scanned systematically, including title, text, illustrations, tables, and references. Each scan is compared, article by article, to the search strategies that the publisher has developed in consultation with the 270 outside experts who form the pool of YEAR BOOK editors. A given article may be reviewed by any number of editors, from one to a dozen or more, regardless of the discipline for which the paper was originally published. In turn, each editor who receives the article reviews it to determine whether or not the article should be included in the YEAR BOOK. This decision is based on the article's inherent quality, its probable usefulness to readers of that YEAR BOOK, and the editor's goal to represent a balanced picture of a given field in each volume of the YEAR BOOK. In addition, the editor indicates when to include figures and tables from the article to help the YEAR BOOK reader better understand the information.

Of the quarter million articles scanned each year, only 5% are selected for detailed analysis within the YEAR BOOK series, thereby assuring readers of the high value of every selection.

The Abstract

The publisher's abstracting staff is headed by a physician-writer and includes individuals with training in the life sciences, medicine, and other areas, plus extensive experience in writing for the health professions and related industries. Each selected article is assigned to a specific writer on this abstracting staff. The abstracter, guided in many cases by notations supplied by the expert editor, writes a structured, condensed summary designed so that the reader can rapidly acquire the essential information contained in the article.

The Commentary

The YEAR BOOK editorial boards, sometimes assisted by guest commentators, write comments that place each article in perspective for the reader. This provides the reader with the equivalent of a personal consultation with a leading international authority—an opportunity to better understand the value of the article and to benefit from the authority's thought processes in assessing the article.

Additional Editorial Features

The editorial boards of each YEAR BOOK organize the abstracts and comments to provide a logical and satisfying sequence of information. To enhance the organization, editors also provide introductions to sections or individual chapters, comments linking a number of abstracts, citations to additional literature, and other features.

The published YEAR BOOK contains enhanced bibliographic citations for each selected article, including extended listings of multiple authors and identification of author affiliations. Each YEAR BOOK contains a Table of Contents specific to that year's volume. From year to year, the Table of Contents for a given YEAR BOOK will vary depending on developments within the field.

Every YEAR BOOK contains a list of the journals from which papers have been selected. This list represents a subset of the nearly 1,000 journals surveyed by the publisher and occasionally reflects a particularly pertinent article from a journal that is not surveyed on a routine basis.

Finally, each volume contains a comprehensive subject index and an index to authors of each selected paper.

The 1995 Year Book Series

Year Book of Allergy and Clinical Immunology: Drs. Rosenwasser, Borish, Gelfand, Leung, Nelson, and Szefler

Year Book of Anesthesiology and Pain Management: Drs. Tinker, Abram, Chestnut, Roizen, Rothenberg, and Wood

Year Book of Cardiology®: Drs. Schlant, Collins, Engle, Gersh, Kaplan, and Waldo

Year Book of Chiropractic®: Dr. Lawrence

Year Book of Critical Care Medicine®: Drs. Parrillo, Balk, Calvin, Franklin, and Shapiro

Year Book of Dentistry®: Drs. Meskin, Berry, Currier, Kennedy, Leinfelder, Roser, and Zakariasen

Year Book of Dermatologic Surgery®: Drs. Swanson, Glogau, and Salasche

Year Book of Dermatology®: Drs. Sober and Fitzpatrick

Year Book of Diagnostic Radiology®: Drs. Federle, Clark, Gross, Latchaw, Madewell, Maynard, and Young

Year Book of Digestive Diseases®: Drs. Greenberger and Moody

Year Book of Drug Therapy®: Drs. Lasagna and Weintraub

Year Book of Emergency Medicine®: Drs. Wagner, Dronen, Davidson, King, Niemann, and Roberts

Year Book of Endocrinology®: Drs. Bagdade, Braverman, Horton, Kannan, Landsberg, Molitch, Morley, Nathan, Odell, Poehlman, Rogol, and Ryan

Year Book of Family Practice®: Drs. Berg, Bowman, Davidson, Dexter, Dietrich, and Scherger

Year Book of Geriatrics and Gerontology®: Drs. Beck, Burton, Goldstein, Reuben, Small, and Whitehouse

Year Book of Hand Surgery®: Drs. Amadio and Hentz

Year Book of Hematology®: Drs. Spivak, Bell, Ness, Quesenberry, Wiernik, and Blume

Year Book of Infectious Diseases®: Drs. Keusch, Barza, Bennish, Gelfand, Klempner, Snydman, and Skolnik

Year Book of Infertility and Reproductive Endocrinology: Drs. Mishell, Lobo, and Sokol

Year Book of Medicine®: Drs. Bone, Cline, Epstein, Greenberger, Malawista, Mandell, O'Rourke, and Utiger

Year Book of Neonatal and Perinatal Medicine®: Drs. Fanaroff and Klaus

Year Book of Nephrology®: Drs. Coe, Favus, Henderson, Kashgarian, Luke, and Curtis

Year Book of Neurology and Neurosurgery®: Drs. Bradley and Wilkins

Year Book of Neuroradiology: Drs. Osborn, Eskridge, Grossman, Hudgins, and Ross

Year Book of Nuclear Medicine®: Drs. Gottschalk, Blaufox, McAfee, Wackers, and Zubal

Year Book of Obstetrics and Gynecology®: Drs. Mishell, Kirschbaum, and Morrow

Year Book of Occupational and Environmental Medicine®: Drs. Emmett, Frank, Gochfeld, and Hessl

Year Book of Oncology®: Drs. Simone, Bosl, Glatstein, Ozols, and Steele

Year Book of Ophthalmology®: Drs. Cohen, Adams, Augsburger, Benson, Eagle, Flanagan, Grossman, Laibson, Nelson, Rapuano, Reinecke, Sergott, Tasman, Tipperman, and Wilson

Year Book of Orthopedics®: Drs. Sledge, Cofield, Dobyns, Griffin, Poss, Springfield, Swiontkowski, Wiesel, and Wilson

Year Book of Otolaryngology–Head and Neck Surgery®: Drs. Paparella and Holt

Year Book of Pain: Drs. Gebhart, Haddox, Jacox, Janjan, Marcus, Rudy, and Shapiro

Year Book of Pathology and Laboratory Medicine: Drs. Mills, Bruns, Gaffey, and Stoler

Year Book of Pediatrics®: Dr. Stockman

Year Book of Plastic, Reconstructive, and Aesthetic Surgery: Drs. Miller, Cohen, McKinney, Robson, Ruberg, and Whitaker

Year Book of Podiatric Medicine and Surgery®: Dr. Kominsky

Year Book of Psychiatry and Applied Mental Health®: Drs. Talbott, Breier, Frances, Meltzer, Schowalter, Tasman, and Yudofsky

Year Book of Pulmonary Disease®: Drs. Bone and Petty

Year Book of Rheumatology®: Drs. Sergent, LeRoy, Meenan, Panush, and Reichlin

Year Book of Sports Medicine®: Drs. Shephard, Drinkwater, Eichner, Torg, Col. Anderson, and Mr. George

Year Book of Surgery®: Drs. Copeland, Bland, Deitch, Eberlein, Howard, Luce, Seeger, Souba, and Sugarbaker

Year Book of Thoracic and Cardiovascular Surgery®: Drs. Ginsberg, Lofland, and Wechsler

Year Book of Transplantation®: Drs. Sollinger, Eckhoff, Hullett, Knechtle, Longo, Mentzer, and Pirsch

Year Book of Ultrasound®: Drs. Merritt, Babcock, Carroll, Fagan, Finberg, and Fleischer

Year Book of Urology®: Drs. DeKernion and Howards

Year Book of Vascular Surgery®: Dr. Porter

1995

The Year Book of SURGERY®

Editor-in-Chief
Edward M. Copeland, III, M.D.

Editorial Board
Kirby I. Bland, M.D.
Edwin A. Deitch, M.D.
Timothy J. Eberlein, M.D.
Richard J. Howard, M.D., Ph.D.
Edward A. Luce, M.D.
James M. Seeger, M.D., F.A.C.S.
Wiley W. Souba, M.D., Sc.D.
David J. Sugarbaker, M.D.

Contributing Editors
Joseph F. Amaral, M.D.
H. Hank Simms, M.D.
Victor E. Pricolo, M.D.

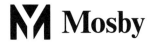 Mosby

St. Louis Baltimore Boston Carlsbad Chicago Naples New York Philadelphia Portland
London Madrid Mexico City Singapore Sydney Tokyo Toronto Wiesbaden

Vice President and Publisher, Continuity Publishing: Kenneth H. Killion
Director, Editorial Development: Gretchen C. Murphy
Assistant Developmental Editor, Continuity: Maria Danan
Acquisitions Editor: Jennifer Roche
Illustrations and Permissions Coordinator: Steven J. Ramay
Manager, Continuity–EDP: Maria Nevinger
Project Manager, Editing: Tamara L. Smith
Senior Project Manager, Production: Max F. Perez
Freelance Staff Supervisor: Barbara M. Kelly
Director, Editorial Services: Edith M. Podrazik, R.N.
Senior Information Specialist: Terri Santo, R.N.
Information Specialist: Kathleen Moss, R.N.
Senior Medical Writer: David A. Cramer, M.D.
Vice President, Professional Sales and Marketing: George M. Parker
Senior Marketing Manager: Eileen M. Lynch
Marketing Specialist: Lynn D. Stevenson

Printed in the United States of America
Composition by Reed Technology and Information Services, Inc.
Printing/binding by Maple-Vail

Mosby–Year Book, Inc.
11830 Westline Industrial Drive
St. Louis, MO 63146

Editorial Office:
Mosby–Year Book, Inc.
200 North LaSalle Street
Chicago, IL 60601
International Standard Serial Number: 0090-3671
International Standard Book Number: 0-8151-7794-1

Table of Contents

Mosby Document Express

Copies of the full text of the original source documents of articles abstracted or referenced in this publication are available by calling Mosby Document Express, toll-free, at **1 (800) 55-MOSBY.**

With Mosby Document Express, you have convenient, 24-hour-a-day access to literally every article on which this publication is based. In fact, through Mosby Document Express, virtually any medical or scientific article can be located and delivered by FAX, overnight delivery service, international airmail, electronic transmission of bitmapped images (via Internet), or regular mail. The average cost of a complete, delivered copy of an article, including up to $4 in copyright clearance charges and first-class mail delivery, is $12.

For inquiries and pricing information, please call the toll-free number shown above. To expedite your order for material appearing in this publication, please be prepared with the code shown next to the bibliographic citation for each abstract.

Journals Represented

Mosby subscribes to and surveys nearly 1,000 U.S. and foreign medical and allied health journals. From these journals, the Editors select the articles to be abstracted. Journals represented in this YEAR BOOK are listed below.

Acta Endocrinologica
American Journal of Clinical Nutrition
American Journal of Emergency Medicine
American Journal of Medicine
American Journal of Pathology
American Journal of Physiology
American Journal of Respiratory and Critical Care Medicine
American Journal of Surgery
American Journal of Surgical Pathology
American Surgeon
Anaesthesia and Intensive Care
Annals of Otology, Rhinology and Laryngology
Annals of Plastic Surgery
Annals of Surgery
Annals of Surgical Oncology
Annals of Thoracic Surgery
Annals of Vascular Surgery
Annals of the Royal College of Surgeons of England
Archives of Otolaryngology-Head and Neck Surgery
Archives of Surgery
British Journal of Radiology
British Journal of Surgery
British Medical Journal
Burns
Canadian Journal of Surgery
Cancer
Cancer Research
Chest
Clinical Investigator
Clinical Transplantation
Critical Care Medicine
Digestive Diseases and Sciences
Diseases of the Colon and Rectum
European Journal of Cancer
European Journal of Plastic Surgery
European Journal of Surgery
Gastroenterology
Gut
Head and Neck
Hepatology
Infection Control and Hospital Epidemiology
International Journal of Radiation, Oncology, Biology, and Physics
Journal of Burn Care and Rehabilitation
Journal of Clinical Oncology
Journal of Emergency Medicine
Journal of Experimental Medicine
Journal of Gerontology
Journal of Laryngology and Otology
Journal of Pain and Symptom Management
Journal of Surgical Oncology

Journal of Surgical Research
Journal of Thoracic and Cardiovascular Surgery
Journal of Trauma
Journal of Vascular Surgery
Journal of the American College of Surgeons
Journal of the American Medical Association
Journal of the Royal College of Surgeons of Edinburgh
Lancet
Laryngoscope
New England Journal of Medicine
Pediatric Nephrology
Pharmacotherapy
Plastic and Reconstructive Surgery
Proceedings of the National Academy of Sciences
Quarterly Journal of Medicine
Radiology
S.A.M.J./S.A.M.T. - South African Medical Journal
Stroke
Surgery
Thorax
Transplantation
Transplantation Proceedings
World Journal of Surgery
Wound Repair and Regeneration

STANDARD ABBREVIATIONS

The following terms are abbreviated in this edition: acquired immunodeficiency syndrome (AIDS), cardiopulmonary resuscitation (CPR), central nervous system (CNS), cerebrospinal fluid (CSF), computed tomography (CT), deoxyribonucleic acid (DNA), electrocardiography (ECG), health maintenance organization (HMO), human immunodeficiency virus (HIV), intensive care unit (ICU), intramuscular (IM), intravenous (IV), magnetic resonance (MR) imaging (MRI), and ribonucleic acid (RNA).

NOTE

The YEAR BOOK OF SURGERY is a literature survey service providing abstracts of articles published in the professional literature. Every effort is made to assure the accuracy of the information presented in these pages. Neither the editors nor the publisher of the YEAR BOOK OF SURGERY can be responsible for errors in the original materials. The editors' comments are their own opinions. Mention of specific products within this publication does not constitute endorsement.

1 General Considerations

Introduction

Cost containment is the buzzword of the 1990s, as is the phrase "shrinking health care dollar." There is little question that too many tests have been ordered for preoperative screening of healthy patients and for routine follow-up of asymptomatic patients with cancer who undergo surgery for cure. Nevertheless, we have tried so hard to get people to "go to the doctor," that it seems a shame now to discourage such behavior. Prevention and early diagnosis are cornerstones of cost containment. Outcomes data and resource consumption are emerging for treatment of elderly patients, emergency medicine, surgical complications, and day-care surgery. Attempts to predict postoperative complications from a set of preoperative data have been undertaken in areas other than nutritional assessment. Certain techniques, such as methods of central venous catheterization, are being reevaluated to correlate cost with the complication rate. In addition, simple observations, such as the increase in experimental wound infection caused by cornstarch on gloves, may result in long-term cost reductions even though powder-free gloves are initially more expensive.

In a study from Vanderbilt University, information from the National Practitioner Data Bank did not identify any measures of quality of clinical care between physicians who are sued frequently and those who are sued infrequently. In fact, many suits arose because of poor communication between physician and patient and a perceived lack of concern and respect for the patient.

The shrinking dollar will decrease or eliminate cross-subsidization of research and education within academic centers unless fewer personnel are employed or salaries are reduced. Retirement has become a topic at national meetings. Many physicians who can retire are doing so at an earlier age rather than tolerate the shifting health care scene. Younger physicians, however, may have to work longer and plan better financially early in their careers to accomplish their monetary goals for retirement. In addition, the necessity to increase surgical volume to maintain income may have a negative effect on surgical education, especially at the junior resident level, where attainment of technical skills is time-consuming. Veteran's Administration (VA) hospitals will become even more important educational affiliates. Quality of care in VA hospitals affiliated with

1

university teaching hospitals is equivalent to nonfederal hospitals. Surgical education may well have improved quality of care in VA hospitals rather than having had a negative effect.

Before mandatory testing of surgeons for HIV infection is legislated, an appropriate disability insurance program should be in place for physicians who have a positive test result. The public is safe, because the risk of a patient contracting AIDS from an infected surgeon appears to be minimal. Some techniques could be altered to protect both patients and surgeons. For example, blunt-tipped needles could be used for abdominal wound closure. A change in suture material as a cost-containment measure, however, may be unwise, because surgeons who are unfamiliar with a new suture or needle may cause more injury to themselves and to the patient.

A potpourri of subjects were selected for this introductory segment because of individual interest in the topics. Is a shortage of organ donors linked to the decrease in autopsy rate? Are so many authors' names on surgical publications necessary? What is the surgical personality and what music, if any, should we listen to in the operating room? Patients always seem to be in pain on emergence from anesthesia. Why not give pain medication at the time of wound closure?

Edward M. Copeland, III, M.D.

Preoperative Laboratory Screening Based on Age, Gender, and Concomitant Medical Diseases

Velanovich V (Madigan Army Med Ctr, Tacoma, Wash)
Surgery 115:56–61, 1994   140-95-1–1

Introduction.—A wide variety of laboratory screening tests that are performed routinely before surgery have come under scrutiny. Some studies have found that the tests are underused once obtained and are neither cost-effective nor predictive of postoperative complications. Patients who were undergoing elective operations were followed to determine the most effective laboratory screening.

Methods.—Five hundred twenty patients who were undergoing elective operations in the general, vascular, thoracic, and head and neck surgical services were included. Data evaluated included patient age, gender, race, American Society of Anesthesiologists physical status classification, ponderal index, and the presence of concomitant respiratory disease, coronary artery disease, and other significant conditions. Preoperative screening included measurement of levels of electrolytes, blood urea nitrogen, creatinine, and glucose; hemogram; nutritional studies; coagulation studies; urinalysis; ECG; and chest radiograph. Results were examined by univariate analysis and by multivariate analysis with stepwise logistic regression.

Suggested Routine Preoperative Screening Based on Associated
Clinical Conditions

Age	Gender	ASA class III and IV
> 30 yr	BUN/creatinine	BUN/Creatinine
ECG	ECG	Glucose
> 60 yr	Chest radiograph	Hemogram
ECG		Nutritional studies
Chest radiograph		Coagulation studies
BUN/Creatinine	**Coronary disease**	ECG
	BUN/Creatinine	Chest radiograph
	ECG	
Respiratory disease	**Malignancy**	**Other heart disease**
Chest radiograph	Hemogram	BUN/Creatinine
	Nutritional studies	ECG
Kidney disease		
BUN/Creatinine		
Glucose	**Diabetes mellitus**	**Vascular disease**
Hemogram	BUN/Creatinine	BUN/Creatinine
	Glucose	ECG
Hypertension	Hemogram	Chest radiograph
Electrolytes	ECG	
Glucose		
BUN/Creatinine		
ECG		

(Courtesy of Velanovich V: *Surgery* 115:56–61, 1994.)

Results.—In univariate analysis, age, gender, and the specific concomitant illness were associated with specific abnormal preoperative laboratory results. Correlations were generally high between the univariate and multivariate analyses. On the basis of findings in this series of patients, only certain preoperative screening tests would by required for certain patients. For those with associated malignancy, for example, the hemogram and nutritional studies would be useful. Glucose, hemogram, blood urea nitrogen/creatinine, nutritional studies, coagulation studies, ECG, and chest radiograph are suggested for patients with American Society of Anesthesiologists class III and IV. Unless otherwise indicated by a specific condition, a chest radiograph is recommended only for patients older than 60 years of age (table).

Conclusion.—Many items included in routine preoperative laboratory testing are neither useful nor cost-effective. Data on patient age, gender, concomitant medical disease, and the type of operation can be used to determine appropriate preoperative laboratory screening. Routine screening preoperative laboratory tests are often not cost-effective in evaluating patients without symptoms and do not necessarily help in assessing perioperative risk.

▶ This study points out what most of us have known for some time: many preoperative studies in asymptomatic, healthy patients who are younger than 70 years of age are of minimal value. We continue to obtain many of these studies for historic reasons, i.e., we ordered the tests during our residency training, or for defensive reasons, i.e., we fear malpractice suits. Enormous savings in health care costs can immediately accrue by reducing preoperative tests and ordering appropriate tests based on the clinical situation rather than tradition.—E.M. Copeland, III, M.D.

Impact of Follow-Up Testing on Survival and Health-Related Quality of Life in Breast Cancer Patients: A Multicenter Randomized Controlled Trial

The GIVIO Investigators (Interdisciplinary Group for Cancer Care Evaluation, Milan, Italy)
JAMA 271:1587–1592, 1994   140-95-1–2

Objective.—Whether a program of very intensive surveillance is worthwhile when following women who have undergone resection of breast cancer was determined in a prospective, randomized trial involving 26 general hospitals in Italy.

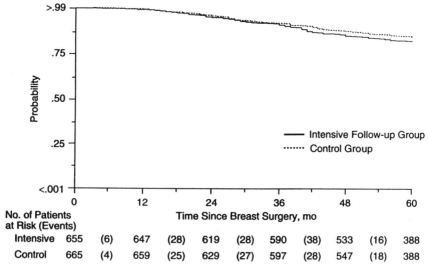

Fig 1–1.—Survival by follow-up regimen. Data are based on 655 patients in the intensive follow-up group who had 132 events of disease and 665 patients in the control group who had 122 events of disease (log rank test = .656; P = .42). (Courtesy of The GIVIO Investigators: JAMA 271:1587–1592, 1994.)

Study Plan.—A total of 1,320 women younger than 70 years of age who had unilateral primary stage I–III breast cancers were included. Six hundred sixty-five women were assigned to have bone scanning, echographic study of the liver, chest roentgenography, and laboratory tests at fixed intervals. The remaining women were seen by a physician at the same intervals but had only those tests that were clinically indicated. Health-related quality of life was assessed using 4 instruments 6 months after randomization, and again after 1, 2, and 5 years. The 2 groups were treated in the same manner. Women with involved lymph nodes received chemotherapy if they were premenopausal or tamoxifen if they were postmenopausal. All patients had mammography annually to detect cancer in the other breast.

Outcome.—More than 80% of women in both groups complied with the assigned follow-up program. Approximately 4 of 5 women in each group were alive after a median follow-up of 6 years (Fig 1–1). Times to recurrence did not differ, and there were no significant group differences in overall health, symptomatic status, emotional well-being, or social functioning. Regardless of group assignment, more than 70% of women said that they wanted to see a physician at frequent intervals and have diagnostic tests, even if they were free of symptoms.

Implication.—Frequent testing has neither an objective nor subjective effect on the quality of life of women who undergo resection of stage I–III breast cancer. Routine medical surveillance is adequate for these patients.

Intensive Diagnostic Follow-Up After Treatment of Primary Breast Cancer: A Randomized Trial
Rosselli Del Turco M, for the National Research Council Project on Breast Cancer Follow-Up (Centro per lo Studio e la Prevenzione Oncologica, Florence, Italy)
JAMA 271:1593–1597, 1994   140-95-1–3

Background.—The survival benefits of early diagnosis of recurrent breast cancer are controversial. The efficacy of various follow-up procedures has been evaluated, but most studies have shown no survival difference with symptomatic vs. asymptomatic detection of recurrences. The most common pattern of initial recurrence is intrathoracic and bone metastases, which can be detected preclinically through periodic 2-view chest radiographs and bone scanning. The efficacy of an intensive follow-up approach including these imaging procedures was evaluated.

Methods.—A total of 1,243 consecutive premenopausal or postmenopausal patients who had undergone surgery for unilateral invasive breast carcinoma were included. None of the women had any evidence of metastases. They were assigned to receive either intensive or clinical follow-up for at least 5 years. Both groups received physical examination every 3 months for the first 2 years and every 6 months thereafter and annual mammography. The intensive follow-up group also underwent 2-view chest radiography and bone scanning every 6 months, on the basis of previous reports that suggested that the lead time gained by these screening tests is no longer than 3–6 months. The clinical follow-up group received no other diagnostic tests unless they had symptoms suggestive of recurrent cancer. The 2 groups were comparable in terms of clinical and prognostic characteristics.

Results.—Compliance with chest radiography and bone scans in the intensive follow-up group exceeded 75%. A total of 393 recurrences, 104 local and 289 distant, were noted during follow-up. Detection of isolated intrathoracic and bone metastases was increased in the intensive follow-up group, 112 vs. 71 cases. There were no differences between groups in metastases at other sites or in local or regional recurrences. The clinical follow-up group had a significantly higher 5-year relapse-free survival rate, although this difference was reduced when both relapses and deaths were included in the analysis. There was no significant difference in overall mortality rates at 5 years: 18.6% in the intensive follow-up group, and 19.5% in the clinical follow-up group.

Conclusions.—For women who undergo surgical treatment for primary breast cancer, intensive follow-up, including chest radiographs and bone scans, increases early detection of metastases. There is no reduction, however, in 5-year mortality rates. These imaging procedures should be performed only in patients with clinical examination findings suspicious for breast cancer recurrence.

▶ In times of medical cost containment, comparative trials to determine intensity of post-treatment follow-up for patients with cancer are extremely valuable. These 2 studies indicated that quality of life and survival were unaffected by detecting metastases when the patient was asymptomatic. In other words, waiting until symptoms developed before searching for metastatic sites gave equally good results when therapy was initiated. Earlier treatment did not result in a survival or quality of life advantage.

Many patients with multiple tumor types undergo more preoperative laboratory tests and roentgenograms than are necessary. For example, a patient with a thin, stage I melanoma needs no search for distant metastases before adequate surgical excision. The money saved by eliminating the unnecessary pre- and postoperative tests that are ordered by both surgeons and our medical colleagues could be staggering.—E.M. Copeland, III, M.D.

Psychological Effects of Routine Follow Up on Cancer Patients After Surgery
Kiebert GM, Welvaart K, Kievit J (Univ of Leiden, The Netherlands; State Univ

Hosp, Leiden, The Netherlands)
Eur J Surg 159:601–607, 1993   140-95-1–4

Background.—The few studies available concerning the effects of routine follow-up on the quality of life of patients with cancer have given conflicting results. The value that patients with cancer place on regular follow-up visits after surgery, the effects regular follow-up visits have on their well-being, and the variables that influence their well-being and attitudes to follow-up visits were assessed.

Methods.—A questionnaire was given to 127 patients who had undergone surgery for cancer. Group 1 included 67 patients who completed questionnaires 1 month before their scheduled follow-up visits. Group 2 included 60 patients who completed a questionnaire while they waited at the surgical outpatient department for their appointment. Group 2 patients were asked to complete another questionnaire 2 weeks later; 46 returned the completed questionnaire. The questionnaire for both groups included 3 sections. The first part assessed clinical and sociodemographic variables. The second part assessed patients' attitudes regarding regular follow up and fear of recurrence. The third part assessed the amount of psychological and physical stress in the preceding 7 days.

Results.—Most patients had a positive attitude about regular follow-up visits and were satisfied with their present schedule of appointments. Both psychological and physical distress were greatest in group 1 and least in group 2 (2 weeks after follow-up). Women reported more psychological distress than men. A lower standard of education and breast cancer in women were associated with more psychological distress. The approaching follow-up visits did not cause an increase in psychological or physical distress. When the results of the examinations and tests done at the follow-up visit gave no cause for alarm, the patients seemed to have a temporary decrease in psychological and physical distress.

Conclusions.—Patients who have undergone surgery for cancer generally welcome routine follow-up visits. A patient's general level of psychological and physical well-being, fear of recurrence, and attitude about follow up are influenced in a positive way by the reassuring effects of the visit. The task of reassuring patients with cancer should become a structural part of routine follow-up visits after surgery.

▶ Follow-up visits will be a target for reduction in managed care programs. Several randomized trials of intense follow-up with multiple radiologic and laboratory tests of asymptomatic patients with breast cancer have not shown a survival advantage for detecting metastases compared with targeted tests for symptomatic metastasis. Therefore, the data may support fewer visits after surgery. Nevertheless, the psychological support provided by frequent follow-up visits must not be overlooked.—E.M. Copeland, III, M.D.

Access and Outcomes of Elderly Patients Enrolled in Managed Care

Clement DG, Retchin SM, Brown RS, Stegall MH (Virginia Commonwealth Univ, Richmond; Mathematica Policy Research, Inc, Princeton, NJ; Univ of Osteopathic Medicine and Health Sciences, Des Moines, Iowa)
JAMA 271:1487–1492, 1994   140-95-1–5

Introduction.—Despite benefits of controlled cost and coordinated care, there is concern that HMO enrollment may limit access to necessary care for elderly patients. Random samples of Medicare beneficiaries from 75 HMOs and Medicare beneficiaries from the same market area receiving fee-for-service benefits were compared.

Methods.—Patients from both groups were interviewed by telephone. Patients with chronic joint pain or acute chest pain were questioned. Respondents were asked whether they saw a physician and then saw a specialist for follow-up. They were also asked whether their response to therapy was monitored and whether follow-up was recommended after the first visit.

Results.—Approximately one third of respondents in each group reported joint pain. Fewer than 10% from either group reported chest pain. Sociodemographics of both groups were similar for both symptoms. Enrollees in an HMO were significantly more likely than persons receiving fee-for-service to visit a physician and have medication prescribed for joint pain but less likely to have joint pain alleviated. Patients who were not enrolled in an HMO and had chest pain were more likely to have a physician visit, be referred to a specialist, have follow-up recommended, and have their progress closely monitored. There were no significant differences in the likelihood of receiving physical therapy for joint pain, having chest pain partially or totally alleviated, undergoing roentgenography, or receiving therapeutic interventions for either symptom.

Conclusion.—Despite differences in access and outcome between the 2 groups, outcomes were similar for 3 of 4 measures examined. Enrollees in an HMO tended to have a less satisfactory outcome for joint pain, but the similarity in the rate of roentgenograms ordered indicates that practice patterns are more similar than might be expected. With the likelihood of managed care increasing, continuous monitoring of access and outcomes is important.

▶ This study has the anticipated outcome: a decrease in both specialty referral and monitored follow-up visits for HMO patients. This result may be appropriate, particularly if outcomes are the same for large patient populations. A disturbing extension of these findings, however, is the potential absence of tertiary referral when indicated. For example, is an HMO general urologist qualified to treat a patient who has a Wilm's tumor when no pediatric surgical oncologist is available in the HMO? Also, can a community hospital provide appropriate care for a patient who has complicated gastrointestinal fistulas? Denial of appropriate specialty care may be the medicolegal "Achilles Heel" of the managed care system.—E.M. Copeland, III, M.D.

Surgical Resource Consumption in an Academic Health Consortium
Muñoz E, Tortella BJ, Jaker M, Sakmyster M, Kanofsky P (Univ of Medicine and Dentistry of New Jersey, Newark)
Surgery 115:411–416, 1994   140-95-1–6

Objective.—In 1992, aggregate health care costs were $850 billion, which represented nearly 14% of the gross national product of the United States. Surgical expenditures account for 30% of all health care outlays. The increasing cost of health care has become a key national issue, leading to the ongoing debate regarding health care reform. The consumption of surgical resources in a consortium of academic medical centers was analyzed.

Methods.—The analysis included 13,600 general surgical patients who were treated at 8 New Jersey teaching hospitals in 1988. Data were drawn from edited, patient-specific data submitted per regulations to the state Department of Health. Same-day surgical procedures were excluded from the analysis. Hospital resource consumption was measured according to length of stay, hospital cost per patient, race, gender, diagnoses and procedure, and mortality rate.

Findings.—Mean hospital cost per patient was approximately $8,200 (Fig 1–2). Mean length of hospital stay was 12 days, the emergency ad-

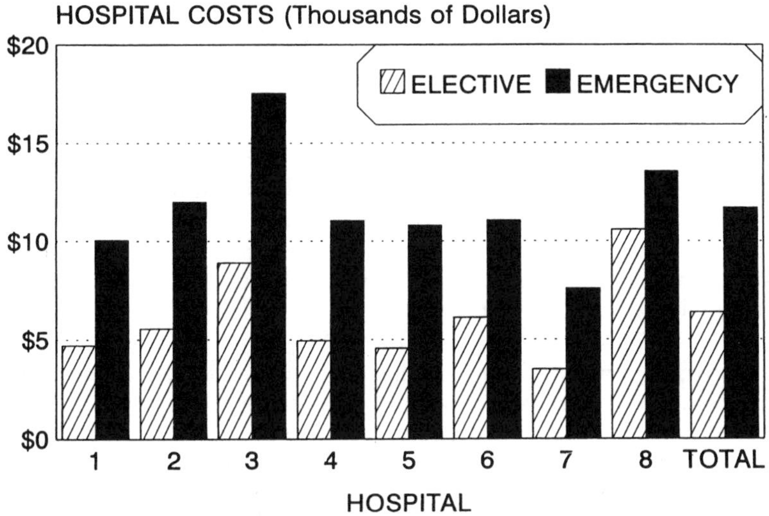

Fig 1–2.—Hospital cost per patient was substantially higher for emergency surgical admissions compared with elective surgical admissions in all 8 hospitals. (Courtesy of Muñoz E, Tortella BJ, Jaker M, et al: *Surgery* 115:411-416, 1994.)

mission rate was 40%, and the mortality rate was 6%. Per-patient costs were $11,700 for emergency admissions vs. $5,800 for nonemergency admissions. Mortality rates were 11% vs. 3%, respectively. Hospital cost per patient was $29,300 for patients who died vs. $6,800 for those who survived; emergency admission rates were 75% vs. 38%.

Conclusion.—Factors associated with higher hospital costs for surgical patients were identified. In particular, the high proportion of emergency admissions among general surgery patients has an important effect. This factor and others must be considered as reimbursement systems change in the coming years. Identification of factors associated with emergency admission and mortality will have an important effect on the health care delivery system.

▶ Cost per emergency admission was nearly twice that for a nonemergency admission and 3 times that for a patient who died. Hospitals that have large emergency departments and provide care for patients with a high severity of disease index will consume a disproportionately high share of the health care dollar. If all hospitals strive to eliminate the high-cost patient, where will patients who have acute or complicated illnesses receive care? Obviously, health care funding agencies need to be aware of these data to distribute properly the health care dollar to appropriate institutions. Such data do lend financial credibility to regionalization of health care. Well-organized hospitals that are staffed properly to handle complicated problems should be able to be economical and could be monitored for fiscal efficiency.—E.M. Copeland, III, M.D.

The Effect of Complications on Length of Stay

McAleese P, Odling-Smee W (Royal Victoria Hospital, Belfast, Northern Ireland)
Ann Surg 220:740–744, 1994　　　　　　　　　　　　　140-95-1–7

Objective.—Hospital length of stay (LOS) and readmission rates were reviewed for patients with and without complications who were admitted to the General Surgical Unit of Royal Victoria Hospital, Northern Ireland, between 1987 and 1990. A numerical scale that could be used to determine increased LOS was devised.

Methods.—The medical records of 5,128 patients who were admitted consecutively with 396 different diagnoses and 228 different types of surgery were retrospectively reviewed. Length of stay, age, type of surgery, and complications were reviewed; patients with and without complications were matched by medical diagnosis and surgical procedure. Specific types of complications were grouped together, and the average was obtained for comparison. A numerical ratio was then allocated to particular types of complications. Readmission rates for complications in patients with a short LOS were also examined.

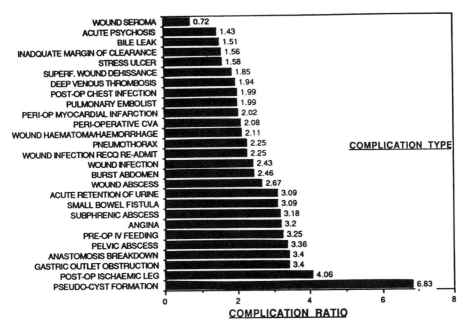

Fig 1–3.—Complication ratio vs. complication type. (Courtesy of McAleese P, Odling-Smee W: *Ann Surg* 220:740–744, 1994.)

Results.—Pressure on beds resulting from increased demand on surgical care decreased hospital LOS. Increased LOS was associated with increased age. The numerical ratio calculated for particular types of complications corresponded to clinical severity. For example, wound seromas did not have an effect on hospital stay, whereas the formation of a pseudocyst did, by a factor of 6.86 (Fig 1–3). In general, complications doubled the average LOS. After the readmission rates for patients with postoperative complications were examined, 7 of the 17 who were readmitted (41%) had been discharged earlier than the average LOS for their diagnoses.

Conclusions.—Length of stay is increased by complications. The complication ratio may be useful when planning discharge. In patients with complications, early discharge may lead to readmission for further treatment.

▶ In Figure 1–3, the complication ratio is obtained by dividing the average LOS with complications by the average LOS without complications (both in days). These data are valuable for an individual hospital when computing budgets for a diagnostic related group if the complication rate for that particular group is known. Likewise, this information helps with discharge planning. For example, if urinary retention can be avoided by a 23-hour hospital stay, rather than immediate discharge, after a hernia repair in an elderly patient, it may be well worth it.—E.M. Copeland, III, M.D.

Outcome After Day-Care Surgery in a Major Teaching Hospital

Osborne GA, Rudkin GE (Royal Adelaide Hosp, South Australia)
Anaesth Intensive Care 21:822–827, 1993   140-95-1–8

Objective.—Because of cutbacks in health care spending, the number of ambulatory surgeries is increasing. Few studies have evaluated the outcome of such surgery. The outcome of ambulatory surgery in the first 6,000 patients treated in a major Australian teaching hospital was measured.

Methods.—Outcome was evaluated in terms of unanticipated hospital admissions, complications, morbidity, recovery time, patient satisfaction, and community support needs.

Results.—Most patients were women, aged 20–29 years. More than 90% were followed by telephone. The most common surgical procedures were oral, gynecologic, ophthalmologic, and orthopedic. Most of the 1.34% unanticipated hospital admissions were related to surgery. Most of the .5% of major complications were related to surgery or to anesthesia. Complications associated with anesthesia were more common with general anesthesia than with local or regional anesthesia, and recovery times were concomitantly longer. Postoperative discomfort consisted primarily of pain, nausea, and vomiting. Recovery times were significantly longer for patients who received general anesthesia for laparoscopic gynecologic procedures than for other procedures. There was no correlation between recovery time and age. After release, as a result of ambulatory surgery, 4% of patients visited a physician and 3.1% visited the hospital emergency department. Most patients were satisfied with the results of ambulatory surgery and the service provided.

Conclusion.—Ambulatory surgery provides an acceptable standard of care to patients.

▶ This is one of the few studies that have evaluated outcome from ambulatory surgery. Take-home analgesics were adequate for 95% of patients, and 98.9% of patients were satisfied with the procedure. The overall complication rate was quite acceptable, and most complications were related to the surgical procedure rather than to anesthesia or to preexisting medical problems (thus, patient complications were under the control of the operating surgeon). One limitation of this study is the young age of the patients, who might be more tolerant of minor complications than an older patient population.—E.M. Copeland, III, M.D.

A Clinical Prediction Rule for Delirium After Elective Noncardiac Surgery

Marcantonio ER, Goldman L, Mangione CM, Ludwig LE, Muraca B, Haslauer CM, Donaldson MC, Whittemore AD, Sugarbaker DJ, Poss R, Haas S, Cook

EF, Orav EJ, Lee TH (Harvard Med School, Boston)
JAMA 271:134–139, 1994   140-95-1-9

Objective.—Postoperative delirium is associated with increased mortality and complication rates, poor functional recovery, and increased length of stay. There is no validated rule for the clinical prediction of delirium in a surgical population. A method of using clinical data that are available before surgery was developed.

Methods.—A total of 1,341 patients who were admitted for major elective general, orthopedic, or gynecologic surgery during a 17-month period were included. Preoperative assessment involved a medical history, physical examination, laboratory testing, and physical and cognitive function tests, including the Specific Activity Scale and the Telephone Interview for Cognitive Status. The Confusion Assessment Method, or data from the medical record or nursing intensity index, was used to diagnose postoperative delirium.

Results.—Postoperative delirium developed in 97% of patients. Factors independently associated with this complication included age 70

Summary of the Clinical Prediction Rule for
Postoperative Delirium

Risk Factor	Points
Age ≥ 70 y	1
Alcohol abuse	1
TICS score < 30*	1
SAS class IV†	1
Markedly abnormal preoperative sodium, potassium, or glucose level‡	1
Aortic aneurysm surgery	2
Noncardiac thoracic surgery	1

Total Points	Risk of Delirium, % §
0	2
1 or 2	11
≥ 3	50

* TICS indicates Telephone Interview for Cognitive Status (scores < 30 suggest cognitive impairment).
† SAS indicates Specific Activity Scale (class IV represents severe physical impairment).
‡ Markedly abnormal levels were defined as follows: sodium, < 130 or > 150 mmol/L; potassium, < 3.0 or > 6.0 mmol/L; or glucose, < 3.3 or > 16.7 mmol/L (< 60 or > 300 mg/dL).
§ Estimates of risk were based on the true incidence of delirium in the validation population.
(Courtesy of Marcantonio ER, Goldman L, Mangione CM, et al: *JAMA* 271:134–139, 1994.)

years or older; self-reported alcohol abuse; poor cognitive status; poor functional status; marked preoperative abnormalities in serum levels of sodium, potassium, or glucose; noncardiac thoracic surgery; and aortic aneurysm surgery (table). These factors were used to develop a simple predictive rule, which was tested in an independent population. By this rule, rates of postoperative delirium were classified as low, 2%; medium, 8% to 13%; or high, 50%. The development of postoperative delirium was associated with increased rates of major complications, longer lengths of stay, and higher rates of discharge to long-term care or rehabilitation facilities.

Conclusion.—This predictive rule can assess a patient's risk of postoperative delirium by using data available before surgery. For patients at high risk, interventions may be able to reduce the risk of postoperative delirium, thereby improving overall surgical outcome.

▶ Predicting postoperative complications from a set of preoperative data is part of the judgment derived through 5 years of surgical residency. Validated rules for prediction of outcome will become especially important for determining the financial risk of any capitated patient population and for assessing the cost of providing surgical care for a set of patients with given preoperative predictors of postoperative complications.

For years, surgical nutritionists have tried to develop preoperative nutritional parameters that dictate the need for total parenteral nutrition on the basis of a reduction in postoperative complications directly attributable to the preoperative use of this method. These validated predictors have not been forthcoming, thus indicating the magnitude of difficulty in developing such a database.—E.M. Copeland, III, M.D.

Comparison Between Peripherally Implanted Ports and Externally Sited Catheters for Long-Term Venous Access
Pullyblank AM, Tanner AG, Carey PD, Guillou PJ, Pearce SZ, Monson JRT (St Mary's Hosp, London)
Ann R Coll Surg Engl 76:33–38, 1994   140-95-1-10

Background.—Some patients with chronic illness require central venous access for long-term IV therapy. The difficulties and complications associated with the maintenance of externally sited catheters have led to the development of totally implantable systems. A recently reported series of 51 patients with a peripheral implantable port for venous access was extended and compared with a series of similar patients with Hickman lines.

Methods.—A consecutive series of 112 patients who had Hickman lines placed in 1988–1989 and a consecutive series of 85 patients who had peripherally implanted ports placed in 1990–1992 were studied. The peripheral port system (PAS Port) was implanted in a basilic vein and was then accessed by percutaneous needle puncture of the septum. With the use of local anesthesia, the port was placed in the antecubital fossa of the nondominant arm. The sensor tip of the port was located by a hand-held locator device (wand) that emitted an electromagnetic field. In 27 patients, the ports were inserted in a ward side room.

Results.—The mean duration of system life for the ports was 194 days. The mean duration for the Hickman lines was 105 days. After port insertion, 2 patients had early complications, and 9 had late complications (total 12.94%, .67/1,000 catheter days). Four of 6 episodes of venous thrombosis were treated successfully with streptokinase, which allowed the port to be left in place. There were no differences in the complication rates between those patients who had ports inserted in the operating room and those whose port was inserted in the ward side room. There were no episodes of catheter occlusion or fluid extravasation, possibly because the port care was supervised by a single, trained user. The Hickman lines were associated with an early complication rate of 10.7% and a late complication rate of 37.6% (3.5/1,000 catheter days). Thirty-two percent of patients required more than 1 Hickman line insertion.

Conclusion.—Peripheral implantable ports are associated with significantly lower complication rates, are more cosmetically acceptable, require fewer maintenance procedures, and impose fewer restrictions on lifestyles than Hickman lines. Peripheral ports have low infection rates and may eliminate some complications, such as pneumothorax and arterial puncture, that are seen with central venous cannulation.

▶ Peripherally implanted ports were reported to have the same efficacy of venous access as central ports. In this study, they had fewer complications associated with long-term use when compared with Hickman catheters. The continuity of care for the peripheral ports was provided by a single, trained nurse, who may represent the sole reason that patients with ports had fewer complications. The placement of peripheral ports does eliminate the need for subclavian venapuncture and all the associated complications. Peripheral ports may be a satisfactory alternative to centrally placed infusion portals.—E.M. Copeland, III, M.D.

A New Hazard of Cornstarch, an Absorbable Dusting Powder

Ruhl CM, Urbancic JH, Foresman PA, Cox MJ, Rodeheaver GT, Zura RD, Edlich RF (Univ of Virginia, Charlottesville)
J Emerg Med 12:11–14, 1994   140-95-1–11

Background.—Years ago, cornstarch replaced talc for use in the manufacture of surgical and examination gloves. Although cornstarch was originally thought to be benign, it has been shown to result in granulomas, adhesions, fibrosis, "starch peritonitis," and fistula formation in the peritoneal cavity. Whether cornstarch impairs local tissue defenses in contaminated wounds was determined.

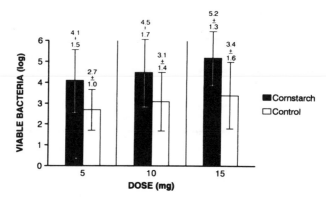

Fig 1–4.—The bacterial count in wounds containing cornstarch were significantly grreater than those of the control wounds subjected to a comparable bacterial inoculum. (Courtesy of Ruhl CM, Urbancic JH, Foresman PA, et al: *J Emerg Med* 12:11-14, 1994.)

Methods.—The effects of a specially processed cornstarch, intended as a glove lubricant, on the resistance of surgical wounds to infection in guinea pigs were measured. A *Staphylococcus aureus* suspension was introduced into each of 2 paravertebral wounds in each animal. One wound was treated with various doses of cornstarch after bacterial contamination: the other received no cornstarch. The wounds were then bandaged. Four days later, the animals were killed, and the inflammatory responses of the wounds were compared.

Results:—The cornstarch-treated wounds showed a significantly greater bacterial concentration than the control wounds (Fig 1–4). Two of 3 cornstarch groups also showed significantly wider indurated margins than the control wounds.

Conclusions.—Cornstarch enhanced bacterial growth and elicited an exaggerated inflammatory response in experimental wounds. Now that powder-free gloves are available, gloves with cornstarch powders should not be used during wound closure. The costs of powder-free gloves should fall as demand increases.

▶ There is little question from this study design that cornstarch was detrimental in experimental wounds. Powder-free gloves are expensive, and gloves are an easy target for cost containment within hospitals. Were cornstarch to be equally detrimental in human beings, powder-free gloves would represent a cost savings in the long run, because of a decrease in cost associated wtih wound complications. Working together, researchers, hospital administrators, clinicians, and epidemiologists must determine which short-term cost-saving goals are appropriate and which ones contribute to more costly complications in the future.—E.M. Copeland, III, M.D.

The Relationship Between Malpractice Claims History and Subsequent Obstetric Care

Entman SS, Glass CA, Hickson GB, Githens PB, Whetten-Goldstein K, Sloan FA (Vanderbilt Univ, Nashville, Tenn; Duke Univ, Durham, NC)
JAMA 272:1588–1591, 1994   140-95-1–12

Purpose.—The National Practitioner Data Bank (NPDB) was formed on the premise that physicians who have been named in malpractice claims or have been disciplined by their peers are more likely to provide substandard care in the future. There is debate, however, regarding the ability of malpractice claims history to predict future quality of care. The relationship between malpractice claims experience and the quality of obstetric care was assessed in a historic cohort of obstetricians.

Methods.—Three hundred fifty-eight Florida obstetricians who were still practicing in 1987 were included. Of these, 133 had never paid a malpractice claim. Of those who had paid claims, 21 who averaged more than .57 claims/yr and made payments greater than average for obstetricians in the state were classified as "high pay," and 21 with a similar frequency of claims but less than average payments were classified as "high frequency." A blinded review was conducted of the medical records of 446 cases from the practices of these physicians, oversampling for adverse outcomes. The quality of clinical care provided in these cases was assessed objectively and subjectively, and the results were compared among the 4 groups.

Findings.—Substandard documentation was 3 times more frequent for cases with adverse outcomes. All 4 groups had a low frequency of unindicated, excessive, or inappropriate testing, including the high-pay and high-frequency groups. Thirty-five percent of cases with adverse outcomes had 1 or more objective errors; however, most of these errors were technical or coincidental in nature. Only 4% were deemed to be related to the outcome. There was no evidence of any threshold of claims experience that stimulated fundamental changes in practice. On subjective review, 15 cases were considered to be of substandard quality, including 8% of those with adverse outcomes and 2% of those with good outcomes. Negative opinions were reached about referral to 4 more physicians who were cited for management errors and 6 more who were cited for overall substandard care.

Conclusions.—Previous malpractice claims experience appears to be unrelated to the technical quality of care delivered by Florida obstetricians. The NPDB and other approaches to identify risk of future clinical errors on the basis of previous malpractice claims may misjudge the likelihood that physicians with previous claims will provide substandard care in the future. The goals of the NPDB may be in the public interest, but the data provided may not reliably identify those physicians who are likely to make errors.

▶ No differences in any of the objective or subjective measures of quality of clinical care were evident among obstetricians who were sued frequently compared with those who had no claims. The incidence of adverse outcomes was the same in both groups, as was the fetal and infant mortality rate. Therefore, in this specific instance, information from the NPDB did not identify obstetricians who might perpetuate substandard care. To some degree, the results of this study are disappointing. Identifying physicians prone to substandard medical behavior would determine a target audience for specific medical education and put some teeth into the requirement of most states for continuing medical education to qualify for relicensure.—E.M. Copeland, III, M.D.

Obstetricians' Prior Malpractice Experience and Patients' Satisfaction With Care
Hickson GB, Clayton EW, Entman SS, Miller CS, Githens PB, Whetten-Goldstein K, Sloan FA (Vanderbilt Univ, Nashville, Tenn; Duke Univ, Durham, NC)
JAMA 272:1583–1587, 1994   140-95-1–13

Background.—Some physicians have a disproportionate number of malpractice suits filed against them. One study found that more than 85% of all malpractice payments for medical specialists were made on behalf of only 3% of that population. Differences between physicians with a high number of claims and those with an average number or no malpractice claims were investigated.

Methods.—In-depth interviews were conducted with women who gave birth in Florida in 1987 to test the hypothesis that physicians' malpractice claims experience is related to patients' satisfaction with care. Obstetricians were divided into 4 groups; those who were sued with high frequency, those who made high payments, those who had no claims, and all others.

Findings.—Women who saw physicians with the most frequent number of claims but not high payments were significantly more likely to report feeling rushed and ignored and never receiving explanations for tests. Women who saw physicians in the high frequency group had twice as many complaints as those who saw physicians who had never been sued. The most common problems described were associated with physician-patient communication.

Conclusions.—Interpersonal factors appear to be strongly associated with malpractice claims experience. Further research is needed to determine whether these factors are as important in other specialties.

▶ Dissatisfied patients most frequently cited problems with communication, i.e., physicians would not offer information or listen. Also, there was a perceived lack of concern and respect for the patient. Many of these physicians had been sued frequently, but little money had changed hands. This study clearly indicates that the number of "nuisance suits" can be reduced by better physician-patient rapport, which may also lower the risk of suit when potential real claims exist.—E.M. Copeland, III, M.D.

Academic Surgical Group Practices at the Dawn of Health Reform
Flint L, Flint CB (Tulane Univ, New Orleans, La)
Ann Surg 220:374–381, 1994   140-95-1–14

Objective.—Health care reform is a market-driven plan that is affecting every aspect of medical care management. The trend is toward prepaid plans with integrated organizations. No one has calculated the costs of this reorganization of the health care system to medical schools, which get 45% of their support from clinical practices. Academic surgical group practices that earned at least $500,000 in 1992 were surveyed to assess vulnerabilities to reimbursement and ability to provide academic support.

Methods.—A 158-question survey was mailed to 100 academic surgical groups.

Results.—Seventy-four surveys, approximately two thirds from public schools, were analyzed. The groups had an average of 41 surgeons and gross revenues of $35 million. Although payer patterns were mixed, 65% of responders had revenue growth during the 1988 to 1992 period (table). Thirteen of 74 practices were HMO-owned, and 42 had satellite clinics. Most responders received more than half their referrals from outside the academic community. More than 27% received significant financial subsidies from teaching hospitals and were larger than groups that did not receive such subsidies. On average, surgeons affiliated with private school received 79% of their income, and surgeons affiliated with public schools received 64%, from the 52% of the gross clinic revenues

---

Patterns of Change in Payers for Academic Surgical Group Practices Having
Complete Payer Mix Data for 1988–1992

Payer	Grew	Declined	Stable
Private (N = 45)	9/45 (20%)	36/45 (80%)	0/45
Medicare (N = 33)	25/33 (76%)	8/33 (24%)	0/33
Medicaid (N = 41)	18/41 (44%)	5/41 (12%)	18/41 (44%)
HMO (N = 28)	20/28 (71%)	3/28 (11%)	5/28 (18%)

Abbreviation: N, number of complete responses.
(Courtesy of Flint L, Flint CB: *Ann Surg* 220:374–381, 1994.)

available for salaries. Clinic income supported 85% of department operations costs, 73% of department staff costs, and 40% percent of research costs. Clinic income is used to support graduate medical education by 69% of groups, resident salaries by 39% of groups, and trainee research costs by 30% of groups.

Conclusion.—Clinical income is used mainly to support academic medicine, but managed care has increased the number of payers whose reimbursement will decrease. Preserving academic group practices is a way to continue the academic support these practices provide.

▶ An investigation of income since 1992 would probably show a decline in gross clinical revenue for most academic departments. A significant portion of faculty salary comes from clinical revenue in both public and private universities. As clinical income falls, an interesting conflict between maintaining salaries for faculty and staff and supporting research and graduate medical education is inevitable.—E.M. Copeland, III, M.D.

Attitudes Toward Retirement: A Survey of The American Surgical Association
Greenfield LJ, Proctor MC (Univ of Michigan Hosps, Ann Arbor)
Ann Surg 220:382–390, 1994   140-95-1–15

Objective.—Although mandatory retirement is prohibited, most surgeons recognize the risks that advanced age places on them, their reputations, and their patients. Some, because of poor insight, financial problems, or lack of alternatives, do not recognize their limitations and continue to operate. There is no accepted way of handling this situation. The results of an attitudinal retirement survey of active, older members of the American Surgery Association were reported.

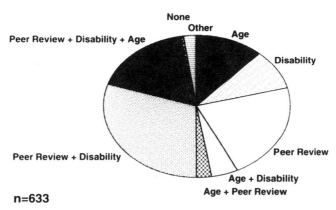

Fig 1–5.—Responses to the question of withdrawing operative privileges showed a majority in favor of peer review or onset of disability rather than age alone. Combination of responses also are shown. (Courtesy of Greenfield LJ, Proctor MC: *Ann Surg* 220:382–390, 1994.)

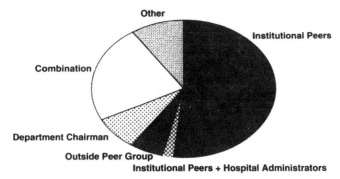

Fig 1–6.—Further response on peer review showed a majority in favor of institutional peers as opposed to an outside group or department chair. (Courtesy of Greenfield LJ, Proctor MC: *Ann Surg* 220:382–390, 1994.)

Methods.—A total of 659 of 882 members responded to the questionnaire.

Results.—Seven percent of responders were younger than 50 years of age, none of whom had retired. Approximately 29% of responders were in the 50–60 age group, with 3% retired, 35% of responders in the 60–70 age group, with 17% retired, and 28% of responders in the 70 plus age group, which had 83% retired. Forty percent of those who reported working at their customary level were older than 60 years of age. In the oldest group, 18% were still operating at a full or reduced level. More than half the responders had no retirement plans. More than three quarters with plans cited post-retirement medical activities. Most believed that withdrawal of operating privileges should be based on peer review or onset of disability, not age (Fig 1–5). Most responders felt institutional peer review was appropriate (Fig 1–6). More than half believed that elimination of mandatory retirement was good.

Conclusion.—A more positive outlook toward retirement is needed. There currently is no mechanism to deal with aging as there is with alcohol or drug abuse. A discreet and objective evaluation process should be developed to enable the removal of surgeons who can place themselves and their patients at risk because of problems related to aging.

▶ Dr. I. S. Ravdin, while chastising me about my lack of interest in medical history, once said, "The closer one gets to being history, the more interest one has in it." The same should be true for retirement, although the results of this study do not indicate it. The need to delay retirement may become more pressing as managed care erodes income. Hopefully, all young surgeons have a financial strategy that will allow voluntary or peer-dictated retirement without undue financial hardship.—E.M. Copeland, III, M.D.

Practice Environment and Resident Operative Experience

Thompson JS, Rikkers LF (Univ of Nebraska, Omaha)
Am J Surg 167:418–422, 1994   140-95-1–16

Objective.—Questionnaires were sent to 100 surgeons to determine how the practice environment and staff perception of required surgical skills affect the level of resident participation in operative procedures.

Methods.—The questionnaires were returned by 72 surgeons. Most respondents were general surgeons (65%), were trained in academic programs (89%), worked regularly with residents (62%), and were less than 15 years out of training (61%). Thirty-four were in private practice, 23 practiced at a university hospital, and 15 were at hospitals directly affiliated with the residency program. Information was gathered on the surgeons' practice environment and their perception of appropriate resident level and required skills for the performance of 20 common general surgery procedures. Four factors—anatomy, suturing, dissection, and judgment—were assessed for each procedure as very important, moderately important, or minimally important.

Results.—Surgeons in private practice and affiliated hospitals were more likely to assign cases to higher level residents than those at the university hospital. Surgeons who worked regularly with residents were

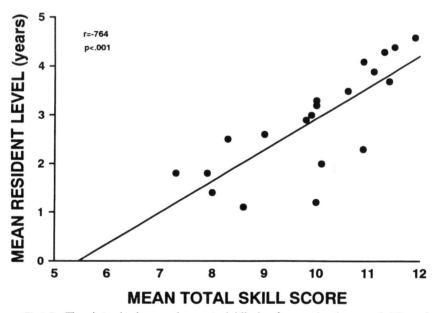

Fig 1–7.—The relationship between the perceived difficulty of a procedure (mean total skill score) and the assignment of resident responsibility (mean resident level) for the 20 procedures. In general, more difficult operations would be assigned to higher level residents. (Courtesy of Thompson JS, Rikkers LF: *Am J Surg* 167:418–422, 1994.)

more likely to assign a lower level resident to a given procedure. Years out of training also influenced resident assignments. Surgeons who were more than 15 years out of training were more likely to assign a higher level resident to procedures. The mean year of assignment ranged from 1.1 years for appendectomy to 4.6 years for pancreaticoduodenectomy. In general, operations viewed as more difficult were assigned to higher level residents (Fig 1-7). The 2 most important factors in determining operative responsibility were anatomy (46%) and judgment (36%); suturing was generally considered the least important factor of those considered. No correlation was observed, however, between assignment of operative responsibility and perception of required skills.

Conclusion.—Factors in the practice environment were more important than the surgical aspects of the procedure in the surgeon's choice of appropriate resident level to perform general surgery procedures. This bias was particularly strong in procedures that involved new technology, such as laparoscopy.

▶ The data contained in this report should be read by all directors of surgical training programs. Assignment of a junior level resident to an older surgeon in private practice will result in minimal practical experience for the resident. The surgeon will let the resident do very little. Save such rotations for more advanced residents. The junior residents will get to do more when scrubbing with young surgeons who have only recently completed their residency training.—E.M. Copeland, III, M.D.

Comparison of Postoperative Mortality and Morbidity in VA and Nonfederal Hospitals
Stremple JF, Bross DS, Davis CL, McDonald GO (Univ of Pittsburgh, Pa; VA Central Office, Washington, DC)
J Surg Res 56:405–416, 1994   140-95-1–17

Background.—In 1991, the Phase III report on the Quality of Surgical Care in the Veterans Administration (VA) was issued to the Congress. The method and results of the report, which compared postoperative morbidity and mortality rates in VA hospitals with those in nonfederal hospitals, were examined.

Methods.—Preliminary VA data were used to devise a list of surgical procedures that included enough patients for a meaningful study. Procedures (e.g., diagnostic and palliative) were deleted from the list if it appeared likely that the patient's death resulted from the underlying condition rather than the surgical procedure. A total of 544,000 patient discharge records (214,000 VA and 330,000 nonfederal) from 1987 through 1988 were studied. The nonfederal records included only men older than 18 years of age who had undergone 1 of 118 surgical procedures or procedure groups. Multivariate analysis methods were used to adjust for the patient characteristics of age, comorbidity, diagnosis, and severity of illness. The Disease Staging method was used to adjust the mortality rate comparisons for the severity of illness.

Results.—For 110 surgical procedures or procedure groups, there were no significant differences in postoperative mortality rates between the VA and nonfederal hospital systems. The VA hospitals showed significantly lower postoperative mortality rates for cervical esophagostomy, endarterectomy, and esophageal anastomosis or esophagocolostomy. The VA hospitals showed significantly higher postoperative mortality rates for suture of ulcer, cholecystostomy, small intestine surgery, colon surgery, and reopening of a recent thoracotomy site. Infection rates were higher in VA hospitals, but respiratory, urinary, and gastrointestinal postoperative morbidity rates were generally lower.

Conclusion.—The postoperative mortality and morbidity rates of the VA hospitals are similar to those in nonfederal hospitals. Many of the differences in mortality rates between the 2 hospital systems are explained by the severity of comorbidity in the VA patients. If comorbidity below the stage 3 level of severity had been included, then even more of the differences might have been explained. The possibility of a link between quality of care and outcome is weakened when mortality rate differences that are based on patients with no comorbidity are not present among patients with serious comorbidity.

▶ Many VA hospitals are either affiliated with, or integrated into, surgical residency training programs. Such affiliations work to equalize the quality of care between teaching institutions and VA hospitals. In this study, 61% of VA hospitals were urban teaching facilities, compared with 15% of nonfederal hospitals. Comorbidity accounted for the reduced survival rate among VA patients in most surgical categories. Affiliations with teaching programs in which major cases, such as esophagectomies, congregate may be responsible for the better survival rate of patients with esophageal disease in the VA hospitals, because the faculties of both institutions are often the same.—E.M. Copeland, III, M.D.

Screening Surgeons for HIV Infection: Assessment of a Potential Public Health Program
Schulman KA, McDonald RC, Lynn LA, Frank I, Christakis NA, Schwartz JS (Georgetown Univ, Washington, DC; Univ of Pennsylvania, Philadelphia)
Infect Control Hosp Epidemiol 15:147–155, 1994   140-95-1–18

Background.—There is currently a heightened concern regarding the appropriate activities of health care providers who are infected with HIV, especially those physicians who do invasive procedures. A model was developed to assess the outcome of a program of testing surgeons for HIV and the risk of HIV acquisition by their patients.

Methods.—Data were developed from a review of the medical literature; subjective probability estimates were used when data were not available. A Monte Carlo simulation model of physician-to-patient transmission of HIV was used to estimate the national annual number of cases of HIV transmission with and without surgeon testing and practice limitations. Three different rates (.15%, .3%, .6%) of physician-to-patient transmission per cutaneous exposure were simulated.

Results.—Assuming a surgeon HIV prevalence of .1% and a surgeon-to-patient transmission rate of .15%, the annual number of transmitted cases would be .5. At the other extreme, assuming a surgeon HIV prevalence of 2% and a transmission rate of .6%, the annual number of transmitted cases would be 36.9. The only published study of HIV infection in surgeons showed a prevalence of .06%. No proven cases of transmission of HIV infection to patients from an infected surgeon have been detected in screening programs that included more than 15,000 patients. A mandatory screening program, after 1 screening cycle, would probably reduce the annual transmissions in the first example to .05 and in the second example to 3.1.

Conclusion.—The risk of a patient acquiring HIV from an infected surgeon during an invasive procedure is very low. The potential costs of such a program would include the costs of testing and counseling, possible decreased patient access to health care, and a disability insurance program for surgeons and trainees. Screening surgeons for HIV infection would be costly and would not completely eliminate the risk to patients. Adequate economic safeguards for surgeons who are infected with HIV to limit their practice voluntarily would require noncancelable, reasonably priced disability and/or life insurance.

▶ Accumulating data have indicated that the risk of a patient contracting AIDS from an infected surgeon is small. This study emphasizes the need for appropriate disability insurance for surgeons who are HIV positive before mandatory testing is legislated.—E.M. Copeland, III, M.D.

Needle Prick Injury to the Surgeon: Do We Need Sharp Needles?
Dauleh MI, Irving AD, Townell NH (Dundee Royal Infirmary, Scotland)
J R Coll Surg Edin 39:310–311, 1994   140-95-1–19

Introduction.—Needle prick injuries to surgeons or assistants carry the risk of transmission of hepatitis or HIV. Despite precautions, the risk of accidental injury still exists. Needle prick injuries and the use of blunt-tip needles for procedures in which an injury is most likely were investigated.

Methods.—All operative procedures during a 6-month period were studied. In the first 253 operations, sharp needles were used. In the remaining 78 procedures, blunt-tip needles were used. Information about glove and skin puncture was recorded. The procedure, sites, and time of needle prick were noted. At the end of each procedure, the gloves were tested for perforations by filling them with water.

Findings.—Forty-eight glove perforations, 22 of which also penetrated the skin, were found. Injuries occurred most frequently to the left hand in right-handed surgeons. Half the perforations occurred during closure of the linea alba. Thirteen perforations occurred during a hernia repair. Blunt-tipped needles were used in 78 operations. Only 2 glove perforations occurred, with no skin penetration. Satisfactory results were achieved for the operations, which were mostly abdominal wound closure and hernia repairs.

Conclusion.—Most perforations of the glove and penetration of the skin occurred during abdominal wound closure and hernia repairs. The use of blunt needles is a practical alternative that can reduce the number of needle prick injuries to the hands of surgeons.

▶ Results of this study indicate that blunt-tipped needles function adequately for abdominal wound closure and hernia repair and reduce the incidence of needle-prick injuries. The use of blunt-tipped needles should be explored in more detail.—E.M. Copeland, III, M.D.

Mechanical Comparison of 10 Suture Materials Before and After In Vivo Incubation
Greenwald D, Shumway S, Albear P, Gottlieb L (Univ of South Florida, Tampa; Univ of Chicago)
J Surg Res 56:372–377, 1994   140-95-1–20

Introduction.—The numerous types of sutures available to the surgeon vary in size, material, design, and behavior. Properties of the various materials used in absorbable and nonabsorbable sutures can be evaluated in many ways. Ten different 2–0 suture materials were tested. Their mechanical properties were catalogued, and their performances over time were compared in an in vivo model.

Methods.—The suture materials evaluated were Dexon, Vicryl, plain gut, chromic gut, polydioxanone (PDS), silk, Maxon, Prolene, nylon, and Ethibond (braided polyester). Nylon, silk, Prolene, and Ethibond are nonabsorbable, and the remaining suture materials are absorbable. Twenty-five individual sutures of each type were randomly selected from single lots taken from current operating room stock. Five of each type were sent to an industrial testing facility for measurement of suture diameter. Ten were tested mechanically until rupture, and 10 were tested after a 6-week period of in vivo incubation in rats.

Results.—Mechanical testing revealed that suture material behaved according to suture design. Braided sutures demonstrated the least compliance, gut sutures were intermediate, and monofilament structures were

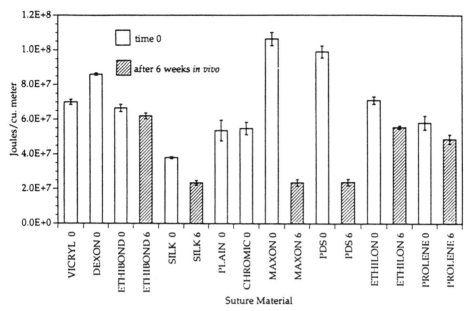

Fig 1–8.—Mean toughness ± SEM of suture material. (Courtesy of Greenwald D, Shumway S, Albear P, et al: *J Surg Res* 56:372–377, 1994.)

the most compliant. The strongest and toughest sutures were Maxon and PDS, which are both monofilament and absorbable; silk was the least strong and the least tough (Fig 1–8). Strain at rupture was greatest for PDS, followed by nylon and Prolene. After 6 weeks of incubation in rats, none of the Vicryl, Dexon, or gut sutures survived with enough structural integrity for testing. All remaining sutures, except for braided polyester, were less strong and less tough with time.

Conclusion.—Undamaged sutures behave differently than sutures stressed or altered in the clinical setting. These data represented the basic mechanical properties of undamaged, untied suture material. Braided sutures demonstrated the greatest degree of resistance to stretch, and monofilament the least, regardless of the chemical composition of the sutures. The only suture to retain all its basic mechanical properties after 6 weeks in vivo was Ethibond.

▶ The results of this study speak for themselves. Surgeons choose a suture material for both strength and stability in wounds. In vivo studies such as these are important to determine whether our needs are being met by the suture materials selected for use.—E.M. Copeland, III, M.D.

A Comparison of Public Attitudes Toward Autopsy, Organ Donation, and Anatomic Dissection: A Swedish Survey

Sanner M (Uppsala Univ, Sweden)
JAMA 271:284–288, 1994   140-95-1–21

Introduction.—Death is an emotionally charged subject. Ideas about death have an important influence on an individual's opinions about

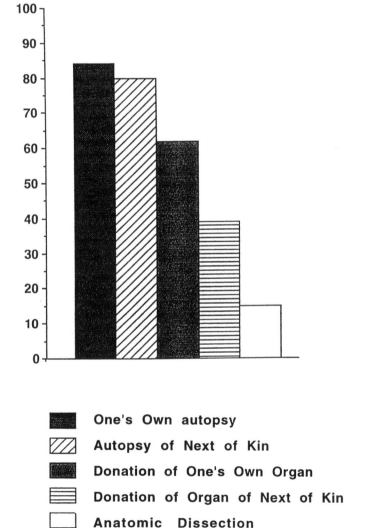

One's Own autopsy

Autopsy of Next of Kin

Donation of One's Own Organ

Donation of Organ of Next of Kin

Anatomic Dissection

Fig 1–9.—Proportion of population that is positive toward various procedures concerning the dead body. (Courtesy of Sanner M: *JAMA* 271:284–288, 1994.)

what might be done with a dead body. There have been no previous studies, however, of public opinion or attitudes toward autopsy and dissection. Reactions to procedures that involve the dead body were assessed. Attitudes about autopsy, organ donation, and donation of the whole body for anatomical dissection were compared.

Methods.—A survey was mailed to an age-stratified, random sample of Swedish residents. The study questionnaire included 24 items designed to assess reactions, including religious and sociodemographic issues, toward autopsy, organ donation, and anatomical dissection. Response rate was 65% in all age groups.

Results.—Eighty-four percent of the respondents reported that they would accept an autopsy for themselves, and 80% would accept one for a close relative. Sixty-two percent of respondents said they would be willing to donate their organs after death, and 39% that they would donate the organs of a family member. Only 15%, however, would consider donating their body for dissection (Fig 1–9). Almost all respondents who accepted dissection also accepted organ donation and autopsy, and almost all who accepted organ donation also accepted autopsy. Respondents who preferred to be cremated after death were more likely to accept organ donation, autopsy, and dissection than those who preferred to be buried. Individuals who did not describe themselves as religious were more likely to have a positive attitude toward organ donation. Approximately two thirds of the respondents expressed some discomfort about autopsy and organ donation. Approximately one third of those willing to undergo autopsy reported fear of not being dead during the procedure. This fear was likely to be shared by individuals who were undecided about organ donation. Women tended to be more sensitive to procedures on the dead body than were men.

Conclusion.—Based on the proportion of individuals who had a positive attitude toward various medical procedures on dead bodies, a scale can be formed with autopsy and dissection at each end point and organ donation in the middle. This scale, which has the characteristics of a Guttman scale, represents a continuum of comfort-discomfort regarding medical procedures after death. Women are more sensitive than men toward operations on their bodies, perhaps because men more often feel called on to accept such procedures.

▶ This study is from Sweden and may not reflect the subjective views of the North American population. If you assume the views to be similar, however, you might wonder why the autopsy rate is low in most academic institutions and why there is a shortage of organ donors. Possibly, we are not asking enough for organ donation or autopsy from our citizens.—E.M. Copeland, III, M.D.

The Contributions of Authors to Multiauthored Biomedical Research Papers

Shapiro DW, Wenger NS, Shapiro MF (Univ of California, Los Angeles)
JAMA 271:438–442, 1994
140-95-1-22

First Authors' Assessments of the Contributions of Authors to Specific Tasks

Task*	All Authors Together (n=1014), %	First Authors (n=184), %	Second Authors (n=175), %	Middle Authors (n=479), %	Last Authors (n=176), %
Initial conception	42	90	34	19	64
Design	47	97	41	24	61
Provision of resources	68	72	62	62	85
Data collection	54	89	62	45	34
Analysis and interpretation of data	52	98	56	30	61
Writing and revision	57	100	55	33	80
Total No. of tasks contributed to					
0 or 1	24	0	17	42	10
2 or 3	32	3	46	40	29
4, 5, or 6	43	97	37	18	61

*For each task, P < .0001 for differences among author positions. (Courtesy of: Shapiro DW, Wenger NS, Shapiro MF: JAMA 271:438–442, 1994.)

Introduction.—Authorship in multiauthored biomedical research papers is under intense scrutiny and debate. Controversies center around standards for authorship, responsibility for fraudulent or invalid research, authorship requirements for promotion and tenure, and order of authorship in relation to contributions made. Two purposes of authorship are to confer credit and to denote responsibility for the research. In the signing of scientific articles, authors add validity and certify the integrity of their work. With the mean number of authors per paper increasing, the central purposes of authorship may no longer be served. A cross-section of the best multiauthored medical research in the United States was surveyed to determine author contributions.

Methods.—Twenty reports of studies with 4 or more authors were sampled from each of the 10 leading biomedical journals. Questionnaires were mailed to the first 3 authors in qualifying studies. Responses from 184 first authors who indicated good or excellent knowledge of contributions of co-authors were used.

Results.—Six major tasks were identified. First authors contributed to 4–6 major tasks in 97% of the studies and to 2–3 tasks in 3% (table). A total of 184 authors (18% of all authors) contributed to only 1 major research task, and 6% of all authors made no substantial contributions to any of the 6 major tasks of the research projects reported. Of those making only 1 contribution, 79% were middle authors, 14% were second authors, and 7% were last authors.

Conclusion.—Order of authorship indicates little about contributions made by any author other than the first author. Contributions of second and last authors were more substantial than those of middle authors but varied greatly. Authors are not listed in decreasing order of the number of tasks they performed. The scientific community needs to consider these findings seriously before the purposes of authorship are lost.

▶ First authors contributed substantially to conception and design of the study and usually did the work leading to the data collected. Last authors contributed to design, because the work was usually done in their laboratories and under their direction. The second authors also were usually a major participant in the work of the study.

The controversial issue is the listing of the remaining authors, who have often provided only patients or limited expertise to a portion of the work. My philosophy is to be inclusive rather than exclusive. However, the lengthy list of authors on many papers today is excessive and detracts from the importance of the contributions made by the major participants.—E.M. Copeland, III, M.D.

Defining the Surgical Personality: A Preliminary Study

Schwartz RW, Barclay JR, Harrell PL, Murphy AE, Jarecky RK, Donnelly MB
(Univ of Kentucky, Lexington)
Surgery 115:62–68, 1994   140-95-1–23

Background.—Most medical schools continue to select students on the basis of intellectual ability or cognitive performance, despite studies that have demonstrated the importance of noncognitive characteristics, such as psychomotor ability and personality or temperament. One problem is a lack of appropriate assessment instruments and test batteries to measure noncognitive attributes. Whether a surgical personality exists was determined, and the temperament and personality traits of physicians who have chosen surgery were described.

Methods.—One hundred ten physicians at the University of Kentucky volunteered for the study. Forty-seven practiced general surgery or a surgical specialty, 28 were primary care physicians, and 35 had chosen a "controllable life-style" specialty, such as anesthesiology, pathology, radiology, and psychiatry. The assessment battery used consisted of 3 inventories: 2 instruments to measure temperament, and 1 to evaluate personality. Participants were also asked to complete a stress inventory.

Results.—Compared with the normative population of the tests, these physicians differed significantly in 11 of 21 factors. As a group, physicians scored significantly better on 9 personality variables: scientific, aesthetic, social, caring, competitive, withdrawn, independent, creative, and

---

Personality/Temperament Characteristics of Surgeons

I. Surgeons tend to score higher than other physicians on the following factors:

    1. Extroverted
    2. Adjusted
    3. Practical
    4. Social
    5. Competitive
    6. Structured
    7. Stable Extrovert
    8. Ratio of inhibition to excitation

II. Surgeons tend to score lower than other physicians on the following factors:

    1. Creative
    2. Withdrawn
    3. Rebellious
    4. Total Stress

(Courtesy of Schwartz RW, Barclay JR, Harrell PL, et al: *Surgery* 115:62–68, 1994.)

---

enterprising. They were significantly less likely to be rebellious or assertive. The 3 broad specialty groups also differed from each other. Surgeons scored highest on extroversion and adjustment and lowest on the creative, withdrawn, and rebellious personality variables. Surgeons scored highest and physicians in controllable lifestyles (i.e., dermatology, pathology) scored lowest on 3 of 4 career/life-style factors: practical, social, competitive, and structured. Temperament proved to be the most powerful discriminator. Surgeons scored highest on both the extroversion factor and the ratio of excitation to inhibition (table).

Conclusion.—Among the physicians evaluated with measures of personality and temperament, surgeons demonstrated the clearest and most consistent profile. Surgeons as a group were extroverted, adjusted, practical, social, structured, and competitive. A reliable assessment of noncognitive factors may predict cognitive and clinical performance successfully.

▶ What else can I say?! This study indicates why so many of my friends are surgeons.—E.M. Copeland, III, M.D.

Effects of Music on Cardiovascular Reactivity Among Surgeons
Allen K, Blascovich J (State Univ of New York, Buffalo)
JAMA 272:882–884, 1994   140-95-1–24

Objective.—There has been no study of the incidence and effect of music in the operating room on patients or surgeons. Other studies have shown, however, that music reduces stress. The effects on surgeons' performance and physiologic responses to music selected by the surgeons or by the experimenters were reported.

Methods.—Fifty males surgeons, aged 31 to 61 years, performed 2 subtraction problems out loud without music and with surgeon-selected and experimenter-selected music. Skin conductance, blood pressure, and pulse rate were monitored. Mathematical speed and accuracy were graded.

Results.—Physiologic responses were highest with no music and lowest during surgeon-selected music. Mathematical speed and accuracy were significantly better with surgeon-selected music.

Comment.—The main benefits of music to the surgeons' psychophysiologic responses and performance were reduced cardiovascular activity and improved task performance. The participants all believed in the benefits of music. The biggest benefit was achieved with surgeon-selected music, regardless of the type of music selected, which supports the value of individual preference.

▶ I do not like music in the operating room. I selected this article for all of you who do.—E.M. Copeland, III, M.D.

Effect of Intraoperative Ketorolac on Postanesthesia Care Unit Comfort

Valdrighi JB, Hanowell LH, Loeb RG, Behrman KH, Disbrow EA (Univ of California at Davis, Sacramento)
J Pain Symptom Manage 9:171–174, 1994   140-95-1–25

Background.—Previous studies have found that ketorolac is an effective analgesic for patients who have moderate pain after surgery. It is not effective as morphine, however, for managing severe pain in the immediate postoperative period. The effectiveness of combined intraoperative ketorolac and opioid analgesics has not been adequately studied. The effects of intraoperative ketorolac on patient comfort in the postanesthesia care unit (PACU) were assessed.

Methods.—Thirty patients who were undergoing general anesthesia for orthopedic or lower abdominal surgical procedures were included in a prospective, randomized, double-blind study. All patients received equivalent doses of intraoperative opioids. At the time of surgical closure, 1 group received 60 mg of IM ketorolac, and the other received 2 mL of normal saline. The patients were followed up to 2 hours in the PACU; at 1 hour after PACU admission, pain was measured on a 100-point visual analogue scale.

Results.—Patients in the control group needed opioids more often and earlier than did those in the ketorolac group. Time to first opioid dose in the PACU was 22 minutes in the control group vs. 76 minutes in the ketorolac group. There was no significant difference in total dosage of postoperative opioids. Pain scores at 1 hour were 36 in the ketorolac group vs. 64 in the control group; there was no difference in time to PACU discharge.

Conclusions.—Intraoperative ketorolac appears to be an effective adjunct in the management of postoperative pain. The analgesic properties of ketorolac may be additive to those of morphine. Because ketorolac acts peripherally, independent of central opioid receptors, it may act synergistically with opioids to interrupt pain transmission.

▶ Pain that develops during emergence from anesthesia in the recovery room is difficult to assess in the semiconscious patient. The administration of ketorolac at the time of wound closure may diminish pain until the patient is awake and conversant, at which time incisional pain can be adequately assessed.—E.M. Copeland, III, M.D.

2 Critical Care

Introduction

The controversy continues. Does the use of inotropes to achieve supranormal oxygen delivery increase survival? How much of the increase in oxygen consumption seen in ICU patients who are treated with adrenergic inotropes to increase oxygen delivery is caused by the thermogenic effects of the inotropes, and how much is caused by previously unmet tissue oxygen needs? These questions are addressed in the first 3 articles in this chapter. On the basis of these and similar studies, the pendulum seems to be swinging away from excessive efforts to increase oxygen delivery and toward a more moderate approach. Thus, when it comes to oxygen delivery, is more better? Maybe, maybe not. On the other hand, there is no doubt that, since its introduction in 1970, the pulmonary artery catheter has changed the approach to bedside hemodynamic monitoring of patients who are critically ill. Surprisingly little information is available, however, to document that the routine use of pulmonary artery catherization improves patient survival. Consequently, a study that documented that information gained via the pulmonary artery catheter increased survival in a subgroup of patients with circulatory shock unresponsive to standard therapy was chosen.

Predicting outcome in patients who are critically ill is assuming increased importance as the entire medical community tries to come to grips with the specter of managed care and the reality of limited resources. Consequently, new and revised mortality models are being developed and tested. One such study found that mortality probability models that accurately predict outcome at admission to the ICU lose their accuracy when applied 48 or 72 hours after admission unless they are modified. Thus, it appears that for a mortality model to maintain its accuracy, it should consider a patient's response to therapy and not be based purely on admission or early values.

The development of nosocomial infections continues to have a significant deleterious effect on the survival of ICU patients, because the mortality risk was 2.48 times higher in patients with nosocomial infection than in noninfected patients. Thus, human and animal studies that evaluate various ways to prevent or limit the consequences of infection continue to be published. For example, in January 1994, an exciting phase II multicenter clinical trial of human recombinant interleukin-1 receptor antagonist (IL-1RA) in the treatment of patients with the sepsis syndrome was published. This study indicated that administration of

IL-1RA was safe and, at higher doses, was associated with a survival benefit. Unfortunately, in June 1994, these encouraging phase II results were not fully validated by the results of the larger phase III clinical trial. That these 2 studies, which were published by the same authors within 6 months of each other, could have such divergent results is, to say the least, perplexing. Perhaps being perplexed is the natural state of events when following the search for the holy sepsis grail. Likewise, recent studies documented that platelet activating factor antagonists decrease certain aspects of the metabolic response to endotoxin in healthy volunteers and might benefit certain subpopulations of patients with severe sepsis. These findings could be viewed with optimism or skepticism; look at the articles and take your choice. In fact, it seems that the intensivists' love affair with steroids has not been extinguished. Or, to paraphrase Mark Twain, news of my demise appears to be premature. Hence, 2 steroid studies were chosen. One study indicates that low-dose steroids attenuates the systemic inflammatory response syndrome in patients with septic shock. A second indicates that steroids may be beneficial in preventing progressive fibroproliferation in late adult respiratory distress syndrome (ARDS).

An interesting approach being tested to improve survival in patients with sepsis is the extracorporeal elimination of circulating endotoxin using polymyxin B-immobilized fibers. The concept behind this therapy is quite simple. If the deleterious effects of gram-negative infection are related to endotoxemia, then removing the endotoxin should result in clinical improvement. On the basis of encouraging results of a pilot clinical study and earlier preclinical studies, it appears that this approach may have potential. The relative merits of sulcrafate vs. H2-blockers in stress ulcer prophylaxis have been hotly debated during the past decade. Recent clinical studies have indicated, however, that the appropriate method of stress ulcer prophylaxis in most ICU patients is neither of the above. Yes, neither acid reduction nor cytoprotection may be required. That is the conclusion of a recent study published in the *New England Journal of Medicine,* which found that stress ulcer prophylaxis is not required in most ICU patients. Another new thought that has gained increased acceptance during the past several years is the use of low-volume, pressure-limited ventilation with permissive hypercapnia in patients with ARDS. Most recently, this approach is supported by a prospective, but uncontrolled, trial in which the use of this ventilatory strategy reduced the mortality rate of patients with ARDS and multiple organ failure by approximately 50% from that predicted by the Acute Physiology and Chronic Health Evaluation II. Sounds good.

Time to switch gears and move from the present to 2 potential buzzwords of the future: heat shock protein and apoptosis. Recognition that the cell contains a number of distinct genetic programs for responding to different insults or stressors has opened a whole new horizon of biology and biologically based therapeutic options. One of the most exciting options involves the biology of the heat shock response and heat shock proteins. Simply stated, cells induced to produce heat shock protein are more resistant to a number of infectious and inflammatory insults. As shown in 2 articles, the induction of the heat shock response improves survival and limits organ injury in animals with otherwise lethal peritonitis. These facts indicate that a strategy of modulating the cells' genetic response may improve survival. Further, because heat shock proteins are induced by fever, and the host's antibacterial systems are more effective at elevated core temperatures, it is time to reconsider the extent to which fever should be "prophylactically" treated. On the other hand, it is also now clear that certain inflammatory stimuli can induce a specific genetic response that will result in programmed cell death. This process has been termed apoptosis. Although speculative, there is some emerging evidence that programmed cell death, or apoptosis, may be an important mechanism of organ failure in systemic inflammatory states. The exact role or relationship of apoptosis to the development of multiple organ failure must await future studies.

The remaining 3 articles deal with a potpourri of topics, ranging from experimental studies that test neutrophil bactericidal permeability increasing protein to clinical studies that investigate the relationship between circulating adhesion molecules and the systemic inflammatory response syndrome. The common element joining these articles is the potential insight they provide into the pathophysiology of sepsis and the systemic inflammatory response syndrome.

Edwin A. Deitch, M.D.

Elevation of Systemic Oxygen Delivery in the Treatment of Critically Ill Patients

Hayes MA, Timmins AC, Yau EHS, Palazzo M, Hinds CJ, Watson D (St Bartholomew's Hospitals at Smithfield and Homerton, London; Charing Cross Hosp, London)
N Engl J Med 330:1717–1722, 1994   140-95-2-1

Background.—To replete tissue oxygen and prevent loss of organ function in patients who are critically ill, an increase in the cardiac index, oxygen delivery, and oxygen consumption to levels that are median maximal values in survivors (> 4.5 L/min/m^2 of body surface area, > 600 mL/min/m^2, and > 170 mL/min/m^2 respectively) has been recommended. The effectiveness of that strategy was evaluated.

Methods.—One hundred nine patients admitted to the ICU for a variety of critical illnesses were studied prospectively. If the cardiac index, oxygen delivery, and oxygen consumption did not reach the aforementioned levels after fluid resuscitation, the patients were randomized to the treatment group, which received dobutamine, 5–200 µg/kg/min, or the control group, which received dobutamine only if the cardiac index was less than 2.8 L/min/m^2.

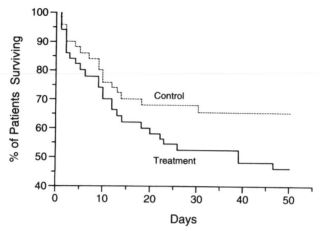

Fig 2–1.—In-hospital survival of patients in the treatment and control groups. (Courtesy of Hayes MA, Timmins AC, Yar EHS, et al: N *Engl J Med* 330:1717–1722, 1994.)

Results.—Nine parents were not randomized because fluid resuscitation achieved the therapeutic goals. Fifty patients were randomized to the treatment group, and 50 patients were randomized to the control group. For cardiac index and oxygen delivery, the 48-hour incremental area under the curve was significantly higher in the treatment group than in the control group. There was no significant difference between the 2 groups for oxygen consumption. All 9 patients that were not randomized survived their hospital stay. Fifty-four percent of the treatment group died while in the hospital, as opposed to 34% of the control group (Fig 2–1).

Conclusion.—Critically ill patients who have had adequate volume replacement and who have sufficient perfusion pressure do not benefit from the use of dobutamine in the ICU to reach target values for cardiac index, oxygen delivery, and oxygen consumption.

▶ It doesn't work and may even be bad. That is the basic conclusion of this randomized trial in which dobutamine was used to help patients reach supranormal levels of oxygen delivery and oxygen consumption. Is this blasphemy, or can it be that supranormal oxygen delivery is not better than normal oxygen delivery in patients who are fully resuscitated? It was never possible to reach the desired levels of oxygen delivery in 35 of 50 patients in the treatment group; in 24 patients in this group, dobutamine-related cardiac adverse events required either discontinuance of the drug or a significant decrease in the dose administered. The authors' observation that the mortality rate of the patients randomized to the supranormal hemodynamic group was higher than that of patients in the control group is important. It underscores the potential danger of trying to drive a physiologic response higher than it can go in ICU patients who are highly stressed.

On the other hand, only 2 of 33 patients who achieved these supranormal levels died. This latter observation supports the idea that the ability of a patient to achieve supranormal indices of oxygen consumption and delivery may be a marker for an intrinsically "healthier" patient with a larger physiologic reserve. It does not mean that driving patients where thay cannot go will be beneficial. The potential dangers of this practice in nonresponders remain to be fully defined. Until then, I advise caution. More may not be better.—E.A. Deitch, M.D.

The Effects of Adrenergic Agents on Oxygen Delivery and Oxygen Consumption in Normal Dogs

Hansen PD, Coffey SC, Lewis FR Jr (Univ of Calif, San Francisco; Henry Ford Hosp, Detroit)
J Trauma 37:283–293, 1994   140-95-2–2

Background.—Patients who have sepsis or are otherwise critically ill are thought to have a supply-dependent relationship between oxygen consumption and oxygen delivery, with consumption continuing to increase with oxygen delivery rather than plateauing as normally occurs. Tissue hypoxia that persists despite above-normal oxygen delivery may be responsible. Adrenergic agents have been given to correct hypoxia by elevating the cardiac output and oxygen delivery. Changes in whole-body

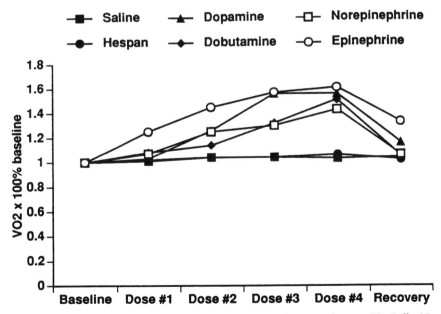

Fig 2–2.—Oxygen consumption times 100% of baseline value. (Courtesy of Hansen PD, Coffey SC, Lewis Jr FR: *J Trauma* 37:283–293, 1994.)

oxygen delivery and oxygen consumption were monitored in dogs that were given physiologic doses of various adrenergic agents.

Methods.—The animals were anesthetized with isoflurane and paralyzed, and body temperature was maintained above 37° C. Oxygen consumption was directly measured after each of 4 incremental doses of dopamine, dobutamine, norepinephrine, and epinephrine and after the animals recovered. The animals also were challenged with a colloidal fluid, 6% Hespan.

Results.—Oxygen consumption increased 43% above baseline after the maximum dose of norepinephrine and 61% after isoproterenol and epinephrine (Fig 2–2). The changes were dose-dependent but consistent at comparable dose levels of all the adrenergic agents. Oxygen delivery increased in a dose-related manner, as much as 150% above baseline with maximal doses. No increase in oxygen consumption was observed in dogs whose oxygen delivery was increased by volume expansion.

Interpretation.—The changes in oxygen consumption and oxygen delivery seen in dogs that are given adrenergic agents resemble those seen in critically ill patients who receive these drugs. The rise in oxygen consumption is probably mediated by β-adrenergic receptors. It results from an increase in metabolism in the whole body rather than an improved oxygen supply to hypoxic tissues. These effects may not benefit patients who are critically ill.

▶ The results of this study speak for themselves. It is possible to produce a pathologic supply-dependent picture of oxygen consumption in otherwise healthy dogs that receive increasing doses of commonly used adrenergic agents. This study therefore supports the authors' hypothesis that the thermogenic effects of adrenergic agents can significantly contribute to the pathologic supply-dependent picture observed in several groups of patients.

In patients with pathologic supply-dependent oxygen consumption who are treated with adrenergic agents, how much of the increase in oxygen consumption is caused by the adrenergic agents and how much is caused by the disease process? Unfortunately, we do not know. Nonetheless, 1 potential approach is to use a nonadrenergic inotropic agent that is not associated with a thermogenic effect. As illustrated in the next article, 1 such agent is amrinone.—E. A. Deitch, M.D.

Thermogenic Effect of Amrinone in Healthy Men
Ruttiman Y, Chioléro R, Revelly J-P, Jeanprêtre N, Schutz Y (Univ Hosp, Lausanne, Switzerland; Univ of Lausanne, Switzerland)
Crit Care Med 22:1235–1240, 1994   140-95-2-3

Background.—Amrinone is a bipyridine derivative that is often used to treat heart failure in patients who are critically ill. It exerts nonadrenergic actions and has both vasodilatory and inotropic effects. Many inotropic

Effect of Progressive Doses of Amrinone on Metabolic and Cardiovascular Variables

Amrinone Infusion Periods (Group 1)

	Preinfusion Baseline	Amrinone 1	Amrinone 2	Amrinone 3
$\dot{V}o_2$ (mL/min)	247 ± 6	252 ± 7	254 ± 7	258 ± 7*
$\dot{V}co_2$ (mL/min)	202 ± 5	207 ± 6	205 ± 620	204 ± 7
Resting metabolic rate (kcal/min)	1.19 ± 0.03	1.22 ± 0.03	1.22 ± 0.03	1.24 ± 0.03*
RQ	0.82 ± 0.02	0.82 ± 0.02	0.81 ± 0.01	0.79 ± 0.02
Rectal temp (°C)	36.6 ± 0.1	36.6 ± 0.01	36.7 ± 0.1	36.7 ± 0.1
HR (beats/min)	58 ± 3	65 ± 3†	69 ± 3†	75 ± 3†
SBP (mm Hg)	120 ± 3	125 ± 3	125 ± 2	123 ± 3
DBP (mm Hg)	72 ± 2	68 ± 2*	67 ± 2*	63 ± 2*
MBP (mm Hg)	86 ± 2	84 ± 28	85 ± 8	83 ± 1
RPP (beats/ min × mm Hg)	6002 ± 221	6873 ± 195‡	6905 ± 80‡	7636 ± 112‡

Note: Values are means ± SEM. Each amrinone infusion period was compared with the preinfusion baseline.
Abbreviations: $\dot{V}o_2$, oxygen consumption; $\dot{V}co_2$, CO_2 production; *RQ*, respiratory quotient; *HR*, heart rate; *SBP*, systolic blood pressure; *DBP*, diastolic blood pressure; *MBP*, mean blood pressure; *RPP*, rate-pressure product.
* $P < .01$.
† $P < .005$.
‡ $P < .05$ vs. control.
(Courtesy of Ruttiman Y, Chioléro R, Revelly J-P, et al: *Crit Care Med* 22:1235–1240, 1994.)

agents, including catecholamines, exert "thermogenic" effects as a result of the direct stimulation of tissue oxygen consumption. The effects of therapeutic doses of amrinone on oxygen consumption and energy metabolism were examined.

Methods.—Ten healthy men, aged 22–35 years, whose body weights ranged from 90% to 121% of ideal were included. Amrinone was given in incremental IV doses, starting with .5 mg/kg followed by 5 μg/kg/min and proceeding to .5 mg/kg followed by 10 μg/kg/min, and finally 1 mg/kg followed by 10 μg/kg/min.

Results.—Heart rate increased in parallel with the dose of amrinone as the diastolic blood pressure decreased significantly (table). The rate-pressure product increased significantly at all infusion rates. Only the highest infusion rate increased oxygen consumption (4.5%) and resting metabolic rate (3.7%) to a significant degree. There were no changes in production of CO_2 or respiratory quotient. Plasma levels of catecholamine were also unchanged, but the level of free fatty acid rose by more than 53% at the highest dose.

Conclusion.—Healthy individuals experience minimal thermogenic and metabolic responses when given therapeutic doses of amrinone. The effects are much smaller than those associated with catecholamines; therefore, the drug may prove advantageous for patients who have severe heart failure.

▶ The importance of this study is that it demonstrates that the thermogenic effect of amrinone is minimal compared with that of adrenergic agents. Thus, although amrinone has less inotropic activity than adrenergic agents, its use may be beneficial in patients with compromised tissue oxygenation in whom supplementary thermogenic stimulation is undesirable.—E.A. Deitch, M.D.

Pulmonary Artery Catheterization in Critically Ill Patients: A Prospective Analysis of Outcome Changes Associated With Catheter-Prompted Changes in Therapy

Mimoz O, Rauss A, Rekik N, Brun-Buisson C, Lemaire F, Brochard L (Université Paris XII, Créteil, France)

Crit Care Med 22:573–579, 1994   140-95-2–4

Background.—The effect of pulmonary artery catheterization on patient improvement has been debated. Misinterpretation of data may lead to inappropriate therapeutic choices and higher morbidity and mortality rates. It has been suggested that the pulmonary artery catheter has been overused and that its limited assistance does not offset associated risks. Physician accuracy in predicating the hemodynamic profiles of patients, associated morbidity, resulting rates of change in therapy, and outcome variations associated with these changes before the insertion of a pulmonary artery catheter were evaluated prospectively.

Methods.—Pulmonary artery catheterizations were performed in 112 patients who did not have acute myocardial infarction. Before catheterization, physicians were asked to predict patients' hemodynamic profiles on the basis of physical examination, laboratory data, radiography, and other diagnostic tools; physicians were then asked to provide a plan for therapy. Patient profiles after catheterization were compared with the predicted diagnoses.

Results.—Physicians correctly predicted hemodynamic profiles in 56% of all patients and in 63% of patients who were in shock and unresponsive to standard therapy. Modifications among hemodynamic profiles varied from 33% to 87%. Two of the 11 patients who had complications required therapy. For all patients, precatheterization characteristics and mortality rates were similar whether or not catheterization caused a change in therapy. For patients in shock who were unresponsive to standard therapy, the mortality rate was significantly lower in those who had a change in therapy after the catheter was inserted, despite identical precatheterization characteristics.

Discussion.—Pulmonary artery catheterization provides data that exceed clinically available information and can induce physicians to change their initial decisions about therapy. The findings suggest a beneficial effect of catheterization on patient outcome. Further studies are needed to confirm the value of catheterization for patients in shock who are unresponsive to standard therapy.

▶ This primarily observational study is one of the few to indicate that use of a pulmonary artery catheter improves survival by facilitating changes in therapy. The article is neither perfect nor definitive. However, because of the ethical constraints of carrying out a randomized trial in which half the patients do not receive a pulmonary artery catheter, it is likely to be as good as we get.

Nonetheless, remember that it is not the catheter that changes clinical outcome but the ability of the physician to interpret the information derived from its use that causes beneficial changes in therapy.—E.A. Deitch, M.D.

Mortality Probability Models for Patients in the Intensive Care Unit for 48 or 72 Hours: A Prospective, Multicenter Study

Lemeshow S, Klar J, Teres D, Avrunin JS, Gehlbach SH, Rapoport J, Rué M (Univ of Massachusetts, Amherst; Tufts Univ, Boston; Mount Holyoke College, South Hadley, Mass)
Crit Care Med 22:1351–1358, 1994   140-95-2–5

Background.—Systems for predicting which ICU patients will die in the hospital have tended to focus on patient characteristics at the time of admission and within the first 24 hours, but later assessments are also important. The Mortality Probability Model (MPM) systems, which are based on both initial and 24-hour evaluations, exhibit good discrimination. Mortality Probability Model systems for predicting hospital mortality after 48 and 72 hours in the ICU were developed.

Methods.—Six adult medical and surgical ICUs participated in a prospective study. Of 6,290 patients who were admitted consecutively, complete data were available for 3,023 patients after 48 hours in the ICU, and for 2,233 after 72 hours. All models included 5 variables that were measured on admission to the ICU, and 8 variables were ascertained every 24 hours.

Findings.—The 24-hour MPM exhibited poor calibration and poor discrimination at 48 and 72 hours. In contrast, the 48- and 72-hour models, which contained the same variables and coefficients as the 24-hour model, calibrated and discriminated well. The later models differ from the MPM_{24} only with respect to their constant terms, which increase to reflect the greater likelihood of death as the ICU stay becomes more prolonged.

Conclusion.—Models designed to estimate mortality risk in ICU patients at a given interval may not be extrapolated to other time periods without being appropriately modified.

▶ Outcomes research is assuming increasing importance because of economic, as well as medical, pressures. Consequently, the ability to assess prognosis throughout a patient's ICU stay and not just at admission is important. The basic message of this study is twofold. First, systems developed to assess prognosis at the time of admission to the ICU lose their accuracy when applied later in the patient's hospital course. Second, these models can be modified to retain their accuracy.

To quote the authors' paraphrase of a common clinical aphorism "if a patient's clinical profile stays the same, he or she is actually getting worse." It's nice to know that this bit of clinical common sense is being applied to the science of prognostication.—E.A. Deitch, M.D.

Influence of Nosocomial Infection on Mortality Rate in an Intensive Care Unit

Bueno-Cavanillas A, Delgado-Rodriguez M, López-Luque A, Schaffino-Cano S, Gálvez-Vargas R (Univ of Granada Hosp, Spain)
Crit Care Med 22:55–60, 1994   140-95-2-6

Introduction.—Nosocomial infection is a common and potentially fatal problem in the ICU. Study of the relationship between mortality and nosocomial infection in ICU patients is complicated by their shared risk factors. The effect of nosocomial infection on mortality in the ICU was investigated. Special attention was given to the potential confounding factors.

Methods.—All 279 patients admitted to the ICU for at least 48 hours during a 16-month period were included. The criteria of the Study on the Efficacy of Nosocomial Infection Control and the Centers for Disease Control and Prevention were used to diagnose nosocomial infections. Admission Acute Physiology and Chronic Health Evaluation (APACHE II) score was assessed, and Therapeutic Intensity Scoring System data were compiled daily.

Findings.—Ninety-three patients had a total of 139 infections. Enterobacteriaceae were the most common organisms isolated, with unidentified organisms being the next most common category. The lower respiratory tract was the most common site of infection, and 79% of infections developed within 1 week of admission. The overall ICU mortality rate was 17%: 28% for those with nosocomial infections, and 11% for those without. The infection-related mortality rate was increased in patients younger than 45 years of age, with a relative risk of 8.35. Patients with respiratory diseases and those with longer ICU stays also had a higher relative risk of mortality. On logistic stepwise regression analysis, which was adjusted for affected organ system, APACHE II score, and therapeutic intensity, risk of death was more than twice as high in patients with nosocomial infection.

Conclusions.—Nosocomial infection doubles the risk of mortality in ICU patients, after adjustment for other factors. The effect is more notable in patients who are younger and less severely ill, probably because patients who are more severely ill die of their underlying disease before infection develops. Patients with respiratory disease are more vulnerable to death from nosocomial infection.

▶ This nicely analyzed, prospective study clearly illustrates that the development of a nosocomial infection remains a major factor in determining survival or death in the ICU. Further, the authors' observation that the development of an infection had the least influence on outcome in patients who were the most severely ill has some interesting implications. First, it highlights the fact that, in these patients, it is the severity of the underlying disease, rather than the development of a subsequent nosocomial infection, that determines the mortality rate. Given this observation, one would be forced to predict that prevention of infection would be of minimal benefit in patients who are the most ill and that the most benefit would be seen in patients with moderate disease in whom prognosis is more favorable. This concept should be kept in mind when assessing the results of studies that evaluate therapeutic maneuvers directed at preventing infection or the consequences of the septic response.—E.A. Deitch, M.D.

Initial Evaluation of Human Recombinant Interleukin-1 Receptor Antagonist in the Treatment of Sepsis Syndrome: A Randomized, Open-Label, Placebo-Controlled Multicenter Trial
Fisher CJ Jr, Slotman GJ, Opal SM, Pribble JP, Bone RC, Emmanuel G, Ng D, Bloedow DC, Catalano MA; the IL-1RA Sepsis Syndrome Study Group (Cleveland Clinic Found, Ohio; Cooper Hosp/Univ Med Ctr, Camden, NJ; Brown Univ, Pawtucket, RI; et al)
Crit Care Med 22:12–21, 1994   140-95-2–7

Introduction. —In sepsis, the release of exogenous microbial components stimulates host inflammatory responses mediated by tumor necrosis factor-α, interleukin-1 (IL-1), and IL-6. Macrophages produce IL-1 receptor antagonist (IL-1RA), which recognizes and binds to both types of IL-1 receptors but has no IL-1 agonist activity, in response to endotoxin and other microbial products. Recombinant IL-1RA has prevented mortality in animal studies of sepsis. The safety, pharmacokinetics, and efficacy of human recombinant IL-1RA was assessed in patients with sepsis syndrome in a phase II study.

Methods.—Ninety-nine ICU patients were included in a prospective, open-label, placebo-controlled study. The patients had sepsis syndrome or septic shock. All received standard supportive care and antimicrobial therapy, as well as escalating doses of IL-1RA or placebo. Treatment began with an IV loading dose of IL-1RA, 100 mg, or placebo. The patients then received a 72-hour IV infusion of either IL-1RA, 17, 67, or 133 mg/hr, or placebo. Treatment groups were compared for 28-day all-cause mortality.

Results.—Treatment with IL-1RA was associated with a dose-dependent survival benefit. Forty-four percent of patients who received placebo died, compared with 32% of those who received the intermediate dose, and 16% of those who received the highest dose. The survival benefit held for the 65 patients who had septic shock at entry and the 45 patients with gram-negative infection.

Treatment with IL-1RA also enhanced survival in patients with an increased concentration of circulating IL-6 of more than 100 pg/mL at entry. In this group, the magnitude of the decrease in IL-6 that occurred 24 hours after therapy was correlated with an increasing dose of IL-1RA. Treatment with IL-1RA was also associated with a significant dose-related reduction in Acute Physiology and Chronic Health Evaluation II score. Plasma clearance of IL-1RA was correlated with estimated creatinine clearance, suggesting that IL-1RA was eliminated by the kidneys. The placebo and active treatment groups were no different in their incidence of adverse effects.

Conclusions.—This phase II clinical study supports the safety and efficacy of human recombinant IL-1RA in patients who have sepsis syndrome. The dose-related survival benefit, which appears to increase with increasing severity of illness, needs to be confirmed in a larger, more definitive clinical trial.

Recombinant Human Interleukin 1 Receptor Antagonist in the Treatment of Patients With Sepsis Syndrome: Results From a Randomized, Double-Blind, Placebo-Controlled Trial
Fisher CJ, for the Phase III rhIL-1ra Sepsis Syndrome Study Group (Cleveland Clinic Found, Ohio)
JAMA 271:1836–1843, 1994   140-95-2–8

Background.—The interleukin-1 receptor antagonist (IL-1RA) is a naturally occurring protein that is produced by macrophages and other cells in response to IL-1, endotoxin, and other microbial substances. Interleukin-1 receptor antagonist binds to IL-1 receptors while exerting no IL-1 agonist activity, and prevents IL-1-mediated cellular responses. A recombinant form of human IL-1RA (rhIL-RA), which has prevented death in animal models of endotoxemia and *Escherichia coli* bacteremia, is now available.

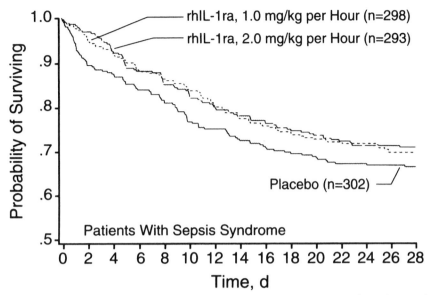

Fig 2–3.—Cumulative survival estimates over 28 days for patients with sepsis syndrome (n = 893) who received placebo or rhIL-1ra in an hourly dose of 1.0 or 2.0 mg/kg. Compared with placebo, mortality was reduced by 9% and 15%, respectively, with the rhIL-1ra hourly dosage regimens of 1.0 and 2.0 mg/kg, although this reduction was not significant (generalized Wilcoxon statistic, P = .22). (Courtesy of Fisher CJ for the Phase III rhIL-1ra Sepsis Syndrome Study Group: *JAMA* 271:1836–1843, 1994.)

Study Plan.—Eight hundred ninety-three patients with sepsis syndrome and septic shock were included in a multicenter, randomized, placebo-controlled, open-label trial of rhIL-1RA. Actively treated patients received an IV loading dose of 100 mg of rhIL-1RA, followed by an infusion of 1 or 2 mg/kg/hr for 72 hours.

Results.—The mortality rate at 28 days was 34% for patients who received placebo, 31% for those who received the lower dose of rhIL-1RA, and 29% for those who received the higher dose (Fig 2–3). In patients who were in shock when admitted to the study, treatment with either dose lowered the point mortality rate at 28 days by 14%. In patients who had dysfunction of 1 or more organs, the higher dose of rhIL-1RA reduced the mortality rate by 10% compared with placebo (Fig 2–4). A significant effect was apparent in patients whose predicted mortality risk was 24% or greater but not in those at lesser risk of dying. Serious adverse effects were comparably frequent in all groups.

Conclusion.—Treatment with rhIL-1RA was not associated with a statistically significant increase in survival time compared with placebo in the primary groups studied. Secondary and retrospective analyses suggest

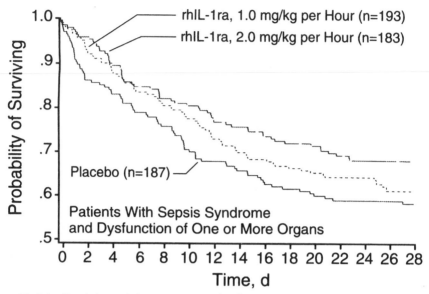

Fig 2–4.—Cumulative survival estimates over 28 days for patients with sepsis syndrome and dysfunction of 1 or more organs at study entry (n = 563) who received placebo or rhIL-1ra in an hourly dose of 1.0 or 2.0 mg/kg. Compared with placebo, mortality was reduced by 7% and 23%, respectively, with the rhIL-1ra hourly dosage regimens of 1.0 and 2.0 mg/kg, although this reduction was not significant (linear dose response, $P = .009$). (Courtesy of Fisher CJ for the Phase III rhIL-1ra Sepsis Syndrome Study Group: *JAMA* 271:1836–1843, 1994.)

that rhIL-1RA may improve survival in patients who have organ dysfunction or a predicted mortality rate greater than 24%.

▶ What can one say when the same investigators publish 2 studies within 6 months of each other and present divergent results? I would have hated to have bought Synergen on the basis of the optimistic open-label phase II study, only to have gone bankrupt when the double-blind phase III study appeared.

Clearly, it is not simple, or is it? The importance of bias in clinical studies continues to be documented and is given great lip service. Because the phase II trial was not blinded, whereas the phase III trial was, that could be the answer. Perhaps. On the other hand, it may be, as the authors suggest, that the population of patients studied was too heterogenous to show an overall improvement in survival and that rhIL-1RA may be effective in certain, well-defined patient subgroups. Time will tell.—E.A. Deitch, M.D.

Platelet-Activating Factor Receptor Antagonist BN 52021 in the Treatment of Severe Sepsis: A Randomized, Double-Blind, Placebo-Controlled, Multicenter Clinical Trial
Dhainaut J-FA, Tenaillon A, Le Tulzo Y, Schlemmer B, Solet J-P, Wolff M, Holzapfel L, Zeni F, Dreyfuss D, Mira J-P, de Vathaire F, Guinot P, BN 52021

Sepsis Study Group (Bourg en Bresse Hosp, France; Bellevue Univ Hosp, France; L Mourier Univ Hosp, Colombes, France; et al)
Crit Care Med 22:1720–1728, 1994   140-95-2–9

Background.—Despite antibiotic treatment, the mortality rate related to severe sepsis approaches 50%. Animal experiments have shown that when inflammatory mediators, such as cytokines or lipid mediators, are blocked, the severity of sepsis decreases. The effect of a natural platelet-activating factor (PAF) receptor antagonist was studied in patients with the sepsis syndrome who received intensive care to determine the safety and efficacy of the drug.

Method.—Two hundred sixty-two patients with documented sepsis syndrome plus either hypotension or toxicity were enrolled in this phase

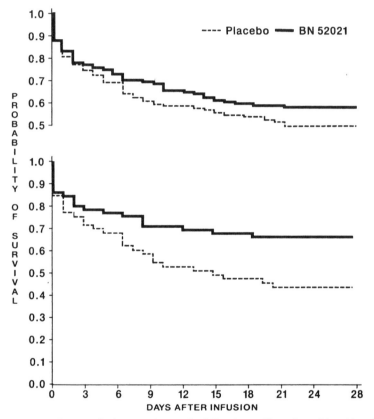

Fig 2–5.—Top, Twenty-eight-day survival curves for 262 patients with sepsis receiving either placebo or platelet-activating factor receptor antagonist (BN 52021), showing an 18% reduction in mortality with BN 52021 treatment (*P* = .17). **Bottom,** Twenty-eight-day survival curves for 120 patients with gram-negative sepsis receiving either placebo or BN 52021, showing a 42% reduction of mortality with BN 52021 treatment (*P* = .01). (Courtesy of Dhainaut J-FA, Tenaillon A, Le Tulzo Y, et al: *Crit Care Med* 22:1720–1728, 1994.)

III study. Patients were randomly assigned to receive an infusion of either 120 mg of the PAF receptor antagonist BN 52021 or a placebo for 15 minutes every 12 hours for 4 days. In addition, the patients received standard intensive care support, including fluids, antibiotic agents, and mechanical ventilation. They were followed for 28 days or until death. A Simplified Acute Physiology Score was determined at enrollment. Vital signs were noted during the first 12 hours after infusion and on days 1, 2, 3, 4, 7, 14, and 28. Data were analyzed with the Mann-Whitney rank-sum test, the Mantel Haenszel chi-square test, the chi-square test, the Kaplan Meier method, and a Cox proportional-hazards model.

Results.—At study end, 66 of 130 patients who received placebo (51%) and 55 of 132 patients who received PAF receptor antagonist (42%) had died. This difference was not statistically significant. The mortality rate was reduced by 18% with BN 52021 treatment (Fig 2–5). The test drug showed higher efficacy in patients with culture-proved gram-negative sepsis than in those with other types of infection. The mortality rate of patients with gram-negative sepsis who received the test drug improved by 42%, but patients with sepsis caused by gram-positive organisms did not improve. When the data from patients with gram-negative sepsis were sorted into subgroups on the basis of the Simplified Acute Physiology Score, mortality was significantly reduced in patients who received the test drug compared with those who received placebo. Resolution of organ failure was significantly higher in the test group. The efficacy of the test drug was higher in patients aged 60 years or older.

Conclusion.—Severely ill patients who have pure or mixed gram-negative sepsis can benefit from treatment with BN 52021. Patients who have sepsis caused by other organisms have little response to BN 52021.

▶ The results of this phase III trial essentially read like the previously published reports on other agents that showed early promise. That is, the PAF antagonist did not improve survival of the total study group that received the drug; by secondary analysis, however, it was found to be effective in certain patient subgroups. These are essentially the same subgroups in which monoclonal antiendotoxin antibodies were found to be effective in retrospective analyses of the original studies. Additional prospective studies that evaluated drug efficacy directly in these subgroups, however, failed to support the initial optimistic conclusions regarding antiendotoxin antibodies. Thus, keeping the results of other sepsis trials in mind, my optimism that PAF antagonists will be found to make a clinical difference is limited. Nevertheless, I am optimistic that combination therapy may be effective when single therapy fails. Therefore, it is important to keep an eye on potential therapeutic options, such as the PAF antagonist.—E.A. Deitch, M.D.

The Metabolic Effects of Platelet-Activating Factor Antagonism in Endotoxemic Man

Thompson WA, Coyle S, Van Zee K, Oldenburg H, Trousdale R, Rogy M, Felsen D, Moldawer L, Lowry SF (New York Hosp–Cornell Univ Med College, New York)
Arch Surg 129:72–79, 1994   140-95-2–10

Background.—Several lines of evidence suggest that the inflammatory phospholipid platelet-activating factor (PAF) may play a critical role in endotoxemia and the sepsis syndrome. The role of PAF in the symptomatic, metabolic, and counter-regulatory hormone responses of endotoxemia in human beings was assessed in a double-blind, placebo-controlled study.

Methods.—Ten healthy male volunteers were studied. Five received the PAF antagonist Ro 24-4736, 10 mg orally, and 5 received placebo. Eighteen hours later, both groups received IV lipopolysaccharide, 4 ng/kg. During the next 24 hours, the 2 groups were compared for vital signs, symptoms, levels of cytokines and hormones, resting energy expenditure, platelet aggregation, and bleeding times.

Results.—The PAF antagonist group had fewer symptoms than the placebo group, including rigors at 1 hour and myalgias at 1–4 hours after administration of lipopolysaccharide. Peak levels of cortisol were 668 nmol/L in the PAF antagonist group vs. 959 nmol/L in the control group. Epinephrine secretion values were 1,057 vs. 2,029 nmol/L, respectively. Pretreatment with Ro 24-4736 yielded almost complete inhibition of PAF-induced platelet aggregation ex vivo. The circulating cytokines tumor necrosis factor-α, interleukin-1β, and interleukin-6 were unchanged, as was the soluble tumor necrosis factor receptor-Is.

Conclusions.—In this model of endotoxemia in human beings, pretreatment with a PAF inhibitor results in attenuation of symptoms and the counter-regulatory hormonal response with no effect on hemodynamics, core temperature, or metabolic rate. The hormonal and symptomatic effects of PAF appear to occur through cytokine-independent mechanisms. The findings support the role of PAF antagonists as an adjunctive treatment to cytokine blockage in patients with gram-negative sepsis.

▶ Studies such as this one, which document that PAF antagonists ameliorate certain aspects of endotoxemia in normal volunteers, have been greeted with great excitement and enthusiasm. It was thought that human studies that showed beneficial physiologic effects of blocking an inflammatory mediator, in combination with encouraging animal work, would allow us to identify clinically useful therapeutic agents. It appears that this may not be the case. We all know the limitations of animal studies and appreciate the aphorism that "the best study of man is man." It also appears, however, that the best study of sick man is sick man. Although studies in healthy volunteers may provide important basic information, we should not let our hopes fool us into thinking that what we observe in these studies of healthy volunteers will be operative in the ICU.—E.A. Deitch, M.D.

Low-Dose Hydrocortisone Infusion Attenuates the Systemic Inflammatory Response Syndrome

Briegel J, Kellermann W, Forst H, Haller M, Bittl M, Hoffmann GE, Büchler M, Uhl W, Peter K, and the Phospholipase A$_2$ Study Group (Ludwig-Maximilians-Universität München, Germany; Städtisches Krankenhaus München-Bogenhausen, Germany; Universität Ulm, Germany)
Clin Investigator 72:782–787, 1994   140-95-2–11

Introduction.—The hypercortisolemia in inflammatory diseases may counteract the overshooting systemic inflammatory response, thereby protecting the host from its own defense reactions. Although levels of cortisol are usually elevated in patients with severe sepsis and septic shock, recent findings have indicated that some patients with septic shock may have relative adrenocortical insufficiency. The effect of low-dose hydrocortisone infusion was evaluated to determine the course of the systemic inflammatory response syndrome.

Methods.—Patients from 7 surgical ICUs were observed. Data from 12 patients who were treated with hydrocortisone were compared with those from 45 cohort patients from other institutions who were not treated with corticosteroids. In the study group, a loading dose of hydrocortisone, 100 mg in 30 minutes, was infused, followed by 10 mg/hr for 14 days. Hemodynamics, vital signs, cardiovascular function, serum chemistry, and inflammatory mediators were measured at appropriate intervals.

Results.—Compared with the external control group, patients in the low-dose hydrocortisone group had significantly decreased febrile response and heart rate and increased mean arterial pressure. In fact, shock reversal occurred in all patients treated with low-dose steroids. Phospholipase A$_2$, C-reactive protein, and neutrophil elastase were measured, and significant decreases in the 2 former inflammatory mediators were noted. On days 7–13 after withdrawal of low-dose hydrocortisone infusion, body temperature, heart rate, and inflammatory mediators increased. Statistical significance was reached for phospholipase A$_2$ and C-reactive protein compared with the external control group.

Conclusion.—Low-dose hydrocortisone infusion attenuates the systemic inflammatory response syndrome in patients with septic shock. A randomized, clinical trial is needed to define the effect of low-dose hydrocortisone infusion on the course and outcome of septic shock.

▶ The authors clearly acknowledge that high-dose glucocorticoids have not been shown to be beneficial in patients with sepsis or septic shock. Low-dose corticosteroid therapy, however, has not been tested. The strength of this study is that the beneficial effects observed with low-dose steroid therapy in patients with septic shock disappeared when the steroids were stopped and were seen again shortly after the steroids were restarted. Note that the dose of steroids used in this preliminary clinical trial was 100- to

200-fold less than that used in previously published clinical trials of steroid therapy in septic shock.

Perhaps there is a role for physiologic doses of steroids.—E.A. Deitch, M.D.

Corticosteroid Rescue Treatment of Progressive Fibroproliferation in Late ARDS: Patterns of Response and Predictors of Outcome
Meduri GU, Chinn AJ, Leeper KV, Wunderink RG, Tolley E, Winer-Muram HT, Khare V, Eltorky M (Univ of Tennessee, Memphis)
Chest 105:1516–1527, 1994   140-95-2-12

Introduction.—Fibroproliferation is fatal in 15% to 40% of patients with late onset adult respiratory distress syndrome (ARDS). Use of IV corticosteroids on such patients has led to significant improvement in lung injury score. How IV corticosteroids act and which factors determine the response to and result of treatment for late onset ARDS were determined.

Methods.—Twenty-five patients who had ARDS and progressive respiratory failure underwent diagnostic bronchoscopic evaluations. Thirteen had open lung biopsies. Corticosteroid treatment was begun an average of 15 days after mechanical ventilation became necessary. Respiratory and cardiovascular parameters, multiple organ failure, systemic inflammatory response syndrome, and type of infection were monitored.

Results.—Nineteen of 25 patients survived. Within 7 days, significant increases were seen in PAO_2: FIO_2. Significant decreases were observed in positive end-expiratory pressure, lung injury score, and minute ventilation. On the basis of response to treatment, patients were classified as rapid, delayed, or nonresponders. The 15 rapid responders improved by day 7, 6 delayed responders improved by day 14, and 4 nonresponders did not improve by day 14. The ICU survival rate for responders (86%) was significantly better than for nonresponders (25%) ($P = .03$).

Discussion.—Histologic differences between survivors and nonsurvivors were significant and included alveolar structure, myxoid type alveolar and interstitial fibrosis, intraluminal bronchiolar fibrosis, and absence of arteriolar subintimal fibroproliferation. Other indicators that differed significantly between survivors and nonsurvivors were presence of liver failure and pattern of physiologic response.

Conclusion.—Early corticosteriod treatment of pulmonary fibroproliferation can be effective. Outcome depends on type of response.

▶ Fibroproliferation is a stereotypical response of the lung to injury and is characterized by deposition of intra-alveolar collagen and production of myofibroblasts. When extensive, this fibroproliferative process can result in severe pulmonary fibrosis that directly contributes to late mortality in a distinct subgroup of patients. Hence, the phase of ARDS characterized by this fibroproliferative response is termed "late ARDS." Because steroids may arrest this fibroproliferative response by modulating macrophage and fibroblast activity, the concept of using steroids in the late phase of ARDS, as was done in this study, appears physiologically sound. All things being equal, on the basis of the encouraging results reported by these authors, the use of methyprednisolone in patients histologically documented to have late ARDS seems reasonable. These patients must be monitored intensively, however, for the development of pneumonia. Finally, I strongly concur with the authors' closing statement that a blinded, randomized study is necessary to confirm the potential benefits of corticosteroid therapy during the proliferative phase of late ARDS.—E.A. Deitch, M.D.

Treatment of Sepsis by Extracorporeal Elimination of Endotoxin Using Polymyxin B-Immobilized Fiber
Aoki H, Kodama M, Tani T, Hanasawa K (Shiga Univ, Japan)
Am J Surg 167:412–417, 1994   140-95-2-13

Introduction.—The mortality rate remains high among patients with septic shock and endotoxemia. Knowledge that polymyxin B (PMX) neutralizes the biological activities of endotoxin has led to the development of a material made of immobilized PMX fibers (PMX-F) for clinical use (Fig 2–6). Polymyxin B fibers consist of a mean of 7 mg of PMX per 1 g of fiber. In preliminary trials, 16 patients with septic multiple organ failure were treated with direct hemoperfusion (DHP) using a PMX-F column.

Patients and Methods.—Most patients were receiving a vasopressor to maintain blood pressure, and many required mechanical ventilation. Nine had peritonitis caused by gastrointestinal perforation. A double-lumen catheter was inserted into the femoral vein for access to blood for DHP with PMX-F adsorbent therapy. The anticoagulant heparin was used in 5 patients, and nafamostat mesilate (NM) was used in 11 patients. Hemodynamic parameters, including heart rate, mean arterial blood pressure, central venous pressure, and cardiac output, were measured. Blood endotoxin concentrations were determined in heparinized blood samples collected before, after 30 minutes of treatment, after DHP treatment, and the next day.

Results.—The 16 patients underwent DHP a total of 29 times. Heparin was used 9 times, and NM was used 20 times. Patients with a systolic pressure of less than 100 mm Hg showed a significant increase from pretreatment level within several hours after the end of DHP. On the next day, 8 patients with a pretreatment mean heart rate of 134 bpm showed a significant decrease to a mean of 122 bpm. Body temperature also decreased significantly in the 11 patients who had a pretreatment body temperature of 38°C or more. The level of endotoxin decreased significantly from 76 pg/mL to 21 pg/mL after 2 hours of DHP. Nine of the

Polystyrene

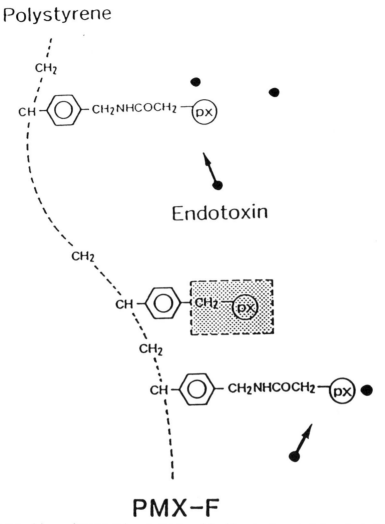

PMX-F

Fig 2–6.—Schema of PMX-F. Polymyxin B is immobilized by using the active halogen in the functional group of the polystyrene based fiber. (Courtesy of Aoki H, Kodama M, Tani T, el al: *Am J Surg* 167:412–417, 1994.)

16 patients were alive 2 weeks after PMX-F therapy, and 7 were discharged from the hospital alive.

Conclusion.—Polymyxin B detoxifies endotoxin but is toxic to the CNS and the kidney. Fixing PMX to polystyrene fibers results in a nontoxic material system. Hemoperfusion using a PMX-F column markedly alleviated symptoms of sepsis syndrome by decreasing the concentration of endotoxin in the blood. The treatment was effective even in patients who did not respond to other methods.

▶ This innovative mechanical approach for removing endotoxin is attractive conceptually. Using PMX=F to reduce the blood level of endotoxin is similar to using a filter to remove dirt and grime from oil in an engine, thereby improving performance. On the basis of encouraging animal preclinical studies and now this uncontrolled pilot clinical study, perhaps it will be possible to cleanse the blood stream of toxic "impurities" mechanically and improve outcome. This approach certainly appears to hold at least as much promise as the use of monoclonal antibodies directed at endotoxin and is likely to be cheaper to boot.—E.A. Deitch, M.D.

Risk Factors for Gastrointestinal Bleeding in Critically Ill Patients
Cook DJ, for the Canadian Critical Care Trials Group (McMaster Univ, Hamilton, Ont, Canada)
N Engl J Med 330:377–381, 1994   140-95-2–14

Objective.—Because measures used to prevent stress ulceration are expensive and may themselves have adverse effects, the frequency of significant gastrointestinal bleeding in critically ill patients was determined.

Study Population.—Consecutive patients older than 16 years of age who were admitted to 4 university-affiliated medical-surgical ICUs during a 1-year period were included. Patients with evidence of upper gastrointestinal bleeding were excluded. Physicians were asked to withhold measures intended to prevent stress ulceration, except in patients with head or burn injuries, organ transplant recipients, and patients in whom peptic ulcer or gastritis had been diagnosed in the previous 6 weeks.

Observations.—Of the 2,252 eligible patients, 674 received prophylaxis against stress ulceration. Their scores on the Acute Physiology and Chronic Evaluation were comparable to those of the other patients, although their mortality rate was higher (16.8% vs. 6.7%). Overall, 33 patients (1.5%) had clinically significant bleeding episodes, defined as overt bleeding with either hemodynamic compromise or a need for transfusion. On multiple regression analysis, the only independent risk factors for clinically important bleeding were prolonged respiratory failure that necessitated mechanical ventilation and coagulopathy. Only 2 of 1,405 patients (.1%) who lacked both risk factors had a clinically significant bleeding episode. Bleeding occurred in 3.4% of patients who were given prophylaxis and in .6% of the others.

Implication.—Because clinically important gastrointestinal bleeding develops in relatively few patients who are critically ill, prophylaxis against stress ulceration may be withheld unless coagulopathy is present or the patient requires mechanical ventilation.

▶ Gastrointestinal bleeding from stress ulcers has largely disappeared from most ICUs as a result of the development and liberal use of effective prophylactic agents. Right—maybe not. This study indicates that the marked decrease in bleeding from stress ulcers may have occurred independently of the use of drug prophylaxis. In fact, only 2 risk factors, respiratory failure and coagulopathy, were associated with an increased risk of stress bleeding, and the incidence of clinically significant bleeding in patients with these risk factors was only 3.7%. Because only 2 of 1,405 patients (.1%) without risk factors had clinically significant bleeding, it is hard to support the notion that all ICU patients require stress ulcer prophylaxis.

Lest one think that the results observed in this study are an aberration, the incidence of clinically significant gastrointestinal bleeding in ICU patients has been found to range from 2% to 3% in many other series. Consequently, there are few hard data to support the routine use of stress bleeding prophylaxis in the ICU.—E.A. Deitch, M.D.

Low Mortality Rate in Adult Respiratory Distress Syndrome Using Low-Volume, Pressure-Limited Ventilation With Permissive Hypercapnia: A Prospective Study

Hickling KG, Walsh J, Henderson S, Jackson R (Christchurch Hosp, New Zealand)

Crit Care Med 22:1568–1578, 1994   140-95-2–15

Introduction.—In a variety of animal studies, it has been shown that controlled mechanical ventilation, with the use of high peak inspiratory pressures, can cause acute lung injury, which appears to result from regional or global lung overdistention. In patients with severe adult respiratory distress syndrome (ARDS), a small amount of aerated lung receives the total ventilation, and overdistention of this aerated lung may occur and result in additional lung injury. There is no definitive evidence, however, that such ventilator-induced lung injury occurs in patients with ARDS. Patients with severe ARDS were evaluated prospectively.

Methods.—Fifty-three patients were managed with a limitation of peak inspiratory pressure to 30–40 cm of H_2O, low tidal volumes (4–7 mL/kg), spontaneous breathing using synchronized intermittent mandatory ventilation from the start of ventilation, and permissive hypercapnia without the use of bicarbonate to buffer acidosis. The hospital mortality rate was compared with that predicted by the Acute Physiology and Chronic Health Evaluation (APACHE) scoring system and the ventilator score.

Results.—The hospital mortality rate was significantly lower than that predicted by the APACHE scores (26.4% vs. 51.3%), even after correcting for the effect of hypercapnic acidosis (26.4% vs. 51.1%). The mortality rate increased with the increasing number of organ failures but was only 43% in patients with 4 or more organ failures, 20.5% with 3 or fewer organ failures, and 6.6% with only respiratory failure. The mean maximum arterial carbon dioxide pressure ($PaCO_2$) was 66.5 torr, and the mean arterial pH at the same time was 7.23. No correlation was seen between the maximum $PaCO_2$ or the corresponding pH and the total respiratory rate at the same time. During mechanical ventilation, no pneumothoraces developed.

Conclusions.—The reduction of regional lung overdistention by the use of low tidal volumes with permissive hypercapnia and limitation of peak inspiratory pressure may reduce ventilator-induced lung injury and improve the outcome in patients with severe ARDS. Without a concurrent control group, these data must be interpreted cautiously.

▶ The results of this prospective but uncontrolled study are consistent with those of several other uncontrolled trials that have suggested that permissive hypercapnia improves survival in patients with severe ARDS. As such, this study supports the new and increasingly popular notion that avoidance of regional lung over distension in patients with ARDS by using small tidal volumes (5–7 mL/kg) and allowing hypercapnia to develop is clinically beneficial.

The basic take-home message of this study is that pressure-limited ventilation may be superior to the more traditional volume-controlled ventilation in patients with ARDS or acute hypoxic respiratory failure.—E.A. Deitch, M.D.

Sodium Arsenite Induces Heat Shock Protein-72 Kilodalton Expression in the Lungs and Protects Rats Against Sepsis
Ribeiro SP, Villar J, Downey GP, Edelson JD, Slutsky AS (Mount Sinai Hosp, Toronto; The Toronto Hosp; Univ of Toronto)
Crit Care Med 22:922–929, 1994   140-95-2-16

Background.—All organisms, including human beings, respond to various stimuli and stresses by synthesizing so–called stress response proteins, or heat shock proteins (HSP). A brief period of warming or heat stress has often been used experimentally to study this phenomenon. Organisms may die when exposed to marked heat stress but survive if given mild heat treatment before exposure. Whether the induction of HSPs by a nonthermal mechanism protects against experimental sepsis was investigated.

Methods.—Adult rats in which sepsis was produced by ligating and perforating the cecum were studied. The animals received either an IV dose of sodium arsenite, 6 mg/kg, or saline in a blinded manner 18 hours before cecal ligation. Heat shock protein–72 was detected in lung tissue by the Western immunoblot technique.

Results.—Injection of sodium arsenite led to production of HSP-72 in the lungs without an elevation of body temperature. Only 6.5% of animals injected with arsenite had died 18 hours after cecal ligation and perforation, compared with 42% of those given saline. Protection was

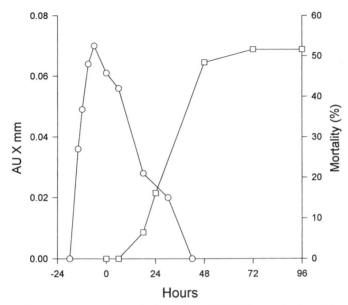

Fig 2–7.—Time-course curve of heat shock protein of 72-kilodalton molecular weight protein expression (*open circles*) in the lungs of sodium arsenite-injected animals was plotted with a mortality curve (*open squares*) from animals injected with sodium arsenite and exposed to cecal ligation and perforation. Note that as heat shock protein expression starts to decrease, mortality rate increases, reaching a peak when heat shock proteins returned to baseline values. AU X*mm*, absorbance unites by millimeter wide. (Courtesy of Ribeiro SP, Villar J, Downey GP, et al: *Crit Care Med* 22: 922–929, 1994.)

evident up to 24 hours after cecal ligation but was no longer significant at 48 hours. Mortality began increasing as the expression of HSP declined (Fig 2–7).

Conclusion.—Stimulation of HSP expression in the lungs of rats protects them against the lethal effects of experimental sepsis.

Induction of the Heat Shock Response Reduces Mortality Rate and Organ Damage in a Sepsis-Induced Acute Lung Injury Model
Villar J, Ribeiro SP, Mullen JBM, Kuliszewski M, Post M, Slutsky AS (Mount Sinai Hosp, Toronto; The Hosp for Sick Children, Toronto; Univ of Toronto)
Crit Care Med 22:914–921, 1994   140-95-2-17

Objective.—A rat model of sepsis was studied to learn whether inducing the formation of heat shock proteins (HSPs) can prevent or reduce organ injury and improve survival.

Methods.—After being exposed to sham or actual heat treatment to raise core body temperature to 41°C, sham or actual peritonitis was induced by cecal ligation and puncture. In addition, the formation of HSP of 70-kD molecular weight (HSP-70) in the lungs and heart was studied by estimating inducible 72-kD HSP messengerRNA by Northern analysis.

Findings.—Nine of 36 unheated rats (25%) had died within 18 hours after cecal ligation and perforation, but all 30 preheated animals had survived. The mortality rates of unheated and heated rats within 1 week of cecal excision and peritoneal lavage were 69% and 20%, respectively. Cecal necrosis developed much more frequently in unheated animals. Those subjected to heat treatment had less evidence of sepsis-induced acute lung injury and liver damage. Levels of HSP-72 peaked 12 hours after hyperthermic stress in the lung and 18 hours after hyperthermic stress in the heart.

Conclusion.—Exposure of rats to heat before induction of sepsis can, through the production of HSP, limit organ damage and promote survival in a model of sepsis-induced acute lung injury.

▶ These 2 articles illustrate that the induction of the heat shock response, either by heating the animals in a chamber or by the administration of sodium arsenite, improves survival and decreases organ injury in a clinically relevant animal model of peritonitis. The mechanism by which a heat shock response improves survival has not been fully elucidated but appears to involve the binding of HSPs to key cellular proteins and enzymes. By binding to these important cellular enzymes during periods of cellular stress, the HSPs prevent these enzymes from being denatured, thereby preventing cell death. Simply stated, by preventing cell death, organ function is preserved, and the host's chance of survival is increased.

Because fever induces the heat shock response, and the host's antibacterial defense systems are more effective at elevated core temperatures, fever appears to be an important host defense mechanism and perhaps should not be treated cavalierly, as is the current policy in most ICUs. My own practice is not to lower the patient's body temperature pharmacologically just because it is elevated. In fact, to the chagrin of my residents, I rarely "treat" a temperature lower than 102° F.—E.A. Deitch, M.D.

Antioxidants Modulate Induction of Programmed Endothelial Cell Death (Apoptosis) by Endotoxin
Abello PA, Fidler SA, Bulkley GB, Buchman TG (Johns Hopkins Univ, Baltimore, Md)
Arch Surg 129:134–141, 1994   140-95-2–18

Background.—Mammalian cells may die by 2 different mechanisms: necrosis or apoptosis (programmed cell death). Porcine endothelial cells sequentially exposed to bacterial endotoxin followed by inducers of the heat shock response die by apoptosis. An in vitro model of the multiple organ dysfunction syndrome, the most common cause of death in the surgical ICU, was described.

Methods.—Several different antioxidants were tested at different concentrations to determine their ability to block apoptosis in cultured porcine endothelial cells. Culture cells were treated with lipopolysaccharide (LPS) for 18 hours. Some cells then were exposed to either heat shock at 43°C or sodium arsenite to induce the heat shock response. Another group of cells was exposed to cycloheximide to interrupt protein synthesis. Various antioxidants were tested for their ability to block apoptosis either before or after LPS application but before sodium arsenite or cycloheximide treatment.

Results.—Apoptosis was blocked by the membrane-permeable, hydroxyl radical scavengers dimethyl sulfoxide and high-dose allopurinol. Apoptosis was also blocked by preventing the generation of hydroxyl radicals, by the chelation of iron with o-phenanthroline. Cell membrane–impermeable hydroxyl radical scavengers (superoxide dismutase, catalase) did not block apoptosis. Hydroxyl radical ablation was only effective when the compounds were administered before the application of LPS.

Conclusions.—The hydroxyl radical may have a role as a nonlethal intracellular signal in endothelial cell apoptosis. The results are consistent with a role for programmed cell death in the pathogenesis of multiple organ dysfunction syndrome. Thus, manipulation of these signals and their effects on gene expression suggests potential new strategies for the prophylaxis and treatment of the multiple organ dysfunction syndrome.

▶ Yes, it is true. Given the right circumstances, cells can and will commit suicide. In certain circumstances, such as during embryogenesis, when certain cell populations must die to allow new populations to emerge, this trait is beneficial. In other circumstances, however, the ability of cells to induce a genetic program leading to cell death can have dire consequences for the host. This important basic science study investigated the mechanisms of programmed cell death, or apoptosis.

In this study, the authors found that endotoxin followed by heat shock resulted in apoptosis. At this point, you may be thinking, Wait a minute, in the 2 studies above, heat shock protected the animals, and now heat shock kills cells. Something does not make sense. The answer is that the cell is a complex place. It turns out that the cellular response to sequential stimuli is not just based on the stimuli, but also on the sequence in which the cell is exposed to the stimuli. Specifically, heat shock before an inflammatory response protects cells, but heat shock after an inflammatory response kills cells. Consequently, it appears that if we wish to shift the balance in favor of cell survival, we may have to intervene to ensure that the sequence of stimuli is beneficial.—E.A. Deitch, M.D.

Human Neutrophil Bactericidal/Permeability-Increasing Protein Reduces Mortality Rate From Endotoxin Challenge: A Placebo-Controlled Study

Fisher CJ Jr, Marra MN, Palardy JE, Marchbanks CR, Scott RW, Opal SM (Cleveland Clinic Found, Ohio; Incyte Pharmaceuticals, Palo Alto, Calif; Brown Univ, Providence, RI; et al)
Crit Care Med 22:553–558, 1994   140-95-2–19

Introduction.—It has been suggested that antiendotoxin immunotherapy can reduce the mortality rate in some patients with gram-negative bacteremia. Because the naturally occurring endotoxin-neutralizing agent bactericidal/permeability-increasing (BPI) protein has potent antimicrobial activity against gram-negative bacteria in vitro, the toxicologic and pharmacologic characteristics of BPI protein were evaluated in a prospective, randomized, placebo-controlled laboratory study.

Methods.—The pharmacokinetics of IV BPI protein were assessed in CD-1 mice, and toxicologic studies were assessed in mice and in Sprague Dawley rats. In both of these species, as well as in New Zealand white rabbits, further studies were performed to assess the ability of IV BPI protein to neutralize endotoxin.

Results.—A single IV bolus injection of BPI protein, 10 mg/kg, caused no changes in hematologic, renal, or hepatic function; activity level; or weight gain during a 1-week period. At the same dose, BPI protein protected all but 1 of 16 mice from a lethal endotoxin challenge, compared with none of a group of saline-treated control mice ($P < .001$). When given up to 1 hour after endotoxin challenge, the protective effects of BPI protein persisted. The induration and dermal necrosis that occurred in the localized dermal Shwartzman reaction were also reduced by BPI protein.

Conclusions.—These animal experiments show that BPI protein is a potent antiendotoxin. It neutralizes endotoxin in vivo and prevents death in animals that are given a lethal endotoxin challenge. Further studies are needed to clarify the potential role of BPI protein as a specific therapeutic agent in human beings.

▶ So, human neutrophil BPI protein protects animals against a lethal endotoxin challenge. Sounds good, but what is BPI protein? It is a natural protein product of neutrophils that has potent antimicrobial and endotoxin neutralizing capacity and may downregulate the biological activity of endotoxin in vivo. Because of these important properties, interest has focused on this natural host defense factor as a potential therapeutic agent in patients with gram-negative sepsis or endotoxemia. In fact, a recent study that involved patients with gram-negative sepsis, as well as normal volunteers injected with endotoxin, demonstrated that the spontaneous production of BPI protein is likely to be inadequate (1). Before BPI protein can be brought to clinical trial, however, it must be tested thoroughly for toxicity and efficacy in relevant animal models. This animal study, although encouraging, does have major limitations. First, BPI protein was only effective when administered in very close (< 60 minutes) temporal association to the endotoxin challenge, a condition not likely to be seen clinically. Additionally, the bolus IV endotoxin injection model used in these experiments is not clinically relevant, and the results of studies that have used this bolus endotoxin model all too frequently have not held up in clinically relevant septic models or in clinical trials. Consequently, further studies in several clinically relevant models of infection are mandatory next steps in the assessment of BPI protein. Until these studies are done, the potential clinical usefulness of BPI protein must remain speculative and unproved.—E.A. Deitch, M.D.

Reference

1. Calvano SE, et al: *Arch Surg* 129:220–226, 1994.

Increased Circulating Adhesion Molecule Concentrations in Patients With the Systemic Inflammatory Response Syndrome: A Prospective Cohort Study

Cowley HC, Heney D, Gearing AJH, Hemingway I, Webster NR (St James' Univ Hosp, Leeds, England; British Bio-Technology Ltd, Oxford, England)

Crit Care Med 22:651–657, 1994   140-95-2-20

Background.—Increased expression of endothelial adhesion molecules is evidence of endothelial activation in experimental animals with the systemic inflammatory response syndrome. Extravasation of activated leukocytes is mediated by adhesion molecules on both endothelial cells and leukocytes and leads to both local tissue damage and systemic inflammatory effects culminating in organ dysfunction.

Method.—Enzyme-linked immunosorbent assays were used to relate soluble derivatives of endothelial adhesion molecules to systemic inflammation and organ dysfunction in a prospective series of 35 patients with the systemic inflammatory response syndrome. Fifteen of these patients had organ dysfunction. Five other patients who were severely ill and 85 healthy individuals were also studied. Levels of soluble E-selectin (sE-selectin), vascular cell adhesion molecule 1, and intercellular adhesion molecule 1 were estimated.

Findings.—Patients with organ dysfunction had significantly higher levels of sE-selectin than did those with either uncomplicated systemic inflammatory response syndrome or other severe illness. All patient groups had elevated levels of vascular cell adhesion molecule 1 and circulating intercellular adhesion molecule 1 compared with control individuals. There was no significant overall difference in mean plasma levels of adhesion molecules between patients who survived and those who died, but no patient whose initial or peak levels of sE-selectin exceeded 36 units/mL survived.

Conclusion.—Estimating circulating levels of adhesion molecules, particularly sE-selectin, may prove helpful in predicting which patients with systemic inflammatory response syndrome will have organ dysfunction.

▶ The take-home messages of this prospective clinical trial are that levels of soluble adhesion molecules are increased in patients with the systemic inflammatory response syndrome and that the highest levels of sE-selectin were observed in the patients with organ failure. This clinical study thus provides important indirect evidence to support the basic concept that endothelial cell activation and injury is involved in the pathogenesis of organ injury.—E.A. Deitch, M.D.

Isolated Pulmonary Infection Acts as a Source of Systemic Tumor Necrosis Factor

Fukushima R, Alexander JW, Gianotti L, Ogle CK (Univ of Cincinnati, Ohio)
Crit Care Med 22:114–120, 1994   140-95-2-21

Background.—Endogenous mediators secreted by the host—particularly such cytokines as tumor necrosis factor (TNF)—appear to mediate many of the biological sequelae of infection. The systemic secretion and effects of TNF have been studied extensively, but the local secretion sites have not. The local secretion of TNF in the lungs was studied as a source of the increased systemic levels of TNF in guinea pigs.

Methods.—Female guinea pigs were presented with an intratracheal challenge of *Escherichia coli*, 10^3 to 10^9. Two and 8 hours later, bacterial colony-forming units in the lung and blood, TNF and prostaglandin E_2 (PGE_2) in the bronchoalveolar lavage fluid, and serum concentrations of TNF were measured.

Results.—Control animals had either very low or undetectable levels of TNF and PGE_2 in bronchoalveolar lavage fluid, whereas the bacteria-challenged animals had high concentrations of both. At 2 hours, levels of TNF in the bronchoalveolar lavage fluid were significantly correlated with serum levels of TNF. Aortic blood showed a significantly higher concentration of TNF than did right atrial blood. At comparable levels of bacterial challenge, TNF in the bronchoalveolar lavage fluid was significantly lower at 8 hours than at 2 hours. However, levels of PGE_2 remained high at 8 hours.

Conclusions.—The lungs may be an important source of TNF in the blood during pulmonary gram-negative infection. The intensity of the infection in its early stages has a major influence on the magnitude of TNF secretion by the lungs. Secretion of TNF appears to be down-regulated within 8 hours after the onset of infection, perhaps by endogenous PGE_2 secretion.

▶ The importance of this study is its demonstration that the lungs, through the local production of TNF, contribute significantly to the increased systemic TNF response observed during pneumonia. The observation that locally produced TNF is released into the systemic circulation helps explain how a localized pulmonary infection (or insult?) can contribute to the development of a systemic septic response, even in the absence of a systemic bacteremia. One logical corollary of this paradigm of a pulmonary-induced systemic inflammatory state would be the local intrapulmonary administration of anticytokine agents to blunt or prevent the development of an uncontrolled systemic inflammatory septic state. Whether this therapeutic approach will prove feasible in the future is unknown but is worthy of pursuit.—E.A. Deitch, M.D.

3   Burns

Introduction

The line separating basic from clinical science continues to narrow. This is true in the field of burn care just as in other areas of medicine. Thus, although the clinical issues in burn care remain focused on such topics as wound healing, infection, nutrition, smoke inhalation, and rehabilitation, the jargon and products of the molecular biological revolution are becoming ever more prominent in the daily care of these and other patients. In fact, the more we learn about the various basic mediators of 1 system, the more we begin to realize that these same mediators influence other systems. For example, it is now well accepted that crosstalk exists between systems once thought to be as distinct as the immune system and the CNS. Recognition of this important concept, in conjunction with rapid developments in molecular biological technology, has resulted in the production and use of factors characterized in 1 system being used to support a second system. This paradigm is well illustrated in a study in which recombinant human growth hormone was used successfully to accelerate wound healing in children with large burns. In a second clinical study, recombinant insulin-like growth factor-1 was found to reduce protein catabolism in patients with major thermal injuries. In a further example of how basic studies help explain clinical observations, a recent study found that interleukin-6 plays a significant role in mediating protein metabolism after thermal injury. Taken together, these studies indicate that, in the future, the line separating basic science from clinical science will continue to blur.

Studies continue to verify the safety of aggressive enteral feeding. Most recently, a randomized clinical trial documented that enteral jejunostomy tube feeding can be continued safely up to and through operative procedures. In fact, the incidence of wound infections was lower in the group that was fed compared with the group of patients whose feedings were withheld. On the basis of these results, the traditional teaching that enteral tube feedings must be discontinued 6 hours or more before surgery should be revisited. Interest in the gut as more than a conduit for nutrients continues, especially because gut barrier failure has been implicated as a predisposing factor in the development of sepsis and multiple systems organ failure. Consequently, 2 articles that examined the pathophysiologic effects of burn injury on gut barrier function were included, as was 1 study that demonstrated that gut barrier function can be modulated hormonally.

The optimal care and therapy of the burn wound continues to be a major focus of interest. One interesting study that appeared this year looked at the long-term consequences of meshed vs. unmeshed skin grafts, as well as the effect of early vs. late grafting of burn wounds on wound contraction. These authors found that the ultimate magnitude of skin graft contraction was less for unmeshed than meshed grafts—a finding that was not too surprising. They also found, however, that skin grafts performed early (within 5 days afterburn) contracted less than skin grafts performed 25–35 days afterburn. This latter observation provides additional support for a policy of early burn wound excision and grafting. Yet, in spite of optimal wound care, the use of pressure garments, and technically satisfactory operative procedure, many patients still have hypertrophic burn scars. Thus, a clinical report that documents that a relatively large percentage of hypertrophic burn scars will respond to intralesional injections with the calcium channel blocker verapamil is potentially exciting. In addition, as reflected by some of the selected articles, work continues on the development of composite skin grafts.

Two studies that dealt with selected pathophysiologic and therapeutic aspects of smoke inhalation were also chosen. The first of these studies characterizes the immense increase in systemic oxygen consumption that occurs after smoke inhalation injury. It also found that positive pressure ventilation can largely eliminate this smoke-induced increased energy expenditure by reducing the work of breathing. The second article examined the therapeutic role of inhaled nitric oxide on pulmonary function in a model of smoke inhalation. On the basis of its apparent clinical usefulness in patients with adult respiratory distress syndrome and other pulmonary disease processes, it is not surprising that inhaled nitric oxide appeared to be physiologically beneficial in this model of smoke inhalation injury. However, because this study only lasted 48 hours, and inhaled nitric oxide did not reduce the histologic extent or magnitude of pulmonary injury, the long-term effectiveness of this therapy is unknown. Although the previous 2 studies dealt with smoke inhalation, it is clear that the lung is also a target organ after isolated cutaneous thermal injury. As discussed in a subsequent article, lung injury after a cutaneous thermal injury appears to occur through leukocyte-mediated endothelial cell injury. This observation, plus those of other studies not included, support the paradigm that immunoinflammatory-mediated tissue and organ injury is important in the pathogenesis of the local and systemic consequences of a major thermal injury.

Studies that investigate the mechanisms behind the impaired immune response observed after thermal injury are yielding important mechanistic information. As outlined in 1 study, it is now possible to begin to determine exactly where, in the cascade of cellular events that are involved in the generation of an immune response, the injury-induced "action" is occurring. As shown in another paper selected, however, one must always correlate the results of tests done in vitro with responses seen in vivo, otherwise false or incomplete conclusions may ensue. Recognition that some of our long-established therapeutic approaches to the care of the patient with burn injury may increase the risk of infection by decreasing immune competence has led us to revisit certain established concepts. One such area is the policy of routine prophylactic transfusions, or when "to transfuse or not to transfuse." On the basis of recent clinical studies, when the goal of transfusion is to maintain the patient's level of hemoglobin in the 10 g/dL range prophylactically, the answer is no.

Although it is easy to focus on the medical aspects of a patient's thermal injury, the psychodynamic and neurophysiologic aspects of this injury continue to demand our attention. In that light, I selected 2 important studies in this area to conclude this year's chapter on Burns. The first article documented the high and frequently unappreciated incidence of significant sleep deprivation after thermal injury. The second article dealt with the long-term effects of thermal injuries on the psychologic well-being and adjustment of both patients and their families.

Edwin A. Deitch, M.D.

Recombinant Human Growth Hormone Accelerates Wound Healing in Children With Large Cutaneous Burns

Gilpin DA, Barrow RE, Rutan RL, Broemeling L, Herndon DN (Shriners Burns Inst, Galveston, Tex; Univ of Texas Med Branch, Galveston)
Ann Surg 220:19–24, 1994   140-95-3–1

Introduction.—In children with severe burn injuries, administration of recombinant human growth hormone (rhGH) may reduce the hypermetabolic period and risk of infection while accelerating the healing of donor sites used for skin grafting. Two different forms of rhGH were examined for their efficacy in healing donor sites in severely burned children. The 2 forms of rhGH used were Protropin, a commercially available product, and Nutropin, which is not yet commercially available. The 2 growth hormone products differ structurally; Protropin includes an N-terminal methionine residue that is not found in Nutropin.

Methods.—Forty-six children with total body surface area burns of greater than 40% and total body surface area full-thickness burns of greater than 20% were included in a double-blind, randomized study of Nutropin. Beginning on the morning of the initial excision, the children received Nutropin or placebo, .2 mg/kg/day by subcutaneous or IM injection. Another 18 children, who did not meet the criteria for receiving Nutropin, received therapeutic Protropin at the same dose. The donor sites, which measured .006 to .010 inches in depth, were harvested and dressed with Scarlet red–impregnated fine mesh gauze. Time to healing of the donor site was defined as the number of days needed before the gauze could be removed without trauma to the healed site.

Results.—Time to donor site healing was 7 days in children who received Nutropin and 6 days in those who received Protropin, compared with 8.5 days in those who received placebo. The reduction in healing time was significant in both of the rhGH groups. Patient subgroups of different ages or times to admission showed no significant differences in healing times. Average length of hospital stay was 40 days for the rhGH groups vs. 55 days for the placebo group.

Conclusions.—Both forms of rhGH can reduce donor site healing time effectively in severely burned children. This is important clinically because the patient's own skin is made rapidly available for harvest and autograft. The results suggest that using rhGH can reduce total length of hospital stay by more than 25%.

▶ This study is important for several reasons, besides its obvious clinical importance. It illustrates that relationships exist among what might be considered otherwise independent systems. Specifically, this study shows that rhGH, which is a product of the pituitary gland that modulates the metabolic response, also modulates wound healing. This study also illustrates how the fruits of molecular biology can have a profoundly important effect on clinical practice.

My enthusiasm for the conceptual significance of this study is not intended to overshadow its practical, clinical importance. By accelerating the healing time of donor sites, not only is the hospital course shortened, but, in my experience, the patients appear to do better. Further, by using rhGH in children who have large burns and limited donor sites, it is frequently possible to use 1.5:1 or 2:1 rather than 3:1 or larger mesh ratios, thereby achieving a superior cosmetic result. In closing, it is important to point out that the role of rhGH in adult patients with burn injury is unclear at present, because there is some evidence that rhGH may not be as effective in adults as children.—E.A. Deitch, M.D.

Insulin-Like Growth Factor-1 Lowers Protein Oxidation in Patients With Thermal Injury
Cioffi WG, Gore DC, Rue LW III, Carrougher G, Guler H-P, McManus WF, Pruitt BA Jr (US Army Inst of Surgical Research, Fort Sam Houston, Tex; Med College of Virginia, Richmond; Univ of Alabama, Birmingham; et al)
Ann Surg 220:310–319, 1994   140-95-3-2

Objective.—Current treatment for patients with burn injury does not include a good method for dealing with the accelerated rate of protein breakdown that accompanies such injury. Although administration of growth hormone shows promise, it fails to restore nitrogen balance to patients who are severely burned and functions as an insulin antagonist. It has been proposed that growth hormone regulates insulin-like growth factor-1 (IGF-1), which is thought to mediate the anabolic effects of growth hormone. The effects of continuous recombinant human IGF-1 infusion on the rate of protein breakdown experienced by patients with burns were evaluated.

Methods.—Blood and urine samples were collected from 8 patients, aged 36–62 years, who were burned on more than 25% of their bodies. Thereafter, each patient received a 3-day IV infusion of IGF-1, 20 μg/kg/hr, a glucose tolerance test, and an infusion of ^{15}N lysine to measure protein oxidation and degradation.

Results.—No patient had hypoglycemia. Serum levels of IGF-1 increased significantly, as did levels of IGF-1 binding proteins 1 and 2. Levels of insulin and C-peptide decreased significantly. Resting energy expenditure did not change. Glucose uptake increased, protein oxidation decreased, insulin secretion responded poorly to glucose challenge, and lysine oxidation decreased significantly.

Conclusion.—These short-term studies show that administration of IGF-1 reduces protein catabolism and is safer than insulin. No serious side effects were associated with the administration of IGF-1. These results indicate that IGF-1 can improve metabolic support in patients with burns and may shorten hospital stays.

▶ Because current nutritional support regimens do not fully reverse net protein catabolism or blunt the increased rate of protein breakdown observed after major thermal injury, more is needed. This clinical study, which documents that the administration of IGF-1 minimizes burn-induced protein catabolism and reduces the loss of lean body mass, is consequently of great clinical interest. Unfortunately, because of several episodes of cardiac arrest and the development of Bell's palsy in other patient groups (AIDS and severe diabetes), IGF-1 has been removed from the market by its manufacturers. Thus, whether IGF-1 will find a place in the treatment of patients with burn injury or other patient groups remains unknown at present. Nonetheless, this study is important because it indicates that the autocatabolic process associated with major burn injury may be reduced therapeutically.—E.A. Deitch, M.D.

Cytokine Response to Burn Injury: Relationship With Protein Metabolism

De Bandt JP, Chollet-Martin S, Hernvann A, Lioret N, Du Roure LD, Lim S-K, Vaubourdolle M, Guechot J, Saizy R, Giboudeau J, Cynober L (Hôpital Saint Antoine, Paris; Hôpital Xavier Bichat, Paris; Hôpital Laennec, Paris)
J Trauma 36:624–628, 1994   140-95-3–3

Purpose.—Several hormones, particularly cortisol, mediate hypercatabolism. Cytokines, which are peptides that are produced mainly by activated reticuloendothelial cells, have been the focus of renewed attention as mediators of the metabolic response to injury. Production of cytokines was evaluated in patients with burn injury according to their extent of injury, and the relationship between the cytokine response and protein metabolism was evaluated.

Methods.—Twelve patients with burn injury were studied 2–21 days after injury. Throughout the healing period, plasma levels of interleukin-1β (IL-1β), tumor necrosis factor-α (TNF-α), IL-6, and markers of protein metabolism were measured. The percentage of surface area burned ranged from 9% to 82%. The pattern of variation in plasma concentrations of cytokines was analyzed, and the relationship between production of cytokines and nutritional status was assessed.

Results.—The most consistently elevated cytokine was IL-6. Maximum concentrations of IL-6 were reached on day 4 and were correlated with the severity of the burn. Levels of TNFα were elevated as well but were not correlated with extent of injury. However, levels of TNF-α on day 7 were 67 pg/mL in patients who had sepsis compared with 20 pg/mL in those who did not. On day 7, cortisolemia was inversely correlated with levels of TNFα but not with levels of IL-6. Positive correlations were noted between levels of IL-6 and protein turnover and catabolism; negative correlations were noted between levels of IL-6 and fibronectin and transthyretin.

Conclusions.—In patients with burn injury, the systemic cytokin response is represented mainly by IL-6. This cytokine appears to be a key mediator of the variations in protein metabolism after burns. Interleukin-6 might represent an index of severity in burn injury. Limiting the effects of this cytokine with specific antibodies might be a useful approach to preventing the complications of burn injury.

▶ It is now clear that the hypermetabolic response to injury or infection is not adequately modeled by changes in traditional stress hormones which indicates that other factors are involved. One such candidate group of mediators is the cytokine. Thus, the relevance of this study is that a relationship is documented between levels of IL-6 and protein metabolism. Although I believe that the authors' assumption that the modulation of circulating IL-6 levels will be beneficial may be too simplistic, their basic observation is of interest and potential importance.—E.A. Deitch, M.D.

Enteral Feeding During Operative Procedures in Thermal Injuries
Jenkins ME, Gottschlich MM, Warden GD (Shriners Burns Inst, Cincinnati, Ohio; Univ of Cincinnati, Ohio)
J Burn Care Rehabil 15:199–205, 1994   140-95-3-4

Introduction.—The hypermetabolism and hypercatabolism that characterizes thermal trauma can result in the catabolism of body tissues if the patient does not receive sufficient nutritional support. Enteral support, however, is traditionally suspended before, during, and after the numerous surgical procedures these patients typically require, which can result in deficiency of calories. The safety of providing continuous intra-operative enteral nutritional support to the small intestine in patients with burn injuries was examined, as were patient outcomes.

Methods.—Eighty patients with burn injuries who required supplemental nutritional support were randomly assigned either to receive intraoperative enteral support (40 patients) or to have enteral support withheld before, during, and after surgery until bowel sounds returned (40 patients). The 2 groups were matched for age, total body surface area injured, smoke inhalation, and postburn admission day. The feeding tubes were positioned in the duodenum. A nasogastric tube was also inserted during surgery for suctioning to prevent reflux and maintain gastric decompression. Caloric requirements were calculated by indirect calorimetry. Serum levels of protein, albumin, prealbumin, transferrin, and IgG were monitored. Infectious complications were identified with regular blood, urine, and sputum cultures.

Results.—The patients who received continual nutritional support underwent 161 surgical procedures; those who had perioperative enteral support withheld underwent 129 surgical procedures. The unfed patients had a consistent and significant caloric deficit and required more supplemental albumin. These patients also experienced significantly more wound infections than those who recceived continuous support. None of the patients aspirated. The 2 groups did not differ significantly in length of stay, incidence of sepsis or pneumonia, or mortality.

Conclusion.—These results indicate that maintaining perioperative enteral nutritional support is safe as long as the feeding tube is positioned in the duodenum and gastric decompression is maintained. Continuous nutritional support was effective in meeting nutritional demand and was asśociated with reduced infection.

▶ The authors conclude that enteral nutrition can be provided safely during the perioperative period and that this approach reduces caloric deficits and the need for exogenous albumin supplementation. This conclusion seems valid, and the nutritional approach has much to commend it. But, there is likely to be more. Looking into the crystal ball, I predict that similar approaches will have direct physiologic benefits that will ultimately be shown to shorten the recovery period and improve clinical outcome.—E.A. Deitch, M.D.

Transport of Fluorescent Dextrans Across the Rat Ileum After Cutaneous Thermal Injury
Berthiaume F, Ezzell RM, Toner M, Yarmush ML, Tompkins RG (Massachusetts Gen Hosp, Boston; Harvard Med School, Boston; Shriners Burns Inst, Boston)
Crit Care Med 22:455–464, 1994   140-95-3-5

Background.—The barrier function of the gut may be impaired by thermal injury and other forms of trauma. In the normal small intestine, macromolecules are generally absorbed very slowly; recent evidence suggests that some trans-cellular pathway may be involved in the transport of macromolecules across the gut mucosa of burned animals. The time course and distribution of macromolecule uptake in the small intestine of rats after cutaneous thermal injury were examined prospectively.

Methods.—Female Sprague-Dawley rats were subjected to scald injuries that covered 20% or 40% of their total body surface area or to a sham injury. Three to 72 hours later, the intestine was cannulated near the distal ileum, and this intestinal loop was filled with physiologic buffer containing fluorescent-labeled dextrans with molecular weights of 3 and 70 kD. After 2 hours of incubation, the tissues were fixed with paraformaldehyde, and cryosections were prepared for examination by laser confocal microscopy.

Results.—Rats with smaller injuries had transient uptake of the 3-kD dextran by the epithelium in focal regions of the ileum. These effects were noted 7–21 hours after injury. Those with large burns had visible epithelial staining within 3 hours, with translocation of the marker to the mesenteric lymphatics and blood vessels. The 70-kD dextran could be seen within the intercellular spaces. The sham-injured rats had little or no epithelial staining.

Conclusions.—A transcellular pathway for the translocation of small macromolecules from the lumen to the mesentery appears to be activated after burn injury in rats. A 20% body surface area burn results in transient uptake of a 3-kD dextran by epithelial cells in the distal ileum. A 40% burn results in rapid uptake of this probe by the gut epithelium and translocation to the lymphatic and blood vessels in the mesentery. The transport of the 3-kD probe across the gut epithelium suggests the presence of a transcellular pathway; a 70-kD dextran can be seen in the intercellular spaces after burn injury.

Differential Changes in Intestinal Permeability Following Burn Injury

Messick WJ, Koruda M, Meyer A, Zimmerman K (Carolinas Med Ctr, Charlotte, NC; Univ of North Carolina, Chapel Hill)
J Trauma 36:306–312, 1994   140-95-3–6

Background.—The predisposition to sepsis and multiple system organ failure (MSOF) in patients who are critically ill has been linked to increased gut permeability (GP). Increased GP to bacteria is referred to as bacterial translocation (BT), a condition that may occur after burn injury, hemorrhagic shock, femoral fracture, and other insults. The mechanism by which BT leads to sepsis and MSOF has not been determined. Whether increased GP is a process that occurs over days and depends on toxin size was investigated.

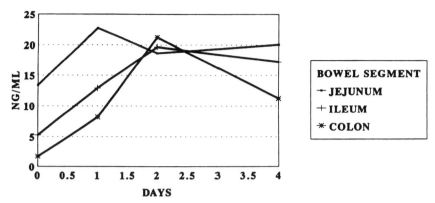

Fig 3–1.—Portal concentration of HRP in burned animals (ng/mL). (Courtesy of Messick WJ, Koruda M, Meyer A, et al: *J Trauma* 36:306–312, 1994.)

Methods.—Scald burn injuries were created in adult male Sprague-Dawley rats. At 4 periods after the injury (16, 24, 48, and 96 hours) the animals were reanesthetized, and the abdomen was opened. Two 10-cm segments of bowel—jejunum, ileum, or colon—were isolated at laparotomy. One bowel segment was infused with fluorescein isothiocyanate-dextran-3 (FDEX; molecular weight, 4,387 d) and a second with horseradish peroxidase (HRP; molecular weight, 40,000 d). After 30 minutes, portal vein blood was aspirated and assayed by spectrophometry for concentrations of FDEX and HRP.

Results.—Portal vein concentrations of FDEX were significantly greater in burned animals than in nonburned controls. Jejunal concentrations of FDEX were not significantly greater than ileal and colonic concentrations at 24 hours but were greater than controls or jejunal concentrations at other times when analyzed separately by Fisher's LSD for post hoc tests. Portal vein concentrations of HRP, the larger probe, were not significantly elevated for any segment above control values. Jejunal permeability to FDEX and HRP (Fig 3–1) increased most at 24 hours. Portal vein concentrations of FDEX based on weight or particle size were significantly greater than concentrations of HRP.

Conclusion.—Burn injury significantly increased the GP of all segments to both FDEX and HRP. The GP was significantly greater for FDEX than for HRP. Jejunal permeability increased most at 24 hours, whereas ileal and colonic GP were higher at days 2 and 4. Gut permeability after burn injury appears to depend on both size and site.

▶ Increased GP and the translocation of enteric bacteria and bacterial products have been implicated in the pathophysiology of sepsis and MSOF, and GP is increased in patients after thermal injury. Consequently, these 2 studies are important because they help define and clarify the pathophysiology of gut barrier failure. In the first study, a novel technique to examine the GP showed that the passage of luminal permeability probes occurred by a transcellular mechanism. The second study illustrated that different segments of the gut lose barrier function to a different degree and that this loss of barrier function is maximal at different times in different segments of the intestine. Although these 2 studies by themselves do not provide enough information to answer the question of why burn injury causes gut barrier failure, they do add further pieces to the puzzle.—E.A. Deitch, M.D.

Bombesin Protects Against Bacterial Translocation Induced by Three Commercially Available Liquid Enteral Diets: A Prospective, Randomized, Multigroup Trial
Haskel Y, Xu D, Lu Q, Deitch EA (Louisiana State Univ, Shreveport)
Crit Care Med 22:108–113, 1994   140-95-3–7

Introduction.—Experimental studies have found that bacterial translocation to the mesenteric lymph nodes is promoted by the oral or IV administration of total parenteral nutrition solutions. Providing bulk-forming dietary fibers, however, can protect against this effect. Whether certain commercially available liquid diets would cause bacterial translocation was investigated. In addition, whether bombesin, an intestinal hormone stimulant, could reduce this diet-induced translocation was examined.

Methods.—Male ICR mice were used in the experiments. The diets tested were Vivonex TEN (diet A), Criticare HN (diet B), and Ensure (diet C). Three groups of mice received 1 of the 3 liquid diets with bombesin, and 3 groups received 1 of the 3 liquid diets without bombesin. Bombesin (or saline) was administered subcutaneously 3 times daily during the 7-day experimental period. A control group of mice was fed

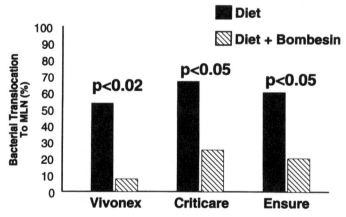

Fig 3–2.—Bombesin reduced the incidence of bacterial translocation to the mesenteric lymph nodes in mice that were fed all three liquid enteral diets. (Courtesy of Haskel Y, Xu D, Lu Q, et al: *Crit Care Med* 22:108–113, 1994.)

rodent chow only. The mice were killed after 7 days, and their organs were removed for bacteriologic culture.

Results.—Mice in all groups gained weight and appeared healthy during the study period. Bacterial translocation occurred consistently in the mesenteric lymph nodes of animals that received liquid diets but was significantly reduced in the groups that received bombesin (Fig 3–2). Bacterial translocation past the mesenteric lymph nodes and loss of mucosal protein content were reduced in all 3 liquid diet groups that were treated with bombesin. Diet-induced cecal bacterial overgrowth, however, was not prevented. The control group that received a chow diet did not exhibit bacterial translocation.

Conclusion.—Certain commercially available enteral liquid diets induce a loss of intestinal barrier function, observed as bacterial translocation. Hormonal modulation of intestinal barrier function with bombesin has a protective effect in diet-induced bacterial translocation. The mechanisms involved in the protective effect of bombesin have yet to be determined.

▶ This article was chosen for 2 reasons. First, the article illustrates that, although enteral feeding is better than parenteral alimentation (especially as far as preserving normal gut barrier function), the optimal commercial enteral diet is still to be defined. Second, by documenting that it is possible to modulate intestinal barrier function hormonally, this article falls within the new field of nutritional pharmacology. In nutritional pharmacology, nutrients and nutrient-related growth factors are used for their nonnutritive effects (e.g., organ support and immune modulation). If clinical studies verify that the parenteral administration of trophic gut factors or hormones, like bombesin, preserve gut function during periods of starvation or stress, an additional page will be added to the emerging chapter on nutritional pharmacology.—E.A. Deitch, M.D.

Contraction and Growth of Deep Burn Wounds Covered by Non-Meshed and Meshed Split Thickness Skin Grafts in Humans
El Hadidy M, Tesauro P, Cavallini M, Colonna M, Rizzo F, Signorini M (Mansoura Univ Hosp, Egypt; Ospedale Niguarda Ca'Granda, Milano, Italy)
Burns 20:226–228, 1994   140-95-3-8

Introduction.—Wound contraction was monitored in patients with burn injury who received either meshed or nonmeshed split-thickness skin grafts.

Management.—Twenty-two male and 16 female patients, aged 3–70 years, were examined. Fifteen patients had greater than 10% total body surface burns. Eighteen patients had their burn wounds excised 2–5 days after injury, whereas 20 underwent surgery 25–35 days after injury. Either

Comparison Between Effects of Meshed and Unmeshed Skin Grafts on Contraction and Growth of Deep Burn Wounds After Early and Late Burn Wound Excision

Early deep burn wounds excision		Late deep burn wounds excision	
Average meshed	*Average unmeshed*	*Average meshed*	*Average unmeshed*
Wounds contracted to a mean wound size of **56%** within **100** days	Wounds contracted to a minimum mean wound size of **64%** within **80 days**	Wounds contracted to a minimum mean wound size of **40.5%** within **100 days**	Wounds contracted to a minimum mean wound size of **51.5%** within **100 days**
Wounds grew back to a mean wound size of **78.5%** within **210 days**	Wounds grew back to a mean wound size of **91%** within **210 days**	Wounds grew back to a mean wound size of **69.5%** within **210 days**	Wounds grew back to a mean wound size of **75.5%** within **210 days**

(Courtesy of El Hadidy M, Tesauro P, Cavallini M, et al: *Burns* 20:226–228, 1994.)

tangential or fascial excision was carried out, followed by grafting with nonmeshed or meshed skin at a ratio of 1:1.5.

Results.—After early excision, wounds covered with meshed grafts contracted to a mean of 56% of the original size, and those covered with nonmeshed grafts contracted to a mean of 64% of the original size. The meshed grafts regrew to a mean size of 78.5%, and the nonmeshed grafts grew back to a mean size to 91%. After late burn wound excision, the wounds covered with meshed grafts contracted to a mean size of 40.5%, and those covered with nonmeshed grafts contracted to a mean of 51.5%. These wounds regrew to mean sizes of 69.5% and 75.5%, respectively. The results are summarized in the table.

Conclusions.—These findings indicate that the timing of the grafting procedure, as well as whether the skin grafts were meshed, influenced the extent of skin graft contraction.

▶ To mesh or not to mesh. To graft early or to graft late. This short study provides a wealth of information regarding these questions. In addition, it documents that maximal graft shrinkage or wound contracture occurs 80–120 days after surgery (depending on the group). This is very important prognostic information, because it can be used to explain to patients what to expect in the future. Further, the observation that wounds grafted early, whether with meshed or unmeshed autograft, had less graft shrinkage than wounds grafted late adds further support for a policy of early burn wound excision and grafting.—E.A. Deitch, M.D.

The Response of Burn Scars to Intralesional Verapamil: Report of Five Cases
Lee RC, Doong H, Jellema AF (Univ of Chicago)
Arch Surg 129:107–111, 1994   140-95-3–9

Objective. —The prevention of hypertrophic scar formation after a burn injury remains a difficult challenge. Hypertrophic scars result from excessive synthesis of the extracellular matrix during wound healing. Recent studies have shown that calcium antagonists retard extracellular matrix production in connective tissue. The effects of intralesional verapamil hydrochloride therapy on scar volume and skin color in patients with burn injury who have hypertrophic scars were assessed.

Patients.—Five patients with hypertrophic burn scars underwent intralesional verapamil therapy on an outpatient basis. Verapamil was administered with a syringe or by pressure injection. The dose per treatment ranged from .1 to .5 mmol/L, and the maximum verapamil dose given per visit was 5 mg. The total number of verapamil treatments varied with each patient. To document the response, photographs were taken of each patient's scar volume and skin color before and after verapamil therapy.

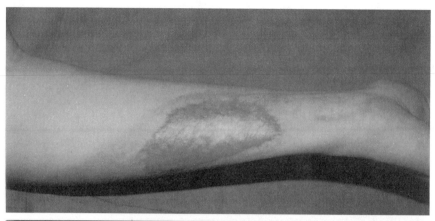

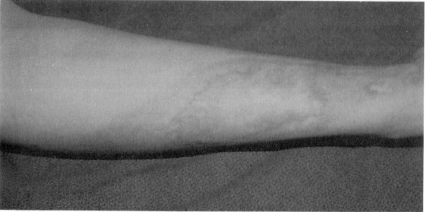

Fig 3–3.—A 17-year-old adolescent with a scar from a high-speed friction burn located on his left medial forearm. *Top,* After 6 months of treatment consisting of wearing a pressure garment, no significant improvement was observed. *Bottom,* After 5 treatments with verapamil hydrochloride over 3 months, the scar was completely flattened and blanched. (Courtesy of Lee RC, Doong, H, Jellema AF: *Arch Surg* 129:107–111, 1994.)

Results.—Intralesional verapamil injections were well tolerated, and there were no complications. Verapamil therapy flattened and faded the scars in 3 patients (Fig 3–3) but did not reduce scar volume in the other 2 patients. All scars became softer and lighter, however, even in the patients whose scar volume was not reduced by the treatment.

Conclusion.—Intralesional verapamil injection in patients with hypertrophic burn scars induces rapid, beneficial effects in some patients. Further studies are needed to assess the overall efficacy of this new treatment modality for scar control.

▶ Although this study includes only 5 patients, it does provide a new method for treating an established and recalcitrant clinical problem. Because this approach makes biological sense, and the potential side effects and complications of intralesional verapamil are minimal, I advise you to try it. I will.—E.A. Deitch, M.D.

Composite Grafts of Autogenic Cultured Epidermis and Glycerol-Preserved Allogeneic Dermis for Definitive Coverage of Full Thickness Burn Wounds: Case Reports

Schiozer WA, Hartinger A, v Donnersmarck GH, Mühlbauer W (Inst of Microbiology, Munich; Klinikum Bogenhausen, Munich)
Burns 20:503–507, 1994   140-95-3-10

Background.—Many patients with extensive, deep burn injuries and other types of wounds have received cultured epithelial grafts (CEG). These grafts have taken well on deep dermal burn wounds, when some patient dermis remains. In full-thickness wounds, however, the take rate has averaged only 16%. Cultured epithelial grafts may require a dermal base to serve as a matrix.

Method.—Missing dermis was replaced with nonviable allogeneic dermis from donor skin preserved in glycerol and overgrafted with autogenic CEG after removing the alloepidermis. Donor skin preserved in 85% glycerol solution is not highly antigenic. In addition, it is sterile, may be stored at room temperature, and is readily available.

Results.—Two patients with deep burns of 55% and 80% of the body surface received composite grafts of auto-CEG on nonviable allogeneic dermis from glycerol-preserved donor skin. Takes of 70% and 77%, respectively, were achieved, and the grafted areas remained stable for 4 and 8 months.

Conclusion.—A composite allo-auto skin replacement appears to be useful in covering extensive full-thickness burn wounds when donor skin is not readily available.

▶ Now that an effective and reliable method of growing keratinocytes has been established, it was hoped that patients with burn injury could undergo grafting with their own skin almost no matter how limited their donor sites were. Although it was possible to use auto-CEG with many patients who had massive burn injury, 1 of 2 problems frequently occurred. The first problem was that the percentage of graft take was quite variable. Second, the long-term quality of a significant percentage of the autografts was poor. These problems seemed to be caused (at least in part) by the absence of a dermal base. Consequently, increasing effort has been directed toward developing composite grafts that are composed of both a dermal matrix and epithelial cells. This brief report describes success with the use of glycerol-preserved donor skin overgrafted with auto-CEGs.

Although the provocative results of this pilot study are too premature to know whether an answer has been found, this study does reflect the direction in which an important aspect of burn care is going.—E.A. Deitch, M.D.

Initial Effect of Smoke Inhalation Injury on Oxygen Consumption (Response to Positive Pressure Ventilation)

Demling R, LaLonde C, Heron P (Brigham and Women's, Boston; Beth Israel, Boston; Children's Hosp, Boston; et al)
Surgery 115:563–570, 1994   140-95-3–11

Purpose.—Systemic oxygen consumption (VO_2) in patients with burn injury appears to be increased during the early postburn period. The addition of smoke inhalation to a body burn further increases early patient instability and mortality. The initial effects of smoke inhalation on VO_2 were measured and the effects of positive pressure ventilation (PPV) on this process were examined.

Methods.—Thirty sheep were insufflated with smoke under short-term general anesthesia to a plasma level of carboxyhemoglobin of 45% and then monitored unanesthetized for 24 hours. After smoke exposure, the sheep were divided into 3 groups: 6 animals were monitored for 24 hours and killed, 6 were placed on PPV during the first 2 hours after smoke exposure, and 6 were placed on PPV on alternating hours beginning at 12 hours after smoke exposure. The remaining 12 animals were used as controls.

Results.—Oxygen consumption was significantly increased during the first 2 hours after smoke inhalation; the mean peak increase was 75% compared with controls. After 12 hours VO_2 increased again; the mean peak increase was 40% compared with controls at 18 hours after the smoke injury. Both increases were attributable to increased oxygen extraction from hemoglobin, rather than to increased cardiac output. The use of PPV during the first 2 hours had no effect on the early increase in VO_2, but arterial oxygenation was significantly improved and shunt fraction was decreased compared with spontaneously breathing animals. The use of late PPV every other hour significantly decreased VO_2 compared with spontaneously breathing animals, with VO_2 returning to baseline levels. However, VO_2 increased again and lung dysfunction increased again within 10 minutes after removal of the ventilator.

Conclusions.—Severe smoke injury alone causes a significant 2-phase increase in systemic VO_2. The early increase is likely caused by the acute release of inflammatory mediators from the airway injury, whereas the late increase is likely caused by the increased work of breathing.

▶ This article sorts out several important physiologic effects of smoke inhalation and helps define the role of PPV. It is impossible to cover all the relevant points raised in this excellent work, so I will just focus on one: oxygen consumption.

As clinicians, we are well aware that thermal injury and smoke inhalation induce a hypermetabolic response. We also know that meeting these increased metabolic needs may be difficult and requires the provision of supranormal levels of calories and protein. What is easy to forget is that therapies directed at lowering the metabolic requirement of these hypermetabolic patients can also be used. This latter concept is well illustrated in this study. The use of PPV not only improved pulmonary function and decreased the shunt fraction but also reduced the level of VO_2 by decreasing the work of breathing. The energy saving effect of PPV was not trivial, nor was the increase in VO_2 induced by the smoke inhalation injury. Specifically, VO_2 increased by 40% in the unventilated sheep after smoke inhalation; this increase could largely be prevented by reducing the work of breathing through mechanical ventilation. In selected instances, the ventilator can be considered an important tool in limiting, and thereby meeting, the energy needs of the patient.—E.A. Deitch, M.D.

The Effect of Inhaled Nitric Oxide on Smoke Inhalation Injury in an Ovine Model

Ogura H, Cioffi WG Jr, Jordan BS, Okerberg CV, Johnson AA, Mason AD Jr, Pruitt BA Jr (US Army Inst of Surgical Research, Fort Sam Houston, Tex)
J Trauma 37:294–302, 1994   140-95-3-12

Background.—The effects of smoke inhalation on the lungs are in part mediated by activated leukocytes and inflammatory cytokines. The inhalation of nitric oxide (NO) reportedly has a selective pulmonary vasodilating action without producing systemic vasodilation. It has been reported to have beneficial effects on patients who have pulmonary hypertension, adult respiratory distress syndrome, chronic obstructive lung disease, or pneumonia. The effects of inhaled NO were studied in a sheep model of smoke inhalation injury.

Methods.—After exposure to smoke generated by burning pine woodchips, groups of animals breathed room air (group 1) or a mixture of room air and 100% oxygen diluted with NO to an inspired concentration of 20 ppm (group 2). In both groups, the inspired oxygen fraction was .21.

Results.—The mean pulmonary artery pressure was significantly higher in group 1 animals than in group 2 animals. A progressive increase in the pulmonary vascular resistance index was seen in control animals only. The mean PaO_2 was consistently higher in animals that breathed NO, and the physiologic shunt was smaller in these animals. The respiratory indices were consistently higher in control animals. There were no significant group differences in static lung compliance, histologic appearance of the lung, or pulmonary resistance at 48 hours between the groups. Group 2 animals had higher arterial levels of arterial nitrate and methemoglobin. The differences in histologic scores of the bronchi and left lower lung parenchyma were not significant.

Implications.—The inhalation of NO significantly lessened the pulmonary arterial hypertension in this ovine model of smoke inhalation injury, with no apparent toxic effects.

▶ Is it time to add smoke inhalation injury to the continuously increasing list of pulmonary disease processes that appear to benefit from inhaled NO? Maybe—however, it is important to point out that, although inhaled NO improved several physiologic parameters, the administration of inhaled NO did not reduce the extent of pulmonary damage. Therefore, whether the beneficial effects of NO will continue past the early smoke inhalation period remains to be defined.—E.A. Deitch, M.D.

Role of Leukocyte Adhesion Molecules in Lung and Dermal Vascular Injury After Thermal Trauma of Skin

Mulligan MS, Till GO, Smith CW, Anderson DC, Miyasaka M, Tamatani T, Todd RF III, Issekutz TB, Ward PA (Univ of Mich, Ann Arbor; Baylor College of Medicine, Houston; Tokyo Metropolitan Inst of Med Science, Japan; et al)
Am J Pathol 144:1008–1015, 1994   140-95-3–13

Introduction.—Second-degree burns of 28% of the total body surface area in rats result in endothelial cell damage both in the injured skin and in the lung 4 hours after thermal trauma. Lung injury secondary to skin burns depends on neutrophils and complements. The role of neutrophils in dermal vascular injury and of adhesion molecules in both dermal and lung vascular injury was studied in rats.

Methods.—Between 25% to 30% of the total body surface area of anesthetized rats was burned. The animals were killed 4 hours later, and blood was analyzed at that time for hemorrhage and permeability indices. In some animals, neutropenia was induced before the thermal trauma with cyclophosphamide to determine neutrophil dependence. To assess the contribution of adhesion molecules in the development of vascular permeability and hemorrhage, antibodies blocking intercellular adhesion molecule-1 (ICAM-1), leukocyte $\alpha4$ and $\beta2$ integrins, and the E-, P-, and L-selectins were injected before the thermal trauma in some animals.

Results.—Vascular permeability was reduced by 44% in the lungs and by 37% in the skin of neutropenic rats. Dermal vascular permeability was significantly reduced in animals that were treated with antibodies to the Mac-1 $\beta2$ integrin complex, ICAM-1, E-selectin, and L-selectin. Antibodies to the leukocyte function-associated antigen 1 (LFA-1) did not significantly affect dermal vascular permeability, and antibodies to very late arising antigen-4 (VLA-4) and P-selectin induced inconsistent reactions. Lung vascular permeability was significantly reduced in the animals treated with antibodies to both the Mac-1 and the LFA-1 $\beta2$ integrin complex, ICAM-1, E-selectin, and L-selectin. Again, the results of anti–VLA-4 and anti–P-selectin injection were inconsistent.

Discussion.—These findings indicate that vascular injury in the skin and lungs of rats 4 hours after a burn depends on neutrophils and is mediated by the Mac-1 (and, in lungs only, LFA-1) $\beta2$ integrin complex, ICAM-1, E-selectin, and L-selectin.

▶ This article emphasizes the roles of injury-induced expression of neutrophil and endothelial receptors in the pathophysiology of neutrophil-mediated dermal and pulmonary vascular injury after a cutaneous burn. This paradigm, in which an insult leads to an inflammatory response and the inflammatory products generated result in vascular and organ injury, is applicable to more than burn injury. It applies to infectious and other inflammatory disease states and is considered a possible mechanism for the development of multiple organ failure. Consequently, it is important for clinicians, as well as researchers, to learn the difference between a selectin and an integrin. Good luck.—E.A. Deitch, M.D.

Altered Gene Transcription After Burn Injury Results in Depressed T-Lymphocyte Activation
Horgan AF, Mendez MV, O'Riordain DS, Holzheimer RG, Mannick JA, Rodrick ML (Harvard Med School, Boston)
Ann Surg 220:342–352, 1994   140-95-3–14

Objective.—Serious burns result in immunologic problems, such as poor production of interleukin-2 (IL-2) or diminished response to T-cell mitogens or antigenic stimulation. Although IL-2 receptor (IL-2R) is one of the main cytokine activators of T cells, and ultimately of protein kinase C (PKC), its mechanism is unclear. Interleukin-2 transcription activators are encoded by the proto-oncogene *c-jun* via the protein product of *c-fos*. The effect of burns on PKC activation was examined in 11 patients and an animal model. In addition, the transcriptional mechanisms responsible for decreased IL-2 messenger RNA expression were determined.

Methods.—Blood was drawn from 11 patients, aged 19–76 years, who had major burns. Peripheral blood mononuclear cells (PBMC) were collected, and proliferative response was measured. A total of 140 male mice were anesthetized and subjected to either a 20% sham injury or scalding injury. Splenocytes from each group were pooled. The IL-2 content of splenocytes and PBMC was determined, and its viability and binding were evaluated. A nuclear transcriptional rate assay was performed on the splenocytes. Expression of IL-2R was assessed with monoclonal antibodies that bound to the p55 and p75 chains of the IL-2R.

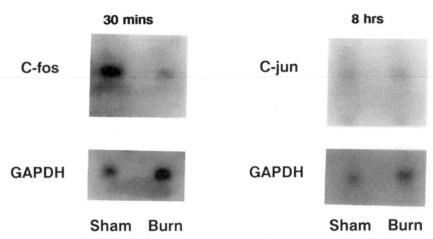

Fig 3–4.—Northern blots of splenocyte RNA from burn and sham burn mice 7 days after burn injury probed for *c-fos* and *c-jun* message. It is apparent that *c-fos* expression is markedly reduced in burn splenocytes, whereas *c-jun* expression is not significantly different from sham burn splenocytes. The glyceraldehyde-3-phosphate dehydrogenase (GAPDH) message is shown as a control (Courtesy of Horgan AF, Mendez MV, O'Riordain DS, et al: *Ann Surg* 220:342–352, 1994.)

Results.—The proliferative response of PBMC to mitogen stimulation, IL-2 production, and mouse splenocyte response was significantly reduced in patients with burn injury and mice. There was no significant difference in either p55 or p75 chain expression between burned patients and controls, which indicated that expression of IL-2R was not altered. There was no significance difference in IL-2 binding between burned patients or mice and controls, although addition of IL-2 to mitogen stimulated cultures of PBMC or splenocytes from burned patients and mice significantly increased proliferative response to mitogens. The messenger RNA expression for IL-2 was significantly decreased in PBMC and splenocytes from burned patients and mice as a result of decreased transcription of IL-2 RNA. Burn injuries altered the expression of *c-fos* but not of *c-jun*. Expression of *c-fos* was significantly decreased in burned mice (Fig 3–4).

Conclusion.—After burn injuries, immunosuppression results from decreased T-cell production of IL-2, which is caused at least in part by inhibition of *c-fos* expression and, consequently, depression of IL-2 gene transcription. Expression and function of IL-2R remain intact.

▶ *c-fos, c-jun,* transcription factor, promoter: What do these terms mean, and do we really need to understand them? Just when we begin to understand the difference between transcription and translation, things seem to get more complicated. Well, the answer is yes. We really do need to understand this new language of molecular biology. As the above article illustrates, it is now becoming possible to determine exactly what is being blocked, impaired, turned off, or regulated at an ever more basic level. Because therapy directed at the machinery of the cell is incipient, knowledge of the basic mechanisms of how a cell regulates its response to specific and different stimuli is likely to become of increasing clinical importance. Don't despair, it is not that difficult. By learning about 20–30 terms, you too can be an expert.

Lesion 1: Activation of the promoter region of a gene is important for that gene to be transcribed (i.e., make messenger RNA). Each promoter region contains binding sites for a number of transcription factors (such as AP-1), which must be occupied for transcription of that gene to occur. In the case of IL-2 messenger RNA production, the products of the 2 proto-oncogenes *c-fos* and *c-jun* dimerize to form the transcriptional activation protein AP-1. Because production of *c-fos* was impaired in the patients with burn injury, the authors concluded that the decrease in production of AP-1 secondary to a failure to induce *c-fos* resulted in decreased IL-2 messenger RNA transcription and, hence, the production of IL-2. Easy, huh?—E.A. Deitch, M.D.

The Humoral Immune Response After Thermal Injury: An Experimental Model
Molloy RG, Nestor M, Collins KH, Holzheimer RG, Mannick JA, Rodrick ML
(Harvard Med School, Boston)
Surgery 115:341–348, 1994   140-95-3–15

Introduction.—Patients with severe thermal injury have major alterations in cell-mediated immunity. Most B-cell responses are regulated by or depend on T-cell help. Although many studies have demonstrated a variety of defects in humoral immunity after thermal injury, the nature of the relationship between the ability to produce antibody in vitro and the subsequent in vivo responses remains to be delineated. The ability of thermally injured mice to initiate, propagate, and maintain a humoral immune response to a T-cell–dependent bacterial antigen after primary and secondary immunization was assessed.

Methods.—Mice were subjected to either hot-water burn injury or sham injury. Primary and secondary humoral immune responses to tetanus toxoid (TT) were assessed for 6 weeks after the actual or sham burns, including determination of serum anti-TT titers and numbers of anti-TT–secreting splenocytes.

Results.—Normal or decreased TT-specific formation of IgM plaque was detected in splenocytes from the burned mice. At the same time, formation of IgG plaque was increased up to 6 weeks after burn injury, indicating a switch from IgM to IgG antibody production. The burn groups, however, had significantly lower serum titers of TT-specific IgG antibody than the sham groups. The discrepancy between enhanced in vitro formation of IgG plaque and impaired levels of TT antibody in vivo was not explained by alterations in serum levels of immunoglobulin.

Conclusions.—Thermal injury appears to result in persistent enhancement of primary and secondary in vitro IgG responses. This murine model shows deficient in vivo IgG responses—particularly after secondary immunization—despite the presence of normal or increased numbers of antigen-specific B cells. Thus, although the mechanisms that produce antigen-specific antibody remain intact after thermal injury, they do not appear to result in increased titers of antigen-specific IgG.

▶ One strength of this article is that it highlights the fact that tests done in vitro may not reflect what is occurring in the live animal or patient. Thus, although important information may be gleaned from studies done in a controlled in vitro environment, one must always remember that things are not as simple as they might seem.—E.A. Deitch, M.D.

Blood Transfusions; For the Thermally Injured or for the Doctor?
Sittig KM, Deitch EA (Louisiana State Univ, Shreveport)
J Trauma 36:369–372, 1994   140-95-3–16

Introduction.—Protocol has historically dictated the administration of blood transfusions when the level of hemoglobin decreased below 10g/dL or the level of hematocrit decreased below 30%. Prophylactic transfusions are not indicated physiologically unless patients with anemia experience cardiopulmonary distress or evidence of inadequate oxygen delivery. In addition, transfusions are intrinsically risky. A comparison was made between policies of selective and routine transfusions in patients with major thermal injuries.

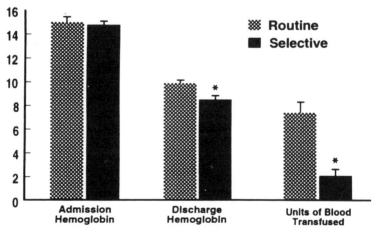

Fig 3–5.—Comparison of admission and discharge hemoglobin levels (g/dL) between the two groups of patients. Data expressed as the mean ± standard error of the mean. *$P < .01$. (Courtesy of Sittig KM, Deitch EA: *J Trauma* 36:369–372, 1994.)

Methods.—Fourteen patients with major thermal injuries (burn size, 28 ± 11% [mean ± SD]) were followed prospectively to determine clinical response to a selective policy of blood transfusions. Transfusions were given when the level of hemoglobin was less than 6 g/dL or patients showed signs of hemodynamic instability. The routine transfusion policy was evaluated by retrospective record review of 38 patients (burn size, 26± 12% [mean ± SD]) with major thermal injury. These patients routinely received blood transfusions to maintain levels of hemoglobin above 9.5–10 g/dL. Both groups had comparable injuries, admission levels of hemoglobin, treatment regimes, surgical procedures, and length of stay.

Results.—Patients in the selective group received 29 units of blood compared with 282 units received by the routine group. Despite this difference, the routine group had only a 16% higher level of hemoglobin at discharge (Fig 3–5). The selective group received 25 of 29 units during surgery, compared with 166 of 282 units in the routine group.

Conclusion.—Patients in the routine group received 3.5 times as much blood as the selective group without apparent clinical benefits. Findings support a policy of selective over routine blood transfusions in patients with major thermal injury. Further study is needed to investigate these recommendations in other patient populations.

▶ This article asks whether the traditional policy of prophylactic blood transfusion to maintain a level of hemoglobin of 10 g/dL is clinically beneficial. The results of this study document that a policy of prophylactic blood transfusions to maintain this arbitrary level was not superior to a selective policy of blood transfusion. Thus, maintaining a patient's level of hemoglobin at 10 g/dL appears to do more for physician anxiety than patient care. Because there are inherent risks of blood transfusion, including the transmission of infection and the induction of an immune compromised state, studies that reevaluate this traditional but unproved clinical practice are worthwhile.

Thus, the answer to the question posed in the title of this paper is that prophylactic blood transfusions are done more for the physician than for the patient.—E.A. Deitch, M.D.

The 1994 Clinical Research Award: A Prospective Clinical Study of the Polysomnographic Stages of Sleep After Burn Injury
Gottschlich MM, Jenkins ME, Mayes T, Khoury J, Kramer M, Warden GD, Kagan RJ (Shriners Burns Inst, Cincinnati, Ohio; Univ of Cincinnati, Ohio; Bethesda Oak Hosp, Cincinnati, Ohio)
J Burn Care Rehabil 15:486–492, 1994   140-95-3–17

Introduction.—Patients with burn injury have been clinically thought to be sleep deprived. In an ICU, the sleep requirement of these patients is a low priority in spite of the influence that sleep deprivation has on

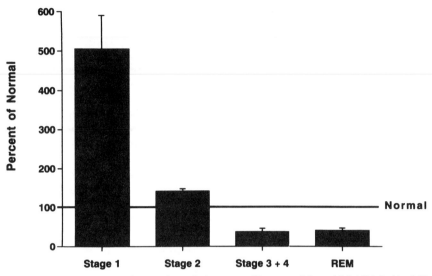

Fig 3–6.—Mean percent of norms for each sleep stage. (Courtesy of Gottschlich MM, Jenkins ME, Mayes T, et al: *J Burn Care Rehabil* 15:486–492, 1994.)

important features of their recovery. The sleep pattern of patients with burn injury was documented.

Methods.—Eleven patients, aged 1.4–16 years, were included. Biweekly 24-hour polysomnographic measurements, including electromyography, electrooculography, and electroencephalography, were recorded. A total of 43 24-hour time periods were studied.

Findings.—The mean burn size was 55%. Total sleep time averaged 625 min/24 hours. Although the total time seemed adequate, there were significant irregularities in the various stages of sleep. The time in stage 3 + 4 sleep and rapid eye movement (deep) sleep was decreased, and the time in stage 1 + 2 (light sleep) was increased (Fig 3–6). During entire 24-hour periods, 40% of patients were lacking stage 3 + 4, whereas 19% were lacking rapid eye movement sleep. All patients demonstrated stage 1 and 2 sleep. This pattern shifted toward more normal patterns over the course of the hospital stay.

Conclusion.—Even though the total sleep time of 10.5 hr/per 24-hour day seems appropriate, the reduction in stage 3 and 4, as well as rapid eye movement, sleep demonstrates that deep sleep is disrupted by thermal injury. Because sleep deprivation can result in adverse physiologic and psychological consequences, these observations suggest that sleep deprivation may play a role in the adverse physiologic consequences of thermal injury.

▶ Sleep deprivation, whether of patients or physicians, is an understudied area. This is especially true, as it has been recognized for a long time that prolonged sleep deprivation can result in ICU psychosis and numerous other physiologic consequences, including alterations in metabolism, impaired wound healing, impaired organ function, and decreased immunity. Yet, in spite of this information and the clinical impression that patients with burn injury, as well as other patients in the ICU, are sleep deprived, almost no hard data are available in this area. Thus, the value of this important study is that it provides some of this missing information.

The authors clarify the apparent paradox of why patients with burn injury appear sleep deprived clinically even though they apparently spend so much of each 24-hour period asleep. The answer is that most of this sleep time is spent in light sleep, and very little time is spent in deep (stages 3 + 4), or rapid eye movement, sleep. This fact is important, as stages 3 + 4 sleep are believed to be the key restorative phases of sleeping, because physiologic changes are associated with these stages of deep sleep. Adequate amounts of rapid eye movement sleep are required to maintain certain mental activities, including memory and learning. In fact, sleep deprivation should be viewed as a specific form of *stress*. As a stressor, it has potentially profound systemic physiologic consequences. Consequently, the results of studies directed at defining better the clinical consequences of sleep deprivation, as well as the development of rapid eye movement and stage 3–4 sleep–promoting therapy, are likely to be of major clinical importance.—E.A. Deitch, M.D.

Parental Well-Being and Behavioral Adjustment of Pediatric Survivors of Burns

Meyer WJ, Blakeney P, Moore P, Murphy L, Robson M, Herndon D (Univ of Texas, Galveston)

J Burn Care Rehabil 15:62–68, 1994   140-95-3-18

Introduction.—Adolescents and children who survive major burns may have a variety of behavioral problems, but standardized tests show that most children adjust well. However, parents usually report more problems for their children than the children report for themselves. The relationship between the problem behaviors of children and the parent's own emotional well-being was examined.

Methods.—Mothers of 38 children with burn injury completed 3 standardized questionnaires: Parental Stress Index (PSI), Child Behavior Checklist, and the Eight State Questionnaire. The children and young adults were aged 4.6–20 years and had 3 distinct burn sizes (15% to 20%, 30% to 50%, and 70% to 100%). The group was further divided into untroubled and troubled by a Child Behavior Checklist total problem T score of 60.

Results.—On most of the scales, the parents were not significantly different from reference populations. The PSI results showed that parents who reported that their children were troubled were themselves stressed, not only by their children's behaviors but also in areas unrelated to their children. The PSI scores were higher for mothers in virtually all categories under the child domain, such as the level for acceptability, demandingness, mood, and reinforcement of the parent. The mothers reported scores in the situational-demographic life stress area that were only one third of those stresses in the reference population. The burn size did not affect differences in the PSI. On the Eight State Questionnaire, the mothers reported feelings of depression and guilt.

Conclusions.—The need for psychological assessment of both children and parents is emphasized. One major reservation about any interpretations of the PSI is that it was originally developed for parents of children younger than 3 years of age; nevertheless the PSI findings are congruent with those of other studies that have used other instruments and techniques to focus on the effects of burns on the parents and the family environment.

▶ Everyone knows that, in case of doubt, it's the parents' fault—so, what's the big deal? The big deal is that in a subgroup of patients with burn injury, especially those who have more than the expected levels of psychosocial stress, the mothers' level of stress appears to be a contributing factor. In fact, this intriguing study documents that a significant percentage of mothers believe that their children have more problems than are perceived by the children or the childrens' teachers. This means that family therapy and individual therapy for the parent are equally important to the well-being and emotional adjustment of the child as is therapy directed at the child. This point should be kept in mind by all of us who care for children who are burned, injured, or chronically ill, because focusing just on the child may not be enough.—E.A. Deitch, M.D.

4 Trauma

Introduction

Because of the impact on patient outcome, the treatment of long bone and pelvic fractures continues to occupy a pivotal place in the care of the blunt trauma patient. Therefore, it behooves all of us, even general surgeons, to pay attention to this field. For that reason, 3 articles (Abstracts 140-95-4–1, 140-95-4–2, and 140-95-4–3) dealing with the operative therapy of femoral shaft fractures and 1 study (Abstract 140-95-4–4) dealing with the role of external fixation of pelvic fractures were chosen for review. One major message of the articles on femoral fractures is that although early operative fracture stabilization benefits most patients, in patients with concomitant lung and, perhaps, head injuries, operative fracture stabilization should be delayed for 2 to 4 days to improve survival. A second message is that immediate external fixation in selected subgroups of patients with pelvic fractures may be of major clinical benefit.

Gizmos, gimmicks, and techniques continue to proliferate and find use in the care of the trauma patient. For example, as illustrated in 2 of the selected articles (Abstracts 140-95-4–5 and 140-95-4–6), video-assisted surgery of trauma patients has expanded from the abdomen to include the treatment of selected thoracic injuries. It is now possible to definitively treat clotted hemothoraces, diaphragmatic injuries, and even empyemas thoracoscopically in many patients, thereby avoiding formal thoracotomies. Diagnostic studies continue to appear indicating that ultrasonography is the optimal initial diagnostic test in patients with blunt abdominal trauma or hemoperitoneum, while CT scan enthusiasts work to refine the prognostic value of CT scans in deciding which patients with solid organ injuries can be safely managed nonoperatively. Diagnostic sonography also appears to be helpful in vascular trauma, since duplex ultrasonographic scanning has been documented to be as successful as arteriography or operative exploration in diagnosing extremity vascular injury in patients with proximity-type injuries. Lastly, because systemic variables of oxygen delivery do not always reflect organ perfusion and these variables fail to reliably identify patients with inadequate organ perfusion, a search for more accurate ways to assess organ perfusion has been in progress over the last decade. One result of this search for the Holy Grail of organ perfusion is the gastric tonometer. By directly assessing the adequacy of gastric blood flow, the gastric tonometer has been touted as the way to monitor organ perfusion and, thereby, serve as an early warning system that things are not right. However, as illustrated in an accompanying article (Abstract 140-95-4-11), there are some technical pitfalls associated with the use of the gastric tonometer that must be guarded against if this technology is to provide accurate information.

A potpourri of articles dealing with clinically relevant and practical topics in trauma care were also chosen. These include 1 article (Abstract 140-95-4-13) documenting the fact that epidural anesthesia improves pain relief and pulmonary function in victims of chest trauma. The second article chosen indicates that aztreonam-based antibiotic therapy is superior to an aminoglycoside-based regimen in patients with penetrating trauma. A study (Abstract 140-95-4-15) verifying the benefits of an operative protocol of abbreviated initial procedures followed by planned reoperations in severely injured patients was selected to highlight this recent advance in the surgical management of the patient with highly lethal injuries. Additionally, because of the importance of the topic, articles dealing with the prevention and early diagnosis of deep venous thrombosis and venous thromboembolism were chosen.

Effort continues unabated in the search for therapeutically effective biological agents that will either improve resistance to infection or beneficially modulate the immunoinflammatory consequences of injury. The first article selected (Abstract 140-95-4-18) tested the protective effect of interferon-γ in a model of intra-abdominal sepsis. Instead of finding that interferon-γ was protective, the opposite was found. Animals that received this biological agent had a higher mortality rate. This study has profound implications, because several multi-institutional trials enrolling hundreds of trauma patients have already been completed and published. Why is it that an animal trial showing the potential dangers of this agent is published only after clinical trials have been published showing that interferon-γ is not beneficial? The answer lies in the fact that many of the basic preclinical studies evaluating potential therapeutic agents used animal models that were not clinically relevant. These clinically irrelevant animal models include lethal models in which the bacteria is administered by IV bolus injection. Thus, in retrospect, it comes as little surprise that therapeutic regimens based on clinically irrelevant models result in clinically irrelevant therapy. Although, to date, the human clinical trials testing various biological agents are not fully encouraging, we are beginning to get a better idea of the various mediators released after trauma and during sepsis. Because good therapy is based on good science and a complete knowledge of disease biology, there remains room for optimism as we continue to unravel the complex biology of the injury and inflammatory responses.

Edwin A. Deitch, M.D.

Incidence, Management, and Outcome of Femoral Shaft Fracture: A Statewide Population-Based Analysis of 2805 Adult Patients in a

Rural State

Fakhry SM, Rutledge R, Dahners LE, Kessler D (Univ of North Carolina, Chapel Hill)
J Trauma 37:255–261, 1994   140-95-4-1

Introduction.—Studies have reported a reduction in complications and mortality when traumatic femur fractures are stabilized early. However, definitions of "early" vary, and the optimal timing of surgical correction is unclear. Some patients are still managed without surgery. The correlations between treatment and outcome were analyzed in a retrospective study of a large group of patients with femoral shaft fractures.

Methods.—Data on all patients who had traumatic femoral shaft fracture injuries were derived from a statewide hospital discharge data base for a 3-year period. The patients were assigned to 2 groups based on an injury severity score (ISS) of $<$ or $\geq$ 15. These 2 groups were then divided into 4 management subgroups: nonsurgical management, surgery within 1 day of admission, surgery within 2–4 days of admission, and surgery more than 4 days after admission. The mortality and the length of stay were analyzed.

Results.—Among the 2,805 patients with femoral shaft fractures, 69% were treated surgically and 31% were managed without operation. Nonsurgical treatment was associated with significantly higher mortality and longer hospital stays than surgical treatment, regardless of the ISS. Among the patients with an ISS of $\geq$ 15, those who had surgery within 1 day of admission had a higher mortality rate than those who underwent surgery within 2–4 days after admission. Otherwise, mortality rates were similar among surgically treated patients. Hospital stays were progressively longer with later surgical stabilization, although they were still usually lower than with nonsurgical management.

Discussion.—The surgical repair of femoral shaft fractures significantly enhanced survival. Surgical delays correlated with longer hospital stays. Patients having surgery immediately after admission had a slightly elevated mortality rate, but surgery performed 2–4 days after admission was associated with optimal survival and length of stay.

▶ This statewide population-based study has much to commend it. By analyzing the results of patients with femoral fractures treated at all 130 acute care hospitals in the state of North Carolina, this study shows that early operative management of femoral shaft fractures improves survival and shortens the hospital stay at rural and community hospitals as well as at trauma centers—an important message for all practicing surgeons.

Additionally, the observation that surgical intervention within the first 24 hours postinjury was associated with a higher mortality rate than surgery at 2–4 days or after 4 days (3.8% vs. 1.8% and 1.5%, respectively) in patients with more severe injuries (ISS $\geq$ 15) is worthy of special attention. In attempting to determine why this may be so, the authors performed subgroup analyses. Based on these analyses, the authors' conclusion that the presence of a severe head or chest injury may be an indication for delaying the repair of the femoral shaft injury for 24–48 hours until these nonbony injuries have been stabilized, seems well justified. This important concept that a 24–48 hour delay in surgical repair of femoral shaft fractures may further improve survival in the subgroup of patients with chest trauma is supported by the following 2 papers.—E.A. Deitch, M.D.

Influences of Different Methods of Intramedullary Femoral Nailing on Lung Function in Patients With Multiple Trauma
Pape H-C, Regel G, Dwenger A, Krumm K, Schweitzer G, Krettek C, Sturm JA, Tscherne H (Hannover Med School, Germany)
J Trauma 35:709–716, 1993   140-95-4–2

Introduction.—Early (< 24 hours) reamed intramedullary femoral nailing appears to be associated with the development of pulmonary complications and subsequent adult respiratory distress syndrome (ARDS) in patients with multiple trauma. Previous studies in an animal model showed that pulmonary dysfunction could be avoided if fracture fixation by a small-diameter nail was performed without prior reaming. Consequently, lung function was compared in 2 groups of patients, 1 with primary femoral nailing with reaming (group RFN) and the other with unreamed femoral nailing (group UFN).

Patients and Methods.—Thirty-one patients were studied, 17 in the RFN group and 14 in the UFN group. The groups were similar in demographic data and had comparable lung function at baseline. All had an Injury Severity Score > 20 but were without severe head or chest trauma. Lung function was assessed by oxygenation ratio and pulmonary hemodynamics by intraoperative pulmonary catheter measurements.

Results.—Lung function remained unchanged intraoperatively in UFN patients; a significant increase in oxygenation ratio was observed postoperatively. A fall in the oxygenation ratio occurred in RFN patients upon reaming of the medullary canal; the oxygenation ratio remained worse than that of the RFN group until day 2 after trauma. In 1 patient in the RFN group, ARDS developed after day 4 and the patient died. Neither group showed changes during or after nailing in positive end-expiratory pressure, respiratory minute volume, maximal inspiratory airway pressure, static compliance, or the ratio of inspiration to expiration. Although pulmonary artery pressure (PAP) did not change during surgery in UFN patients, it increased significantly (from a mean of 27.2 mm Hg to 36.3 mm Hg) upon reaming in RFN patients. In RFN patients, PAP normalized 1 hour after nail insertion. In RFN patients, the platelet count decreased from a mean of $123 \times 1,000/\text{mL}$ on admission to 87.8 $\times 1,000/\text{mL}$ at day 2 after surgery. A rise occurred after day 3 after surgery.

Conclusion.—Patients with multiple trauma who underwent intramedullary nailing with reaming of the medullary canal had a significant impairment of oxygenation. Unreamed intramedullary stabilization of the femur did not adversely affect the lung in patients with the same overall degree of injury. Thus, by using the technique of unreamed femoral nailing, it may be possible to provide primary intramedullary stabilization without the risk of impairing lung function and predisposing to the development of ARDS.

▶ Over the last 5 years, the group from the Hanover Medical School in Germany have made many significant contributions to our understanding of why pulmonary function deteriorates and why the incidence of ARDS and the mortality rate increase in certain groups of trauma patients undergoing immediate intramedullary stabilization of femoral shaft fractures. In this study of trauma patients, the authors verify previous animal studies indicating that intramedullary femoral reaming and nailing adversely affects lung function and that this deterioration in lung function can be prevented by using an unreamed technique of femoral fracture stabilization.

The clinical implications of this study for the care of the trauma patient are significant. The authors have provided us with an alternative approach to fracture stabilization that is not associated with the development of pulmonary dysfunction. However, further study is needed to determine whether this unreamed approach is equally effective in patients with chest trauma. Until then, we should continue to be cautious regarding immediate (within 24 hours) femoral fracture stabilization in patients with concomitant significant chest trauma.—E.A. Deitch, M.D.

Intramedullary Pressure Changes and Fat Intravasation During Intramedullary Nailing: An Experimental Study in Sheep
Wozasek GE, Simon P, Redl H, Schlag G (Univ of Vienna; Ludwig Boltzmann Inst for Experimental and Clinical Traumatology, Vienna)
J Trauma 36:202–207, 1994   140-95-4–3

Introduction.—Embolization of bone marrow is a danger inherent in intramedullary nailing of long bone fractures in patients with multiple injuries. An investigation was done to determine the severity of fat intravasation in the blood during intramedullary reaming and nailing and to ascertain whether it is paralleled by a rise in intramedullary pressure (IMP) and echocardiographic changes.

Methods.—Sixteen healthy female adult mountin sheep were divided into 2 groups and intramedullary reaming and nailing was performed. Pressure transducers were implanted to measure IMP. The right femur and tibia in group I ($n = 12$) and both tibias in group II ($n = 4$) were nailed. In group I, infiltration of fat globules during intramedullary nailing was assessed by a scoring system using the Gurd blood test. In group II, 2-dimensional graded echocardiography was used.

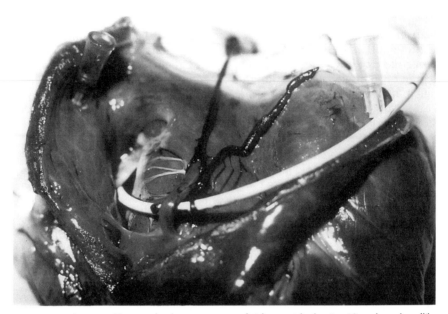

Fig 4–1.—Autopsy with opened pulmonary artery and right ventricle showing 10-cm-long threadlike embolus between pulmonary catheter and papillary muscle. (Courtesy of Wozasek GE, Simon P, Redl H, et al: *J Trauma* 36:202–207, 1994.)

Results.—Intramedullary reaming procedures caused great rises in IMP. Nailing was associated with minimal increases in IMP. Blood samples collected from the pulmonary artery for the Gurd test 60 sec after peak pressures had 49% positive tibial findings compared with 86% positive findings with sonographic monitoring. Echocardiography showed maximum infiltration of particles occurred at the time the nail was driven in, which was also the time of minimal IMP rise. At autopsy, a 10-cm–long threadlike embolism was found between the pulmonary catheter and papillary muscle (Fig 4–1).

Conclusion.—Fat and bone marrow intravasation occurred at the time of intramedullary nailing and was independent of IMP rise. Early lung failure remains a major threat in this process.

▶ This experimental study and the accompanying figure graphically illustrate the potential hazards of intramedullary reaming and nailing. By pinpointing the time of maximal fat and bone marrow emboli as occurring during the period of nailing, the authors provide further evidence in support of delaying nailing in the patient subgroups discussed in Abstracts 140-95-4–1 and 140-95-4–2.—E.A. Deitch, M.D.

Acute Mortality Associated With Injuries to the Pelvic Ring: The Role of Early Patient Mobilization and External Fixation

Riemer BL, Butterfield SL, Diamond DL, Young JC, Raves JJ, Cottington E, Kislan K (Med College of Pennsylvania, Pittsburgh)
J Trauma 35:671–675, 1993   140-95-4–4

Introduction.—Fatal pelvic ring injuries are frequently accompanied by significant bleeding. External fixation is 1 of the methods used to control bleeding. It also relieves pain, allowing patients to be mobilized to an upright chest position. The mortality rate among 605 patients with pelvic ring injuries was studied retrospectively.

Methods.—Three time periods were compared: (1) 1981, preprotocol, with 2 external fixators applied on days 2 and 4 after injury; (2) 1982, transitional, with orthopedic trauma service begun; and (3) 1983 to 1988, protocol in place, with immediate external fixation for mobilization to an upright position in all patients with pelvic ring injury. Injury Severity Scores (ISSs) were used to describe severity of injury and statistically predict mortality.

Results.—Of 61 preprotocol patients, 16 (26%) died, 15 of 68 patients (22%) died in the transitional period, and 30 of 476 patients (6%) died after protocol was started (table). Mean ISSs were comparable for all 3 groups. The most significant change in mortality rate was a decrease of 43% to 14% from 1981 to 1983 through 1988 that occurred in patients who had closed head injuries and pelvic ring injury. There was also a significant drop in the mortality rate during the same period in patients with pelvic ring injury who were hypotensive. Mortality rates did not change from 1981 to 1983 through 1988 in patients with similar ISSs who had multiple blunt injuries but no pelvic ring injury. Use of external fixation for pelvic ring injury went from 3% in 1981 to 31% in 1983 through 1988.

Statistical Analysis of Mortality of Patients With Pelvic Ring Injuries

Variable	Year			Significance
	1981	1982	1983-1988	
Number of patients	61	68	476	
Average ISS	22	26	23	NS
Number of external fixators*	0	12 (18%)	146 (31%)	0.0001
Number of deaths	16 (26%)	15 (22%)	30 (6%)	0.0001

*Two fixators applied at days 2 and 4 as reconstructive procedures.
(Courtesy of Riemer BL, Butterfield SL, Diamond DL, et al: *J Trauma* 35:671–675, 1993.)

Conclusion.—External fixation significantly decreases mortality rates in patients with pelvic ring injury. This procedure should be considered resuscitative, not reconstructive, in patients with this type of injury.

▶ The major concept stressed in this retrospective clinical study is that the external fixation and orthopedic stabilization of pelvic fractures should be viewed as part of patient resuscitation. This is especially true in hemodynamically unstable patients with pelvic fractures, as well as in patients with structurally unstable pelvic fractures. The technique of external fixation of the pelvis has many advantages. It is generally effective in limiting bleeding, helps to control pain, can be performed quickly and, if done percutaneously, does not require general anesthesia or a trip to the operating room. Thus, the approach of external pelvic fracture fixation in selected patients with pelvic fractures has much to commend it.—E.A. Deitch, M.D.

Preliminary Report on Videothoracoscopy in the Evaluation and Treatment of Thoracic Injury

Smith RS, Fry WR, Tsoi EKM, Morabito DJ, Koehler RH, Reinganum SJ, Organ CH Jr (Univ of California, Davis-East Bay, Oakland)
Am J Surg 166:690–695, 1993   140-95-4–5

Background.—When bleeding or clotted hemothorax persists after placement of a chest tube, thoracotomy is often considered to be necessary. Thoracoscopy has proved useful in detecting diaphragmatic injuries before serious complications develop, but it has not been widely used in trauma care.

Objective.—A· prospective trial was undertaken to learn whether videothoracoscopy is useful in evaluating patients with chest injuries and in preventing formal thoracotomies.

Patients.—Thoracoscopy was performed in 24 patients having a mean age of 32 years, all but 2 of them males. Twenty-two patients had penetrating injuries, and 2 had blunt injuries. Nine patients would otherwise have undergone thoracotomy for clotted hemothorax. Ten patients were suspected of having diaphragmatic injuries, and 5 had ongoing bleeding. Videothoracoscopy was done under general anesthesia using double-lumen endotracheal tube.

Results.—Videothorascopy altered management in 15 of the 24 patients (63%) by precluding the need for formal thoracotomy or celiotomy. Clotted hemothorax was successfully removed in 8 of 9 patients. Diaphragmatic laceration was confirmed in 5 of 10 patients and ruled out in 4 others. One patient did not tolerate unilateral lung ventilation. Four small diaphragmatic lacerations were repaired thoracoscopically. A lacerated intercostal artery was identified in all 5 patients who were continuing to bleed. Bleeding was controlled by diathermy and/or thoracoscopic suturing in 3 patients, whereas 2 required open thoracotomy.

Conclusion.—Videothoracoscopy should be used more widely in patients with thoracic injuries. It would seem to be the best way of evaluating patients who are suspected of having diaphragmatic injury.

▶ The importance of this article is that it provides solid clinical data indicating that videothoracoscopy is effective in both the diagnosis and treatment of selected thoracic injuries. One important point stressed in this article is that hemothorax evacuation is more effective when thoracoscopy is performed early (within 10 days) rather than late and that an early thorascopic approach to clot removal is an effective way to prevent the development of late empyema formation. The authors also stress that conventional rather than laparoscopic instruments are more effective in disrupting and removing clot. Based upon this report, other studies, and experience at my institution, thoracoscopy appears to be an effective early tool in the management of selected patients with thoracic trauma.—E.A. Deitch, M.D.

Thoracoscopic Drainage and Decortication as Definitive Treatment for Empyema Thoracis Following Penetrating Chest Injury

O'Brien J, Cohen M, Solit R, Solit R, Lindenbaum G, Finnegan J, Vernick J
(Thomas-Jefferson Univ, Philadelphia; Crozer Chester Med Ctr, Upton, Pa)
J Trauma 36:536–539, 1994   140-95-4–6

Background.—The development of video-endoscopic equipment and techniques has led to a revolution in the management of intrathoracic diseases. The use of these new methods in carrying out thoracic drainage and decortication as a definitive treatment for empyema thoracis after penetrating chest trauma was reviewed.

Method.—Over a 9-month period, 8 patients were treated for empyema thoracis resulting from penetrating chest trauma (either a gunshot or a stab wound). The associated injuries included spinal cord injury with neurologic deficit, liver and diaphragmatic injury, and subclavian and carotid injury. All patients had a hemothorax or pneumothorax first treated with closed tube thoracostomy in the emergency department. All 8 patients had empyema, and thoracoscopic drainage and decortication were subsequently performed.

Results.—In all 8 patients, the thoracoscopic technique brought a complete resolution of the empyema. Chest tubes were removed after 2–25 days (median, 8.5 days), and the postoperative length of stay was a median of 19 days. The surgical procedure took an average time of 110 minutes. The estimated blood loss was between 100 and 250 mL for 7 patients; 1 patient lost 2,800 mL. Six patients had organisms cultured and the organisms obtained included 4 *Staphylococcus* (1 methicillin-resistant *Staphylococcus aureus*) and 1 each of *Proteus, Streptococcus,* and a diphtheroid. Two patients required additional thoracoscopic interventions for the treatment of a persistent air leak and the lysis of adhesions for a trapped lung.

Conclusion.—Thoracoscopic drainage and decortication offer a safe and practical alternative to thoracotomy as definitive treatment of empyema thoracis after a penetrating chest injury.

▶ The concept of avoiding a thoracotomy by video-assisted thoracoscopy is emotionally attractive in patients with empyemas. This paper would imply that the procedure is relatively easy, but that may not be the case when a true rind has formed and this peel must be removed from the lung. Because a relatively large percentage of this small series had parapneumonic empyemas, in which the extent of the pulmonary reaction is limited, more data are needed regarding patients with more extensive disease to verify the authors' optimistic conclusions and results. Will this procedure truly be effective in the majority of patients with established empyemas? Let's hope so!—E.A. Deitch, M.D.

The Role of Ultrasonography in Blunt Abdominal Trauma: Results in 250 Consecutive Cases

Goletti O, Ghiselli G, Lippolis PV, Chiarugi M, Braccini G, Macaluso C, Cavina E (Univ of Pisa, Italy)

J Trauma 36:178–181, 1994

140-95-4-7

Background.—An adequate diagnostic approach is crucial in the management of blunt abdominal trauma victims. The accuracy of ultrasound

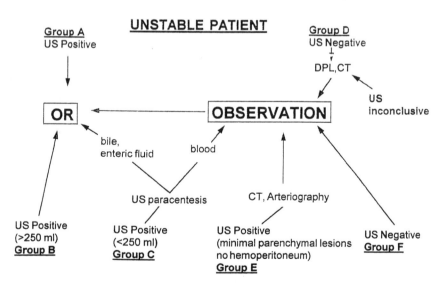

Fig 4–2.—Diagnostic and therapeutic algorithm for blunt abdominal trauma. (Courtesy of Goletti O, Ghiselli G, Lippolis PV, et al: *J Trauma* 36:178-181, 1994.)

in detecting abdominal lesions and free fluid collections was investigated.

Methods.—Two hundred fifty patients were included. The role of associated ultrasound–guided paracentesis in doubtful cases and in patients referred for nonoperative treatment was of special interest.

Findings.—The ultrasound had an overall sensitivity of 98% in detecting free fluid collection. Its specificity was 99% and the positive predictive value was 100%. Overall sensitivity, specificity, and positive predictive values were, respectively, 93%, 99%, and 93% in spleen injuries; 80%, 100%, and 100% in liver injuries; and 100%, 100%, and 100% in kidney lesions. On the basis of ultrasound–guided paracentesis findings, 3 stable patients underwent celiotomy.

Conclusion.—Ultrasonography is the preferred diagnostic approach for patients with blunt abdominal trauma (Fig 4–2). This technique is versatile, sensitive, repeatable, and feasible at the bedside. It also allows the performance of a guided paracentesis.

▶ In contrast to the United States, in Europe, ultrasonography has become the standard diagnostic test in patients with blunt abdominal trauma and is routinely used in emergency rooms. The figure above illustrates the authors' diagnostic and therapeutic ultrasonographic algorithm. Basically, unstable patients with free fluid collections (group A) or patients with free intra-abdominal fluid collections estimated to be 250 cc or more (group B) were taken immediately to surgery. Otherwise, as shown in this figure, further diagnostic tests or observation only was used. As documented in the abstract, this approach was very accurate; the overall accuracy of diagnostic ultrasonography was comparable to CT.

One might ask, If the accuracy of ultrasonography is comparable to CT, why not use CT? The answer is that diagnostic sonography can be performed in the emergency room in just a few minutes (average time to perform the procedure in this study was 4 minutes). The advantage of keeping potentially unstable trauma patients in the emergency area where they can be effectively monitored rather than having them in the bowels of the radiology department is not trivial. However, it is important to note that ultrasonography is not reliable in patients with intestinal perforation or large retroperitoneal hematomas (1).

Thus, on balance, it does appear that ultrasonography does have some major advantages over CT scanning in patients with blunt abdominal trauma. Consequently, diagnostic ultrasonography is being used in an increasing number of trauma centers in the United States.—E.A. Deitch, M.D.

Reference

1. Glaser K, et al: *Arch Surg* 129:743–747, 1994.

Ultrasonography for the Evaluation of Hemoperitoneum During Resuscitation: A Simple Scoring System

Huang M-S, Liu M, Wu J-K, Shih H-C, Ko T-J, Lee C-H (Natl Yang-Ming Med College, Taipei, Taiwan, Republic of China)
J Trauma 36:173–177, 1994   140-95-4-8

Purpose.—Intra-abdominal bleeding results in persistent hypovolemic shock in about 10% of patients with blunt abdominal trauma; these patients need urgent laparotomy. The physical examination and radiographic and laboratory data in this situation are unreliable. Some centers routinely use ultrasound for the evaluation of hemoperitoneum in patients with blunt abdominal trauma. The reliability of a new ultrasound scoring system for rapid estimation of the amount of hemoperitoneum was examined.

Methods.—In the first stage of the prospective study, the ultrasound scoring system was developed by examining 10 patients before and after infusion of 1,000 mL of diagnostic fluid into the abdominal cavity. Various locations were scored for the presence of fluid on ultrasonography, and the points were summed to obtain a ultrasound score ranging from 0 to 8. Patients with a score of 3 or above were estimated to have at least 1,000 mL of intra-abdominal free fluid. The utility of the score was then evaluated in 49 patients with blunt abdominal trauma with hemoperitoneum on their initial ultrasound evaluation.

Results.—Twenty-five patients had an ultrasound score of 3 or above, and all but 1 of this group required therapeutic laparotomy. Of the remaining 24 patients, who had an ultrasound score of less than 3, only 9 required laparotomy. Defining an ultrasound score of 3 or above as an indication of hemoperitoneum, the sensitivity was 84%; specificity, 71%; and accuracy, 71%.

Conclusion.—For patients with blunt abdominal trauma, ultrasonography is an effective screening test for hemoperitoneum and for estimation of the amount of blood lost. The ultrasound score can be very helpful during the resuscitation process. Patients with an ultrasound score of 3 or above should have urgent laparotomy; those with a score of less than 3 who are hemodynamically stable can have further evaluation and be considered for nonsurgical treatment.

▶ This article was chosen to illustrate the point that work is being carried out to verify and quantitate the findings on ultrasound. Although the results of this study have only modest clinical implications, the study does reflect an area in which there is significant activity. Although I am somewhat skeptical of this approach, stay tuned.—E.A. Deitch, M.D.

Is Computed Tomographic Grading of Splenic Injury Useful in the Nonsurgical Management of Blunt Trauma?

Kohn JS, Clark DE, Isler RJ, Pope CF (Maine Med Ctr, Portland)
J Trauma 36:385–389, 1994   140-95-4-9

Objective.—Aided by the use of CT scanning, trauma surgeons have found that surgery for blunt splenic injury is often unnecessary for adult and pediatric patients in stable condition. Reports have disagreed as to whether the initial CT findings can predict the outcome of nonsurgical management in patients with splenic injury. The authors addressed this question in an evaluation of their experience with nonsurgical management of blunt splenic injury.

Methods.—The experience included 37 adult patients and 33 children or adolescents with blunt splenic injury who were managed nonsurgically. This decision was made on the basis of published clinical criteria, without consideration of the CT appearance of the spleen. Delayed surgery was needed in 7 patients, all of whom recovered after total splenectomy; the nonsurgical approach was, thus, considered to have failed in these patients. The CT scans of all 70 patients were examined in blinded fashion by 2 radiologists who graded them according to 3 published scoring systems.

Results.—Failure of nonsurgical management was no more likely in patients with higher grades of splenic injury on CT evaluation. Of 10 patients who had very high scores on each of the published scales, 9 were successfully managed without surgery. Another 3 patients with very low scores required emergency surgery. Nonsurgical management was more likely to fail in patients with an elevated Injury Severity Score. The nonsurgical approach did not fail in any patient younger than age 17 years.

Conclusion.—In appropriately selected patients with blunt splenic injury, observation without surgery is safe, regardless of the magnitude of the injury on CT scans. Clinical criteria—including the patient's age and associated injuries—should be used in deciding whether to perform early exploration. Although CT scanning can accurately identify splenic injury in patients with blunt trauma, it cannot predict clinical outcome.

▶ This article was chosen for its reality testing. As much as we might hope that we can unequivocally decide which patients with splenic injuries will require operative intervention based on the CT appearance of the spleen, this does not appear to be the case. In other words, a picture may be worth a thousand words, but the words are not always correct. Thus, this article highlights the importance of a certain degree of skepticism.—E.A. Deitch, M.D.

The Success of Duplex Ultrasonographic Scanning in Diagnosis of Extremity Vascular Proximity Trauma

Fry WR, Smith RS, Sayers DV, Henderson VJ, Morabito DJ, Tsoi EK, Harness JK, Organ CH Jr (Univ of Calif, Davis–East Bay)
Arch Surg 128:1368–1372, 1993   140-95-4-10

Background.—Although duplex scanning has numerous advantages in the diagnosis of extremity vascular proximity trauma, few studies have addressed its correlation with other methods and none have reported its use in the actual diagnosis of venous injuries. The value of duplex scanning in the initial assessment of vascular proximity trauma was examined in a prospective study.

Methods.—Duplex scanning was compared with arteriography or operative exploration in 200 patients with 225 extremity injuries. All patients were seen at an urban trauma center with vascular proximity injury or diminished pulse strength in the injured extremity. After the first 50 cases, the remainder were evaluated by duplex scanning alone, with other diagnostic methods being used when the duplex scan suggested the presence of an injury.

Results.—In the first 50 cases, duplex scanning demonstrated a sensitivity and specificity of 100%, compared with arteriography and operative exploration. In the subsequent 175 injuries, duplex scanning detected 19 arterial injuries. Seventeen of these were confirmed by angiography or operative exploration, or both (table). There was 1 false positive result—a spasm of the superficial femoral artery detected on arteriography. An additional 7 unsuspected venous injuries were diagnosed as well.

Conclusion.—The safety and efficacy of duplex scanning as a noninvasive method for initial evaluation of possible extremity vascular proximity injury have been documented. At this trauma center, duplex scanning is now the diagnostic test of choice in the initial evaluation of vascular proximity injuries when distal extremity blood flow is present.

Results on Duplex Scans, Compared With Those on Arteriography and Operative Exploration, or Both

Arteriography/Operative Exploration Results	Duplex Scanning Results	
	Positive	**Negative**
Positive	36	0
Negative	1	31

(Courtesy of Fry WR, Smith RS, Sayers DV, et al: *Arch Surg* 128:1368–1372, 1993.)

▶ The results of this study speak for themselves. I agree with the authors that because of its safety and the fact that it is noninvasive, duplex scanning appears to be the preferred initial diagnostic test in patients with vascular proximity injuries. In addition, duplex scanning is accomplished with a portable machine, and in patients with other potential injuries, this is of major importance.—E.A. Deitch, M.D.

Gastric Tonometry Supplements Information Provided by Systemic Indicators of Oxygen Transport
Chang MC, Cheatham ML, Nelson LD, Rutherford EJ, Morris JA Jr (Vanderbilt Univ, Nashville, Tenn)
J Trauma 37:488–494, 1994   140-95-4-11

Objective.—Standard techniques for evaluating perfusion status may not provide the best indication of progressive shock or lack of oxygen in tissues. The results of gastric tonometry measurements of the degree of visceral perfusion were documented.

Methods.—Twenty critically ill trauma patients (mean age, 44 years) were monitored at 1, 2, 4, 8, 16, and 24 hours. Systemic hemodynamics and oxygen transport were measured with a radial arterial catheter and an oximetry pulmonary artery catheter. Arterial pH was measured, and base deficit and lactate levels were calculated. Gastric intramucosal pH was measured.

Results.—Six patients died. All received ventilatory support. Systemic hemodynamic and oxygen transport variables did not correlate with gastric intramucosal pH (pHi). Poor visceral perfusion was significantly as-

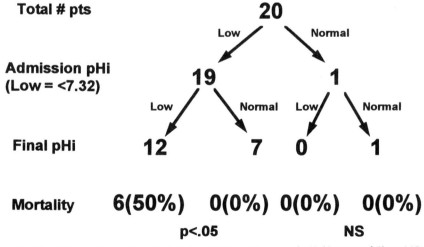

Fig 4–3.—Patient outcome shown by initial and 24-hour intramucosal pH. (Courtesy of Chang MC, Cheatham ML, Nelson LD, et al: *J Trauma* 37:488–494, 1994.)

sociated with organ dysfunction and failure, because the patients with a low pHi on admission who did not respond to therapy within 24 hours had a higher mortality rate (Fig 4–3) and a higher incidence of organ dysfunction (2.6 vs. .6 organs/patients). By logistic regression, the only variables statistically associated with mortality were pHi, base deficit, and mixed venous oxygen saturation.

Conclusion.—Although the study was small, the results indicate that measurements of gastric intramucosal pH in critically ill trauma patients after 24 hours of treatment provides prognostic information not available from standard measurements of oxygen transport.

▶ Not only does the controversy continue but over the last decade a new player has been added. The controversy is twofold. First, can we accurately identify patients who have inadequate organ perfusion in spite of traditionally adequate levels of volume resuscitation, and, secondly, can this information be used to improve survival or limit organ dysfunction? The new player is gastric tonometry and the results of this study—as well as other, but not all, studies on gastric tonometry—indicate that serial measurements of gastric mucosal pH might identify patients at increased risk of sustaining organ failure and dying. To an optimist, this would indicate that direct measurements of the adequacy of organ perfusion (the stomach) is the missing link preventing us from being able to determine exactly which patients would require increased levels of oxygen delivery and that this knowledge will result in improved survival rates.

Will gastric tonometry be a reliable yardstick on which to base therapeutic decisions or will it, like other variables used in the past, have its Achilles heel? Some say yes, some say no. I say maybe. Nonetheless, the idea is good and worthy of continued pursuit. Let's keep our fingers crossed and hope.—E.A. Deitch, M.D.

Saline PCO_2 Is an Important Source of Error in the Assessment of Gastric Intramucosal pH
Takala J, Parviainen I, Siloaho M, Ruokonen E, Hämäläinen E (Kuopio Univ, Finland)
Crit Care Med 22:1877–1879, 1994   140-95-4–12

Introduction.—There are a variety of variables that can affect the interpretation of gastric intramucosal pH. An added source of variance is the blood gas analyzer itself. Four different analyzers were tested for their accuracy in determining saline PCO_2.

Methods.—Saline partial pressure of carbon dioxide (PCO_2) was determined by 4 different blood gas analyzers: Ciba-Corning 238 pH/blood gas analyzer, ABL-520 blood gas system, the Nova Stat Profile 4 analyzer, and the IL-1302 blood gas analyzer. In 20 blood samples from patients, the mean difference in blood PCO_2 was .8. Saline samples were balanced

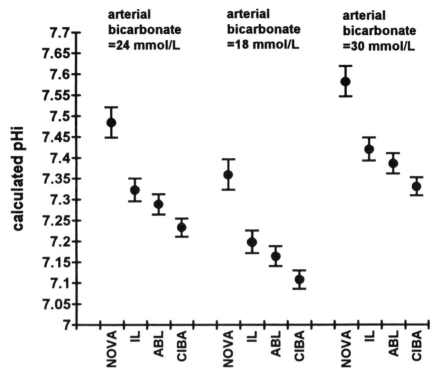

Fig 4–4.—*Abbreviations:* NOVA, Stat Profile 4 analyzer (Nova Biomedical); *IL*, IL-1302 blood gas analyzer (Instrumentation Laboratories); *ABL*, ABL-520 blood gas system (Radiometer); *CIBA*, 238 pH/blood gas analyzer (Ciba Corning). Calculated gastric intramucosal pH (pHi) corresponding to the mean P_{CO_2} and its 95% confidence limits, as measured by 4 blood gas analyzers using saline ampules with a P_{CO_2} of 45 torr (6kPa), assuming arterial bicarbonate concentrations of 18, 24, and 30 mmol/L. (Courtesy of Takala J, Parviainen I, Siloaho M, et al: *Crit Care Med* 22:1877–1879, 1994.)

for 20 minutes in gas mixes of CO_2 and nitrogen to obtain P_{CO_2} levels of 30, 45, and 68 mm Hg. Bias, the mean difference between the measured and reference values, and precision, the standard deviation of the bias, were determined. The effect of buffering the solution was also evaluated.

Findings.—Measurement bias increased with the higher P_{CO_2} levels. The Nova analyzer underestimated P_{CO_2} by 50% to 60%, whereas the other analyzers underestimated the P_{CO_2} by 5% to 19%. The bias was reduced in all analyzers with the use of a buffer (Fig 4–4). At 45 mm Hg, a difference in gastric pH of .06 pH units can be detected by all the analyzers except the Nova analyzer.

Conclusion.—Both the analyzer and the PCO_2 level are sources of error in the assessment of gastric intramucosal pH. It is not valid to compare values obtained on separated analyzers.

▶ This straightforward article documents the effect of different blood gas analyzers on the accuracy of the PCO_2 and pH measurements. Therefore, the message is clear and of major practical importance: Know the limits of the systems used in your hospital.—E.A. Deitch, M.D.

Prospective Evaluation of Epidural Versus Intrapleural Catheters for Analgesia in Chest Wall Trauma
Luchette FA, Radafshar SM, Kaiser R, Flynn W, Hassett JM (State Univ of New York at Buffalo)
J Trauma 36:865–870, 1994   140-95-4-13

Objective.—Blunt chest trauma can cause serious ventilation problems and a great deal of chest pain. Therefore, determination of optimal methods of pain relief are important.

Methods.—Nineteen patients aged 18 to 80 with multiple injuries, including chest trauma, were enrolled in a prospective study in which they received bupivacaine either through epidural or intrapleural catheters. Pulmonary function and pain relief were monitored.

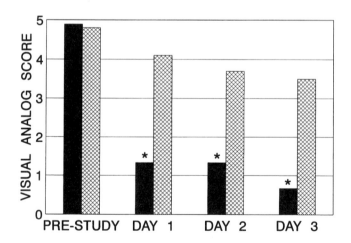

■ EPIDURAL ▨ INTRAPLEURAL

Fig 4–5.—Pain with movement or coughing was significantly less throughout the study in the epidural group. *Analysis was performed with paired Student's *t* tests and significance at $P < 0.05$. (Courtesy of Luchette FA, Radafshar SM, Kaiser R, et al: *J Trauma* 36:865–870, 1994.)

Results.—Ten patients received intrapleural catheters and 9 received epidural catheters. The patients receiving continuous epidural bupivacaine had significantly less pain (Fig 4–5). Additionally, the patients receiving epidural analgesia had significantly increased tidal volumes and negative inspiratory pressures as compared with the patients receiving intrapleural bupivacaine. Mild hypotension, which was easily corrected, was a common complication in patients with epidural catheters.

Conclusion.—Epidural analgesia is superior to intrapleural block in controlling pain and maintaining normal pulmonary function.

▶ The value of good pain relief in preventing pulmonary complications in patients with chest trauma is well known, because pain-induced pulmonary splinting leads to decreased ventilation and atelectasis. In fact, all of us have seen patients in whom pain-related pulmonary splinting led to serious complications such as hypoxia or pneumonia. Consequently, this study, by prospectively documenting the superiority of epidural analgesia, is worthy of note, although one must be wary of the initial hypotension observed when these patients received their initial bolus dose of epidural bupivacaine.—E.A. Deitch, M.D.

Superiority of Aztreonam/Clindamycin Compared With Gentamicin/Clindamycin in Patients With Penetrating Abdominal Trauma

Fabian TC, Hess MM, Croce MA, Wilson RS, Wilson SE, Charland SL, Rodman JH, Boucher BA (Univ of Tenn, Memphis; Wayne State Univ, Detroit, Mich; Univ of California, Irvine; et al)
Am J Surg 167:291–296, 1994   140-95-4–14

Introduction.—Treatment of patients who survive the initial impact of penetrating abdominal trauma must focus on preventing infection. After prompt, definitive surgery, antibiotic regimens are instituted that can control both anaerobic organisms and Enterobacteriaceae. Combined gentamicin and clindamycin has been the standard regimen for both treatment and prevention of infection. However, a newly approved drug, aztreonam, has a prolonged half-life and may, therefore, be superior to gentamicin in preventing infection in these patients. A multicenter, prospective, a double-blind trial compared the efficacy, safety, and pharmacokinetics of aztreonam and clindamycin with those of gentamicin and clindamycin.

Methods.—Adult patients with penetrating abdominal wounds were randomly assigned to receive either aztreonam and clindamycin (A/C) or gentamicin and clindamycin (G/C). Patients in the G/C group received gentamicin, 5 mg/kg, in 3 doses during the first 24 hours and subsequent doses to maintain standardized serum levels of 2–8 μg/mL. Patients in the A/C group received 2 g of aztreonam every 8 hours. All patients were given 900 mg of clindamycin every 8 hours. The patients without colon injury were given antibiotics for 24 hours; patients with colon injury were given antibiotics for 4 days. Drug concentrations and pharmacokinetics were studied in serum samples from the patients and from healthy volunteers. Episodes of wound infection, intra-abdominal infection, or necrotizing fasciitis were considered antibiotic failures.

Results.—There were 36 evaluable patients in the G/C group and 37 in the A/C group. Patients in the 2 groups had comparable degrees of injury, incidence of colon wounds, and transfusion requirements. Antibiotic failures occurred in 8 patients and included 2 wound infections, 4 intra-abdominal abscesses, 1 diffuse peritonitis, and 1 necrotizing fasciitis. All of the failures occurred in patients with hollow viscus injuries. Most antibiotic failures (7 of 8) occurred in the patients treated with G/C. Patients in the A/C group had shorter hospital stays. The atreonam half-life was increased in patients with penetrating abdominal trauma, compared to healthy volunteers, and was particularly prolonged in patients with colon injury.

Discussion.—Antibiotic regimens including aztreonam produce improved outcomes compared with those including gentamicin. It appears that the prolonged half-life of aztreonam accounts for its superior clinical efficacy, because therapeutic concentrations of gentamycin were not maintained in several patients.

▶ This well-controlled trial indicates that specific antibiotic choice does make a difference. In an era in which antibiotic proliferation is uncontrolled and the differences between many regimens are more apparent than real, it is important to be reminded that not all antibiotic regimens are equally effective.—E.A. Deitch, M.D.

Planned Reoperation for Trauma: A Two Year Experience With 124 Consecutive Patients
Hirshberg A, Wall MJ Jr, Mattox KL (Baylor College of Medicine, Houston; Ben Taub Gen Hosp, Houston)
J Trauma 37:365–369, 1994   140-95-4–15

Introduction.—A strategy of planned reoperation is being increasingly used in caring for critically injured patients. Because many of these patients are not likely to survive a major operation, the alternative is to control bleeding and take any other supportive measures that are necessary, warm and resuscitate the patient, and perform a definitive repair when the patient has become functionally stable.

Objective.—The results of this strategy were examined in 124 trauma patients who, in a 2-year period, underwent nondefinitive surgical procedures for injuries of the trunk. A majority had penetrating injuries that most often involved the abdomen alone or both the abdomen and chest.

Initial Management.—Indications included the inability to control bleeding directly; a need to end surgery in a patient who was hypother-

Techniques Used at Initial Operation	
Indication	Number of Patients
Packing	109
Gastrointestinal interruption	27
Temporary urinary control	8
Stapled lung resection	9
Rapid vascular control	18
Rapid skin closure	108
Temporary plastic bag	20

(Courtesy of Hirshberg A, Wall MJ Jr, Mattox KL: *J Trauma* 37:365–369, 1994.)

mic or had a coagulopathy; and massive visceral edema that prevented formal closure of the abdomen or chest. A variety of initial operative methods were used (table).

Reoperation.—Seventy-three patients lived and underwent a total of 101 reoperations. The initial reoperation was planned in 52 patients, whereas 21 were treated for bleeding or abdominal compartment syndrome. Fourteen injuries were missed. The overall mortality rate was 58%. The best results were achieved when an early decision was made to end the initial procedure and when planned reoperation was carried out.

Conclusion.—It is expected that as more trauma surgeons adopt a policy of planned reoperation, the indications will be more precisely defined and salvage rates will improve.

▶ When is it time to quit in patients with severe truncal trauma? In most trauma patients, the answer to this question is quite simple: After bleeding has been definitively controlled and visceral injuries have been fixed. However, in some patients, this approach is not possible, and the best one can do is pack off areas of bleeding and control intestinal contamination. In fact, based on this clinical report and several others in the literature, this approach of an initial abbreviated laparotomy followed by a later planned reoperation has become almost standard policy for the cold, coagulopathic, hypotensive trauma victim in most trauma centers. I know that in my practice this approach has been valuable in the treatment of nontrauma as well as trauma patients. I strongly advise those of you who have not adopted this approach to seriously consider trying it if the proper clinical occasion should arise.—E.A. Deitch, M.D.

Prevention of Venous Thromboembolism in Trauma Patients

Knudson MM, Lewis FR, Clinton A, Atkinson K, Megerman J (Univ of California, San Francisco; Henry Ford Hosp, Detroit; Kendall Healthcare Products Company, Mansfield, Mass)

J Trauma 37:480–487, 1994   140-95-4–16

Objective.—Because trauma patients are at significant risk of thromboembolic complications, a prospective study of 400 such patients was undertaken at an urban trauma center to evaluate 2 methods of preventing deep venous thrombosis (DVT).

Study Plan.—Adult patients, excluding pregnant women, were categorized according to whether they could receive heparin or wear compression boots and stocking, and then randomized to 1 of these treatments or to a control group. Heparin was given subcutaneously in a dose of 500 units at 12-hour intervals. Thigh-length sequential gradient pneumatic leg compression devices (SCDs) were used.

Results.—Of 251 patients who completed the study, DVT developed in 15 (6%), and in 2 others, pulmonary embolism developed without evidence of DVT. One of the latter patients died. Six of the patients with DVT received anticoagulant therapy without complications, and 2 received a vena caval filter. Risk factors for thromboembolism included prolonged bed rest and blunt (as opposed to penetrating) trauma. Patients 30 years of age and older and those with pelvic or lower limb fractures also were at increased risk. Low-dose heparin did not effectively prevent thromboembolism, and SCDs were protective only in patients with neurotrauma.

Recommendations.—The SCDs are still recommended for use in trauma victims when risk factors for thromboembolism, especially neurologic injury, are present. Other patients should be monitored by duplex venous examination to detect clinically silent DVT.

▶ This is an important article. It documents that in up to 6% of trauma patients—even including those patients receiving prophylactic treatment—DVT develops and that 13% of patients with DVT have a pulmonary embolism. Although only 1 of the 251 patients enrolled in this study died of a pulmonary embolism, if one considers the large number of at risk trauma patients admitted to hospitals each year, it is clear why pulmonary embolism is considered to be 1 of the most common preventible causes of death in trauma patients.

A prospective study of venous thromboembolism after major trauma published after this article was chosen further defines the risk of DVT and lethal pulmonary embolism (1). In this study, proximal DVT developed in 18% of the patients, and 1% of the entire patient population died from pulmonary emboli. For these reasons and because compression therapy and subcutaneous heparin either cannot be used or are not effective, many trauma surgeons seriously consider prophylactically placing Greenfield filters in high-risk patients. I know I do.—E.A. Deitch, M.D.

Reference

1. Geerts WH, et al: N Engl J Med 331:1601–1606, 1994.

Hypercapnia: Is There a Cause for Concern?

Simon RJ, Mawilmada S, Ivatury RR (New York Med College, Bronx, NY)
J Trauma 37:74–80, 1994   140-95-4–17

Introduction.—Evidence that mechanical ventilation–induced barotrauma may contribute to pulmonary dysfunction in patients with acute respiratory distress syndrome (ARDS) has led to the development of alternate methods of ventilation. Most of these alternate methods of mechanical ventilation result in hypercapnia. Because hypercapnia has a number of negative effects, these new ventilatory modalities have had limited acceptance.

Methods.—Twelve patients with severe pulmonary dysfunction, defined as peak inspiratory pressure (PIP) $\geq$ 45 cm H_2O or an arterial blood partial pressure of oxygen/fraction of inspired oxygen (PaO_2/FIO_2) ratio $\leq$ 250 were treated by inverse ratio ventilation with low tidal volumes in an attempt to limit barotrauma. The systemic effects of this hypercapnia-inducing ventilatory regimen on neurologic status, cardiac function, and cellular oxygen utilization was assessed.

Results.—The mean peak arterial blood partial pressure of carbon dioxide ($PaCO_2$) was 63.3 mm Hg and reached as high as 96 mm Hg. Hypercapnia was maintained for 2–12 days. Six of the 12 patients survived; the 6 nonsurvivors died of multiple system organ failure (4 patients) or respiratory insufficiency (2 patients). Chest tube insertion was required in only 1 patient, a nonsurvivor. There were no differences between survivors and nonsurvivors for peak $PaCO_2$ values, cardiac output, or cellular oxygen utilization adequacy. Neurologic function was unaffected in the survivors. The nonsurvivors had higher indices of lung injury and were less able to compensate for respiratory acidosis.

Discussion.—Moderate levels of hypercapnia may be safely used in most patients with severe pulmonary dysfunction, although permissive hypercapnia is not indicated for patients with intracranial hypertension. The efficacy of ventilation methods still need to be studied to determine which technique is most effective in patients with severe pulmonary dysfunction.

▶ The ventilatory management of patients with ARDS continues to mature. Recognition that iatrogenic barotrauma caused by standard methods of ventilatory support (i.e., high tidal volumes and peak end-expiratory pressure) may be playing a major role in the pathogenesis of ARDS, has resulted in certain conceptual modifications in our thinking. One concept that has emerged is that our fear of hypercapnia is not fully warranted, and, thus, it may not be wise to adjust the ventilatory settings to maintain normocarbia at the expense of inducing barotrauma. Because barotrauma has been correlated with elevated PIP, ventilatory maneuvers that reduce PIP—such as reducing the tidal volume or lengthening the time period over which the tidal volume is delivered (inverse ratio ventilation)—are being increasingly used clinically.

Consequently, this small retrospective study was chosen, because it, like other recent studies, indicates that our fear of hypercapnia may be largely unwarranted, and it provides an opportunity to address the basic rationale for this ventilatory approach. It is important to state at the onset that this study does not answer the question of whether ventilatory maneuvers associated with permissive hypercapnia will be beneficial. Prospective studies will be required to answer that question.

In summary, this study is important because it addresses the basic concept that patients with pulmonary failure who are ventilated in such a manner that high airway pressures are produced will eventually have potentially life-threatening complications of barotrauma, including pneumothoraces and progression of pulmonary injury. Because once barotrauma has developed, it is very difficult to treat, our goals should focus on its prevention.—E.A. Deitch, M.D.

Interferon-Gamma Increases Mortality Following Cecal Ligation and Puncture

Miles RH, Paxton TP, Dries DJ, Gamelli RL (Loyola Univ, Maywood, Ill; Chicago Med School, East Chicago, Ill)
J Trauma 36:607–611, 1994   140-95-4–18

Background.—Major trauma is associated with a significant elevation in the number of circulating macrophages together with a decline in T-helper cells. Both monocyte production of interleukin-1 and T-cell synthesis of interferon-γ (IFN-γ) are greatly reduced. Whether mortality from intra-abdominal sepsis might be reduced by the administration of IFN-γ was determined.

Methods.—A septic focus was created in 50 male BDF mice using cecal ligation and puncture (CLP). Immediately after the procedure, the animals received IFN-γ (100–22,500 U) or vehicle control subcutaneously via the right flank, with normal saline given subcutaneously dorsally for resuscitation. Injections were continued daily until the animal died or to postoperative day 7. In a second set of experiments, daily injections of vehicle control or IFN-γ (100 U) were administered to 60 mice 24, 48, or 72 hours before CLP.

Results.—None of the doses of IFN-γ administered immediately after CLP yielded any survival benefit. Mortality was increased in the IFN-γ group vs. the vehicle control group in a dose-dependent fashion. At day 4 post-CLP, survival was 70% in control animals, 50% in the 100 U IFN-

Mortality Curve

Cecal Ligation and Puncture
Gamma Interferon vs. Control

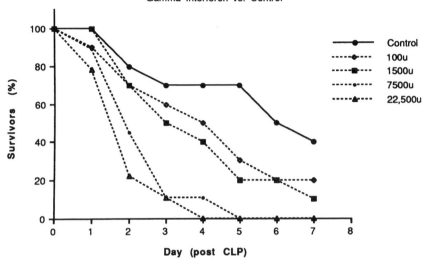

Day (post CLP)

Fig 4–6.—Mortality curve for CLP mice administered IFN-γ immediately postprocedure and then daily in doses ranging from 100 U to 22,500 U compared with vehicle control. All animals surviving to day 7 were classified as long-term survivors. Number = 10 in all groups at the onset of experiments (day 0). All groups were found to have a statistically different mortality curve from the control (P < .05). (Courtesy of Miles RH, Paxton TP, Dries DJ, et al: *J Trauma* 36:607–611, 1994.)

γ group, 40% in the 1,500 IFN-γ group, and 10% in the 7,500 IFN-γ group; no animals were alive in the 22,500 IFN-γ group. IFN-γ–treated animals had a lower survival rate than controls in all of the recorded time points (Fig 4-6). With pretreatment, mortality was comparable to that of controls in all sets of experiments with a single exception. Overall survival at 7 days was higher for animals pretreated with IFN-γ 24 hours before CPL, although the difference was not statistically significant.

Conclusion.—Late infections and their sequelae remain the leading cause of death in critically injured surgical patients. Levels of IFN-γ are depressed in patients with traumatic injury, suggesting a role for this lymphokine in injury-related immunocompetence. Yet treatment with IFN-γ did not confer protection in this experimental model of sepsis and was even found to have a negative effect on survival.

▶ This experimental study in a clinically relevant animal model has profound implications. First, it suggests that just because a biological agent is decreased in certain clinical situations does not mean that replacing it will of necessity be beneficial. The idea that "If it is low, raise it" and "If it is high, reduce it," while conceptually attractive, may not only be too simplistic but may even be hazardous to the health of our patients. It is just such a simplistic approach, supported by clinically irrelevant animal and in vitro studies, that has led to the initiation of several poorly conceived clinical trials involving a number of biological agents. Secondly, it highlights the point that the timing of drug administration as well as the condition of the patient may determine whether the biological agents exerts a beneficial or harmful effect. As far as IFN-γ is concerned, it appears that providing the agent in the immediate preseptic period may be good, but if this narrow preseptic temporal window is missed, bad things may happen.—E.A. Deitch, M.D.

Cytokine, Complement, and Endotoxin Profiles Associated With the Development of the Adult Respiratory Distress Syndrome After Severe Injury
Donnelly TJ, Meade P, Jagels M, Cryer HG, Law MM, Hugli TE, Shoemaker WC, Abraham E (Univ of Calif, Los Angeles; King-Drew Med Ctr, Los Angeles; Scripps Research Inst, La Jolla, Calif)
Crit Care Med 22:768–776, 1994   140-95-4–19

Introduction.—Studies suggest that interleukin (IL)-6, tumor necrosis factor (TNF)-α, IL-1β, endotoxin, and complement fragments are involved in the development of adult respiratory distress syndrome (ARDS) in traumatically injured patients. The sequence and pattern of release of these components immediately after injury, however, have not been characterized. Plasma concentrations of these mediators in patients who have received traumatic injuries were examined.

Methods.—Plasma samples were obtained every 4 hours from 15 patients with an Injury Severity Score of > 25. Hemodynamic and oxygen metabolism factors were measured in 7 patients with ARDS and 8 non-ARDS patients, aged 24–47 years, without lung injury. In patients with ARDS, immunologic assays were used to determine TNF-α, IL-6, IL-8, IL1β, endotoxin, C3a, and C4a.

Results.—Three patients with ARDS and 7 non-ARDS patients survived. There was a significant decrease in oxygenation and the arterial blood partial pressure of oxygen/fraction of inspired oxygen (PaO_2/F_{IO_2}) ratio and a significant increase in shunt fraction, mean pulmonary arterial pressure, and central venous pressure for patients with ARDS. Interferon-8, C3a, and C4a concentrations were significantly increased in patients with ARDS 16 hours after injury. No patients had detectable levels of circulating IL-8, TNF-α, or endotoxin.

Discussion.—None of the mediators studied here showed changes that would indicate the onset of ARDS. Severe oxygenation impairment appeared at 4 hours post injury, long before systemic release of inflammatory mediators.

Conclusion.—Measurement of inflammatory mediators is not predictive of the development of ARDS in patients with traumatic injury.

▶ This article was chosen because it illustrates the poor predictive power of circulating immunoinflammatory factor levels in determining which patients with major injuries will sustain ARDS. Based on clinical studies such as this one and the fact that cytokines exert their effects locally and are not normally present in the plasma, plus experimental studies in sepsis models documenting that tissue and plasma levels of cytokines such as TNF do not correlate (1), it is not surprising that the interpretation of plasma concentrations of inflammatory mediators is so difficult. What this means is that better methods of quantitating and assessing the biological consequences of putative inflammatory substances are needed. Just measuring circulating levels of these factors is not fully adequate. As will be illustrated in Abstracts 140-95-4–20 and 140-95-4–21, one recent approach is to measure circulating levels of various cytokine and adhesion molecule receptors.—E.A. Deitch, M.D.

Reference

1. Hadjiminas DJ, et al: *J Surg Res* 56;549–555, 1994.

Trauma Causes Sustained Elevation of Soluble Tumor Necrosis Factor Receptors

Cinat ME, Waxman K, Granger GA, Pearce W, Annas C, Daughters K (Univ of California-Irvine, Orange)
J Am Coll Surg 179:529–537, 1994   140-95-4–20

Introduction.—The systemic effects of tumor necrosis factor (TNF) are thought to be modulated by soluble tumor necrosis factor receptors (sTNF-R), whereby its interaction with target organs and binding to serum TNF are prevented. Recent studies have shown that the early release of the soluble forms of the 55 and 75 kd membrane receptors for TNF are caused by traumatic injury. The magnitude and duration of the TNF receptor elevation after trauma and whether the levels of sTNF-R correlate with the severeity of injury and outcome were investigated.

Methods.—One hundred patients who arrived in the trauma center from August through November 1992 were evaluated (74 male patients and 26 female patients with a mean age of 29.44 years). Twenty patients died and 80 survived. Most patients had multiple injuries. Serum samples were drawn from these patients within 1 hour after injury; this was continued for as long as 15 days. Sera from 24 healthy volunteers were obtained and used as normal controls. The samples were analyzed by using polyclonal enzyme-linked immunosorbent assays for TNF and the levels of sTNF 55 and 75 kd receptors.

Results.—Within 1 hour of injury, trauma caused immediate elevation of the levels of both receptors, and they remained elevated for as long as 15 days after injury. The TNF was not measurable. Late variations in the levels were related to complications, such as hypoxia, infection, and sepsis. In critically ill patients and nonsurvivors, the levels were significantly more elevated. In normal control patients, the mean values for 55 and 75 kd sTNF-R were 640 and 2,187 pg per mL, respectively. In the injured patients, the mean sera levels upon arrival at the trauma center were 1,924 and 4,231 pg per mL, respectively. Typically, receptors were elevated immediately upon arrival at the emergency department. During initial resuscitation, the levels declined, followed by a second increase within 1 to 4 hours.

Conclusion.—After trauma, in the absence of measurable TNF, the levels of sTNF-R are significantly elevated. The extent of the elevation seems to depend on the severity of the injury and complications. Further studies are needed to explain the mechanism and biological importance of sTNF-R release after trauma.

▶ Failure of circulating cytokine levels, such as TNF, to correlate with clinical outcome is apparent in this study as well as in Abstract 140-95-4–19. Although premature, the strategy of measuring sTNF-R levels as a surrogate marker for TNF activity appears to hold some promise, as shown in this study. One strength of this paper is that 100 patients were studied. Because such a large number of patients were studied, the likelihood of the authors' conclusion that sTNF-R levels may be of prognostic importance is increased. This point is of potential importance, because in the next abstract (140-95-4–21), in which only 13 patients were studied, sTNF-R levels did not predict in which patients multiple organ failure would develop, although the levels were higher in the patients with multiple organ failure.—E.A. Deitch, M.D.

Elevated Levels of Soluble ICAM-1 Correlate With the Development of Multiple Organ Failure in Severely Injured Trauma Patients
Law MM, Cryer HG, Abraham E (Univ of California, Los Angeles)
J Trauma 37:100–109, 1994   140-95-4–21

Introduction.—Neutrophils, because of their role in inflammatory tissue destruction, have been implicated in the pathogenesis of multiple organ failure (MOF). They are influenced by proinflammatory cytokines, such as tumor necrosis factor (TNF)-α and the interleukins (ILs). A method for measuring the level of shed endothelial cell adhesion molecules for neutrophils (sICAM-1) was recently developed. It was hypothesized that serum concentrations of IL-6, IL-8, soluble TNF-α receptor (sTNF$_r$), and sICAM-1 may predict the development of MOF in patients with severe multiple trauma.

Methods.—Critically ill, multiply injured trauma patients with an Injury Severity Score of at least 25 were studied. Plasma specimens were assayed for IL-6, IL-8, sTNF$_r$, and sICAM-1 before, at, and after resuscitation. Organ dysfunction was assessed to identify patients with MOF.

Results.—Thirteen patients were studied; 6 patients had MOF develop. The mean levels of IL-6 were higher in the MOF patients than in the other group before resuscitation, then decreased. Both early and late mean levels of IL-8 were elevated in the MOF patients compared with non-MOF patients. However, there were wide variations in the levels of both interleukins in both groups, making differences not statistically significant. The mean levels of sTNF$_r$, although elevated in all the patients, remained consistent throughout the observation period in the non-MOF patients but increased in the MOF patients; however, the differences were not statistically significant. The mean sICAM-1 values were within the normal range before and at resuscitation in the non-MOF patients and rose slightly thereafter. In the MOF patients, the initial sICAM-1 value was slightly higher than in the non-MOF patients, but rose precipitously during and after resuscitation, showing significant differences between the groups. The MOF score correlated significantly with the sICAM-1 levels at and after resuscitation and the late sTNF$_r$ values.

Conclusion.—These data suggest that sICAM-1 values may predict the development and severity of MOF in severely, multiply injured patients. The finding of increased levels of sICAM-1 in MOF patients supports the hypothesized role of increased leukocyte-endothelium adhesion in the development of MOF. Further study of the pathophysiologic mechanisms by which ICAM-1 operates may suggest preventive strategies.

▶ One of the major reasons that this clinical study was chosen was that the results indicate that endothelial cell activation is up regulated shortly after injury and that the extent of endothelial cell activation/injury may be important in the pathogenesis of end-organ injury that leads to MOF. This notion is supported by the observed pattern of sICAM-1 release into the circulation and the fact that there was a correlation between the absolute level of sICAM-1 and the severity of subsequent MOF. Now, why is that important? It is important because there are a number of agents being tested that can modify endothelial cell injury/activation and, thereby, potentially limit end-organ dysfunction.—E.A. Deitch, M.D.

5 Infection

Introduction

Infections acquired in the hospital continue to be a source of morbidity and death in both patients and health care workers. Patients can acquire infections from other patients, from health care workers, or as a result of invasive procedures. Health care workers can also acquire infections from patients. In response to the publicity that occurred when a dentist infected 6 of his patients, the Centers for Disease Control and Prevention proposed in 1991 that all health care providers who perform "exposure-prone" invasive procedures undergo testing for HIV. The first paper, Abstract 140-95-5-1, discusses the high cost of preventing infections that surgeons or dentists might transmit to patients in hospitals. Yet, there are no documented HIV infections of patients occurring as a result of transmission by physicians or dentists in the hospital setting.

The second paper, Abstract 140-95-5-2, documents that surrogate testing for hepatitis C by the use of alanine aminotransferase testing and antibodies to hepatitis B core antigens was effective in preventing hepatitis C transmission before a test for hepatitis C became available.

Two articles deal with bloodstream infections. The first, Abstract 140-95-5-3, discusses the high cost of nosocomial bloodstream infections in surgical intensive care units, not only in dollars but also in terms of morbidity and mortality.

The second, Abstract 140-95-5-4, discusses *Candida* sepsis in compromised surgical patients and reviews the high mortality rate of these infections, especially for those patients in the intensive care unit. Catheter sepsis, Abstract 140-95-5-5, continues to plague hospitals. Now with parenteral nutrition and intravenous antibiotic therapy being given to outpatients, catheter-related sepsis will be seen more and more in the home care setting. This article stresses the necessity for rigorous asepsis in placement of these catheters and strict adherence to protocols in caring for these patients at home.

A valid method of judging how "sick" patients with peritonitis and other surgical infections are has long been sought by surgeons and others who seek to be able to validly compare 1 study with another. This study from Germany, deals only with patients with peritonitis, whereas many currently used studies (e.g., the APACHE scoring system) were not designed originally for patients with intra-abdominal infections but rather were established in another clinical setting. This peritonitis index may be the most valid method for comparing these complicated patients.

Hyperbaric oxygen has long been used for treating necrotizing soft-tissue infections (Abstract 140-95-5-7); proving that it is better than standard treatment is difficult, however. No prospective randomized study has ever been (and probably could be) done. This article is a multicenter review of the treatment of hyperbaric oxygen in soft tissue infections and comes out in favor of hyperbaric treatment.

It is frequently difficult to differentiate between acute appendicitis and pelvic inflammatory disease in women of childbearing age (Abstract 140-95-5-8). This article by Webster et al. sought originally to determine whether such a differentiation could be done by reviewing the clinical presentation. Their conclusion is that such a differentiation cannot be effectively carried out.

Endotoxin is an important mediator in patients with sepsis and multiple organ failure. A novel approach uses an extracorporeal device to reduce or eliminate endotoxin from the circulation (Abstract 140-95-5-9). Although most of the patients included in this article survived, it is difficult to know the role of the filtration system in leading to that survival.

Bacterial translocation can be demonstrated in the blood of solid organ donors who presumably have an intact gastrointestinal mucosa (Abstract 140-95-5-10). This article thus provides further evidence that bacterial translocation can indeed occur. The role of bacterial translocation in the pathogenesis of disease, however, still remains unsettled. Finally, an article from India (Abstract 140-95-5-11) discusses surgical problems that can be encountered in patients with *Salmonella* infection. These infections are seen relatively uncommonly in the United States, but they are the most common bacteria causing mycotic aneurysms.

Richard J. Howard, M.D., Ph.D.

The Cost-Effectiveness of HIV Testing of Physicians and Dentists in the United States

Phillips KA, Lowe RA, Kahn JG, Lurie P, Avins AL, Ciccarone D (Univ of Calif, San Francisco; Univ of Calif, Berkeley)
JAMA 271:851–858, 1994   140-95-5-1

Objective.—Testing of health care workers for HIV is a controversial issue. In 1991, the Centers for Disease Control (CDC) issued recommendations for health care workers who perform invasive procedures. Congress has since mandated that states adopt equivalent guidelines. A study compared the cost-effectiveness of several options for one-time HIV testing of physicians and dentists.

Methods.—The options considered were mandatory testing of all physicians and dentists, mandatory testing only of those who perform inva-

Results for Surgeons and Other Physicians

Prevalence and Risk	Total Costs, in Millions of $*	No. of Patient Infections Averted	Cost per Infection Averted, $*	Incremental Cost per Infection Averted (Compared With Current Testing), $*†
Medium seroprevalence (0.4%) and medium transmission risk (0.00002)				
Increased voluntary testing	28.1	9.6	2 931 000	1 208 000
Mandatory with inform patients	28.4	20.8	1 361 000	395 000
Mandatory with restriction of practice	27.9	25.0	1 115 000	291 000
Mandatory with exclusion	27.8	26.1	1 065 000	271 000
Mandatory testing of all physicians with exclusion	51.6	26.1	1 979 000	1 372 000
Low prevalence (0.05%)	17.7	3.1	5 659 000	1 802 000
High prevalence (1%)	45.3	62.5	725 000	162 000
Low transmission risk (0.0000014)	30.6	2.2	13 757 000	4 495 000
High transmission risk (0.00016)	23.0	66.1	348 000	36 000
Low prevalence and low transmission risk	18.0	0.2	89 874 000	29 807 000
High prevalence and high transmission risk	(2.6)	465.5	(6000)	(81 000)

Note: All results shown are for mandatory testing of surgeons only with restrictions of practice, except as noted.
*Costs are rounded to the nearest thousand. Costs in parentheses are net savings.
†Incremental costs per infection averted are calculated by comparing the policy option to current levels of voluntary testing. For comparison, the number of infections occurring over 7 years, at medium prevalence and medium transmission risk, is calculated to be 21.9 with current levels of testing and 26.3 with no testing.
(Courtesy of Phillips KA, Lowe RA, Kahn JG, et al: JAMA 271:851-858, 1994.)

sive procedures (surgeons and dentists), increased voluntary testing with interventions or inducements, and continued voluntary testing with no change in current policies. For health care workers testing HIV positive, mandatory or voluntary exclusion from practice, restriction from performing invasive procedures, or requirements to inform patients of serostatus were considered. Testing cost data were obtained from the CDC.

Results.—One-time mandatory testing of surgeons and dentists with mandatory restriction of those who test HIV-positive is always more cost-effective than other options, but costs per infection averted and incremental costs vary tremendously under different assumptions. Mandatory testing of all surgeons might avert 25 infections at a total cost of $27.9 million, or $1,115,000 per infection averted, and an incremental cost of $291,000 per infection averted compared with current levels of voluntary testing. The incremental cost-effectiveness per patient infection averted increases to $29,807,000 for a low seroprevalence and low transmission risk, to a savings of $81,000 per infection averted for a high seroprevalence and high transmission risk (table).

Conclusions.—The cost-effectiveness of HIV testing policies is highly sensitive to seroprevalence and transmission risk. The findings of this analysis neither justify nor preclude a mandatory testing policy.

▶ The 1991 proposal by the CDC recommending that all health care workers who perform invasive procedures undergo testing for HIV and hepatitis was opposed by many medical groups and was never put into effect. From time to time, other groups recommend testing of physicians, especially surgeons and dentists, for blood-borne infection. This paper attempts to estimate the cost of preventing a single case of HIV through one-time mandatory testing of all surgeons. The conclusion that testing of surgeons might avert 25 HIV infections and cost $27.9 million dollars, or $1,115,000 per infection, is their best estimate from current data. The mathematical model that they used is highly sensitive to seroprevalence rates among surgeons and to transmission risk. Both of these numbers, however, have an extremely low level of confidence. For instance, they use .4% as the HIV seroprevalence rate in surgeons, based on the CDC data of HIV seroprevalence among health care workers. This number assumes that the seroprevalence rate in surgeons is identical to that in all health care workers. Two studies that actually tested surgeons for HIV seroprevalence found seroprevalence rates to be only one fourth of that (1). The estimated risk of transmission of HIV from an infected surgeon to a patient (0.00002) may also be too high. Except for a single dentist in Florida transmitting HIV to 6 of his patients, there is not 1 other case of even suspected transmission from a surgeon or dentist to a patient. The CDC has investigated the Florida dentist thoroughly, and no mechanism of transmission could be found. Many now suspect that the dentist intentionally infected his patients. Thus, even with what may be a high estimate of seropositivity among surgeons and infection risks, the cost of preventing a single case of HIV in patients is extremely high. If the model uses a low seroprevalence rate .05% among surgeons, the cost per infection averted increased to $5,659,000. It is likely that a surgeon eventually will transmit HIV to 1 of his patients; we do not live in a risk-free world. But certainly the risk is so low that testing surgeons for HIV cannot be justified, and this model only tests surgeons 1 time. No one has addressed how often surgeons should be tested. Certainly one-time testing is not sufficient if a surgeon operates on patients with HIV or engages in risky behavior. He or she could become infected after initially testing negative. How often should a surgeon be tested? It seems to be the logical conclusion that surgeons should not be tested.—R.J. Howard, M.D., Ph.D.

Reference

1. Panlilio AL, et al: *J Am Coll Surg* 180:16–24, 1995.

Safety of the Blood Supply: Surrogate Testing and Transmission of Hepatitis C in Patients After Massive Transfusion

Morris JA Jr, Wilcox TR, Reed GW, Hunter EB, Wallas CH, Steane EA, Shotts SD, Vitsky JL (Vanderbilt Univ, Nashville, Tenn; American Red Cross, Tennessee Valley Region, Nashville, Tenn)
Ann Surg 219:517–526, 1994   140-95-5–2

Objective.—An increasing number of trauma victims are surviving massive injuries today, in part by receiving multiple transfusions. Despite modern screening methods, post-transfusion hepatitis still poses a significant risk. A study was designed to show whether the frequency of post-transfusion hepatitis C would decline when blood donors were screened for both alanine aminotransferase (ALT) and antibody to hepatitis B core antigen (Core).

Study Population.—Among 8,765 patients admitted to a level I trauma center in 1985–1990 were 221 who received more than 20 units of packed red blood cells, whole blood, or both. Ninety-one of them lived to be discharged from the hospital, and 69 patients constituted the study group. These patients had been exposed to 4,987 units, for an average of 72 units per patient. Thirty-eight patients had received more than 50 units of exposure, and 11 patients had received more than 100 units.

Findings.—Sixteen of the 69 study patients (23%) tested positive for hepatitis C virus (HCV) by Chiron second-generation recombinant immunoblot assay (RIBA) (Fig 5–1). Six of those patients had elevated ALT levels. More than half the patients were positive for cytomegalovirus. Six patients were Core-positive and 1 tested positive for syphilis, but none of the patients were positive for HIV-1, HTLV type 1, or hepatitis B surface antigen. Six patients were positive for antibody to hepatitis B core antigen, and 3 of them also were RIBA-positive. Three of 9 HCV-positive patients who were followed up had persistently elevated liver enzymes. The sole liver biopsy demonstrated chronic persistent hepatitis. The calculated risk of post-transfusion hepatitis C per unit of exposure decreased from 1.52% to .239% after the advent of ALT/Core testing.

Conclusion.—The risk of transmitting hepatitis C is not great enough to preclude massive transfusions in victims of massive trauma.

▶ After testing became available for hepatitis B, physicians realized that most cases of post-transfusion hepatitis were due to non-A, non-B hepatitis. Because no direct test for non-A, non-B hepatitis was available, testing for ALT or antibodies to Core was used as surrogates for non-A, non-B hepatitis. This study is a retrospective review of the effectiveness of that testing. It showed that testing and eliminating blood that had elevated ALT levels or antibodies to Core reduced the risk of post-transfusion non-A, non-B hepatitis from 1.5% to .239%. The great majority of non-A, non-B hepatitis is due to HCV. In 1991, direct testing for antibody to HCV became available and currently, all donor units are tested. This study does confirm that the blood sup-

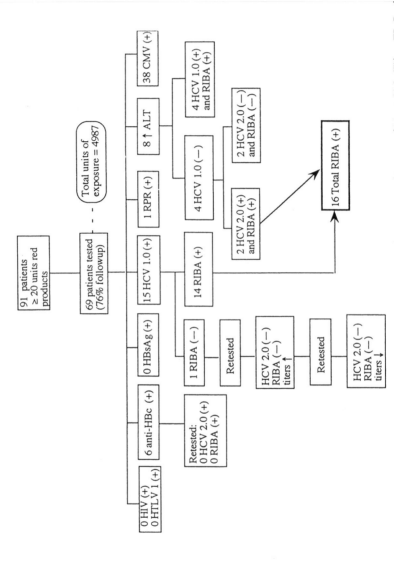

Fig 5-1.—Flow diagram showing that 16 of 69 patients had posttransfusion hepatitis C by RISA assay. (Courtesy of Morris JA Jr, Wilcox TR, Reed GW, et al: *Ann Surg* 219:517-526, 1994.)

ply is safe, and that the American blood-banking system continues the ongoing effort of providing a safe blood supply.—R.J. Howard, M.D., Ph.D.

Nosocomial Bloodstream Infection in Critically Ill Patients: Excess Length of Stay, Extra Costs, and Attributable Mortality
Pittet D, Tarara D, Wenzel RP (University of Iowa, Iowa City; Hôpital Cantonal Universitaire de Genéve)
JAMA 271:1598–1601, 1994   140-95-5-3

Objective.—The risk of nosocomial bloodstream infections is high in surgical intensive care units (SICUs). An assessment of the excess length of stay, extra costs, and mortality attributable to nosocomial bloodstream infections in SICU patients was conducted in a pairwise-matched, case-control assessment.

Subjects.—Between July 1, 1988 and June 30, 1990, 97 of 4,002 patients admitted to the SICU had nosocomial bloodstream infections. Controls were matched for primary diagnosis at admission, age, sex, length of stay before the day of infection in cases, and total number of discharge diagnoses. Matching was successful for 89% of the cohort, providing 86 matched case-control pairs.

Results.—A total of 107 episodes of nosocomial bloodstream infection occurred, for an infection rate of 2.7 per 100 admissions. The most frequent pathogens were coagulase-negative staphylococci, *Staphylococcus aureus,* and enteric gram-negative rods. Crude mortality rates were 50% in cases and 15% in controls, for an estimated attributable mortality rate of 35% (95% confidence interval [CI], 25%–45%). The estimated risk ratio for death was 3.1 (95% CI, 1.78–6.15). The overall excess length of total hospital stay attributable to infection was 14 days (40 days for cases vs. 26 days for controls), and even longer, 24 days, when only the 41 matched pairs who survived the infection were considered. The median length of SICU stay attributed to infection doubled from 7 days in control to 15 days in cases. Furthermore, the survivors accounted for 95% of the total number of extra days attributable to infection. The extra cost attributable to infection was about $1.7 million, or an average of $40,890 per patient.

Conclusion.—In critically ill patients, nosocomial bloodstream infections cause excess mortality and significantly prolong SICU and hospital lengths of stay, as well as significant economic burden.

▶ This article documents what we have already suspected—nosocomial bloodstream infections in SICUs are associated with a high mortality rate, increased length of stay, and extra costs. The increased average cost of $40,890 per patient is very high and most likely reflects how much more ill these patients were than control patients. Preventing nosocomial bloodstream infections could greatly lower the cost for patients in the ICU. Yet, it is somewhat disappointing that studies such as these seldom provide (and they never were intended to) useful clues on how to prevent these infections.—R.J. Howard, M.D., Ph.D.

Candida Sepsis in Surgical Patients
Eubanks PJ, de Virgilio C, Klein S, Bongard F (Harbor-Univ of California Los Angeles Med Ctr, Torrance)
Am J Surg 166:617–620, 1993   140-95-5-4

Introduction.—The incidence of candidemia has increased in surgical patients during recent years. It remains difficult to detect *Candida* infections, despite extensive investigation of serodiagnostic tests. The perioperative risk factors contributing to the death of patients with positive blood cultures for *Candida* species were identified retrospectively.

Patients and Methods.—Microbiological laboratory records at the study institution were reviewed for the period from 1981 to 1990. Transplant recipients were excluded. Survivors and nonsurvivors among all surgical patients with positive *Candida* blood cultures were compared for their medical history, treatment, clinical course, type of surgery, and other variables. All patients had received amphotericin B, 500–1,000 mg, as determined by the individual clinical course.

Results.—Forty-six patients, 26 men and 20 women, were identified during the study period. Twenty-six of those patients with positive *Candida* blood cultures had initially undergone celiotomy and a gastrointestinal procedure. There were 26 deaths, for an overall mortality of 57%. Nonsurvivors were older on average than survivors (54.9 vs. 42.5 years). Both hepatic failure and dialysis-dependent renal insufficiency were significantly correlated with mortality. The 19 patients who required pressor support for postoperative hypotension and the 14 patients in whom adult respiratory distress syndrome developed had increased mortality (74% and 79%, respectively). Survivors and nonsurvivors did not differ significantly with regard to sex, blood transfusions, steroid use, pneumonia, gastrointestinal bleeding, or early institution of antibiotic therapy in the emergency room. Bacterial septicemia developed in 26 of the 46 patients and was preceded by or concomitant with the onset of fungal sepsis in 88%. The most commonly isolated *Candida* species was *Candida albicans* (65%).

Conclusion.—All of the patients in this series had received at least 1 week of IV treatment with antibiotics and 96% had a central venous catheter, both factors that have been associated with *Candida* proliferation. The risk of mortality was higher in older patients and in those with multiple organ dysfunction. Oral antifungal agents are recommended for all postoperative patients and surveillance cultures for those who are critically ill.

▶ Fungal infections are most commonly seen in compromised hosts, whether the immunocompromise is due to burn, injury, trauma, immunosuppressive drugs, or other causes. This study investigates *Candida* septicemia in nonimmunosuppressed surgical patients. This study found, as have earlier reports, that previous antibiotic therapy seemed to be a predisposing cause of *Candida* infections. A high mortality rate is common in patients with fungal infections, especially those in the ICU. Whether *Candida* infections occur in septic patients or in patients who are likely to die anyway, and how much these organisms contribute to death is still unsettled. In this series, organ dysfunction was significantly correlated with death. The dilemma with *Candida* and other opportunistic infections is how to diagnose them early. Serologic studies are unreliable and frequently, cultures with these organisms can be found at postmortem examination. Solomkin (1) found that culturing *Candida* from 3 sites, even though none was from a deep site or bloodstream, was evidence of disseminatioin and provided justification for antifungal therapy. The place of antifungal prophylaxis in susceptible patients has not been established.—R.J. Howard, M.D., Ph.D.

Reference

1. Solomkin JS, et al: *New Horizons* 1:202–213, 1993.

Incidence and Management of Catheter-Related Sepsis in Patients Receiving Home Parenteral Nutrition
Williams N, Carlson GL, Scott NA, Irving MH (Univ of Manchester, England)
Br J Surg 81:392–394, 1994   140-95-5–5

Background.—Catheter-related sepsis is the most common cause of morbidity and hospital readmission in patients receiving home parenteral nutrition (HPN). The incidence and management of this formidable clinical problem were investigated.

Method.—Fifty patients with a median age of 43 years each received a median duration of 48 months of HPN. All central lines were inserted by a member of the staff using local anesthesia, and the subsequent use and care of the catheter was carried out by specialist nurses until patients were instructed in the principles of asepsis and catheter-handling protocol. Patients were formally assessed before being considered competent to manage the central lines at home.

Results.—Thirteen episodes of bacterial catheter sepsis occurred in 12 patients. The median interval between catheter insertion and the development of sepsis was 22 months. A single organism, *Staphylococcus*, was found to be the most common source of infection. Two patients had multiple organisms cultured, and the catheters were removed. In 4 cases of bacterial catheter sepsis, the catheter was successfully salvaged by an antibiotic-fibrinolytic "lock" technique. Ten cases of exit-site sepsis were recorded in 8 patients. The median interval between catheter insertion and the development of sepsis in those patients was 25 months. All were managed by elective catheter replacement. Seventeen of the 50 patients had 23 episodes of septic complications from the central venous catheter, representing an overall incidence of 1 episode per 113 patient months of HPN.

Conclusion.—Although catheter sepsis remains a significant cause of morbidity in patients receiving parenteral nutrition, the principles of strict adherence to protocol, rigorous asepsis, inviolate catheter use, and meticulous care are relatively successful in reducing its incidence and subsequent morbidity.

▶ Catheter-related sepsis continues to be a problem in patients being treated with parenteral nutrition. With more patients receiving HPN, the necessity for preventing these infections is paramount. All investigators who study catheter-related sepsis stress the importance of rigorous asepsis when placing these catheters and in caring for these catheters on a day-to-day basis. Having protocols for placing and caring for catheters can help to reduce the incidence of infection.—R.J. Howard, M.D., Ph.D.

Prediction of Outcome Using the Mannheim Peritonitis Index in 2003 Patients

Billing A, Fröhlich D, Schildberg FW, and the Peritonitis Study Group (Ludwig-Maximilians-Universität München)

Br J Surg 81:209–213, 1994   140-95-5–6

Background.—Several classification systems for scoring the severity of peritoneal inflammation have been proposed. Of those, the Mannheim peritonitis index is the easiest to use. The reliability of the Mannheim peritonitis index was assessed and its predictive power when applied to different populations examined.

Methods.—The Mannheim peritonitis index consists of 8 risk factors of previously validated prognostic relevance, with a weighting according to the predictive power. The data on all 8 risk factors are collected during the first laparotomy, thus enabling immediate classification of disease severity. Seven surgical centers in Europe contributed Mannheim peritonitis index scores for 2,003 patients. Only patients for whom information on all 8 risk factors was available were included in the analysis.

Results.—The prevalence of risk factors varied considerably between centers. For a threshold index score of 26, the sensitivity was 86%, the specificity 74%, and the accuracy 83% for predicting death from peritonitis. The mean mortality rate was 2.3% for patients with a score less than 21, 22.5% for patients with scores from 21 to 29, and 59.1% for patients with scores greater than 29 (Fig 5–2).

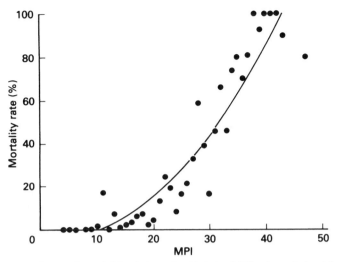

Fig 5–2.—Mortality rate for each Mannheim peritonitis index (MPI) value, calculated from all patients, with best-fit polynomial curve. (Courtesy of Billing A, Fröhlich D, Schildberg FW, et al: *Br J Surg* 81:209–213, 1994.)

Conclusions. —The Mannheim peritonitis index is a reliable system for classifying disease severity in patients with peritoneal inflammation, but its predictive power needs to be further increased.

▶ For years surgeons have been seeking a scoring system that would permit valid grading of the severity of intra-abdominal infections. Because the extent of these infections varies so widely, it is difficult to compare the results of studies. Peritonitis from a ruptured appendix generally leads to a vastly different outcome than peritonitis from colon perforation. Yet both patients may be included in studies of peritonitis. Although a variety of scoring systems are available to judge how "sick" a patient may be, none previously was designed specifically for peritonitis. The most popular scoring system is the acute physiology and chronic health evaluation (APACHE) system of Knaus. But this system was designed as a prediction of mortality rate for patients in an ICU setting. Other scoring systems (e.g., the Injury Severity Score) were designed for trauma patients. The Mannheim Peritonitis Index discussed in this paper allows scoring to be done after the first operation, and thus permits an early prediction of outcome. This scoring system is not new. It was based on data from patients treated between 1963 and 1979 and was developed by discriminant analysis of 17 possible risk factors. Eight of these risk factors were prognostic and were weighted according to their predictive power. This paper is used to evaluate mortality rates in patients with peritonitis. The correlation between score and mortality rate is as good as any system currently available. Because the Mannheim Peritonitis Index is not calculated until after the first operation, and because most antibiotic and other trials required randomization before the first operation, it may not be useful in these studies.—R.J. Howard, M.D., Ph.D.

A Multicenter Review of the Treatment of Major Truncal Necrotizing Infections With and Without Hyperbaric Oxygen Therapy

Brown DR, Davis NL, Lepawsky M, Cunningham J, Kortbeek J (Univ of British Columbia, Vancouver, Canada; Vancouver Gen Hosp, BC; Univ of Calgary, Alta, Canada)
Am J Surg 167:485–489, 1994   140-95-5-7

Background.—The use of hyperbarix oxygen (HBO) in treating major necrotizing infections is controversial. Although it is generally considered an important adjunct to surgery and antibiotics in the treatment of clostridial myonecrosis, its use in other necrotizing infections, such as synergistic gangrene, Fournier's gangrene, and nonclostridial myonecrosis, is not universally recommended. An investigation of the extent to which HBO therapy affects patient outcome was undertaken.

Method.—A retrospective review (1980 to 1992) of the medical records of 54 patients with major truncal necrotizing infections was carried out. Thirty patients were treated with HBO therapy, and 24 were treated without HBO therapy. Outcome in terms of mortality, length of hospital and ICU stay, duration of antibiotic therapy, and number and type of operations was compared between the 2 groups.

Results.—The HBO-treated group was found to be younger and tended to experience more clostridial infections than the non–HBO-treated patients. No significant differences were seen in the length of hospital or ICU stay in the 2 groups. Neither was the duration of antibiotic treatment significantly different. The HBO-treated group, however, underwent significantly more operations than the non–HBO-treated group (97 vs. 41). The HBO group received 71 operative debridements, compared with 31 in the non-HBO group. Laparotomy was carried out in 20 patients in the HBO-treated group, compared with only 10 of the non–HBO-treated group. The mortality rate was slightly higher in the non–HBO-treated group—10 of 24, compared with 9 of 30 in the HBO-treated group—although this difference was not statistically significant.

Conclusion.—This study failed to demonstrate that HBO therapy brings a significant reduction in mortality in the treatment of major truncal necrotizing infections. However, the apparent selection bias and the trend toward increased survival in the HBO-treated group, although not statistically significant, justify the continued use of HBO in these patients. Future research in this area should comprise a multicenter prospective study to obtain a database from which to evaluate the outcome of patients treated for these infections.

▶ This article reflects some of the difficulties in *proving* HBO therapy is better than standard treatment for necrotizing soft tissue infections or other conditions other than decompression illness and carbon monoxide poisoning. This retrospective review found no statistical difference in mortality rates between the HBO group and the non-HBO group. Nevertheless, the authors held that the increased survival in the HBO-treated group (12%) justified the continued use of HBO therapy. This nonrandomized, retrospective review involved only 54 patients who must have varied markedly from each other. It is impossible to have a controlled, randomized trial because these patients are so few and because they vary so much in their diseases. The HBO-treated group might have survived better, in fact, because they were younger and they underwent more operative debridements. The decision to use HBO therapy was based on the preference of the physician. However, it is always difficult to discern the bases on which physicians might have elected to use HBO. What were their criteria to use it for some patients and not for others? One might guess that the sickest patients were given HBO therapy, and hence the increased survival may have some meaning. But there is no way to confirm that from this paper. Hyperbaric oxygen therapy remains an unproved adjunct to surgical debridement, the sine qua non of treating necrotizing soft tissue infections.—R.J. Howard, M.D., Ph.D.

Differentiating Acute Appendicitis From Pelvic Inflammatory Disease in Women of Childbearing Age

Webster DP, Schneider CN, Cheche S, Daar AA, Miller G (Chicago College of Osteopathic Medicine; St. Catherine's Hospital, Kenosha, Wis)
Am J Emerg Med 11:569–572, 1993   140-95-5–8

Introduction.—Because the appendix is close to the uterus and the ovary and fallopian tube on the right side, inflammation of reproductive structures may produce symptoms that suggest acute appendicitis. At least one fourth of women who are thought to have appendicitis are instead found to have pelvic inflammatory disease (PID).

Objective.—Clinical findings that can help distinguish between acute appendicitis and PID were sought in 81 ovulating women who had histologically documented appendicitis and 71 others with a final diagnosis of PID.

Findings.—Patients in the 2 groups were similar in age. Those with appendicitis were more often anorectic and less often described urinary symptoms or a vaginal discharge. The patients with PID were much more likely to have had PID previously. They also were more likely to have tenderness outside the right lower quadrant and on movement of the cervix. A vaginal discharge and positive urinalysis were more frequent in women with PID. Appendicitis occurred throughout the menstrual cycle, whereas PID tended to occur in the menstrual and follicular phases and was infrequent in the second half of the cycle.

Conclusion.—Although there are differences in the findings between women with acute appendicitis and those with PID, the distinction still is difficult.

▶ Although some clinical findings differ between acute appendicitis and PID, the differences could not be used to distinguish these 2 frequently confused entities in women of childbearing age. The proportion of patients with right lower quadrant tenderness, rebound tenderness, adnexal masses, or rectal tenderness was not significantly different between the 2 groups. These are the most frequently helpful physical findings. Thus, in the end, and as the authors acknowledge, the distinction is still difficult. The likelihood of decreasing the incidence of performing operations for suspected appendicitis and finding pelvic inflammatory disease is low.—R.J. Howard, M.D., Ph.D.

Treatment of Sepsis by Extracorporeal Elimination of Endotoxin Using Ploymyxin B-Immobilized Fiber

Aoki H, Kodama M, Tani T, Hanasawa K (Shiga Univ of Med Science, Japan)
Am J Surg 167:412–417, 1994   140-95-5–9

Introduction.—Mortality remains high among patients with septic shock and endotoxemia. Knowledge that polymyxin B (PMX) neutralizes the biological activities of endotoxin led to the development of a material made of immobilized PMX fibers (PMX-F) for clinical use. This material, PMX-F, consists of a mean of 7 mg of PMX per 1 g of fiber. In

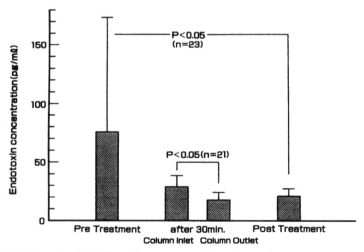

Fig 5–3.—In samples that had an endotoxin concentration of 9.8 pg/mL, the mean value was 76 ± 95 pg/mL before DHP. This level significantly decreased to 21 ± 7 pg/mL immediately after DHP ($P < .05$). The concentration was 30 ± 10 pg/mL at the inlet and 20 ± 6 pg/mL at the outlet ($P < .05$). (Courtesy of Aoki H, Kodama M, Tani T, et al: *Am J Surg* 167:412-417, 1994.)

preliminary trials, 16 patients with septic multiple organ failure were treated with direct hemoperfusion (DHP) using a PMX-F column.

Patients and Methods.—Most of the patients were receiving a vasopressor to maintain blood pressure, and many required mechanical ventilation. Nine had peritonitis resulting from gastrointestinal perforation. A double-lumen catheter was inserted into the femoral vein for access to blood for DHP with PMX-F adsorbent therapy. Anticoagulants used were heparin in 5 patients and nafamostat mesilate (NM) in 11 patients. The hemodynamic parameters measured included heart rate, mean arterial blood pressure, central venous pressure, and cardiac output. Blood endotoxin concentrations were determined in heparinized blood samples collected before, after 30 minutes of treatment, after DHP treatment, and on the next day.

Results.—The 16 patients underwent DHP a total of 29 times. Heparin was used 9 times and NM 20 times. Patients with a systolic pressure of less than 100 mm Hg showed a significant increase from pretreatment levels within several hours after the end of DHP. On the next day, 8 patients with a pretreatment mean heart rate of 134 bpm showed a significant decrease to a mean of 122 bpm. Body temperature significantly decreased as well in the 11 patients with a pretreatment body temperature of 38°C or more. The endotoxin level decreased significantly from 76 pg/mL to 21 pg/mL after 2 hours of DHP (Fig 5–3). Nine of the 16 patients were alive 2 weeks after PMX-F therapy, and 7 were discharged from the hospital alive.

Conclusion.—Polymixin B detoxifies endotoxin, but it is toxic to the CNS and the kidney. Fixing PMX to polystyrene fibers results in a nontoxic material system. Hemoperfusion using a PMX-F column markedly alleviated symptoms of sepsis syndrome by decreasing the endotoxin concentration in the blood. The treatment was effective even in patients who had failed to respond to other methods.

▶ This is a novel approach to neutralize the biological activities of endotoxin in 15 patients with sepsis and multiple organ failure. Although the endotoxin levels decreased from 76 pg/mL to 21 pg/mL after 2 hours (a statistically significant decrease), we do not know whether it was a biologically meaningful difference. Even though 9 of the 16 patients survived, a figure the authors claim is much higher than that reported with conventional treatment of septic multiple organ failure, one cannot make a definitive statement of efficacy until a controlled trial is done.—R.J. Howard, M.D., Ph.D.

Translocation of Bacteria and Endotoxin in Organ Donors
van Goor H, Rosman C, Grond J, Kooi K, Wübbels GH, Bleichrodt RP (Univ Hosp Groningen, The Netherlands; Twenteborg Hosp Almelo, The Netherlands)
Arch Surg 129:1063–1066, 1994   140-95-5–10

Number of Donors With Positive Culture Specimens and Isolated Bacteria

Culture Specimen	Positive Culture Specimens	No. of Organ Donors			Identical Rods Also in Small Bowel	
		Isolated Bacteria				
		Gram-negative	Gram-positive	Both	Yes	No
Mesenteric lymph nodes	11	1	6	4	9	2
Lung	7	1	6	0	5	2
Liver	2	2	0	0	2	0
Spleen	5	1	4	0	4	1
Peripheral blood	1	0	1	0	1	0
Portal blood	0	0	0	0	0	0
Abdominal fluid	0	0	0	0	0	0

(Courtesy of van Goor H, Rosman C, Grond J, et al: *Arch Surg* 129:1063–1066, 1994.)

Objective.—It has been proposed that translocation of intestinal bacterial and endotoxin absorption occur in critically ill patients with an anatomically intact gastrointestinal tract and that this phenomenon contributes to the development of multiple organ failure. Because the integrity of the bowel in critically ill patients cannot be verified, an attempt was made to determine if bacterial translocation and endotoxin absorption occur in critically ill organ donors with intact gastrointestinal tracts.

Patients.—Thirteen men and 8 women who were multiple organ donors with a mean age of 26 years were studied. The patients died after a median hospital stay of 1.9 days. Blood samples, abdominal fluid, bowel contents, mesenteric lymph nodes, and organs were cultured, and plasma endotoxin levels were measured.

Results.—Bacteria were cultured from specimens obtained from 14 (67%) organ donors (table). The bacteria isolated in 81% of the blood culture specimens were identical to those isolated from the bowel content. Endotoxin was found in 53% of abdominal fluid samples, 19% of peripheral blood samples, and 10% of portal blood samples. None of the organ donors had anatomical abnormalities of the bowel wall.

Conclusions.—Bacterial translocation and endotoxin absorption are common in critically ill organ donors. These events may adversely affect organ function in organ transplant recipients and other critically ill patients.

▶ Much has been made of the role of bacterial translocation in the pathogenesis of infections and human disease, especially in severely ill or severely injured patients. Although apparently easily demonstrated in animals, it is much less easily demonstrated in humans, and its role is still unknown. This paper shows that bacterial translocation can be demonstrated in a high percentage of organ donors who were severely ill, yet presumably had an intact gastrointestinal mucosa. One of the problems with previous studies has been the question of whether the gastrointestinal mucosa was indeed intact. Although this paper confirms that bacterial translocation does occur, its role in the pathogenesis of infections is still uncertain.—R.J. Howard, M.D., Ph.D.

Unusual Manifestations of Salmonellosis: A Surgical Problem
Lalitha MK, John R (Christian Med College & Hosp, Vellore, Tamil Nadu, India)
Q J Med 87:301–309, 1994   140-95-5–11

Objective.—Endemic salmonellosis is a major health problem in India. A retrospective review of the prevalence, predisposing factors, and clinical presentation of unusual salmonella infections requiring surgery was carried out. Of 6,250 cases of salmonellosis recorded, 100 required surgical intervention in addition to medical therapy.

Results.—Thirty-one of the 100 cases in which surgery was required involved the hepatobiliary system, and 10 more involved other intra-abdominal infections. Fifteen patients had soft tissue infections, with the most common manifestation being superficial abscesses of the skin (7), parotid (2), thyroid (2), breast (1), inguinal node (1), branchial sinus (1), and injection site (1). Three patients had arterial infections. Two men and 2 women had genital infections: 1 was a case of salmonella infection in a preexisting hydrocele, and another was an epididymo-orchitis with a loculated salmonella infection. Infection was also seen in a preexisting ovarian cyst in a patient with endometriosis. Bone and joint infections were found in 15 patients; the knee, shoulder, and the hip being the most common sites. The salmonella serotypes most frequently encountered were *Salmonella typhi* (3) and *S. typhimurium* (36), followed by *S. paratyphi* (15).

Conclusion.—A wide spectrum of salmonella infections other than enteric fever may occur. Microbiological evaluation of appropriately obtained specimens in such pyogenic infections is required, particularly in the setting of unusual pyogenic infections in the immunocompromised. The emergenc of multidrug-resistant salmonellae has led to the development of new quinolone antibiotics to replace trimethoprim-sulfamethoxazole and chloramphenicol. Surgical treatment should be considered in cases of deep-seated infections, as well as in immunosuppressed patients.

▶ Although infections with *Salmonella* are uncommon in this country, information regarding 100 patients with *Salmonella* infection requiring surgical intervention was collected during a 12-year period at Christian Medical College and Hospital in Vellore, India. These infections may be seen in certain immunosuppressed patients in the United States, and *Salmonella* is the most common bacterial infection causing mycotic aneurysms. *Salmonella* is commonly found in the gastrointestinal tracts of chickens in this country and can contaminate their eggs. Humans can ingest *Salmonella* with improperly cooked eggs and may become infected by this route. Surgeons should be aware of infections that can be caused by these organisms.—R.J. Howard, M.D., Ph.D.

6 Transplantation

Introduction

Two much awaited papers were published on the results of prospective randomized trials comparing tacrolimus (FK506) with cyclosporine in liver transplant recipients (Abstracts 140-95-6-1 and 140-95-6-2). Both studies involved more than 500 patients each, and both showed surprisingly similar results: there was no statistical difference with respect to graft outcome in either group and only minor differences in side effects and complications. A randomized study was also published that compared OKT3-based immunoprophylaxis with cyclosporin in liver transplant recipients (Abstract 140-95-6-3). Although there were fewer early rejection episodes and fewer septic complications in patients who completed the 14-day course of OKT3, there was no difference in long-term graft or patient survival. Two papers addressed alcohol and liver disease. The first is from Austria and discusses a high recidivism rate for patients undergoing liver transplantation for alcoholic cirrhosis (Abstract 140-95-6-4). The authors of this study, however, did not require any abstinence from alcohol before transplantation, something that most United States' centers require. The other paper (Abstract 140-95-6-5) attempted to create a model for survival in patients with alcoholic liver disease, similar to the male model for predicting survival in patients with primary biliary cirrhosis. The authors demonstrated that patients with low or medium risk factors did not benefit from liver transplantation, whereas high risk patients did much better with liver transplantation. Third-party pairs will demand more proof of efficacy in the future, such as in the type of study published here. Along the same lines, complications are a major problem after liver transplantation, yet there is no standard method for categorizing them. One paper by Clavien et al. (Abstract 140-95-6-6) attempts to provide an exhaustive classification system for liver transplant complications. This detailed system can be applied to patients at most transplant centers and serves as a basis for comparison among these centers.

Biopsy has been the gold standard in diagnosing kidney transplant rejection. Rush et al. did protocol biopsies in a series of patients and found that 30% of patients with stable renal function who underwent biopsies 1–3 months after transplantation and whose creatinine had not risen more than 10% had histologic evidence of rejection (Abstract 140-95-6-7). Although the authors felt obliged to treat all of these patients, an interesting study (which the authors proposed to carry out) would be to randomize patients with normal renal function whose biopsies demonstrate rejection to treatment or no treatment. A study published by Ramos and other members of the patient care and education committee of the American Society of Transplant Physicians describes how individual transplant centers evaluate patients before kidney transplantation (Abstract 140-95-6-8). Inasmuch as there was nothing in this study to indicate that 1 method of preoperative evaluation was better than another, it does allow individual centers to know what the majority of transplant centers in the United States are doing.

Virtually no individual transplant center performs enough pediatric renal transplants to be able to do valid comparisons. For that reason, the North American Pediatric Renal Transplant Cooperative Study, a multicenter cooperative group, was formed (Abstract 140-95-6-9). This publication is a compilation of immunosuppressive protocols and outcome results in these highly diverse transplant centers. No attempt at a controlled clinical trial was done, but these centers were able to gather a large number of both cadaveric and related transplants, permitting some conclusions to be drawn about the efficacy of different immunosuppressive protocols.

Although several studies have been published about the results of transplantation among older patients, few have accumulated the experience of the University of Minnesota (Abstract 140-95-6-10). This paper discusses the results of renal transplantation among 138 patients older than age 60. Transplantation in these patients can be safely carried out, and the results are comparable to younger patients, except that the mortality rate is somewhat higher as would be expected in older patients. Two common methods are used for performing ureteroneocystostomy in renal transplant centers: the Ledbetter-Politano technique and the extravesicle (Lich) technique (Abstract 140-95-6-12). The authors found no significant difference with either technique in the series of patients operated on by several surgeons. This study was not randomized, but the number of complications was not statistically different, even though the urinary leak rate was approximately twice as high for the Lich technique.

A study from Northeast Ohio found that with the current UNOS matching system giving weight to tissue typing, African-Americans were not disadvantaged when receiving transplants compared with Caucasians. A matching system that gave more weight for waiting time would not result in a higher rate of transplantation (Abstract 140-95-6-13). This finding is somewhat surprising, because any system that gives preference for tissue matching would seem to disadvantage African-Americans.

With the shortage of organs suitable for transplantation becoming ever more acute, transplant surgeons are wondering whether donors previously thought to be unsuitable might not be appropriate for transplantation. Many authors have discussed whether kidneys from donors positive for hepatitis C should be used for transplantation. Kiberd et al. (Abstract 140-95-6-14) addressed this question based on the quality-adjusted life years in patients receiving these kidneys. They concluded that patients with hepatitis C might appropriately be given transplants from donors with hepatitis C rather than simply discarding these organs. Another method to increase the donor supply is to use O-haplotype match-related grafts (Abstract 140-95-6–15). The results of O-haplotype match-related grafts were comparable to 1-haplotype match-related grafts but not as good as 2-haplotype match-related grafts.

An update of the Pittsburgh experience with intestinal transplantation was discussed in 1 article by Abu-Elmagd et al. (Abstract 140-95-6–17). Although these patients had many complications, prolonged hospitalizations, and high costs, total parenteral nutrition was eventually discontinued in all patients. It is a continuing promise that further refinements will make intestinal transplantation available to more potential recipients. As health maintenance and managed care organizations come to dominate medicine, we will become more cognizant of the necessity to hold down costs. An economic analysis by Evans et al. (Abstract 140-95-6–18) studies hospital costs for patients having lung transplantation. These data provide a benchmark to which other centers can compare themselves. The data were for transplants done at 27 centers in 1988, so the data are old, and appropriate adjustments for inflation will have to be made to arrive at the current charges.

Specific immunologic unresponsiveness has always been the Holy Grail of transplantation. The most recent method for attempting to induce tolerance is injection of the donor's antigens (frequently as a source of intact cells), into the thymus gland of potential recipients. The paper by Sayegh attempts to delineate the mechanism of this tolerance in rats (Abstract 140-95-6–19). Whether this method will ever become clinically applicable is uncertain, although investigators are currently attempting to induce some form of at least limited tolerance by administering bone marrow cells to recipients of organ transplants.

Richard J. Howard, M.D., Ph.D.

A Comparison of Tacrolimus (FK 506) and Cyclosporine for Immunosuppresion in Liver Transplantation

Klintmalm GB, for The US Multicenter FK506 Liver Study Group (Baylor Univ Med Ctr, Dallas, Tex)
N Engl J Med 331:1110–1115, 1994   140-95-6–1

Purpose.—Tacrolimus, also known as FK 506, is a macrolide compound isolated from *Streptomyces tsukubaensis* that has potent immunosuppressant activity in solid-organ transplants. It is about 100 times more potent than cyclosporine, on which most immunosuppressant regimens for liver transplantation are based. The safety and efficacy of tacrolimus- and cyclosporine-based immunosuppression for primary liver transplantation were compared in an open-label, multicenter, randomized trial.

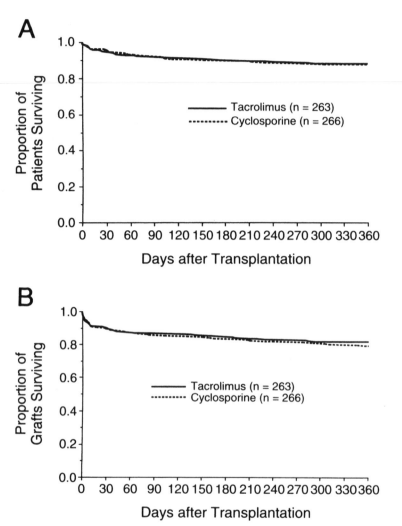

Fig 6–1.—Kaplan-Meier estimates of patient survival (**A**) and graft survival (**B**) in the tacrolimus and cyclosporine groups. (Courtesy of Klintmalm GB, for The US Multicenter FK506 Liver Study Group: N Engl J Med 331:1110–1115, 1994.)

Methods.—The subjects were 478 adults and 51 children (12 years of age or younger) who were receiving their first liver transplant at 1 of 12 United States' centers. The oral tacrolimus dose began at .15 mg/kg every 12 hours to a maximum of .6 mg/kg/day orally. The tacrolimus regimen also included hydrocortisone plus prednisone when tolerated in adults and prednisone in children. The cyclosporine-based regimens varied by center. Patient and graft survival were assessed at 1 year; acute rejection, corticosteroid-resistant rejection, and refractory rejection were assessed as secondary end points.

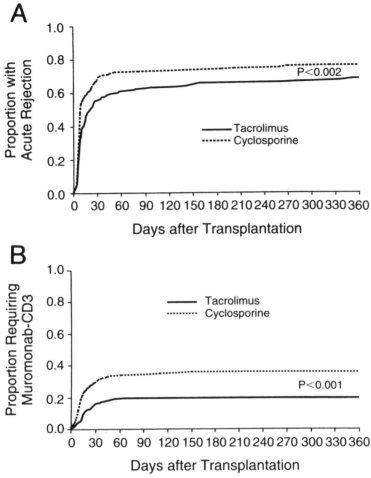

Fig 6–2.—Kaplan-Meier estimates of patients with acute rejection (**A**) and patients requiring muromonab-CD3 for corticosteroid-resistant rejection (**B**) in the tacrolimus and cyclosporine groups. (Courtesy of Klintmalm GB, for The US Multicenter FK506 Liver Study Group: N *Engl J Med* 331:1110–1115, 1994.)

Results.—One-year actuarial patient survival rates, based on Kaplan-Meier analysis, were 88% in both groups (Fig 6–1). Graft-survival rates were 82% for tacrolimus and 79% for cyclosporine. Acute rejection was significantly less common with tacrolimus than with cyclosporine at 154 vs. 173 patients (Fig 6–2), as were corticosteroid-resistant rejection at 43 vs. 82 patients, and refractory rejection at 6 vs. 32 patients. Adverse events—mainly nephrotoxicity and neurotoxicity—required withdrawal from the study in 37 patients in the tacrolimus group vs. 13 in the cyclosporine group.

Conclusions.—In patients undergoing primary liver transplantation, tacrolimus- and cyclosporine-based immunosuppressive regimens yield similar results in terms of both patient and graft survival. Acute, corticosteroid-resistant, and refractory rejection are significantly less common with tacrolimus; however, adverse reactions requiring drug discontinuation are more common with tacrolimus. Tacrolimus is effective in treating refractory rejection in patients treated with cyclosporine-based immunosuppression, helping to reduce the need for secondary transplantation.

Randomised Trial Comparing Tacrolimus (FK506) and Cyclosporin in Prevention of Liver Allograft Rejection

European FK506 Multicentre Liver Study Group (King's College School of Medicine and Dentistry, London)

Lancet 344:423–428, 1994   140-95-6-2

Purpose.—Preliminary studies have shown that tacrolimus (FK506) is a potent immunosuppressant that effectively prevents and reverses rejection in organ transplant recipients. The efficacy and safety of tacrolimus-based and conventional cyclosporine-based immunosuppressive regimens after liver transplantation were compared.

Patients.—Of 529 patients aged 18–70 years who were having primary liver transplantation at 8 European centers, 264 were randomly allocated to receive tacrolimus plus low-dose corticosteroids and 265 were allocated to receive a site-specific cyclosporine regimen. Rejection rates, infection rates, patient survival, and graft survival were analyzed at 12 months.

Results.—Tacrolimus was associated with a significant reduction in the incidence of acute, refractory acute, and chronic rejection episodes despite significantly lower use of corticosteroids (Fig 6–3). Fifty-one patients in the tacrolimus group experienced an acute rejection episode within 7 days of transplantation compared with 84 patients in the cyclosporine group. Most acute rejection episodes occurred within the first 4 weeks. The infection rate was also lower in patients treated with tacrolimus. Patient survival and graft survival did not differ significantly between the 2 treatment groups. All patients had adverse events; impaired renal function was the most serious complication. In all, 76 patients treated with tacrolimus and 64 treated with cyclosporine had to be withdrawn from the study because of severe adverse events.

Conclusions.—Tacrolimus has advantages over cyclosporine in terms of lower rejection rates and lower corticosteroid requirements. No side effects uniquely attributable to tacrolimus were reported.

▶ These 2 papers, 1 from Europe and 1 from the United States, describe randomized, controlled trials comparing tacrolimus (FK506) with cyclospo-

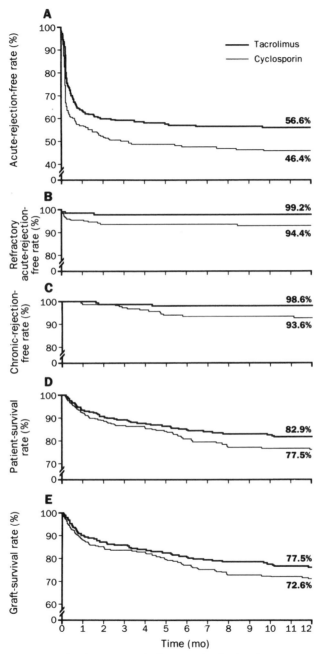

Fig 6–3.—Outcome rates (Kaplan-Meier method) expressed as freedom from rejection or as survival. **A,** acute rejection; **B,** refractory acute rejection; **C,** chronic rejection; **D,** patient survival; **E,** graft survival. For clarity, percentages shown are 12-month figures. Note truncated vertical axes. (Courtesy of: European FK506 Multicentre Liver Study Group: *Lancet* 344:423–428, 1994.)

rine-based immunosuppression to prevent graft rejection in liver transplant recipients. Both studies are large and include more than 500 patients. Both show surprisingly similar results. Although the incidence of acute corticosteroid-resistant and chronic rejection was lower in patients treated with tacrolimus than in those receiving cyclosporine-based regimens, the overall patient and graft survivals were not significantly different. In addition, the total dose of steroids was lower in patients receiving tacrolimus than in those with cyclosporine-based immunosuppressive drugs. This later finding may have led to the lower incidence of infectious complications in the tacrolimus group. The smaller doses of steroids in patients treated with tacrolimus may have been responsible for the lower infection rate. Although the European study showed comparable safety profiles, they did show more renal impairment and neurologic complications and disturbances of glucose metabolism in the tacrolimus group. These studies demonstrate that tacrolimus is as effective, although not more so than cyclosporine, in achieving satisfactory patient and graft survival in liver transplant recipients, even though it appears to result in fewer rejection episodes. With the outcome of both treatment groups so similar, one might hope that tacrolimus would be marketed so that its cost would be lower than cyclosporine, a major long-term problem for solid-organ recipients. Unfortunately, this does not seem to be the case.—R.J. Howard, M.D., Ph.D.

A Randomized Trial of OKT3-Based Versus Cyclosporine-Based Immunoprophylaxis After Liver Transplantation: Long-Term Results of a European and Australian Multicenter Study

Farges O, Ericzon BG, Bresson-Hadni S, Lynch SV, Höckerstedt K, Houssin D, Galmarini D, Faure J-L, Baldauf C, Bismuth H (Hôpital Paul Brousse, Villejuif, France; Huddinge Hospital, Sweden; Centre Hopitalier Universitaire Jean Minjoz, Besancon, France; et al)
Transplantation 58:891–898, 1994   140-95-6–3

Objective.—A prospective multicenter trial was begun in Europe and Australia in 1988 to compare a 2-week course of OKT3, combined with azathioprine and steroids, with standard triple therapy in patients given a first orthotopic liver transplant.

Study Plan.—Forty-six patients were randomized to receive OKT3 for 2 weeks in conjunction with steroid treatment and azathioprine. Cyclosporine was phased in starting on day 11. The OKT3 was given by IV push in a dose of 5 mg daily (2.5 mg daily for patients weighing less than 30 kg). Fifty control patients received standard triple therapy, which included cyclosporine in a dose of 3 mg/kg.

Results.—The OKT3 was withdrawn from 5 patients because of adverse effects, and 7 other patients did not receive the full course of treatment. Acute rejection occurred marginally more often in control patients than in those given OKT3 in the first year (75% vs. 67%). Fewer patients in the OKT3 group had multiple rejection episodes. In all, 7% of patients required retransplantation because of rejection in the first year of follow-up. Renal function was significantly better in OKT3 recipients, but there was no significant difference in the frequency of graft nonfunction at 4 years. More patients in the control group had severe infections.

Conclusion.—Immunoprophylaxis based on OKT3 is a safe alternative to cyclosporine-based management in patients given a first liver transplant.

▶ This study did show that OKT3-based immunoprophylaxis of liver transplantation resulted in decreased incidence of rejection, improved renal function during the second postoperative week, and fewer septic complications in patients who completed the full 14-day course. However, as in previous studies comparing OKT3 and other immunoprophylaxis regimens, there was no improvement in patient or graft survival. It is not surprising that the authors achieve a better graft survival in that current results with cyclosporine-based immunosuppression were already quite good, and any incremental increase is more difficult to achieve. Even if there were a difference, it is likely that this study would not have found it because of the small number of patients in each group. One rarely finds discussions of these statistical considerations either in the methods section or in the results of the paper. This and many other clinical reports lack the power to find a difference even if 1 exists. Although the authors state that further trials should be aimed at assessing the overall cost-effectiveness of prophylaxis, it is too bad that cost data were not included in this study, because the authors could have analyzed cost of liver transplantation in these 2 groups. I believe the greater cost of OKT3 prophylaxis would require substantially improved graft and/or patient survival or a significantly decreased hospital stay (thus lowering costs) to justify its use.—R.J. Howard, M.D., Ph.D.

Efficacy of Liver Transplantation for Alcoholic Cirrhosis With Respect to Recidivism and Compliance
Berlakovich GA, Steininger R, Herbst F, Barlan M, Mittlböck M, Mülbacher F
(Univ of Vienna)
Transplantation 58:560–565, 1994   140-95-6-4

Objective.—Many liver transplant centers are hesitant to place alcoholics with end-stage liver failure on waiting lists for orthotopic liver transplantation (OLT) because alcoholics have a high rate of recidivism and comply poorly with the required immunosuppressive therapy. Survival data and lifestyle changes of alcoholic liver transplant recipients were examined to evaluate the importance of these factors in OLT.

Methods.—Fifty-eight alcoholic liver transplant patients, 27 to 66 years of age, received questionnaires that addressed health habits, socioeco-

% Freedom of Recidivism

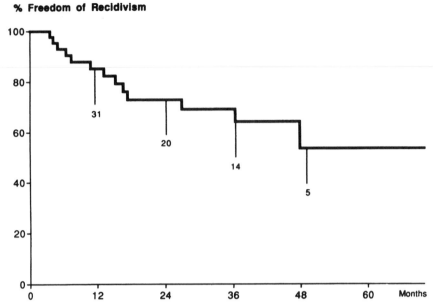

Fig 6–4.—Probability of overall patient alcoholism recidivism ($n = 44$). Numbers below the graph indicate patients at risk; SE > 10% at 45 months. (Courtesy of Berlakovich GA, Steininger R, Herbst F, et al: *Transplantation* 58:560–565, 1994.)

nomic status and changes, and compliance with immunotherapy. A total of 44 patients survived at least 3 months.

Results.—A total of 77% of the patients had a Child's score of C, and 23% had a score of B. Survival rates at years 1, 2, and 5 were 71%, 66%, and 63%, respectively. Average survival times was 78 months, whereas the corresponding actuarial survival time was 42 months. In 86% of the deaths, patients had a Child's score of C. Fourteen patients resumed drinking, most within 2 years of receiving the transplant (Fig 6–4). Liver function returned to normal after patients stopped drinking. None of the social or lifestyle factors analyzed were predictive of alcoholic relapse. After surgery, significantly more patients were able to work, were married, and were socially active than before surgery. Of the 13 acute rejection episodes, there was no significant difference between patients who returned to drinking and patients who did not.

Conclusion.—There was a high recidivism rate in this study. However, previous alcohol abuse did not compromise success of the transplant or compliance with therapy requirements.

▶ This study from Austria finds a high (31%) recidivism rate among 58 patients transplanted for end-stage liver disease due to alcoholic cirrhosis. Centers vary widely on their approach to the alcoholic patient. Some require prolonged abstinence from alcoholism and participation in a rehabilitation program, whereas others have no or minimal requirements for abstinence before transplantation is considered. This program from Vienna did not require any abstinence from alcohol before transplantation. That, possibly, may be responsible for the high recidivism rate in this study. The problem with having too long a period of abstinence before being considered for transplantation is that many of these patients will die first. Some programs in the United States that give transplants to alcoholic patients with a minimum requirement of abstinence have found a very small rate of return to drinking. The issues of whether or not and when to transplant patients with liver failure from alcoholic cirrhosis are not settled.—R.J. Howard, M.D., Ph.D.

Evaluation of Efficacy of Liver Transplantation in Alcoholic Cirrhosis By a Case-Control Study and Simulated Controls

Poynard T, for a Multi-Centre Group (Groupe Hospitalier Pitié Salpêtrière, Paris)

Lancet 344:502–507, 1994   140-95-6–5

Objective.—The usefulness of liver transplantation in patients with alcoholic cirrhosis was compared with simulated and matched controls who were treated conservatively.

Patients.—Between 1983 and 1992, 169 patients with alcoholic cirrhosis underwent primary liver transplantation in 1 of 12 French centers. Their 2-year survival was compared with a matched control group of 169

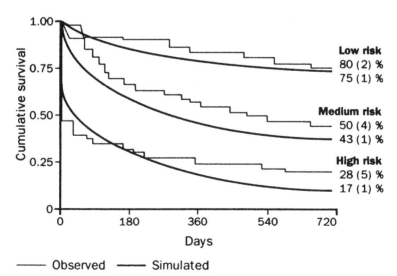

Fig 6–5.—Internal validation of the Beclere model. Actual Kaplan-Meier and predicted survival curves for risk tertiles for the 772 cohort patients with alcoholic cirrhosis. There was a significant difference between the survivals according to the risk group but no significant difference between actual and predicted survival in each risk group. (Courtesy of Poynard T, for a Multi-Centre Group: *Lancet* 344:502–507, 1994.)

patients with similar age, severity of alcoholic cirrhosis, and bleeding history and a simulated control group of 169 patients whose theoretical survival was determined in a cohort of 797 patients with alcoholic cirrhosis (Fig 6-5).

Results.—At 2 years, the actual survival rate was 73% (confidence interval, 67%–79%) for transplanted patients, 67% for matched controls, and 67% for simulated controls; the differences among groups were not significant. When prognostic factors were considered, transplantation exhibited a borderline independent, significant prognostic value. The 2-year survival rate for patients with severe liver disease was 64%, which was significantly higher than that in matched controls (41%) or simulated controls (23%). Such a beneficial effect was not evident in patients with less severe cirrhosis.

Conclusion.—Liver transplantation increases the 2-year survival of patients with severe alcoholic cirrhosis. The role of liver transplantation in patients with less severe disease should be further evaluated in nonrandomized, controlled studies with longer follow-up or randomized trials.

▶ This article creates a model for survival in patients with alcoholic liver disease that is similar to the Mayo model for predicting survival in patients with primary biliary cirrhosis. The authors then use this model to compare the efficacy of transplantation in these individuals. Patients undergoing liver transplantation did much better than matched patients who did not receive liver transplantation if they were high risk patients. However, there was little difference between transplanted patients and matched controls who did not have transplantation if they were medium risk or low risk patients. More and more third-party payers will demand proof of efficacy of treatments. Studies such as this, which attempt to establish models for predicting survival in certain patient groups and studying the efficacy of treatment of those patients, are needed for many therapies and interventions.—R.J. Howard, M.D., Ph.D.

Definition and Classification of Negative Outcomes in Solid Organ Transplantation

Clavien P-A, Camargo CA Jr, Croxford R, Langer B, Levy GA, Greig PD (Univ of Toronto; Duke Univ Med Ctr, Durham, NC)
Ann Surg 220:109–120, 1994   140-95-6–6

Background.—Despite the increasing popularity of organ transplantation seen in the last decade, the procedure is still associated with considerable mortality and morbidity. Negative outcomes of solid organ transplantation were identified, and a new classification of complications by severity was proposed. After specific complications of orthotopic liver transplantation (OLT) were defined, results, risk factors, and prognostic scores for transplantation were evaluated in 215 consecutive OLTs done at the University of Toronto.

Method.—On the basis of previous definitions and classification of complications for general surgery, a new method of classification for transplantation in 4 grades was suggested. The results, including risk factors, of the first 205 OLTs done at the University of Toronto were then assessed using the new classification.

Results.—Of the 215 patients having OLT, all but 2 (99.1%) experienced at least 1 complication. Ninety-two percent of patients who survived more than 3 months had grade 1 (minor) complications. Nearly three quarters of the patients (74%) had grade 2 (life-threatening) complications, and 30% had grade 3 complications (residual disability or cancer). Twenty-nine percent had grade 4 complications (retransplantation or death). Grade 1 complications usually include steroid-responsive rejection (69% of patients) and minor infections. Grade 2 complications included infection that required antibiotic agents or invasive procedures (64% of patients), postoperative bleeding that required more than 3 units of packed red blood cells (35%), primary dysfunction (26%), and biliary disease that was treated with antibiotic agents or invasive procedures (18%). Among the grade 3 complications, renal failure was the most common, which is defined as a permanent increase in serum creatinine levels greater than twice the values before transplantation (11% of patients). Grade 4 complications leading to death or retransplantation were, in many cases, caused by infection (14%) and primary dysfunction (11%). The last 50 patients having transplantation had significantly fewer grade 1 and 2 complications than the first 50 patients. This was partly due to the improved medical status of the patients at the time of surgery. Univariate and multivariate analyses of risk factors showed that grade 1 complications could be predicted by donor obesity; grade 2 complications tended to occur after the donor liver was rewarmed for more than 90 minutes; and grade 3 and 4 complications were best predicted by the Acute Physiology and Chronic Health Evaluation II scoring system and donor cardiac arrest.

Conclusion.—This study provided a definition of negative outcomes and a classification of complications after solid organ transplantation. The use of the classification in OLT provides a better appreciation of the morbidity of the procedure, decrease in the number of some complications, and the opportunity to analyze risk factors and test prognostic scoring systems. This evaluation was done from a medical perspective; further studies from the patient perspective are now required to assess and standardize quality of life and patient satisfaction.

▶ This paper was selected because it provides a useful basis for categorizing complications after liver transplantation. It was adapted from another scheme the authors devised for complications after surgery (1). This system can allow complications to be compared from 1 study to another and from 1 center to another. It can also be adapted for heart transplantation and for kidney transplantation. Most managed care providers focus on low-cost, good graft survival, and low complication rates. Schemes such as this should facilitate data comparison among centers.—R.J. Howard, M.D., Ph.D.

Reference

1. Clavien P-A, et al: *Surgery* 111:518–526, 1992.

Histological Findings in Early Routine Biopsies of Stable Renal Allograft Recipients

Rush DN, Henry SF, Jeffery JR, Schroeder TJ, Gough J (University of Manitoba Health Sciences Centre, Winnipeg, Canada; University of Cincinnati Hospital, Ohio)
Transplantation 57:208–211, 1994   140-95-6–7

Background.—The availability of renal ultrasound and spring-loaded biopsy "guns" has made renal allograft biopsy a safe procedure. The histologic findings of allograft biopsies from clinically stable renal transplant patients, in whom biopsies were carried out monthly for the first 3 months post-transplant were compared to a cohort of clinically unstable patients. Serum interleukin-2 receptor (sIL-2R) levels were also monitored because an increase has been associated with clinical rejection episodes.

Method.—Thirty-one consecutive patients who had undergone renal transplants participated. The patients were treated with triple therapy comprising (CsA) azathioprine, and prednisone. They were considered stable if their serum creatinine levels had not increased by more than 10% in the previous 14 days and if there had been no increase in the immunosuppression regimen during the same time period. Patients were considered unstable if the creatinine had risen above 10% for at least 2 days in the previous 14 days or had been treated for presumed rejection. Core biopsies were performed on all patients at 1, 2, and 3 months post-transplant using an automated biopsy "gun." Serum interleukin-2 receptor levels were measured within 72 hours of biopsy.

Results.—A total of 70 biopsies were carried out, of which 53 satisfied the inclusion criteria. Twenty-nine biopsies were obtained from clinically stable allografts, of which 9 showed histologic evidence of rejection that could not have been predicted from pretransplant (HLA mismatch, panel-reactive antibody titer) or post-transplant (cyclosporine and sIL-2R levels) variables. Patients with rejection on biopsy were treated with methylprednisolone, followed by high doses of oral steroids. Follow-up biopsies carried out 1 month later in 7 rejection patients showed an improvement in 3, and persistent rejection in another 3. There were 10 follow-up biopsies in the nonrejection group, which showed normal or "borderline" findings in 8 patients and chronic changes in 2.

Conclusion.—Histologic evidence of allograft rejection was revealed in one third of renal biopsies obtained from patients with stable graft function in the first 3 months after transplant. The significance of these early, subclinical rejection episodes is unknown, and a further controlled study is being carried out to investigate their effect on long-term graft histology and function.

▶ Biopsy has always been regarded as the gold standard in diagnosing rejection in kidney transplant recipients, and the serum creatinine is the most clinically useful test. Yet, 30% of patients with stable renal function who were biopsied 1–3 months post-transplant and whose creatinine had not risen more than 10% in the 2 weeks before the biopsies had histologic evidence of rejection. The authors felt obliged to treat all patients who showed histologic rejection because the degree of rejection mimics that of patients with clinical rejection (elevated creatinine). The authors are now conducting a randomized study to investigate whether treating subclinical rejection that is detected by routine allograft biopsy has a beneficial effect on long-term renal allograft histology and function. Such a study will certainly be welcome. If treating histologic rejection in the absence of clinical rejection does not result in a beneficial effect on histology or function, then perhaps we should regard histology as the copper standard rather than the gold standard.—R.J. Howard, M.D., Ph.D.

The Evaluation of Candidates for Renal Transplantation: The Current Practice of U. S. Transplant Centers
Ramos EL, Kasiske BL, Alexander SR, Danovitch GM, Harmon WE, Kahana L, Kiresuk TJ, Neylan JF (Univ of Florida, Gainesville; Univ of Minnesota, Minneapolis; Univ of Texas Southwestern, Dallas; et al)
Transplantation 57:490–497, 1994   140-95-6–8

Background.—Candidates for kidney transplantation are routinely evaluated for medical, social, and psychological factors that may affect successful outcomes. A survey of all U.S. centers that participate in the United Network for Organ Sharing was conducted by the Patient Care and Education Committee of the American Society of Transplant Physicians to determine similarities and differences in evaluation and selection processes. The primary goal was not to dictate practice guidelines or policy, but rather to describe current practices and define areas for further investigation.

Findings.—The survey response rate was 81% (147/182). The response to each question was evaluated according to the specialty of the individual completing the questionnaire, as well as the type and size of the center. University-based and larger centers reported acceptance of more medically complicated patients. Eighty-three percent indicated that attendance to dialysis was an important determinant of compliance after transplantation. No specific upper age limits for transplantation were set by 66% of the centers. In 56% of the centers, patients with chronic active hepatitis in the setting of hepatitis B antigenemia were excluded.

TABLE 1.—Cardiovascular Evaluation

Number of centers (% centers responding)

	Stress—thallium	Coronary angiogram	Cardiac echo
Symptomatic patients*	131 (89%)	123 (84%)	90 (61%)
Asymptomatic older patients†	98 (67%)	11 (7%)	34 (23%)
All diabetic patients	125 (86%)	22 (15%)	48 (33%)
Asymptomatic patients with risk factors‡	101 (69%)	12 (8%)	8 (5%)
No specific policy	37 (26%)	11 (7%)	46 (31%)

* Symptoms: angina for stress—thallium; positive stress test for coronary angiogram.
† > 52 ± 7 years for stress—thallium; > 57 ± 5 years for coronary angiogram; > 52 ± 6 years for cardiac echo.
‡ Risk factors: history of myocardial infarction, smoking history, hypertension, hyperlipidemia.
(Courtesy of Ramos EL, Kasiske BL, Alexander SR, et al: *Transplantation* 57:490–497, 1994.)

TABLE 2.—Blood Transfusion Policy

Number of centers (% centers responding)

	Cadaver transplants	LURT
Transfusions not required	111 (79%)	68 (57%)
Historical transfusions (> 1 year) accepted	19 (14%)	7 (6%)
Transfusions required within 1 year of activation (PRA <10%)	4 (3%)	6 (5%)
Transfusions required within 1 year of activation (any PRA)	3 (2%)	9 (8%)
No specific policy	4 (3%)	29 (24%)

Abbreviations: LURT, living-unrelated renal transplants; PRA, peak reactive antibody.
(Courtesy of Ramos EL, Kasiske BL, Alexander SR, et al: *Transplantation* 57:490–497, 1994.)

Fifty percent of the centers reported having no specific policy for evaluating hepatitis C antibody-positive patients, whereas 54% indicated that hepatitis C antibody-positive donors were excluded. An abdominal ultrasound examination was obtained for all patients undergoing transplant evaluation in 34% of the centers. Eighty-nine percent of the centers also performed a stress thallium test when evaluating symptomatic patients with suspected coronary artery disease, and 15% reported routine use of coronary angiography for all diabetic patients (Table 1). Finally, 79% of the centers did not require preoperative blood transfusions for recipients of cadaveric kidney (Table 2).

Conclusions.—U.S. transplant centers lack uniformity in their evaluation and selection of patients for renal transplantation. This diversity is particularly noteworthy in the areas of viral hepatitis, cardiovascular disease, and noncompliance. Further investigations of these topics are recommended. Findings may serve to facilitate patient placement on transplant lists and minimize cost and inconvenience to the population with chronic renal failure.

▶ This survey of most of the nation's kidney transplant centers can help individual centers know where they are in relation to the rest of the country as far as evaluation of potential kidney transplant recipients. There is nothing in this paper that indicates that 1 approach is correct and another is incorrect. It does let each center know where it is in relation to the rest of the country.—R.J. Howard, M.D., Ph.D.

Maintenance Immunosuppression Therapy and Outcome of Renal Transplantation in North American Children — A Report of the North American Pediatric Renal Transplant Cooperative Study

Tejani A, Stablein D, Fine R, Alexander S (State Univ of New York Health Science Ctr, Brooklyn; The EMMES Corp, Potomac, Md; Univ of Texas Southwestern Med Ctr, Houston)

Pediatr Nephrol 7:132–137, 1993   140-95-6–9

Introduction.—The frequency of the combined use of prednisone, cyclosporine, and azathioprine for immunosuppressive therapy after renal transplantation has steadily increased since 1985. However, the necessity of using triple therapy in patients receiving living-related donor (LRD) kidneys is not certain. The association between immunosuppressive regimen and graft outcome was determined in pediatric patients receiving either cadaver or LRD kidneys.

Methods.—Records of 568 patients receiving cadaver kidney transplants and 492 LRD recipients from 74 health centers were evaluated for graft outcome for 1–6 months after transplantation. Only patients younger than 18 years of age were included in the study. Three immunosuppressive regimens had been used: prednisone and azathioprine (PA); prednisone and cyclosporine (PC); and prednisone, cyclosporine, and azathioprine (PCA). The influence of immunosuppressive therapy on graft outcome was determined.

Results.—Among the patients receiving cadaver kidneys, the rate of graft rejection within 30 days was higher with PA than with either PC or PCA, as was hospitalization for rejection within 6 months, the hemolytic uremic syndrome, hypertension, and administration of antibiotic agents. The rate of graft rejection at 6 months was 33% for PA, 15.3% for PC, and 8.3% for PCA. Patients receiving PA were hospitalized for an average of 15.5 days during the first 6 months compared with 6 and 9.5 days for those receiving PCA and PC, respectively. Serum creatinine concentrations at 30 days were lowest in the PCA group. Smaller differences were seen among patients receiving LRD kidneys. Hospitalization duration and the rate of hospitalization for graft rejection were highest in the PA group. Graft failure was 8.3% for PA, 0% for PC, and 3.7% for PCA. No differences were seen between serum creatinine concentrations in the PC and PCA groups.

Conclusions.—The PA combination is a poor therapeutic choice after either cadaver or LRD kidney transplantation. The PCA combination is superior to both PA and PC in patients receiving cadaver kidneys. In LRD recipients, PCA and PC are both superior to PA, but no benefit was seen in the use of PCA rather than PC.

▶ Although comparative trials of adult recipients of kidney transplants with different immunosuppressive protocols are available, virtually none are available of pediatric transplant recipients because no center performs enough pediatric transplants. For this reason, the North American Pediatric Renal Transplant Cooperative Study, which has 24 participating transplant centers, collects extensive data on renal transplantations performed on children younger than age 18 at institutions in the United States and Canada. This historical, nonrandomized review compares 3 immunosuppressive protocols in children. The study was able to accumulate a large number of recipients of cadaveric renal transplants (586) and LRD transplants (492 recipients). Only a small number in both groups (36 in the cadaveric and 78 in the related transplants) received PA alone. Furthermore, 74% of recipients of cadaveric grafts and 64% of recipients of related grafts received triple therapy. The combination of PC with or without azathioprine was superior to PA alone in both cadaveric and related renal transplantation. Triple therapy was superior to both PA or PC for recipients of cadaveric kidneys. There were fewer graft failures and fewer other adverse effects, such as rejection and hospitalization. It is surprising that as late as 1990 20% of institutions were still not using triple therapy for either cadaveric or LRD transplants.—R.J. Howard, M.D., Ph.D.

Renal Transplantation for Patients 60 Years of Age or Older: A Single-Institution Experience

Benedetti E, Matas AJ, Hakim N, Fasola C, Gillingham K, McHugh L, Najarian

JS (University of Minnesota, Minneapolis)
Ann Surg 220:445–460, 1994   140-95-6–10

Background.—The advent of cyclosporine-based immunosuppressive protocols has decreased the risk of renal allograft rejection in patients older than 45 years of age. Accordingly, the question of whether older patients should be rejected as candidates for transplant on the basis of age alone must be reexamined. Outcomes of kidney transplants in patients older than age 60 were examined.

Methods.—Medical records of all patients receiving kidney transplants from January 1, 1970 through December 31, 1993 at the study institution were reviewed. Outcomes including patient and graft survival, hospital length of stay, incidence of rejection and rehospitalization, and the causes of graft loss were compared for patients between 18 and 59 years of age and those 60 years of age and older. Surviving patients 60 years old and older were also asked to complete an outcome survey.

Results.—During the study period, 2,828 adults received 3,103 kidney transplants, of which 138 transplants were for individuals 60 years of age or older. During the precyclosporine era, only 18 patients 60 years old or older received transplants, and patient and graft survival rates were significantly worse than those of patients 45 years old or younger. One hundred-eight individuals, 60 years or older, have received transplants since the cyclosporine protocols have been in use. Recipient and graft survival rates were similar to those 18–59 years of age until 3 years post-transplant, at which time mortality increased for the older patients. Graft survival was similar for both groups when deaths were censored. Longer initial hospitalizations were required by those 60 years of age or older, but they had fewer rejection episodes and fewer rehospitalizations than the younger patients. Quality-of-life scores for surviving transplant recipients age 60 or older were similar to national norms.

Conclusions.—Kidney transplantation is successful in patients aged 60 years and older. Even though most patients had extrarenal disease at the time of transplantation, it was not a predictor of outcome and should not be used to exclude older patients from eligibility for renal transplantation. Post-transplant quality of life is similar to their peers in the U.S. population.

▶ In the early days of kidney transplantation, most transplant centers had an arbitrary age cut-off for transplantation. Patients who were older were thought to be too high risk to undergo renal transplantation. As transplant surgeons became more skilled at preventing and treating complications associated with transplantation and immunosuppression, the age at which transplantation could be safely done gradually increased. (The increasing age limit of transplantation also parallels the increasing age of transplant surgeons, who most likely thought that at age 50, 55, or 60 years, they themselves were not too old to undergo a transplant.) The findings of this study from the

University of Minnesota matches those of most other studies that discuss transplantation in older individuals. These patients die at a higher rate (older people die at a higher rate than younger people), but their graft survival rates are similar to younger individuals if patients who die with function are censored from the data. The causes of death in older individuals were more likely to be from malignancy and nonviral infections, although the incidence of myocardial infarction was similar between older and younger patients.

Like many other facets of medicine, this study demonstrates that many of our preconceived ideas (in this case, that some patients are too old to be transplanted) are incorrect when actually submitted to a clinical trial. Many other medical and surgical "truths" should no doubt be subjected to actual clinical trial, or possibly discarded.—R.J. Howard, M.D., Ph.D.

Cyclosporine Pharmacokinetics and Variability From A Microemulsion Formulation: A Multicenter Investigation in Kidney Transplant Patients
Kovarik JM, Mueller EA, van Bree JB, Flückiger SS, Lange H, Schmidt B, Boesken WH, Lison AE, Kutz K (Phillips University of Marburg, Germany; Brothers of Charity Hosp, Trier, Germany; Central Hosp, Bremen, Germany)
Transplantation 58:658–663, 1994   140-95-6–11

Background.—Considerable clinical research has attempted to describe the pharmacokinetics of cyclosporine since its introduction in transplantation medicine. Pilot study data from an earlier investigation, regarding the steady-state pharmacokinetics and tolerability of a microemulsion formulation of cyclosporine, was studied further to confirm findings.

Methods.—Clinically stable renal allograft recipients 18 years of age and older who had received cyclosporine orally for at least 6 months were enrolled at 3 centers. For at least 2 weeks before the investigation period, all patients were given the same commercially prepared cyclosporine with the individualized total daily dose divided into 2 equal doses given every 12 hours. The 8-week study period was divided into 4 sequential 2-week periods. During period I, patients entered the study on the stable, individualized twice-daily dosage regimen of the commercial cyclosporine. They were changed over to the microemulsion formulation during period II at the same dose as at study entry. Dosages were titrated if necessary to provide comparable steady-state trough concentrations as at study entry during period III. Reinstitution of the commercial formulation occurred during period IV.

Results.—Fifty-five patients completed the study, and all tolerated both study drug formulations well. No cyclosporine dose adjustments were required by 52 of 55 patients at any time during the study to maintain trough concentrations in the target range. Trough concentrations were significantly higher after the conversion to microemulsion formulation although, clinically, concentrations remained in the target therapeu-

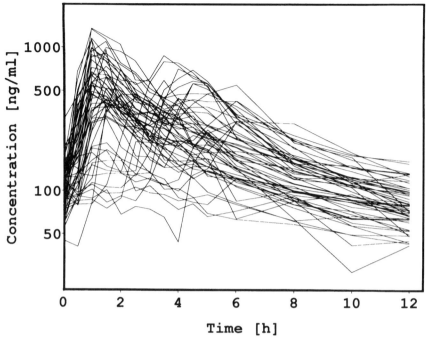

Fig 6–6.—Synoptic view of the steady-state cyclosporine concentration-time profiles of 55 stable kidney transplant patients receiving individualized doses of the commercial formulation in study period I. (Courtesy of Kovarik JM, Mueller EA, van Bree JB, et al: *Transplantation* 58:658–663, 1994.)

tic range. Absorption-related pharmacokinetic differences between the formulations were evident as manifested by a faster rate and extent of cyclosporine absorption from the microemulsion formulation. Maximum blood concentration increased on average of 59% and occurred about 1 hour earlier, with the area under the blood concentration-time curve over a steady-state dosing interval increasing an average 30% (Figs 6–6 and 6–7). Intraindividual variability was significantly reduced with the microemulsion formulation.

Conclusions.—A milligram-to-milligram conversion from the current commercial formulation to the microemulsion formulation was well tolerated and is an appropriate initial changeover in this population.

▶ This study compares the pharmacokinetics of cyclosporine and cyclosporine in a microemulsion formulation (Sandimmune Neoral). This new formulation does not depend on emulsification for absorption, inasmuch as it is already emulsified. Because of this new formulation, the time to maximum concentration is decreased and the area under the curve is increased for similar doses. Also, intraindividual variability is reduced. This new formulation should allow more dependable cyclosporine levels to be achieved in transplant recipients.—R.J. Howard, M.D., Ph.D.

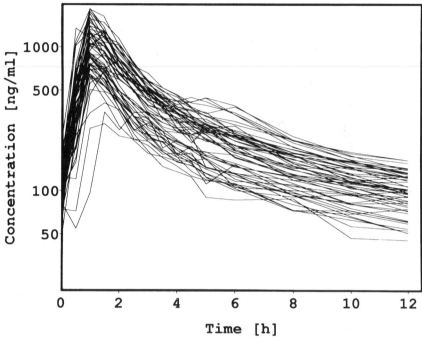

Fig 6–7.—Synoptic view of the steady-state cyclosporine concentration-time profiles following the change over to the microemulsion formulation in study period II. (Courtesy of Kovarik JM, Mueller EA, van Bree JB, et al: *Transplantation* 58:658–663, 1994.)

Trial of Intravesical Versus Extravesical Ureteroneocystostomy in Renal Transplant Recipients

Jindal RM, Carpinito G, Bernard D, Schmitt G, Idelson B, Joshi P, Hakaim A, Cho SI (Boston Univ Med Ctr; Boston VA Med Ctr)
Clin Transplant 8:396–398, 1994   140-95-6–12

Background.—During renal transplantation, the donor ureter is anastomosed to the recipient bladder by a variety of techniques. Classically, the intravesical Leadbetter-Politano (LP) technique is used. It has a high success rate in correcting vesicoureteral reflux; however, serious complications such as stenoses or leaks continue to result in significant morbidity. Many transplant centers have explored the use of extravesicular ureteroneocystostomy (Lich technique) for ureteric implantation in renal transplant recipients. The results comparing complication rates of the LP and Lich techniques were analyzed.

Methods.—One hundred eighty-five patients underwent transplantation and were followed up for complications. The trial was conducted between January 1987 and August 1991 with continued follow-up. The Lich group included 69 transplant recipients and the LP group had 116.

The mean age of the patients in the Lich group was 52 years vs. 44 years for the LP group. In the Lich group, 38% of the patients were diabetic compared with 6% of the LP group.

Findings.—A statistical difference in overall incidence of urologic complications was not seen. Stenosis was seen in none of the Lich group and 3 patients in the LP group. Leaks occurred in 3 patients who had the Lich procedure and 1 who had LP. No difference in the incidence of rejection episodes or infection was seen, and graft and patient survival was comparable.

Conclusion.—Although the complication rates of the 2 techniques are comparable, the extravesicular Lich technique is simple and offers avoidance of a separate cystostomy, reducing trauma to the bladder and postoperative bleeding. This technique involves a short, single bladder incision. The LP procedure provides a longer course of the ureter, making it vulnerable to ischemia and consequent stenosis or necrosis. Despite the lack of statistical evidence, the Lich technique appears to be superior to LP in avoiding ureteric stenoses and is recommended as the procedure of choice.

▶ This noncontrolled trial finds no statistical difference in the incidence of urologic complications in transplant recipients who have ureteroneocystostomy done by the intravesical LP technique or the extravesicle Lich technique. The authors do not provide details on the method of selecting 1 procedure rather than the other. Presumably, it was the choice of the surgeon performing the transplant procedure. Despite the lack of any statistically significant difference in the rate of urinary applications (even though the urinary leak rate was approximately twice as high for the Lich technique as for the LP technique), the authors conclude that the Lich technique appears to be better because it avoids a separate cystostomy, thereby reducing trauma to the bladder and postoperative bleeding. This conclusion *may* be correct. It is unfortunate, however, that the authors provide no data to substantiate their conclusion, and we are left with their testimony alone. It appears from this and other studies that both techniques are acceptable for performing ureteroneocystostomy in that there is little to recommend 1 over the other.—R.J. Howard, M.D., Ph.D.

Effect of HLA Matching on Organ Distribution Among Whites and African-Americans

Zachary AA, Braun WE, Hayes JM, McElroy JB, Novick AC, Schulak JA, Sharp WV (Cleveland Clinic Found, Ohio; Univ Hosps of Cleveland, Ohio; St Elizabeth's Hosp, Youngstown, Ohio; et al)
Transplantation 57:1115–1119, 1994   140-95-6–13

Background.—About 1 in 3 individuals awaiting cadaver kidney transplantation in the United States are African-Americans, but they receive only 1 of 5 transplants. Some of the disparity may reflect incompatibility of antigens, which are distributed differently in African-Americans and North American whites. An effect of HLA matching on organ allocation has been suggested but not definitively demonstrated.

Objective.—The allocation of 185 cadaver kidneys was examined under 2 systems: the current United Network for Organ Sharing (UNOS) point system, and a variant that assigns more points for waiting time than the system previously used by UNOS.

Findings.—The racial makeup of the donor pools and recipient waiting lists was the same for both periods studied. The proportion of African-Americans undergoing transplantation increased from 29% to 34% under the current UNOS point system, which gave more weight to HLA matching. Under this system, 6 of 8 kidneys from African-American donors were given to African-American recipients, compared with only 2 of 8 under the variant system.

Implications.—The current UNOS point system of allocating cadaver kidneys does not disadvantage African-American patients. It appears necessary to increase donations by African-Americans and to continue to use HLA matching as a key criterion for organ distribution.

▶ Although African-Americans comprise one third of patients awaiting cadaveric transplantation, they receive only 20% of the transplants. Many have thought this disparity reflected the frequency distributions of HLA antigens in the African-American and Caucasian populations. Because relatively more donors are Caucasian, any sharing system that favors tissue matching is bound to result in more whites being transplanted than African-Americans. The authors tested this hypothesis in the Northeast Ohio Transplant Group. They compared the UNOS matching system with an alternative that assigns more points for waiting time. The authors found that the models suggest that African-Americans are more likely to receive transplants with the current UNOS system than with a variant that assigns more points for waiting time, at least in Northeastern Ohio transplant programs. Nevertheless, with the current allocation scheme, which gives so much weight to HLA matching, African-American patients on the cadaveric waiting list will most likely continue to be transplanted at a lower rate than Caucasians.—R.J. Howard, M.D., Ph.D.

Should Hepatitis C–Infected Kidneys Be Transplanted in the United States?
Kiberd BA (Queen's Univ, Kingston, Ont, Canada)
Transplantation 57:1068–1072, 1994   140-95-6–14

Background.—Most transfusion-associated liver disease is believed to be caused by hepatitis C virus (HCV) infection. Patients with end-stage renal disease have a high prevalence of HCV infection. Liver failure is an important cause of late mortality in long-term renal transplant recipients.

Model Input Values

Events	Probabilities	Range
Donor anti-HCV test positive	0.04	0.02–0.04
Donor true HCV infection	0.02	0.005–0.02
Symptomatic acute hepatitis infection (D+/R−)*	0.25	0.10–0.50
Symptomatic chronic liver disease (D+/R−)	0.50	0.25–1.00
Patient survival year 1	0.94	0.90–0.95
Subsequent years	0.962	0.95–0.98
Allograft survival year 1	0.80	0.75–0.85
Subsequent years	0.945	0.90–0.95
Patient survival (year 7 onward) with chronic liver disease (D+R−)	0.866†	0.72–0.90

Events	Costs (U.S. $)	Range
HCV test	50	50–200
Dialysis	32,000	32–48,000
Transplant year 1 (including organ)	84,000	64–94,000
Transplant year 2 or more	7,000	6–12,000
Transplant or dialysis, additional annual cost with acute or chronic liver infection (D+/R−)	2,000	2–3,000
Death	5,000	1–10,000

Outcomes	QALY probabilities	Range
Dialysis	0.41	0.41–0.56
Functioning transplant	0.74	0.60–0.85
Cirrhosis/acute/chronic active hepatitis with functioning transplant	0.41	0.35–0.60
Chronic liver disease on dialysis	0.36	0.00–0.36

* Symptoms of acute hepatitis were limited to 1 year.
† Annual survivial rate with chronic liver disease 10% lower than normal (.90 × .962 = .866).
(Courtesy of Kiberd BA: *Transplantation* 57:1068–1072, 1994.)

The economic impact of the following 3 organ allocation options was examined based on donor and recipient HCV status: (1) discard all kidneys from HCV-positive donors; (2) screen all donors and transplant infected organs into HCV-positive recipients only; (3) ignore HCV status and transplant without screening.

Methods.—A cost-utility analysis was done using best-estimate probabilities, costs, and patient outcomes derived from the literature (table). The patient outcome unit of measure was the quality-adjusted life year (QALY). The software package, Lotus 1-2-3, release 3.1, was used to carry out all calculations on a personal computer.

Results.—The cost per QALY was calculated to be $77,650 per QALY for dialysis; $33,260 per QALY for transplantation; and $38,850 per QALY for transplantation using a kidney donor who was positive for HCV, whereas the recipient was negative. Assuming a potential to transplant 8,100 kidneys per year during the next 20 years, transplanting kidneys from HCV-infected donors only into HCV-infected recipients was shown to be most cost-effective, producing 47,203 QALYs at a cost of $1.572 billion.

Conclusions.—A consistent policy related to the use of donor kidneys that may potentially be infected with HCV is needed. Discarding all kidneys from donors that are HCV positive is expensive and reduces patient outcomes. The potential risks and benefits of receiving infected organs should be fully explained to patients before they are asked for informed consent for kidney transplant surgery.

▶ Whether to use kidneys from HCV-positive donors is controversial. Between 1.8% and 14% of donors are HCV positive. Roth (1) found that when 48 kidneys from HCV-positive donors were transplanted, only 3 recipients had evidence of viral transmission, but most were not tested preoperatively. Thirteen patients (28%) had evidence of liver disease but only 5 were HCV positive. Other analysts (2, 3) have found a higher rate of transmission; thus different authors disagree on whether HCV-positive donor kidneys should be used for transplantation. This paper investigates different alternatives based on the cost per QALYs. Although the data can be argued because they are numbers obtained from the literature, and a QALY is based on patient's perception, the authors found that transplanting kidneys from HCV-positive donors into positive recipients produces the most QALYs, whereas transplanting these kidneys into any recipient produced the lowest cost. As the authors recognize, there may be other unrecognized costs such as are associated with legal and ethical issues. Furthermore, the increased cost from discarding all positive donor kidneys is small (less than 1%), compared with the entire Medicare end-stage renal disease program costs. Different programs are responding in different ways, and the issues still remain unsettled.—R.J. Howard, M.D., Ph.D.

References

1. Roth D: *Ann Intern Med* 117:470, 1992.
2. Pereira BJG: *N Engl J Med* 325:454, 1991.
3. Tesi RJ: *Transplantation* 57:826, 1994.

Successful Long-Term Outcome with 0-Haplotype-Matched Living-Related Kidney Donors

Jones JW Jr, Gillingham KJ, Sutherland DER, Payne WD, Dunn DL, Gores PF, Gruessner RWG, Najarian JS, Matas AJ (University of Minnesota, Minneapolis)

Transplantation 57:512–515, 1994   140-95-6–15

Rationale.—Although the list of those awaiting cadaver kidney transplantation continues to grow, the number of available living-donor transplants has not appreciably increased. Willing relatives often are turned away because of a poor HLA ABDR match with the recipient. This situation encouraged a policy of accepting the 0-haplotype-match (0-HTM) living-related donor.

Study Population.—The outcome of renal transplantation was examined in 352 adult patients given primary living-related donor kidneys since 1985. The 44 0-HTM transplants were compared with 92 2-HTM and 216 1-HTM cases. Primary cadaver kidney transplants were given to 362 adult patients in the same period.

Management.—Recipients of living-donor organs received triple immunosuppressive therapy consisting of cyclosporine, azathioprine, and prednisone. The cadaver kidney recipients were transfused preoperatively and subsequently treated sequentially with prednisone, azathioprine, and antilymphoblast globulin.

Results.—Patients in the 2-HTM group had significantly better survival than the cadaver kidney recipients at 6 years (97% vs. 76%). The 1-HTM and 0-HTM groups both had a survival rate of 81%. Graft survival at 6 years did not differ significantly between the various HTM groups, but the 1-HTM and 2-HTM recipients had better graft survival than the cadaver kidney recipients. Both the 1- and 2-HTM groups had relatively fewer rejection episodes in the first year than patients in the 0-HTM and cadaver kidney groups. Readmissions and time in the hospital were least in the 2-HTM group, but the differences were not significant. There were no substantial group differences in serum creatinine levels.

Conclusion.—The use of kidneys from living-related donors is clearly advantageous regardless of the extent of haplotype matching.

▶ Because of the ever-increasing shortage of organs suitable for transplantation, transplant surgeons are using related and cadaveric donors that only a few years ago were deemed to be unsuitable for transplantation. Surprisingly, many of these kidneys are turning out to be appropriate for transplantation when actually tried clinically, which gives an indication of how poor many of our preconceived ideas can be. This study from Minnesota argues that 0-haplotype kidneys from related donors have graft survival comparable to 1-haplotype matches. The graft survival curves between 0- and 1-haplotype matches do not differ and are both above that of cadaveric grafts. 0-haplotype-related grafts should certainly be used more widely.—R.J. Howard, M.D., Ph.D.

The Crossmatch in Renal Transplantation: Evaluation of Flow Cytometry as a Replacement for Standard Cytotoxicity

Scornik JC, Brunson ME, Schaub B, Howard RJ, Pfaff WW (Univ of Florida, Gainesville)

Transplantation 57:621–625, 1994   140-95-6–16

Background.—Many transplantation laboratories use the flow cytometry (FC) crossmatch in addition to the standard complement-dependent cytotoxicity (CDC) crossmatch for evaluating donor-recipient compatibility. The possibility of using FC as the definitive crossmatch for cadaveric donor renal transplantation has not previously been examined.

Patients.—Crossmatches by FC and CDC were done for 230 patients who received renal transplants. Crossmatch results were available for 132 patients evaluated for cadaveric donor transplantation.

Results.—When the T-cell crossmatch was negative by FC, it was always negative by CDC. When the T-cell crossmatch was positive by CDC, it was also positive by FC, but several cases that were T-cell-

Number of Positive CDC T- and B-Cell
Crossmatches According to Flow
Cytometry Results

Flow cytometry results*		n	CDC-positive cases	
T cell	B cell		T cell	B cell†
Negative	Negative	150	0	4
Negative	Positive	27	0	10
Positive	Negative	28	1	7
Positive	Positive	59	19	21
Total		264	20	42

* Positive flow cytometry results: T cells, normal serum: patient's serum ratio > 2; B cells, normal serum: patient's serum ratio > 3.
† Positive B-cell crossmatches by CDC are considered only when the T-cell crossmatch by CDC is negative.
Abbreviations: CDC, complement-dependent cytotoxicity.
(Courtesy of: Scornik JC, Brunson ME, Schaub B, et al: *Transplantation* 57:621–625, 1994.)

negative by CDC were positive by FC. The ability to predict a positive CDC B-cell crossmatch by FC followed a similar trend, but many cases that were B–cell-positive by CDC were negative by FC (table). To better predict a positive CDC crossmatch, the amount of antibody was considered. The probability of a positive T-cell CDC crossmatch increased as the FC reactions became quantitatively stronger. Actual graft survival rates were 85% for all patients, 83% for FC-positive patients, and 86% for FC-negative patients.

Conclusions.—The FC crossmatch may become the definitive crossmatch test because it provides a higher degree of confidence than does the CDC test in defining borderline results.

▶ Flow cytometry crossmatching is faster and less subject to technician interpretation than standard CDC testing. It can be used as a final test for 80% of transplants (unsensitized first transplant recipients who have a negative test and sensitized or second transplant recipients who have a positive test). Further refinements may make this test suitable for all testing and allow it to completely replace CDC testing. Getting the results of crossmatching earlier has decreased the cold ischemic time.—R.J. Howard, M.D., Ph.D.

Three Years Clinical Experience with Intestinal Transplantation
Abu-Elmagd K, Todo S, Tzakis A, Reyes J, Nour B, Furukawa H, Fung JJ, Demetris A, Starzl TE (Univ of Pittsburgh Med Ctr, Pa)
J Am Coll Surg 179:385–400, 1994   140-95-6–17

Background.—Until recently results of the sporadic attempts at intestinal transplantation were discouraging. The superior therapeutic efficacy of the new immunosuppressive drug FK 506 has rekindled interest in small bowel and multivisceral transplantation.

Patients.—The patient population included 21 adults, 19–58 years of age and 22 children, .5–15.5 years of age. Indications for intestinal transplantation included short bowel syndrome, intestinal insufficiency, and malignant tumors with or without associated liver disease. Fifteen patients were given intestinal allografts (Fig 6–8), 21 received hepatic and intestinal allografts, and 7 were given multivisceral allografts that contained at least 4 organs. Thirteen grafts contained the ascending and right transverse colon. Five of the 7 patients given multivisceral allografts had been on total parenteral nutrition (TPN) for 1–132 months before their operation. Intravenous FK 506, steroids, and prostaglandin E1 administration were started during the operation; enteral FK 506 was started 1–2 weeks after transplantation.

Results.—After a follow-up period of 6–39 months, there were 30 survivors, 29 of whom still had their grafts. Those who received isolated intestinal allografts had the most rapid recovery and resumption of diet and the highest 3-month survival (100%) and graft survival (88%) rates.

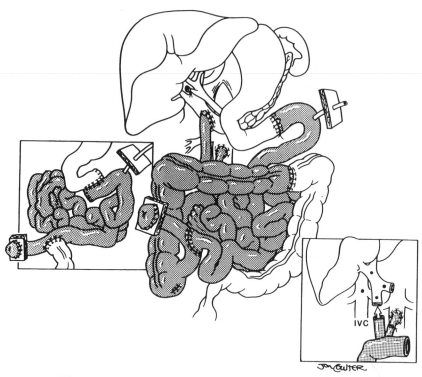

Fig 6–8.—*Abbreviation:* IVC, inferior vena cava. Isolated intestinal transplantation including one half of the colon (**main figure**) or the small intestine only (**left insert**) is shown. Graft venous outflow is drained end-to-side (**main figure**) or end-to-end (**right insert**) into the host portal system. (Courtesy of Abu-Elmagd K, Todo S, Tzakis A, et al: *J Am Coll Surg* 179:385–400, 1994.)

However, the isolated intestine was more prone to rejection so that by the end of the first 2 postoperative years, multivisceral transplantation had the best survival rate (86%). Only 2 patients with combined liver and intestinal grafts did not experience any episodes of graft rejection. Most patients were able to discontinue TPN.

Conclusions.—Although the survival rates achieved with these 3 intestinal transplant procedures are reason for optimism, the high complication rate, the enormous effort and expense it took to care for these patients, and the exorbitantly high threat of rejection that remained despite heavy immunosuppression preclude the widespread use of these procedures at this time.

▶ This article is a further discussion of the Pittsburgh experience with intestinal transplantation. The initial summary of the clinical experience from Pittsburgh was presented in the 1993 Yearbook of Surgery (1). This paper details that experience in 43 patients. Although accompanied by many complications, prolonged hospitalization, and high costs, the transplant group from

Pittsburgh has showed that intestinal transplantation is clinically possible. Total parenteral nutrition was discontinued in all recipients 18–210 days after transplantation. We are not told whether and, if so, how many patients required supplemental intravenous nutrition in addition to oral or tube feedings. Intestinal transplantation is an exciting new area of transplantation. Several hurdles remain to be overcome, but the continued effort of centers such as this will achieve success in the long run.—R.J. Howard, M.D., Ph.D.

Reference

1. Todo S, et al: *Ann Surg* 216:223–234, 1992.

An Economic Analysis of Heart-Lung Transplantation: Costs, Insurance Coverage, and Reimbursement

Evans RW, Manninen DL, Dong FB (Mayo Clinic, Rochester, Minn; Battelle-Seattle Research Ctr, Seattle)
J Thorac Cardiovasc Surg 105:972–978, 1993   140-95-6–18

Purpose.—Because heart-lung transplantation is still considered an experimental procedure, relatively few are done. The lack of available donors is one of the main constraints. The National Cooperative Transplantation Study Group analyzed the hospital charges for heart-lung transplantation and the experience of transplantation centers with insurance reimbursement.

Methods.—The 3 primary elements of transplantation costs are hospital charges, professional fees, and costs of donor organ acquisition. The reimbursement part of this analysis included only hospital data because reimbursement status for physician fees was difficult to assess. In 1988, 27 heart-lung transplantation centers in the United States did 72 procedures. Complete financial data from the date of transplantation until hospital discharge were available for 42 patients.

Results.—The total median charge for a heart-lung transplantation was $134,881, of which $98,127 was for hospital charges and $12,028 was for donor acquisition costs. The average hospital stay was 31 days. Charges widely varied, with total charges for 50% of the patients ranging from $99,535 to $216,639 and organ procurement charges ranging from $5,149 to $38,000 (table). More than 78% of the procedures included in this analysis were paid for by private insurers; for 84.6% of cases, reimbursement exceeded 90% of all billed charges.

Conclusions.—Although the future of heart-lung transplantation is still more uncertain than that of any other solid organ transplant procedure, the data on insurer reimbursement are encouraging.

▶ As managed care organizations become responsible for more patients, cost data will be as important as results in selecting which transplant centers survive. This paper provides information on the cost of lung transplantation

Organ Procurement Charges in the United States, 1988

Transplant procedure	Minimum	25th percentile	Costs (in 1988 dollars) 50th percentile (median)	75th percentile	Maximum
Kidney	682	9,979	12,290	16,000	87,629
Heart	390	9,859	12,578	16,124	60,000
Liver	4,775	12,808	16,281	21,496	65,652
Heart-lung	5,149	9,934	12,028	16,750	38,000
Pancreas	585	9,600	15,400	24,685	32,952

(Courtesy of: Evans RW, Manninen DL, Dong FB: J Thorac Cardiovasc Surg 105:972–978, 1993.)

in 1988 at 27 transplant centers. Since that time, many other centers have begun doing lung transplantation. The authors use hospital charges rather than hospital costs. They recognize that hospital costs represent the true expense of a procedure rather than charges, which represent the cost of doing the procedure and any mark-up. In many instances, it can be difficult to find a logical relationship between the 2. When dealing with managed care organizations, hospitals must bid down the charge for doing a given procedure.

Their interest in deciding how much they must charge for a procedure is what their true costs are, not what their charges may have been.

These data do provide some benchmark to which other centers can compare themselves. Unfortunately, the data are several years old and adjustments will have to be made for inflation to arrive at current charges. In addition, the success rate is higher and length of stay is generally lower since 1988. The charge for lung transplantation appears to be consistent and compares favorably with charges for other organ transplant procedures.—R.J. Howard, M.D., Ph.D.

Mechanisms of Acquired Thymic Unresponsiveness to Renal Allografts: Thymic Recognition of Immunodominant Allo-MHC Peptides Induces Peripheral T Cell Anergy

Sayegh MH, Perico N, Gallon L, Imberti O, Hancock WW, Remuzzi G, Carpenter CB (Brigham and Women's Hosp, Boston; Harvard Med School, Boston; Mario Negri Inst, Bergamo, Italy; et al)
Transplantation 58:125–132, 1994   140-95-6–19

Background.—The thymus is the key element in acquiring tolerance to self. A single intrathymic injection of synthetic 24mer peptides, representing full sequences of the hypervariable domain of WF class II major histocompatibility complex (MHC) molecules, has induced donor-specific unresponsiveness to WF rat renal allografts in adult Lewis (LEW) rat recipients. This effect was prevented by recipient thymectomy within a week after the injection. The peripheral T cells of long-term survivors exhibited antigen-specific hyporesponsiveness in the mixed lymphocyte reaction (MLR) test.

Objective.—The mechanisms underlying the acquired thymic tolerance induced by processed MHC allopeptides were examined both in vivo and in vitro.

Findings.—The LEW rats given intrathymic injections of nonimmunogenic peptides rejected their renal allografts within 6–10 days, whereas those given immunogenic peptides were alive after more than 100 days with normal allograft function. The T cells from tolerized animals exhibited antigen-specific hyporesponsiveness in the MLR within a week after allograft transfer. Immunohistologic study of allografts from tolerized animals demonstrated markedly reduced mononuclear cell infiltration and no evidence of tubulitis a week after engraftment. Staining for inflammatory cytokines and alloantibodies was markedly reduced compared with acutely rejecting grafts. Recombinant IK-2, given systemically from the day of transplantation, prevented the development of tolerance. No such effect was seen when interleukin-2 was given 4–6 weeks after transplantation or when thymectomy was done after 2 weeks.

Clinical Implications.—The human thymus involutes in adult life, but it may continue to host the cells that recognize injected alloantigen and induce systemic unresponsiveness. A precise understanding of the cellular interactions that promote specific anergy might help in developing methods to induce tolerance in transplant recipients without having to operate on the thymus.

▶ Many investigators observed that direct inoculation of donor cells into the thymus can lead to specific tolerance of subsequent organ allografts. This paper attempts to find the mechanism of specific tolerance by demonstrating tolerance to synthetic peptides corresponding to the hypervariable domain of class II MHC in rats. Injection of these peptides into the thymus of rats led to tolerance of renal allografts, but administration of nonimmune peptides did not. Studies such as this are a step toward working out the mechanism of specific tolerance. Whether they will eventually have clinical applicability and allow specific immunologic unresponsiveness—the Holy Grail of clinical transplantation—remains to be seen.—R.J. Howard, M.D., Ph.D.

7 Endocrinology

Introduction

The first paper (Abstract 140-95-7–1) presents a practical application of genetic testing that permits identification of patients at risk for medullary thyroid carcinoma. The authors performed prophylactic thyroidectomy in these patients. The promise of genetic testing is great, but it does raise many ethical questions. Articles continue to be published about the newest method of scanning for parathyroid adenomas by using T-99M-Sestamibi (Abstract 140-95-7–2). This localization method is more sensitive and specific than other previously used localization methods. Another paper attempts to evaluate the cost-effectiveness of preoperative localization studies (Abstract 140-95-7–3). According to this article, despite the accuracy of current methods of localization, they are not as reliable as a skilled parathyroid surgeon. This article suggests that their increased costs do not contribute to the likelihood of finding glands at the operating table in patients having an initial operation for hyperparathyroidism. This evaluation, of course, assumes that the parathyroidectomy is performed by a surgeon skilled and experienced in parathyroid surgery. Probably most parathyroidectomies in this country are not done by these surgeons, but rather by general surgeons in the community who only occasionally perform parathyroidectomies. For these surgeons, localization studies might be helpful.

Three papers (Abstract 140-95-7–5 through Abstract 140-95-7–7) find that a majority of patients with primary hyperparathyroidism who are poor risks for surgical intervention can be successfully treated with alcohol injection into the parathyroid adenoma or by angioablation when a parathyroid exploration has failed. These methods appear to be safe and effective.

Needle aspiration cytology can be used to evaluate thyroid nodules (Abstract 140-95-7–8). The ability to use cytology to follow-up with these patients depends on how skillful the cytologist is. This article shows that in their hands, fine-needle aspiration biopsy is highly predictive of future biological behavior. The extent of resection in patients with papillary thyroid cancer has long been debated (and no doubt will continue to be). Very often, long-term follow-up studies are not available. The paper by Mazzaferri (Abstract 140-95-7–9) provides data that suggest patients with tumors larger than 1.5 cm were more likely to survive if they had more aggressive surgery. This paper is 1 of the longest follow-ups of patients with papillary thyroid cancer. A paper by Coburn et al. (Abstract 140-95-7–10) examines patients with recurring thyroid cancer and argues strongly for ^{131}I scanning to allow early detection and treatment of recurrence or metastases. The paper by Degroot et al. (Abstract 140-95-7–11) stresses that previous classifications for thyroid cancer do not segregate low-risk patients from some high-risk patients. In reviewing their patients, they also find that aggressive surgery is a main indicator of survival after a diagnosis of thyroid cancer.

Laparoscopic surgical techniques can safely be applied to adrenalectomy (Abstract 140-95-7–12). A paper by Gagner et al. finds that adrenalectomy was unsuccessful in only 1 of 25 patients in whom it was attempted. Concomitant procedures can also be performed in these patients. We usually think that bilateral adrenalectomy with corticosteroid replacement should be curative for patients with Cushing's syndrome. In fact, follow-up studies show that these patients frequently have long-term problems (Abstract 140-95-7–13). These problems may reflect the imperfect replacement patients have with synthetic corticosteroids. Survival is poor in patients with adrenal adenocarcinoma, even in those in whom resection was thought to be complete (Abstract 140-95-7–14). Adrenal adenocarcinoma is uncommon; it took 40 years for a cancer center to accumulate 53 cases. Tumors are frequently detected late because they produce poorly defined, vague symptoms. Many tumors are not detected until they are already large and distant metastases for local spread has occurred.

Richard J. Howard, M.D., Ph.D.

Predictive DNA Testing and Prophylactic Thyroidectomy in Patients at Risk for Multiple Endocrine Neoplasia Type 2A

Wells SA Jr, Chi DD, Toshima K, Dehner LP, Coffin CM, Dowton SB, Ivanovich JL, DeBenedetti MK, Dilley WG, Moley JF, Norton JA, Donis-Keller H (Washington University School of Medicine, St. Louis, Mo; Nippon Medical School, Tokyo; St. Louis VA Med Ctr, St. Louis, Mo)
Ann Surg 220:237–250, 1994   140-95-7–1

Background.—The occurrence of medullary thyroid carcinoma, pheochromocytoma, and hyperparathyroidism characterizes multiple endocrine neoplasia type 2A (MEN 2A). The disease has an autosomal dominant inheritance pattern with virtually all affected patients having medullary thyroid carcinoma, a uniformly malignant endocrinopathy. Members of 7 kindreds with MEN 2A were evaluated by using haplotype studies, direct mutation analysis, and biochemical testing.

Methods.—A polymerase chain reaction-based genetic test for the 19 known RET mutations in MEN 2A was designed. By using genetic markers flanking the MEN 2A marker locus, haplotypes were also constructed. Before and after provocative testing, plasma calcitonin concen-

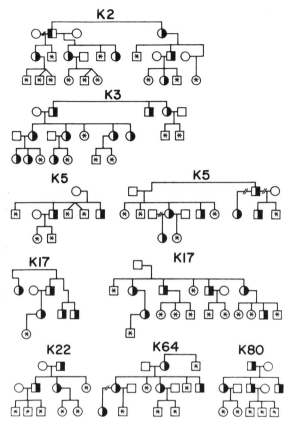

Fig 7–1.—Structure of the family segments selected from 7 kindreds (K2, K3, K5, K17, K22, K64, and K80) with multiple endocrine neoplasia type 2A (MEN 2A). Each *square* represents a male and each *circle,* a female. The *half filled symbols* represent kindred members with proved clinical diagnosis of MEN 2A. *Asterisks* represent kindred members who are at risk for inheriting MEN 2A. (Courtesy of Wells SA Jr, Chi DD, Toshima K, et al: *Ann Surg* 220:237–250, 1994.)

trations were determined. Kindred members' unaffected spouses (n = 26) served as controls.

Results.—Forty-eight of the 132 members of the 7 kindreds with MEN 2A had an established diagnosis and 58 were at 50% risk of inheriting the disease (Fig 7–1). Of the 58 at risk, direct DNA testing and haplotype analysis showed that 21 had inherited mutation in the RET protooncogene associated with MEN 2A. Nine of those 21 had elevated plasma calcitonin concentrations. Thirteen of the 21 (6 with normal and 7 with elevated calcitonin) agreed to immediate thyroidectomy. Pathologic examination demonstrated C-cell hyperplasia with or without medullary thyroid carcinoma in each of the 13 patients. No metastases were found in the patients and postoperative stimulated plasma calcitonin levels were normal.

Conclusions.—Direct genetic testing in MEN 2A has simplified the management of kindreds with this disease and established the place of preventive thyroidectomy in this familial cancer syndrome.

▶ This paper demonstrates the power of modern genetic testing. These authors were able to identify patients who had inherited the RET proto-oncogene associated with MEN 2A. Based on this genetic analysis, they recommended that these patients undergo thyroidectomy even though there were no other indications that suggested medullary thyroid carcinoma. With powerful tests such as this, patients destined to have inherited neoplastic disease can undergo prophylactic surgery so that the tumors never develop. Studies like these represent the beginning of modern genetics applied to surgical therapy. Yet, genetic testing (for the presence of genes that indicate increased propensity for cancer or other diseases, for instance) is already creating ethical issues. What if insurance companies require such testing before issuing policies? What if prospective spouses require testing before agreeing to marriage? These are only some of the questions raised by genetic testing.—R.J. Howard, M.D., Ph.D.

Preoperative Imaging of Abnormal Parathyroid Glands in Patients With Hyperparathyroid Disease Using Combination Tc-99m-Pertechnetate and Tc-99m-Sestamibi Radionuclide Scans

Wei JP, Burke GJ, Mansberger AR Jr (Med College of Georgia, Augusta)
Ann Surg 219:568–573, 1994 140-95-7–2

Objective.—Radiologic localization of abnormal parathyroid glands is difficult because of problems with visualizing adenomas outside the area of exploration or glandular hyperplasia. Recently, 2 new techniques have been developed, using the new radionuclide technetium (Tc)-99m-sestamibi alone, which is more sensitive for adenomas than for hyperplastic glands, or in combination with iodine-123. The imaging effectiveness of a combination of Tc-99m-pertechnetate and Tc-99m-sestamibi was investigated in preoperative localization of abnormal parathyroid glands.

Correlation of Tc-99m-Sestamibi Localization of Parathyroid Glands With Surgical and Pathologic Findings

Histology	True (+)	True (−)	False (+)	False (−)
Adenomas	12	0	1	1
Normal	0	25	0	0
Hyperplastic	35	0	0	11
Carcinoma	1	0	0	0

(Courtesy of Wei JP, Burke GJ, Mansberger AR Jr: *Ann Surg* 219:568–573, 1994.)

Methods.—A total of 30 patients, aged 28–88 years, with confirmed primary, secondary, and tertiary hyperparathyroid disease had combined sequential Tc-99m-pertechnetate and Tc-99m-sestamibi scans, with the latter image being subtracted from the former. Seven patients had associated renal failure.

Results.—Thirteen of 23 patients with primary disease had solitary adenomas and 25 normal glands within the surgical exploration field. Adenomas were significantly larger than normal glands. Ten of these patients had diffuse hyperplasia, and 22 hyperplastic glands were found. The subtraction scans localized 12 of 13 solitary parathyroid tumors, missing a small adenoma (table). No normal glands were imaged. The sensitivity and specificity for adenoma detection was 92% and 100%, respectively, with a positive predictive value of 100%. In patients with diffuse hyperplastic glands, 37 of 47 abnormal glands were detected by subtraction scanning. These glands were significantly larger than nonimaged glands. Sensitivity for hyperplastic glands was 79% with a positive predictive value of 100%.

Conclusion.—Although Tc-99m-pertechnetate and thallium-201 are the most common radionuclides used, they are not sufficiently sensitive for preoperative use. Technetium-99m-pertechnetate and Tc-99m-sestamibi subtraction scanning is sensitive to solitary parathyroid adenomas and hyperplastic glands but does not always localize diffuse hyperplastic glands.

▶ A new scanning method, with TC-99m-sestamibi (in this case with TC-99m-pertechnetate) to localize abnormal parathyroid glands gave the best results of published localization methods (sensitivity, 92%; specificity, 100%). The test is not as good for localizing hyperplastic glands (sensitivity, 70%; positive predictive value, 100%). Nevertheless, even this diagnostic test cannot locate diseased parathyroid glands as well as an experienced parathyroid surgeon. Whether localization studies should be used before parathyroidectomy depends in large part on the skill of the surgeon. Localization studies for parathyroid glands continues to be the subject of numerous studies published every year. In 1994 alone, at least 18 studies on parathyroid localization using TC-99m-sestamibi were contained in Medline. The final place of parathyroid localization remains unsettled. It is most useful for patients who have already had surgery and for surgeons who do not regularly perform parathyroid surgery (which probably includes most of the general surgeons in the United States).—R.J. Howard, M.D., Ph.D.

Cost-Effectiveness of Preoperative Localization Studies in Primary Hyperparathyroid Disease

Roe SM, Burns RP, Graham LD, Brock WB, Russell WL (Univ of Tennessee, Chattanooga)
Ann Surg 219:582–586, 1994   140-95-7–3

Background.—Preoperative localization studies are frequently advocated in patients with primary hyperparathyroid disease (PHPT) to identify and locate abnormal parathyroid glands. Although these studies may lead to an accurate identification of abnormal glands, it is unclear whether they bring improvement in surgical cure or long-term morbidity. A quantitative evaluation of the cost of preoperative localization studies was attempted by investigating their success and cost-effectiveness.

Method.—A retrospective review was carried out of 113 patients who underwent initial cervical exploration for PHPT between August 1981 and October 1993. Twenty-four of these patients had surgery without preoperative localization studies, and the remaining 89 had 132 noninvasive preoperative localization studies. Age, sex, type, and number of preoperative localizing studies, postoperative calcium levels, and operative time were analyzed. Postoperative morbidity and surgical results were also assessed. Parathyroid disease identified during surgery was recorded and compared with preoperative localization site predictions. The total cost of each of the various localization studies was assessed and a statistical analysis of operative times was carried out.

Results.—In 23 of the 24 patients (96%) who had surgery without preoperative localization studies, disease was identified and normal calcium levels were achieved after surgery. Eighty-seven of the 89 patients (98%) who had preoperative localization studies were surgically cured. The sensitivity of localization studies was found to be highest with thallium-technetium scintiscanning (60%), followed by ultrasound (33%), and magnetic resonance imaging (18%). Specificity rates for these tests were 94%, 96%, and 97%, respectively. The positive predictive value was 79% for thallium-technetium scintiscanning, with an overall accuracy of 85%. The average cost of localization studies was $901 per patient. The mean operating time did not differ significantly between patients who underwent localizing studies and those who did not.

Conclusion.—The results of this study indicate that preoperative parathyroid localization studies do not improve parathyroid localization or cure rate in patients with PHPT. Neither do they reduce operating time. Such tests are not cost-effective and are best reserved for those patients with recurrent or persistent PHPT who need further surgical intervention.

▶ Every year several articles are published that discuss the use of preoperative localization studies in patients with parathyroid disease. Virtually all findings conclude that localization studies have an accuracy rate of approximately 85%, but that it is below the 96%–98% accuracy of knowledgeable parathyroid surgeons. Few have evaluated the cost of doing these studies. This study shows that the cost of such studies was high and resulted in no increased accuracy in localization compared with a skilled surgeon. Furthermore, localization studies were not very helpful in patients who had multigland disease. What this and other studies have not taken into account, however, is the skill of the surgeon. This and virtually all studies published on preoperative localization are done in centers where skilled parathyroid surgeons are available. The dilemma is that most parathyroid operations in this country are probably performed at community hospitals where surgeons cannot specialize in endocrine surgery. Community hospital surgeons individually probably do only a small number of parathyroid operations. For those surgeons who do not regularly perform parathyroidectomies, localization studies may be helpful.—R.J. Howard, M.D., Ph.D.

Functional Recovery of the Parathyroid Glands After Surgery for Primary Hyperparathyroidism
Bergenfelz A, Valdermarsoon S, Ahrén B (Lund University, Sweden)
Surgery 116:827–836, 1994   140-95-7-4

Introduction.—Serum levels of parathyroid hormone (PTH) decline rapidly when a parathyroid adenoma is excised but reportedly recover within 72 hours. It is not clear, however, how the parathyroid glands function in the immediate postoperative period in patients with primary hyperparathyroidism (pHPT).

Objective and Methods.—The effects of high and low serum calcium levels of the serum PTH were examined 1 and 4 days postoperatively in 6 patients with pHPT caused by a parathyroid adenoma. Seven healthy individuals also were studied. Patients underwent ethylenediaminetetraacetic acid (EDTA) infusion tests and also were given an oral load of 1.5 g of elemental calcium.

Results.—Serum levels of intact PTH and ionized calcium decreased rapidly after excision of the parathyroid adenoma. All patients had normal levels of PTH on the second postoperative day. The nadir of serum ionized calcium was reached on the fourth day. The increased set point characteristic of pHPT was no longer noted the first day after surgery. The PTH level was normally suppressed by calcium on the second day, but increased suppressibility was evident on the fifth postoperative day. On EDTA infusion testing, the secretory reserve of PTH increased postoperatively. An increased level of intact PTH still was induced by hypocalcemia a year postoperatively.

Implications.—Parathyroid function rapidly returns to normal after removal of a parathyroid adenoma that has caused pHPT. Suppressibility of PTH secretion may be increased in the immediate postoperative period, and patients tend to have an exaggerated calcemic response to an oral calcium load.

▶ Secretion of PTH by normal parathyroid glands is suppressed in patients with parathyroid adenoma. This paper demonstrates that PTH secretion is still suppressed 1 day after surgery but recovers very rapidly after excision of the adenoma. Further, without the presence of an adenoma, the increased setpoint of PTH normalizes on the first postoperative day. Although the amount of PTH after EDTA infusion testing did not differ on the fifth postoperative day compared with results 1 year later or for healthy subjects, the relative increase of serum levels of PTH during the EDTA infusion test did not normalize until after the fifth postoperative day. This normal responsiveness to calcium occurs extremely early after parathyroidectomy in patients with a functioning parathyroid adenoma.—R.J. Howard, M.D., Ph.D.

Results of Ultrasonically Guided Percutaneous Ethanol Injection Into Parathyroid Adenomas in Primary Hyperparathyroidism
Vergès BL, Cercueil JP, Jacob D, Vaillant G, Brun JM, Putelat R (Univ Hosp, Dijon, France)
Acta Endocrinol 129:381–387, 1993   140-95-7–5

Introduction.—Surgery may sometimes be inadvisable in high-risk patients with primary hyperparathyroidism. An alternative treatment for patients unable to undergo surgery consists of ultrasonically guided ethanol injection. The advantages and limitations of this new procedure were evaluated in a group of 13 patients.

Patients and Methods.—Patients selected for ultrasonically guided percutaneous ethanol injection of parathyroid adenomas ranged in age from 66 to 98 years. The volumes of the parathyroid tumors ranged from .11 to 4.18 mL. Local anesthesia was used, and a 20-gauge needle was inserted into the tumor under complete ultrasound control. The solution was injected (.5-1 mL of 95% ethanol) when the needle tip was seen inside the parathyroid tumor. One to 8 injections were performed in each patient. The injections were given 3 to 8 days apart when 2 or more were required. Total success after treatment consisted of complete normalization of calcium and parathyroid hormone (PTH) levels.

Results.—The ultrasound-guided ethanol injection treatment was totally successful in 7 patients who had undergone 1 to 3 injections. Plasma calcium and PTH levels remained normal during a median follow-up period of 28 months. Four patients had a partial success, showing significant clinical improvement and normal plasma calcium levels, yet persistent elevated PTH levels remained during a median follow-up period of 20 months. The ethanol injection treatment failed in 2 patients, both of whom subsequently underwent surgery (Fig 7–2).

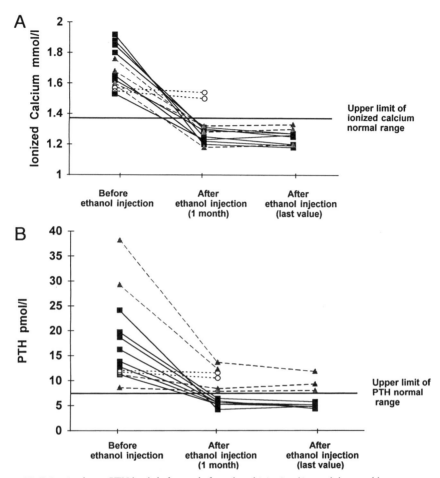

Fig 7–2.—A, plasma PTH levels before and after ethanol injection (1 month later and last measurement) in the 13 patients: (*solid square*) patients with "total success"; (*solid triangle*) patients with "partial success"; (*open circle*) patients with "failure". **B,** plasma-ionized calcium levels before and after ethanol injection (1 month later and last measurement) in the 13 patients: (*solid square*) patients with "total success"; (*solid triangle*) patients with "partial success"; (*open circle*) patients with "failure". (Courtesy of Vergès BL, Cercueil JP, Jacob D, et al: *Acta Endocrinol* 129:381–387, 1993.)

Conclusion.—Ultrasonically guided percutaneous injection of ethanol was found to be a useful alternative for patients with primary hyperparathyroidism who have contraindications for surgery. The treatment was generally well tolerated. Transient dysphonia, observed in 4 patients, was the only side-effect. Necrosis of the tumor must be total for a successful outcome. Plasma calcium and phosphorus levels are significantly reduced 48 hours after successful injections. Tumor size does not appear to affect outcome.

Reexploration and Angiographic Ablation for Hyperparathyroidism

McIntyre RC Jr, Kumpe DA, Liechty RD (Univ of Colorado Health Sciences Ctr; Veterans Affairs Hosp, Denver)
Arch Surg 129:499–505, 1994   140-95-7–6

Background.—Many reviews have defined the causes of failed initial surgery for primary hyperparathyroidism. Although the reasons for failure are well documented, persistent and recurrent hyperparathyroidism continues to be a clinical problem. The causes of initial failure, the accuracy of preoperative localization tests, the role of angiographic parathyroid ablation, and the safety and efficacy of reexploration for hyperparathyroidism were investigated.

Methods.—Forty-two patients undergoing reexploration or angiographic ablation for hyperparathyroidism were assessed retrospectively. Follow-up ranged from 1 month to 13 years. In preoperative localization studies, the cervical approach was used when the abnormal gland was suspected of being in the neck or the mediastinum superior to the aortic arch. Sternotomy was used for deeper mediastinal glands unresectable through a cervical approach. Angiographic ablation of mediastinal glands was done with contrast administration after a catheter was wedged into the selective feeding artery.

Findings.—Initial failure resulted from mediastinal glands in 18 patients, surgeon inexperience in 12, supernumerary glands in 6, and other anatomical anomalies. Hyperplasia accounted for hyperparathyroidism in 26% of the patients and adenomas in 74%. Preoperative localization studies included technetium-Tc-99m-sestamibi scanning, with a sensitivity of 86%; technetium-thallium scanning, with a sensitivity of 67%; arteriography, with a sensitivity of 63%; and venous sampling, with a sensitivity of 52%. Computed tomography had a sensitivity of 42%, MRI, 33%; and ultrasonography, 27%. In 89% of 27 patients undergoing reexploration, hypercalcemia resolved. Localization results were negative in all 4 patients in whom failures occurred. Angiographic ablation succeeded in 67% of 6 patients. One patient in whom ablation failed had successful mediastinal exploration. Hypoparathyroidism occurred in 14.3%. There were no cases of recurrent nerve injury.

Conclusions.—In this series, the most common causes of initial failure were ectopic mediastinal glands and incomplete surgical exploration. The technetium-Tc-99m-sestamibi scan is the most sensitive preoperative localization study. Angiographic ablation of parathyroid tissue is most effective for patients who are poor surgical candidates and for avoiding mediastinum sternotomy. Reexploration and angiographic ablation were associated with a high success rate with acceptable morbidity and mortality.

▶ Persistent or recurrent hyperparathyroidism after initial parathyroid exploration remains 1 of the more frustrating problems for surgeons. Although the use of preoperative localization studies might be abated before initial parathyroid exploration, they are clearly warranted before reexploration. This article demonstrates that, in the hands of skilled radiologists and surgeons, the majority of individuals with persistent or recurrent hyperparathyroidism can be rendered normally calcemic either by surgery or by angiographic ablation. The most common cause for failure was mediastinal glands. The second most common cause was incomplete initial exploration with failure to identify enlarged glands in their normal anatomical position. This series from a referral center is highly selected in that the most common cause for persistent or recurrent hyperparathyroidism was the presence of mediastinal glands, whereas incomplete primary neck exploration is usually the cause of persistent disease.—R.J. Howard, M.D., Ph.D.

Acute Change in Parathyroid Function in Primary Hyperparathyroidism Following Ultrasonically Guided Ethanol Injection Into Solitary Parathyroid Adenomas
Karstrup S, Hegedüs L, Holm HH (University of Copenhagen, Herlev, Denmark; University of Odense, Denmark)
Acta Endocrinol 129:377–380, 1993   140-95-7-7

Background.—Primary hyperparathyroidism is usually treated operatively, but not all patients are suitable candidates for surgery, and some may refuse the operation. An alternative approach is to inject ethanol under ultrasonographic guidance to inactivate hyperactive parathyroid tumors.

Series.—Parathyroid function was monitored in 7 consecutive women with biochemically documented primary hyperparathyroidism who were treated by ultrasonically guided chemical parathyroidectomy. All had a single parathyroid tumor. Three of the patients refused operative treatment, and 3 others required prompt lowering of the serum calcium because of severe hypercalcemic symptoms. One patient had recently experienced cardiac arrest and failed to respond to bisphosphonate infusion.

Treatment.—Under ultrasound guidance using a 7-MHz sector scanner, an individualized dose of 96% ethanol was injected up to 3 times at 24-hour intervals. Treatment ceased when the serum ionized calcium returned to normal or when complications developed.

Results.—In 6 of 7 patients, the serum ionized calcium became normal within 5 days of initial treatment. Normal serum parathyroid hormone levels were achieved after a median time of 24 hours. The 1 patient who continued to be hypercalcemic then accepted neck surgery and was found to have 2 adenomas, only 1 of which had been detected by ultrasound.

Conclusion.—It is possible to rapidly control the serum ionized calcium and parathyroid hormone levels in patients with primary hyperparathyroidism by injecting the adenoma with ethanol under ultrasound guidance.

▶ The last three articles find that the majority of patients who have primary hyperparathyroidism and who are poor risks for surgical intervention may be successfully treated with alcohol injection into the parathyroid adenoma or by angioablation in those who have failed parathyroid exploration. Most patients were completely cured or improved (they had normal calcium levels but had slightly elevated PTH levels). Successfully treated patients required no more than 3 injections of alcohol. A small number of patients had temporary dysphonia, in most only during injection. Vocal cord paralysis did not occur in any patient. We are not told how many patients may be potential candidates for alcohol injection. Presumably, the tumor has to be successfully located by ultrasonography for the patient to be considered for this treatment. Although this method is not new, it can provide an alternative for patients not amenable to surgical therapy. If it is as successful as the authors indicate, why not consider a trial of it as primary therapy for all patients, saving surgery only for those who continue to have hypercalcemia after alcohol injection? The authors do not address this point, but a clinical trial would be interesting.—R.J. Howard, M.D., Ph.D.

Fate of Untreated Benign Thyroid Nodules: Results of Long-Term Follow-Up

Kuma K, Matsuzuka F, Yokozawa T, Miyauchi A, Sugawara M (Kuma Hosp, Kobe, Japan; Kagawa Med School, Japan; VA Med Ctr, West Los Angeles; et al)

World J Surg 18:495–499, 1994   140-95-7–8

Purpose.—The fate of benign thyroid nodules has not been well studied. How benign thyroid nodules change over time was investigated.

Methods.—Of 532 patients who had had benign aspiration biopsy cytology of their thyroid nodules between 1981 and 1983, 134 agreed to return for a repeat examination. Palpation of the thyroid nodules was carried out by the same 2 thyroidologists who had done the initial examination. All patients underwent ultrasonography and fine-needle aspiration biopsy (FNAB) to examine the nature of the nodules. Ultrasound-guided FNAB was carried out only in patients with small nodules, multiple nodules, or cystic nodules associated with papillomatous proliferation.

Results.—Fifty-five patients with distinctly palpable single nodules underwent FNAB and 61 had ultrasound-guided FNAB (Fig 7–3). At the initial examination, there were 86 single nodules, 14 multiple nodules, and 34 cystic nodules. At follow-up 9–11 years later, more than 99% of the benign nodules were still benign and about 92% had no change in cytologic classification. There was only 1 case (.9%) of thyroid cancer in a nodule previously diagnosed as benign. The most striking finding was

Benign thyroid nodules class 2 by aspiration biopsy cytology

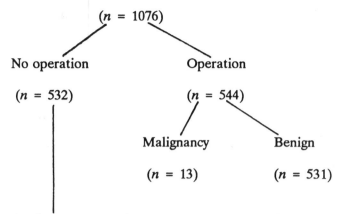

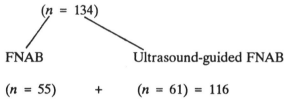

Fig 7–3.—Changes in aspiration biopsy cytology from class 2 to other classes 9–11 years later. (Courtesy of Kuma K, Matsuzuka F, Yokozawa T, et al: *World J Surg* 18:495–499, 1994.)

that 45 nodules had disappeared and 25 had become smaller. Those changes occurred most often among cystic nodules, of which nearly 80% had either decreased in size or disappeared.

Conclusions.—Most biopsy-proved benign thyroid nodules remain benign for a prolonged period. A nodule that has increased in size at follow-up must be reassessed to determine the need for surgical treatment.

▶ It is reassuring that thyroid nodules that were thought to be benign and followed up without medical or surgical treatment turned out to be benign when reexamined 9–11 years later by FNAB. Only 1 of 134 biopsy specimens showed cancer. Eleven of these 134 patients were operated on because of suspicion of malignancy; only 3 had carcinoma. Thus, the authors demonstrate that FNAB is highly predictive of future biological behavior. They selected patients with benign thyroid nodules by aspiration biopsy who were not candidates for surgery. One wonders whether the 3 patients who demonstrated carcinoma when the thyroid nodules were eventually removed had the carcinoma present on the original FNAB, and it was missed because of a stamping error or misinterpretation of the cytology. This question, of course, remains unanswered. What the study does show is the safety of following up thyroid nodules that are shown to be benign by fine needle aspiration biopsy. It shows that more than 99% of benign thyroid nodules remain benign, mirroring the findings of others (1).—R.J. Howard, M.D., Ph.D.

Reference

1. Grant CS, et al: *Surgery* 106:1980, 1989.

Long-Term Impact of Initial Surgical and Medical Therapy on Papillary and Follicular Thyroid Cancer

Mazzaferri EL, Jhiang SM (Ohio State University Coll of Medicine, Columbus)
Am J Med 97:418–428, 1994   140-95-7–9

Background.—Little information is available regarding the long-term outcomes of medical and surgical treatment of thyroid cancer. Outcome data regarding the cohort of patients reported in this study have been collected since 1962. Analysis of this data illuminates the long-term consequences of initial therapy.

Methods.—All patients treated in either US Air Force medical facilities or Ohio State University hospitals for either papillary or follicular thyroid cancer since 1950 have been followed up prospectively through mail and telephone questionnaires. When tumor recurrence or death occurred,

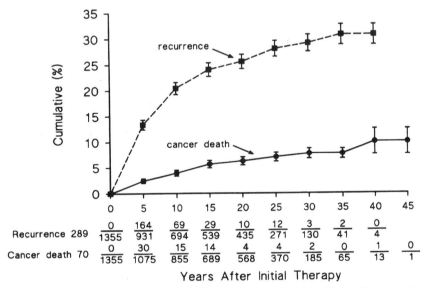

Fig 7–4.—Tumor recurrence and cancer deaths. Numerators are number of events during, and denominators the number of patients at the beginning of each time interval. *Vertical bars* represent standard errors. (Courtesy of Mazzaferri EL, Jhiang SM: *Am J Med* 97:418–428, 1994.)

follow-up information was also gathered by letters to attending physicians. All data were gathered through December 31, 1993.

Results.—The cohort comprised 1,355 individuals—1,077 with papillary and 278 with follicular cancer. Sixty-nine percent of the cohort was female. The first treatment for all but 7 occurred between 1950 and 1993, and the mean age at initial treatment was 35.7 years. Median follow-up was 15.7 years. The survival rate was 76% after 30 years; the recurrence rate was 30%, and the cancer death rate was 8% during the same period (Fig 7–4). Patients younger than 40 years had the lowest mortality rate and recurrences were most frequent at the extremes of age. In a Cox regression model that excluded those who had distant metastases at the time of diagnosis, the likelihood of cancer death was increased by age greater than 40 years, tumor size greater than or equal to 1.5 cm, local tumor invasion, regional lymph-node metastases, and delay in therapy. With the same regression model, the likelihood of cancer mortality was reduced by female sex, surgery more extensive than lobectomy, and ^{131}I plus thyroid hormone therapy. Tumor histologic type did not affect cancer mortality. Iodine 131 therapy by itself given to ablate normal thyroid gland remnants or as cancer therapy significantly reduced cancer recurrence and cancer mortality.

Conclusions.—Tumor features and initial therapy have long-term implications that are independent of the patient's age. Total thyroid ablation is not routinely necessary in tumors smaller than 1.5 cm that are completely confined to the thyroid. Patients with larger tumors or those that are multicentric, metastatic, or invasive have significantly improved outcomes in terms of both recurrence and mortality when ^{131}I therapy is combined with near-total or total thyroidectomy.

▶ Few studies have such a long-term follow-up of such a large group of patients with follicular or papillary thyroid carcinoma as this. This study clearly shows that for tumors larger than 1.5 cm, more aggressive surgery including total thyroidectomy or near-total thyroidectomy is associated with a lower mortality rate. The authors considered patients to have died of cancer only if the death certificate, hospital, family, or attending physican letters so indicated. Some cancer deaths might have been missed using these criteria. Overall, 215 (16%) of the patients could not be contacted and were considered lost to follow-up. We do not know, of course, whether these patients had recurrent tumors or died of their cancer, something that might have influenced the authors' results. This study provides 1 of the most detailed, long-term analyses of a large group of patients with papillary or follicular thyroid cancer.—R.J. Howard, M.D., Ph.D.

Recurrent Thyroid Cancer: Role of Surgery *Versus* Radioactive Iodine (I[131])

Coburn M, Teates D, Wanebo HJ (Brown Univ, Providence, RI; Univ of Virginia Med Ctr, Charlottesville)
Ann Surg 219:587–595, 1994   140-95-7-10

Objective.—Well-differentiated thyroid cancer has a very good prognosis with expected 10-year survival rates of 90% or greater. However, survival rates for patients with recurrences after curative treatment are much lower. Iodine 131 scanning can detect recurrent disease before it becomes clinically evident. Survival rates of patients with recurrences of well-differentiated thyroid cancer diagnosed exclusively by I[131] scanning were compared with those in whom cancer was diagnosed by clinical examination.

Methods.—Between 1956 and 1990, 382 patients were given a diagnosis of well-differentiated thyroid carcinomas and 74 of them (19.5%) had recurrences. Of the 74 recurrences, 28% were local, 53% were regional, and 6% were locoregional. Of the patients whose recurrence was detected by I[131] scanning, only 9.5% had persistent disease or were dead of disease, compared with 54% of those with clinically detected recurrences. Iodine 131 ablation in 20 patients with scintigraphically detected recurrences resulted in salvage of 18 (90%) patients. Surgery alone in 21 patients with clinically detected recurrences salvaged 12 (57%) patients. The addition of I[131] ablation to surgery in 15 patients with clinically detected recurrences salvaged only 3 patients (20%) (Fig 7–5). All patients

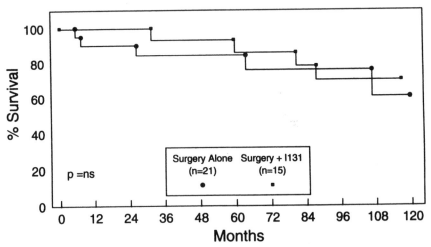

Fig 7–5.—The comparison of treatment outcomes in patients with clinical recurrences treated by surgery vs. surgery plus I[131] with no significant difference in overall survival. (Courtesy of Coburn M, Teates D, Wanebo HJ: *Ann Surg* 219:587–595, 1994.)

with distant recurrences have died of their disease, regardless of treatment.

Conclusions.—The prognosis for patients with distant metastatic recurrences of thyroid cancer detected clinically is poor. Local and regional recurrences detected exclusively by I[131] scanning have a better prognosis than if clinically detected.

▶ This paper reviews 74 patients with recurrent thyroid cancer detected during an 18-year period. All patients with distant metastases died. Those with local or regional recurrence could be salvaged, especially if their recurrences were detected with ^{131}I scanning as opposed to clinical examination. Of the detected recurrences, 50% occurred less than 2 years after initial treatment. Although the results of this paper argue strongly for ^{131}I scanning, the authors do not address the issues of which patients should have it when after initial treatment should scanning be done, and how often should it be performed.—R.J. Howard, M.D., Ph.D.

Does the Method of Management of Papillary Thyroid Carcinoma Make a Difference in Outcome?
DeGroot LJ, Kaplan EL, Straus FH, Shukla MS (The University of Chicago)
World J Surg 18:123–130, 1994   140-95-7–11

Background.—A previous study reviewed the data on a group of 269 patients with papillary thyroid carcinoma during a period of 12 years, showing that the major predictors of adverse outcome were increasing extent of spread of disease at time of first diagnosis, increasing age at diagnosis, and increasing size of the primary lesion. Using the same data,

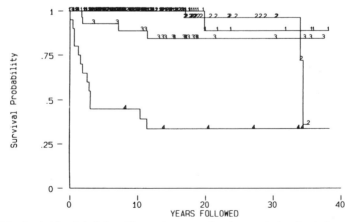

Fig 7–6.—Survival by clinical class. The numbers appearing above each class line indicate the duration of follow up of individual cases in each of the four clinical classes. (Courtesy of DeGroot LJ, Kaplan EL, Straus FH, et al: *World J Surg* 18:123–130, 1994.)

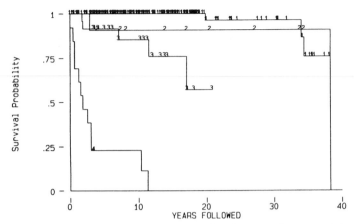

Fig 7-7.—Survival by the American Joint Commission class. (Courtesy of DeGroot LJ, Kaplan EL, Straus FH, et al: *World J Surg* 18:123–130, 1994.)

whether a prognostic classification scheme can be used to predict an appropriate surgical approach, what the effect of treatment is on prognosis, and if patients with an "excellent" prognosis benefit from more extensive surgery and ^{131}I ablation was determined.

Method.—Data were used from the previous study of 269 patients with papillary thyroid carcinoma treated at the University of Chicago since the early 1970s.

Results.—Prognostic classification schemes developed by the American Joint Commission, Cady et al., Hay et al., the European Thyroid Association, and the study's own clinical class scheme each divided patients into risk category groups (Figs 7-6, 7-7). However, all systems failed to segregate some apparently low-risk patients who eventually died of thyroid carcinoma. Considering the excellent, but not perfect, precision of the prognostic schemes, the need for detailed pathologic analysis, and, ideally, postoperative thyroid scanning, it was concluded that the prognostic classification schemes do not permit the decision regarding extent of surgery. Significantly fewer deaths and recurrences were seen in patients who were operated on by 3 experienced surgeons at the University of Chicago than in patients operated on by other surgeons and not routinely ablated. However, when groups were restricted to those consisting only of patients who underwent more extensive surgery, postoperative ^{131}I ablation, or both, little difference was seen between the 2 groups. This finding suggested that the difference in prognosis, comparing patients treated at the University of Chicago and those treated elsewhere, was principally because of the routine use of more extensive surgery and postoperative radioactive iodide ablation. An excellent prognosis was seen in patients under 45 years, with intrathyroidal disease or positive neck nodes and tumors less than 2.5 cm in diameter. The use of ^{131}I ablation was related to a significant reduction in recurrences.

Conclusion.—These data support the use of lobectomy plus contralateral subtotal lobectomy or near-total thyroidectomy in treating thyroid cancers larger than 1 cm in size and in patients aged 45 years or older. They also suggest that the use of ^{131}I postoperatively provides the best prognosis in terms of reduction in deaths and recurrences.

▶ The authors find that previous classification systems for thyroid cancer do not segregate some "low-risk" patients who will still die of their thyroid cancer. The argument is that the main indicator of survival after thyroid cancer is aggressive surgical therapy with or without ^{131}I ablation. This paper adds yet another argument for more aggressive surgical therapy in patients with papillary thyroid carcinoma.—R.J. Howard, M.D., Ph.D.

Early Experience With Laparoscopic Approach for Adrenalectomy
Gagner M, Lacroix A, Prinz RA, Bolté E, Albala D, Potvin C, Hamet P, Kuchel O, Quérin S, Pomp A (Hôtel-Dieu de Montréal, Quebec, Canada)
Surgery 114:1120–1125, 1993   140-95-7-12

Objective.—Because conventional operative approaches to adrenalectomy may cause considerable incisional pain when incisions are close to the intercostal nerves, a laparoscopic method was developed and performed 25 times on 22 patients.

Technique.—For left-sided adrenalectomy, the patient is placed in the lateral decubitus position and insufflation of CO_2 begins in the subcostal region, inflating the abdomen to 15 mm Hg. A 30-degree-angle laparoscope with a diameter of 10 mm is used, with four 11-mm trocars placed subcostally, in the flank, and dorsally. It is necessary to mobilize the splenic flexure of the colon and the lateral part of the abdominal wall, using endoscopic scissors and a laparoscopic dissector. The posterolateral attachments of the spleen are dissected to expose the upper renal pole, and the spleen is retracted medially by grasping the splenic ligament, revealing the adrenal gland. The inferior part of the organ is dissected last. A drain is left in place for 12 hours. In removing the right adrenal gland, the perinephric fat is dissected superiorly and close to the vena cava after dissecting the right triangular ligament of the liver to expose the cava. The superior and anterior aspects of the adrenal gland are dissected first, and the inferior pole last. Care is needed to avoid tearing the lateral branches of the vena cava.

Results.—All but 1 of the 25 laparoscopic adrenalectomies were successful. Three patients had bilateral procedures, and 2 operations were done for Cushing's disease. The unsuccessful procedure involved a 15-cm angiomyolipoma. The mean operating time was 2.3 hours. Patients were in the hospital for a median of 4 days. Half the patients had undergone previous abdominal surgery, which did not interfere with the laparoscopic procedure. Two patients required blood transfusion postoperatively, and there was 1 case each of colonic pseudo-obstruction, urinary tract infection, and incisional hematoma. Nine other procedures were performed at the time of adrenalectomy.

Conclusions.—Laparoscopic adrenalectomy is a minimally invasive procedure and, for this reason, patients may be willing to undergo it sooner when a nodule is found on CT examination. Most adrenal lesions may be removed by laparoscopy using a flank approach with the patient in the lateral decubitus position.

▶ This and several other recently reported articles indicate that laparoscopic surgical techniques can safely be applied to adrenalectomy. The only 1 of the 25 patients in whom adrenalectomy was unsuccessful had an extremely large (15 cm) tumor. Injury to other organs did not occur in this series. Concomitant procedures were performed in 9 patients, including a periaortic node dissection for a 3-cm node between the aorta and vena cava behind the head of the pancreas in a patient with bilateral malignant pheochromocytoma.—R.J. Howard, M.D., Ph.D.

Long-Term Outcome of Bilateral Adrenalectomy in Patients With Cushing's Syndrome
O'Riordain DS, Farley DR, Young WF Jr, Grant CS, van Heerden JA (Mayo Clinic and Found, Rochester, Minn)
Surgery 116:1088–1094, 1994   140-95-7–13

Background.—Despite considerable evolution in the treatment of Cushing's syndrome during the past 40 years, bilateral adrenalectomy retains an important role in its treatment. Yet little information is avail-

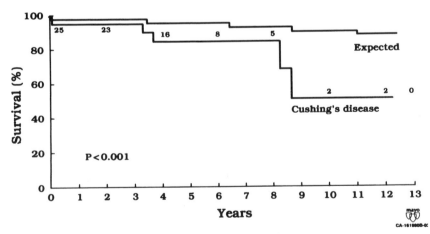

Fig 7–8.—Cumulative survival (Kaplan-Meier) of 25 patients undergoing bilateral adrenalectomy for Cushing's disease compared with expected survival. (Courtesy of O'Riordain DS, Farley DR, Young WF Jr, et al: *Surgery* 116:1088–1094, 1994.)

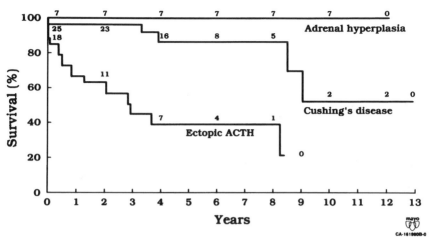

Fig 7–9.—Cumulative survival (Kaplan-Meier) dividing patients undergoing bilateral adrenalectomy into 3 major etiologic groups. (Courtesy of O'Riordain DS, Farley DR, Young WF Jr, et al: *Surgery* 116:1088–1094, 1994.)

able on the long-term consequences of total adrenalectomy. The long-term outcomes of bilateral adrenalectomy in patients with Cushing's syndrome were examined.

Methods.—Medical records were reviewed of all patients undergoing bilateral adrenalectomy for Cushing's syndrome at the Mayo Clinic between 1980 and 1991. All living patients were interviewed a minimum of 2 years after their surgery.

Results.—The records of 50 patients were reviewed, and all 33 of the patients still living at the time of the study consented to interviews. Interviews were conducted at a median of 62 months after surgery. Patients reported a high incidence of chronic physical problems including chronic fatigue, nausea and vomiting, and hypotension and syncope, with only 10 individuals (30%) remaining free from significant symptoms on long-term follow-up. Three patients were hospitalized a total of 9 times with acute steroid insufficiency. Among the 12 patients reporting a total of 16 surgical procedures during follow-up, none reported steroid-related complications. All 50 patients undergoing bilateral adrenalectomy had a cumulative survival rate of 86% at 1 year, 77% at 3 years, and 70% at 5 years. Individuals with Cushing's syndrome had significantly worse survival rates compared with expected survival (Fig 7–8). There were significant differences between major etiologic subgroups in 5-year survival rates: 100% in individuals with adrenal hyperplasia; 86% for those with Cushing's syndrome; and 39% for patients with ectopic adrenocorticotrophic hormone production (Fig 7–9).

Conclusions.—Although effective and necessary in a select group of patients with Cushing's syndrome, bilateral adrenalectomy is associated with occasional morbidity and mortality consequent to adrenal insufficiency. An active, long-term program of postoperative rehabilitation is essential for all patients undergoing adrenalectomy.

▶ Although bilateral adrenalectomy for Cushing's syndrome with replacement of corticosteroids should be curative of this disease, patients so treated do, in fact, have many long-term symptoms related to imperfect steroid replacement therapy. The chronic physical problems these patients have may represent the imperfect adrenocortical balance that can be achieved with replacement therapy with exogenous steroids compared with functioning intact adrenal glands. There were no deaths among patients with adrenal hyperplasia, whereas those with ectopic adrenocorticotrophic hormone production or Cushing's disease were more likely to have neoplastic disease outside the adrenal glands. Nine of the 15 late deaths were due to benign or malignant neoplasms in other endocrine glands.—R.J. Howard, M.D., Ph.D.

Adrenal Adenocarcinoma: A Review of 53 Cases
Zografos GC, Driscoll DL, Karakousis CP, Huben RP (Roswell Park Cancer Inst, Buffalo, NY)
J Surg Oncol 55:160–164, 1994   140-95-7–14

Introduction.—Because adrenal carcinomas are relatively uncommon and may reach a considerable size without clinical evidence of disease, diagnosis is often made at an advanced stage. All cases of adrenal adenocarcinoma seen at the study institution during the past 40 years were reviewed for presenting signs and symptoms, biochemical, hormonal, and radiographic changes, surgical treatment, survival, and metastatic sites.

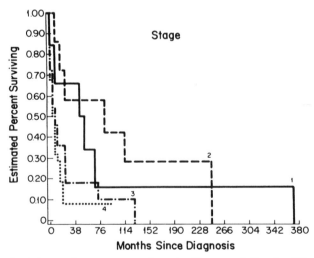

Fig 7–10.—Survival according to stage at diagnosis. (Courtesy of Zografos GC, Driscoll DL, Karakousis CP, et al: *J Surg Oncol* 55:160–164, 1994.)

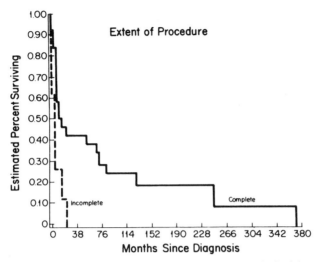

Fig 7–11.—Survival according to type of resection (complete or incomplete) of the primary tumor. (Courtesy of Zografos GC, Driscoll DL, Karakousis CP, et al: *J Surg Oncol* 55:160-164, 1994.)

Patients and Methods.—A total of 53 patients, 30 men and 23 women, with a median age of 51 years, were treated for adrenal carcinoma between 1950 and 1990. Tumors were classified as "functioning" if there was clinical evidence of endocrine disease. Tumor staging was based upon size, nodal status, local invasion, and metastases.

Results.—The primary location of the tumor was the left adrenal gland in 32 patients and the right adrenal gland in 19; 2 patients had synchronous bilateral involvement. Median diameter was 14 cm for right adrenal tumors and 11 cm for left adrenal tumors. Twenty-nine patients were stage IV at diagnosis, with positive nodes and local invasion or distant metastases (Fig 7-10). Flank pain was the most common symptom. The median time between first symptoms and diagnosis was 8 months. Diagnosis was made incidentally in 16 of 32 patients for whom this information was available. Nineteen patients had endocrine manifestations from functioning tumors. Arteriography had the highest sensitivity (95%) of various radiographic localization techniques, followed by CT (94%), ultrasound (92%), and intravenous pyelography (81%). Forty-three patients underwent 1 or more operations, and 21 were found to have extra-adrenal extension of the tumor. Complete surgical removal of all gross tumor was possible in 24 patients. Overall median survival was 8 months (Fig 7-11). Only 3 of the 53 patients are alive, 1 with disease 6 years after diagnosis and 2 who are free of disease at 8 and 13 years after diagnosis.

Conclusion.—Adrenocortical carcinoma accounts for only .02% of all cancers. Diagnosis is often delayed until metastasis is present. The key to cure is early and complete resection of the tumor. Factors significantly related to survival were detection at an early stage and completeness of the surgical procedure.

▶ It took 40 years for a cancer center to accumulate 53 cases of adenocarcinoma, an indication of its rarity. The most important prognostic indicator of survival was completeness of resection. But even in those patients thought to have complete resection, survival was poor. These tumors present with poorly defined symptoms of flank and abdominal pain, and frequently the diagnosis is delayed. In this series, the mean delay was 21 months (median, 8 months). During the 40 years, no doubt, the method of diagnosis and treatment of this disease has changed. Although arteriography was the most sensitive of the diagnostic tests used, most likely it was used early in the series before ultrasonography and CT scanning were available. Intravenous pyelography and arteriography probably were used much less frequently in patients operated on in the later part of this series. Similarly, the 4 operative deaths may have occurred early in the series. With better trained surgeons and better blood replacement, the mortality rate may well be lower in patients operated on more recently. The patients are not divided according to the period in which they had surgery. Similarly, whereas complete resection was most correlated with survival, we are not told whether patients operated on more recently were more likely to undergo complete resection. One would suspect that more complete surgical resections would be attempted in patients undergoing operation in the later part of this series.—R.J. Howard, M.D., Ph.D.

8 Nutrition and Metabolism

Introduction

THE METABOLIC RESPONSE TO CATABOLIC DISEASE STATES

Surgeons care for patients who undergo major operations and sustain life-threatening insults such as injury, sepsis, and cancer. Although the magnitude and temporal nature of such stresses can be quite variable, the regulation of the body's response to these insults is, in many ways, quite similar. It is becoming increasingly apparent that many, if not all, of the physiologic, metabolic, and immunologic responses to trauma, infection, and cancer are not mediated by bacteria, their toxins, or directly by tumor cells, but instead by a group of host-derived polypeptide molecules that have collectively been called cytokines. Elaboration of these cytokine signals may be stimulated by several stimuli including bacteria, endotoxin, necrotic tissue, and tumor growth. These molecules work together with classic stress hormones and with other humoral mediators to orchestrate and coordinate the cellular response to critical illnesses.

The genes that encode the synthesis of these key signal proteins allow the body to respond to infectious, inflammatory, and malignant insults with remarkable resilience. From a teleologic standpoint, these responses are designed to benefit the organism, enhance recovery, and assure a relatively speedy return to health. From an evolutionary standpoint, these biological responses are the result of a process that favors survival of the fittest in the struggle to preserve the species. Ironically, these polypeptide mediators, which clearly orchestrate many of the appropriate and beneficial responses to these catabolic diseases (i.e., fever, tachycardia, acute phase protein synthesis), can also initiate detrimental physiologic responses (hypotension, organ failure, cachexia, and death). One school of thought is that cytokines are produced locally within tissues and are designed to control cellular metabolism in a paracrine or autocrine fashion; only when there is excess production leading to spillover into the systemic circulation are their effects harmful. Currently, 1 of the exciting areas in nutritional research relates to methods of modulating the production of these cytokines using dietary manipulations.

RETHINKING OUR PERSPECTIVE OF THE GUT

Traditionally the gut has been viewed as an organ of quiescence or inactivity during sepsis or after major surgery or accidental injury. This concept of bowel inactivity has evolved for several reasons: 1) ileus is often present and nasogastric decompression is frequently necessary; 2) the gastrointestinal (GI) tract is often unused or unusable for nutrition in critically ill patients; 3) laboratory tests for the serial monitoring of "gut function" are currently unavailable; and 4) the surgeon's attention is often directed toward other organs that are prone to failure such as the kidneys, lungs, and heart. Historically, the intestine has ranked low on the problem list of critically ill surgical patients.

Despite this traditional view, newer evidence has reshaped our thinking about the role of the gut in seriously ill patients. For example, carefully performed studies in both animals and patients have documented that the intestine activity metabolizes both circulating and luminal substrate. In contradistinction to the view that the intestine serves only as a conduit for the absorption of food, it is now apparent that the enterocytes also metabolize and shuttle substrates, indicating that the gut also behaves as a central metabolic processing station. The GI tract also produces a vast array of gut peptides, so-called GI hormones, that exert trophic effects such that intestinal epithelial cell growth and turnover are stimulated—this helps maintain mucosal integrity. The production of these peptides is strongly influenced by the presence or absence of luminal nutrients, and their exogenous administration has been shown to enhance mucosal proliferation and villous morphology.

The mucosa of the entire gastrointestinal tract also acts as a barrier to luminal bacteria and their toxins. The mucous layer contiguous with the brush border of the enterocytes serves as 1 level of protection, whereas the tight junctions that "lock" the enterocytes together act as another. In addition, the gut-associated lymphoid tissue located in the bowel wall processes antigens that cross this mucosal barrier. Although these functions remain intact in healthy individuals and in most patients, it has been demonstrated that this barrier may become compromised after a variety of "stress insults" leading to a breakdown of the gut mucosal barrier.

MICROBIAL TRANSLOCATION

Microbial translocation can be defined as the passage of both viable and nonviable microbes (bacterial, yeast, viruses) and microbial products (endotoxin) across an anatomically intact barrier. Studies in animals that have examined the mechanism by which translocation occurs have demonstrated that both small and large microbes can translocate directly through the morphologically intact enterocytes. Substances such as endotoxin and cholera toxin have been shown to disrupt the interepithelial tight junctions, thereby widening paracellular channels and facilitating the passage of certain macromolecules.

Studies in humans, however, are not quite as clear-cut. Although it has been shown that intestinal permeability is increased in burn patients, in patients receiving total parenteral nutrition, and in volunteers receiving endotoxin, it has been more difficult to demonstrate the presence of bacteria in the portal blood of critically ill patients. Moore and colleagues (1) studied 20 severely injured trauma patients, 30% of whom went on to have multiple organ failure. The incidence of positive portal vein blood cultures during the first 5 days after injury was less than 2%, and most of these were thought to be contaminants. Endotoxin was not detectable in the portal blood, and cytokine levels, although elevated, were similar in portal venous and systemic blood. Thus, although most authorities would agree that the gut barrier function may be compromised in critically ill patients, this may not be manifested as positive blood cultures.

STRATEGIES USED TO MAINTAIN GUT MUCOSAL BARRIER FUNCTION

Strategies used to maintain gut barrier function have focused on 3 general approaches: 1) the use of enteral nutrition; 2) the use of anabolic agents (growth hormone, gut peptides); and 3) the use of specific mucosal nutrients (glutamine). Knowing that gut function is related to gut nutrition, it is not surprising that the best single way to maintain a healthy gut is to provide enteral nutrition to critically ill patients whenever feasible. Early feeding after a burn injury has been shown to be beneficial in terms of reducing the hypermetabolic response, decreasing the incidence of translocation, and preserving intestinal morphology. Several studies in injured patients have demonstrated the superiority of enteral nutrition over parenteral nutrition (or no nutrition) in terms of reducing major complications.

A number of growth factors may assist in preserving gut integrity in critically ill patients. Bombesin, a gut peptide analogous to gastrin-releasing peptide, has been shown to play a key role in the development of the GI tract. Chu and colleagues (2) demonstrated that the administration of bombesin to animals with methotrexate-induced enterocolitis resulted in an increase in mucosal weight, DNA content, and protein content. Mortality from methotrexate was significantly diminished when bombesin was given. Along these lines, growth hormone is another compound that may improve gut function. Growth hormone works in large part through the production of insulin-like growth factor-1 (IGF-1). Studies by Huang et al. (3) revealed that IGF-1 reduced gut atrophy and diminished bacterial translocation after burn injury.

Administering specific nutrients is yet another strategy that has been used in an attempt to improve gut function in critically ill patients. Glutamine, the most abundant amino acid in the body and a key gut fuel, is absent from commercially available total parenteral nutrition (TPN) solutions and is present in relatively low amounts in most enteral diets. Because glutamine is essential for gut function and metabolism, and because glutamine depletion is characteristic of catabolic patients, several investigators have evaluated the effect of providing exogenous glutamine to patients. The best study to date examining its impact on gut function is by van der Hulst and colleagues (4). These investigators randomized 20 surgical patients requiring TPN to a standard formula or a glutamine-enriched solution. Using the nonabsorbable sugars, lactose and mannitol, the authors reported a marked increase in mucosal permeability in patients receiving standard TPN for 12 days. In contrast, no increase in barrier function was noted in the glutamine group. Simultaneously, mild villous atrophy was noted in patients receiving the standard formula, but no change in villous height was observed when glutamine was provided. These clinical improvements are consistent with a role for glutamine in preserving mucosal structure and function during the administration of TPN.

Wiley W. Souba, M.D., Sc.D.

References

1. Moore FA, Moore EE, Poggetti R, et al: Gut bacterial translocation via the portal vein: A clinical perspective with major torso trauma. *J Trauma* 31:629–638, 1991.
2. Chu KU, Higashides, Evers BM, et al: Bombesin improves survival from methotrexate-induced enterocolitis. *Ann Surg* 220:570–577, 1994.
3. Huang KF, Chung DH, Herndon DN: Insulin-like growth factor 1 (IGF-1) reduces gut atrophy and bacterial translocation after severe burn injury. *Arch Surgery* 128:47–53, 1993.
4. van der Hulst RRWJ, van Kreel BK, von Meyenfeldt MF: Glutamine and the preservation of gut integrity. *Lancet* 341:1363–1365, 1993.

Metabolic Aspects of the Catastrophic State

Superior Nitrogen Balance After Laparoscopic-Assisted Colectomy

Senagore AJ, Kilbride MJ, Luchtefeld MA, MacKeigan JM, Davis AT, Moore JD (Ferguson-Blodgett Digestive Disease Inst, Grand Rapids, Mich; Michigan State Univ, East Lansing; Cook County Hosp, Chicago; et al)
Ann Surg 221:171–175, 1995   140-95-8-1

Background.—A significant advantage of early resumption of enteral nutrition after gastrointestinal surgery is early positive nitrogen balance. The use of enteral feeding tubes to accomplish early feeding in patients undergoing laparotomy is uncomfortable and associated with a variety of mechanical and infectious complications; the cost of the solutions and increased nursing care is an additional problem. Nitrogen balance after laparoscopic-assisted colectomy was compared with that after open colectomy in a prospective study.

Methods.—There were 19 patients; 10 had open colectomy and 9 had laparoscopic-assisted colectomy. Postoperatively, assessment of nitrogen intake and 24-hour urine collections were performed and total urinary urea nitrogen and urinary 3-methylhistidine were analyzed.

Results.—In patients who underwent laparoscopic-assisted colectomy, time to passage of flatus, resumption of oral intake, and first bowel movement were significantly earlier. Also, operative time was longer, hospital stay was significantly shorter, total hospital charges were lower, and Karnofsky performance scores were significantly higher. Pneumonia and wound infections occurred only in patients with open colectomy; also, blood loss was higher and incidence of infectious complications was significantly higher in patients with open colectomy. Between the 2 groups, urinary nitrogen losses were similar, but patients with laparoscopic-assisted colectomy achieved superior nitrogen intake earlier and also achieved net positive nitrogen balance significantly earlier. Urinary loss of 3-methylhistidine was similar in the 2 groups.

Conclusion.—These results are similar to the best results from nasojejunal tube feeding without intubation or increased nursing care. Patients undergoing laparoscopic-assisted colectomy can resume early enteral nutrition without intubation. Improved nutritional support may contribute to a lower incidence of septic complications in these patients. Laparoscopic-assisted colectomy offers a significant nutritional advantage over standard laparotomy and may lower the cost of care.

▶ We have generally assumed that functional recovery after an operative procedure is paralleled by a normalization of altered biochemical indices. Indeed, Senagore and colleagues have demonstrated that nitrogen balance is improved in patients undergoing laparoscopic colectomy compared with those having standard "open" resections. This improvement in nitrogen balance correlated with a faster recovery—previous studies have shown that such patients return to work sooner. In addition to a diminution in the stress response, such patients are able to resume normal food intake much sooner—both of these occurrences contributed to the improved nitrogen balance observed. Moreover, hospitalization was shorter and complications were diminished in the laparoscopic colectomy group, and these improvements translated into cost savings. Should further studies demonstrate that laparoscopic colectomy does not negatively impact survival or tumor recurrence, the economics will drive the use of "minimally invasive surgery" in the care of these patients.—W.W. Souba, M.D., Sc.D.

Aging Exaggerates Glucose Intolerance Following Injury
Watters JM, Moulton SB, Clancey SM, Blakslee JM, Monaghan R (Univ of Ottawa, Canada; Ottawa Civic Hosp, Canada)
J Trauma 37:786–791, 1994   140-95-8–2

Introduction.—After traumatic injury, patients often have changes in carbohydrate metabolism, including hyperglycemia and glucose intolerance. These changes also occur as a response to normal aging. The inter-

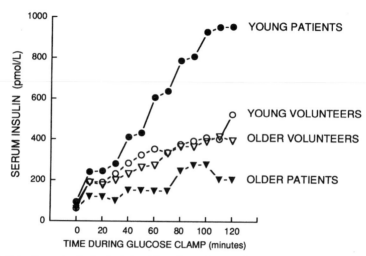

Fig 8–1.—Serum insulin levels during 2-hour hyperglycemic glucose camp in young and older patients and volunteers. (Courtesy of Watters JM, Moulton SB, Clancey SM, et al: *J Trauma* 37:786–791, 1994.)

action of aging and injury may magnify the difficulty of providing adequate nutritional and metabolic care of elderly patients who have had trauma. To test this hypothesis, insulin responses and whole body glucose uptake were studied in young and older patients who have had trauma and healthy volunteers.

Methods.—Two-hour hyperglycemic glucose clamp studies were performed in stable and fully resuscitated patients with trauma and healthy, active volunteers either younger than age 30 or older than age 60. Blood and urine samples were also obtained during the testing period for analysis of plasma insulin, C-peptide, and glucagon levels, and urine glucose, C-peptide, and cortisol levels. Patients with known metabolic dysfunction, pregnancy, or Glasgow Coma Scale scores below 14 at admission were excluded.

Results.—The younger and older patients with trauma had comparable Injury Severity Scores and underwent glucose studies on similar postinjury days. At baseline, urine cortisol and plasma glucose and glucagon levels were higher in patients than in volunteers but did not differ between age groups. During the steady-state period, plasma glucose levels were higher in both injured and older patients, compared with healthy and younger patients, respectively. In response to glucose infusion, serum insulin and C-peptide level increases were related both to injury and to age (Fig 8–1). Changes in urine glucose and cortisol levels were related to injury but not to age. Whole body uptake of exogenous glucose was reduced in patients compared with volunteers, and in older compared with younger groups.

Discussion.—Aging significantly affects glucose homeostasis after injury, mainly because of reduced insulin secretion and exogenous glucose disposal. These findings have important implications for the use of glucose as the principal calorie source in critically ill or injured elderly patients.

▶ Watters and colleagues have shown that aging has a major impact on postinjury glucose metabolism, being associated with exaggerated glucose intolerance and a diminished insulin response to glucose infusion. Although the study does not provide detailed insights into the mechanism of peripheral insulin resistance, it does suggest that, in older patients, insulin responsiveness to a glucose challenge is about half of that of young patients. As many as one third of patients hospitalized for treatment of injuries are older than 60 years of age and the length of hospitalization for such individuals is longer than for younger patients. The use of glucose as a principal calorie source during nutritional support may be more limited in acutely ill elderly patients and potentially more dangerous. Blood glucose levels should be monitored closely, and a reduction in the rate of administration of glucose may be necessary. Administration of insulin to control glucose in the physiologic range may be of benefit to these individuals.—W.W. Souba, M.D., Sc.D.

Modulation of Cellular Proliferation Alters Glutamine Transport and Metabolism in Human Hepatoma Cells

Bode BP, Souba WW (Harvard Med School, Boston)
Ann Surg 220:411–424, 1994   140-95-8–3

Introduction.—Hepatoma cells transport glutamine 10–30 times faster than normal hepatocytes. Additionally, hepatoma cells express 2 disparate proteins to fulfill their heightened need for glutamine. The effects of attenuation of cellular proliferation on glutamine transport and metabolism were examined in hepatoma cells.

Methods.—Proliferation rates, glutamine transport, and glutaminase activities were determined in human hepatoma cell lines HepG2, Huh-7 and SK-Hep. These were ascertained in the presence and absence of chemotherapeutic agents novobiocin and butyrate, as were the transport activities of alanine, arginine, and leucine. Glutaminase activity was determined for normal hepatic tissue, then compared with that in hepatoma cells.

Results.—Glutaminase activities were 6 times higher than the activity found in a normal human liver. Although there were differences in proliferation rates, glutaminase activities were similar in HepG2, Huh-7, and SK-Hep. Hepatomas expressed the kidney-type isozyme. Normal hepatocytes expressed liver-specific glutaminase. Cellular proliferation was inhibited and glutamine transport and glutaminase activity were reduced by more than 50% after 48 hours in SK-Hep cells when treated with butyrate and novobiocin. The slower-growing and more differentiated

HepG2 and Huh-7 cell lines required 72 hours to attenuate glutamine uptake by 30% and 50%, respectively. A 30% to 60% attenuation of transport of alanine, arginine, and leucine was noted in the treatment of all 3 cell lines when novobiocin and butyrate were combined.

Conclusion.—Marked increases in glutamine transport and metabolism characterize hepatocellular transformation. Glutamine transport and metabolism are attenuated by inhibition of cellular proliferation. Inhibition of cellular proliferation similarly affects amino acid transporters.

▶ The process of tumorigenesis in this study was associated with a marked increase in cellular proliferation and a simultaneous 15- to 30-fold increase in the uptake of glutamine to support intermediary metabolism, protein synthesis, and nucleotide biosynthesis. The molecular events involved in the regulation of this marked increase in glutamine transport are unclear. Moreover, the fate of the transported glutamine has not been well studied. Although hepatomas are likely to use glutamine as a preferential fuel, it is unlikely that the metabolic rate of these malignant cells is increased many-fold. Thus, the additional glutamine taken up may be used to replenish tri-carboxylic (TCA) cycle intermediates that are siphoned off rapidly by these metabolically active cells to support the synthesis of key molecules. Evidence for this is the sixfold increase in glutaminase activity and the expression of the high affinity kidney-type glutaminase that is not expressed in normal hepatocytes. This enzyme converts glutamine to glutamate, which can subsequently enter the TCA cycle at the level of α-ketoglutarate. Preventing the malignant cell from taking up glutamine or blocking its intracellular metabolism may have therapeutic possibilities.—W.W. Souba, M.D., Sc.D.

Injury-Induced Inhibition of Fat Absorption
Carter EA, Tompkins RG (Harvard Med School, Boston; Massachusetts Gen Hosp, Boston)
J Burn Care Rehabil 15:154–157, 1994   140-95-8-4

Background.—Thermal injury transiently reduces the uptake of various nutrients; inhibits the synthesis of DNA, RNA, and protein in the gut mucosa; and impedes barrier function. In addition, plasma triglyceride levels increase after burn injury. The clearance of triglycerides from the plasma is reduced because of an inhibitory effect of burn injury on lipoprotein lipase. It is possible that lipase in the intestinal brush border, which hydrolyzes triglyceride to free fatty acids and is required for absorption of triglycerides, might also be inhibited.

Objective and Methods.—The absorption and oxidation of enterally administered ^{14}C-palmitate triglyceride were estimated in thermally injured rats. Lipase activity in the brush border and the small bowel and colonic content of fat also were determined. The animals were subjected to a full-thickness 20% body surface injury.

Results.—The absorption of labeled triglyceride and the production of $^{14}CO_2$ were reduced by half 18 hours after thermal injury. Brush border lipase activity also was reduced by 50%.

Conclusion.—Burn injury appears to render the intestine unable to properly absorb fat. Inhibition of intestinal lipase activity may be at least partly responsible.

▶ The authors have shown that intestinal fat absorption is diminished after burn injury. How soon after injury this alteration begins to become apparent and when it abates is unclear from the study. Nonetheless, an impairment in intestinal fat absorption suggests that enteral diets fed to burn patients should contain appropriate fuels, especially in view of recent investigations that have shown the benefits of immediate enteral nutrition after thermal injury. Decreasing the fat content and increasing the carbohydrate calories in the diet fed to burn patients is implied from this work.—W.W. Souba, M.D., Sc.D.

Starvation Induces Differential Small Bowel Luminal Amino Acid Transport
Sarac TP, Souba WW, Miller JH, Ryan CK, Koch M, Bessey PQ, Sax HC (Univ of Rochester, New York; Massachusetts Gen Hosp, Boston)
Surgery 116:679–686, 1994   140-95-8-5

Introduction.—Studies have shown that different dietary amino acids have specific roles in small intestinal transporter protein activity, nutrient absorption during normal feeding, and metabolic responses to stress.

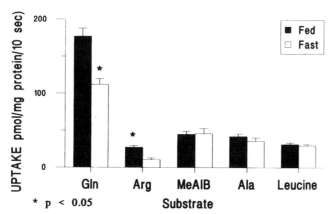

Fig 8–2.—Effects of 72-hour fasting on active amino acid transport in brush border membrane vesicles (BBMV). Jejunal BBMV from control (Fed) and fasted rabbits were incubated with 100 μmol/L of glutamine (Gln), arginine (Arg), alanine (Ala), methylamino-isobutyric acid (MeAIB), and leucine amino acid uptake buffer for 10 seconds. Values are mean ± SEM from 4 separate BBMV preparations. (Courtesy of Sarac TP, Souba WW, Miller JH, et al: *Surgery* 116:679–686, 1994.)

However, small intestinal amino acid transport during fasting has not been characterized. Using an animal model, amino acid transport in the brush border membrane vesicles (BBMV) was studied during nutrient deprivation.

Methods.—Fourteen New Zealand white rabbits were fasted for 72 hours, and another 12 rabbits were allowed ad libitum feeding. The jejunum was removed, and BBMV were prepared from mucosal scrapings and purified. The uptake of radiolabeled glutamine, alanine, leucine, arginine, and methylamino-isobutyric acid by the BBMV was measured by rapid mixing filtration.

Results.—Fasting resulted in an average weight loss of 138 g and also caused significant reduction in villous height. Nutrient deprivation significantly inhibited the transport of glutamine and arginine, while having no effect on the uptake of methylamino-isobutyric acid, alanine, and leucine by the BBMV (Fig 8-2). Glutamine transport was reduced at each of the tested substrate concentrations in the animals that were fasted.

Discussion.—The activities of certain, but not all, carrier proteins were blunted in the small intestine of animals deprived of nutrients. The nutritive transport decreased and gluconeogenic precursor transport was maintained. This differential transport activity response to fasting may cause some of the food intolerance experienced by patients after prolonged bowel rest, which is common in surgical and critically ill patients.

Growth Hormone Enhances Amino Acid Uptake by the Human Small Intestine
Inoue Y, Copeland EM, Souba WW (Univ of Florida, Gainesville; Massachusetts Gen Hosp, Boston; Harvard Med School, Boston)
Ann Surg 219:715–724, 1994   140-95-8-6

Background.—The administration of growth hormone (GH) to malnourished or catabolic surgical patients improves protein gain and muscle strength. It is not known whether these anabolic effects are partially attributable to the effect of GH on nutrient uptake from the gut. The luminal transport of amino acids and glucose in the small intestine was studied in patients given GH.

Methods.—Twelve adult patients without weight loss or clinically significant organ dysfunction were randomly divided into 3 groups and treated for 3 days preoperatively. Five patients received high-dose GH (.2 mg/kg daily), 2 patients received low-dose GH (.1 mg/kg daily) subcutaneously, and 5 control patients received no GH. Segments of jejunum were obtained from 4 patients and ileum from 8 patients. Brush border membrane vesicles (BBMVs) were prepared by differential centrifugation. A rapid mixing/filtration technique was used to measure carrier-mediated transport of glutamine, leucine, alanine, arginine, MeAIB (methyl α-aminoisobutyric acid), and glucose by BBMVs.

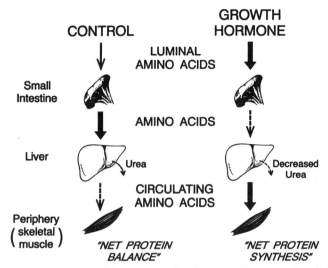

Fig 8–3.—Interorgan amino acid flows in control and GH-treated patients. Growth hormone increases amino acid uptake by the small intestine while reducing hepatic plasma membrane transport activity. This reduces the rate of hepatic ureagenesis and provides additional circulating amino acids to support protein synthesis in skeletal muscle. (Courtesy of Inoue Y, Copeland EM, Souba WW: *Ann Surg* 219:715–724, 1994.)

Results.—Amino acid transport rates in both the ileal and jejunal BBMVs were not significantly increased by low-dose GH treatment. However, high-dose GH treatment caused a generalized 20% to 70% increase in amino acid transport. Glucose transport was not affected. The results of the GH treatment were the same in the ilium and jejunum. The increased transport of leucine and glutamine was caused by a 50% increase in carrier V_{max}, suggesting the brush border membrane had an increased number of functional carriers. The total rates of amino acid uptake from the small intestinal lumen of GH-treated patients were increased by 35% (Fig 8–3). The results are consistent with other studies showing that GH redistributes the flow of amino acids to support peripheral tissue anabolism.

Conclusions.—Growth hormone enhances the uptake of amino acids from the small intestine. These amino acids provide energy and precursors for protein synthesis in the gut mucosa and substrate for anabolism in peripheral tissues. Additional studies are needed to define any beneficial effect of combining GH and aggressive enteral feeding in critically ill patients.

▶ Inasmuch as the bowel plays a major role in absorbing nutrients, surgeons have become interested in gut physiology and have done a number of studies to investigate how this role can be supported. Sarac and colleagues demonstrated that fasting results in a decrease in the activities of several brush border amino acid transport proteins. These proteins reside in the brush border membrane of the enterocytes and serve to bind luminal amino acids and translocate them into the cytoplasm of the cell. A diminished activity is consistent with a reduced number of transporters—such a response is appropriate when luminal substrate is not provided. The gut responds to the presence or absence of luminal nutrients by up-regulating or down-regulating transport activity. In response to feeding, for example, transport activity can be stimulated. Clearly, an increase in transport is required to deliver luminal nutrients into the portal circulation. Feeding the gut stimulates it to maintain its functions, 1 of which is to serve as an organ of nutrient uptake. This transport function of the gut mucosa may be further amplified by using trophic agents such as GH. Although GH has been shown to stimulate protein synthesis and wound healing, Inoue and colleagues showed that it also stimulates amino acid and glucose transport by the human small intestine. Such nutrients serve as precursors to support protein synthesis and energy metabolism. The combination of growth hormone and luminal nutrition may work synergistically to enhance nutrient absorption by the small intestine. These observations have important clinical implications in surgical patients.—W.W. Souba, M.D., Sc.D.

---

³¹P Magnetic Resonance Spectroscopy Demonstrates Expansion of the Extracellular Space in the Skeletal Muscle of Starved Rats

Mizobata Y, Rounds JD, Prechek D, DeRosa E, Wilmore DW, Jacobs DO (Brigham and Women's Hosp, Boston; Harvard Med School, Boston)
J Surg Res 56:491–499, 1994   140-95-8-7

Objective.—Because starvation significantly changes the distribution of water in the body, its effects on both water distribution and cellular energy metabolism in skeletal muscle were studied in rats by ³¹P magnetic resonance spectroscopy (MRS).

Methods.—Two ³¹P MRS-visible water space markers were used to quantify the volumes of intracellular and extracellular water in gastrocnemius muscle samples from male Wistar rats. Dimethyl methylphosphonate (DMMP) was used as a marker of total body water, and phenylphosphonate (PPA) was used as a marker of extracellular water. Studies were repeated after starvation or ad lib feeding for 4 days. Muscle water

TABLE 1.—In Vitro Substrate Concentrations

	Control	Starvation
ATP (μmole/g wet wt)	6.81 $\pm$ 0.24	7.33 $\pm$ 0.28
Protein (mg/g tissue)	301.4 $\pm$ 12.2	153.6 $\pm$ 17.4*
Creatine (μmole/g wet wt)	14.70 $\pm$ 1.02	19.10 $\pm$ 0.96*

Note: Data are means $\pm$ SEM
* $P < .01$ vs. Control by ANOVA
(Courtesy of Mizobata Y, Rounds JD, Prechek D, et al: *J Surg Res* 56:491–499, 1994.)

TABLE 2.—Changes in High-Energy Phosphate Ratios and pH

	Control		Starvation	
	Day 0	Day 4	Day 0	Day 4
PCr/ATP	4.10 ± 0.04	4.11 ± 0.06	4.09 ± 0.06	$3.61 \pm 0.06^{*}\dagger$
PCr/P_i	11.9 ± 0.59	13.3 ± 0.94	13.1 ± 1.22	$10.1 \pm 0.47^{*}\dagger$
ATP/P_i	2.89 ± 0.15	3.24 ± 0.14	3.21 ± 0.29	2.80 ± 0.22
pH_i	7.22 ± 0.01	$7.19 \pm 0.01\dagger$	7.24 ± 0.01	$7.18 \pm 0.01\dagger$
pH_e	7.33 ± 0.02	7.32 ± 0.03	7.38 ± 0.01	$7.30 \pm 0.02\dagger$

Note: Data are means $\pm$ SEM. Data were analyzed by ANOVA repeated measures, LSD.
Abbreviations: PCr, phosphocreatine; *pH_i,* intracellular pH; *pH_e,* extracellular pH
* $P < .01$ vs. Control
$\dagger P < .01$ vs. Day 0
(Courtesy of Mizobata Y, Rounds JD, Prechek D, et al: *J Surg Res* 56:491–499, 1994.)

spaces also were estimated using the chloride method and Nernst's equation.

Results.—Muscle water content, determined by drying, was comparable in the starved and fed animals. In vivo measurements of DMMP relative to all MRS-visible phosphates also indicated similar total water space in the 2 groups, but starvation significantly increased the ratio of PPA to DMMP from .67 to .87. Expansion of the extracellular space was associated with contraction of the intracellular compartment in starved rats. Similar changes were documented in vitro by the chloride method (Table 1). The ratio of phosphocreatine to adenosine triphosphate (ATP) decreased in starved animals (Table 2), and was inversely related to change in the PPA/DMMP ratio.

Conclusion.—Starvation appears to change the distribution of water in skeletal muscle tissue in association with depletion of energy stores.

▶ A vascular permeability defect, manifested as "third-spacing," is a characteristic clinical feature of critically ill patients. Changes in the distribution of body water and various ions are important to consider when evaluating the effects of various stresses on a cell and the efficacy of therapeutic interventions designed to improve cellular health. For example, there is good evidence that the cellular hydration state is an important factor controlling protein turnover, and that cellular shrinkage alone may be sufficient to trigger the net breakdown of intracellular protein. Magnetic resonance spectroscopy is an accurate, noninvasive technique that can be used to measure: 1) changes in water distribution and pH; 2) intracellular and extracellular sodium; 3) chemical reaction rates (including ATP synthesis and breakdown); 4) changes in free ADP and energy status; and 5) cellular function and ATP turnover. In this study, Mizobata and associates have shown that starvation alters the distribution of water within skeletal muscle and that these changes are related to the depletion of energy stores. Magnetic resonance spectroscopy is a noninvasive technique that is likely to be used clinically to evaluate the energy and hydration state of surgical patients.—W.W. Souba, M.D., Sc.D.

Specific Nutrients

Contrasting Effects of Identical Nutrients Given Parenterally or Enterally After 70% Hepatectomy

Delany HM, John J, Teh EL, Li C-S, Gliedman ML, Steinberg JJ, Levenson SM (Albert Einstein College, The Bronx, NY; Montefiore Med Ctr, The Bronx, NY)
Am J Surg 167:135–144, 1994   140-95-8–8

Hypothesis.—Nutritional care is a key aspect in the care of patients who require major hepatic resection due to primary or metastatic malignancy, or in the course of repairing a liver injury. Clinical experience suggested that prolonged parenteral nutrition has adverse effects on patients undergoing major resections of liver tissue compared with enteral nutrition.

Objective.—The effects of total parenteral nutrition (TPN) and total enteral nutrition (TEN) were compared with those of standard oral feeding in rats subjected to 70% hepatic resection.

Methods.—The jugular vein was catheterized, and a gastrostomy catheter was placed at the time of liver resection. A formula designed to approximate normal intake was administered at half-strength on the first day, three-fourths strength on the second day, and full strength thereafter. The diet included a 20% fat emulsion and provided 216 kcal/kg daily. The surviving animals were killed 7 days postoperatively.

Results.—Mortality in the first postoperative week was 68% in the TPN group, but only 9% in the TEN and standard feeding groups. Among animals that survived, those in the TPN group had the lowest serum albumin and bilirubin levels and the highest wet weight of regenerated liver. Nevertheless, TPN recipients had very low levels of glycogen in their livers and decreased amphophylic hepatocyte cytoplasm. Their spleens were twice the size of those in the other groups. Mortality was high whether the fat emulsion was given as a daily bolus or through IV, and even if it was omitted (Fig 8–4). When the caloric content of the TPN formula was varied, an increasing intake correlated with higher mortality rates. None of the TEN recipients died.

Conclusion.—Rats undergoing a large hepatic resection do best when fed enterally and when given a caloric load that can be managed by the remaining liver tissue.

▶ This simple but well-done study indicates that TEN is superior to TPN after major hepatic resection. The authors administered identical solutions enterally and parenterally to allow comparison of the route of administration on outcome. A similar study was done 15 years ago by Kudsk (1) and colleagues. They demonstrated that rats subjected to an intraperitoneal injection of hemoglobin and *Escherichia coli* had an enhanced survival rate when

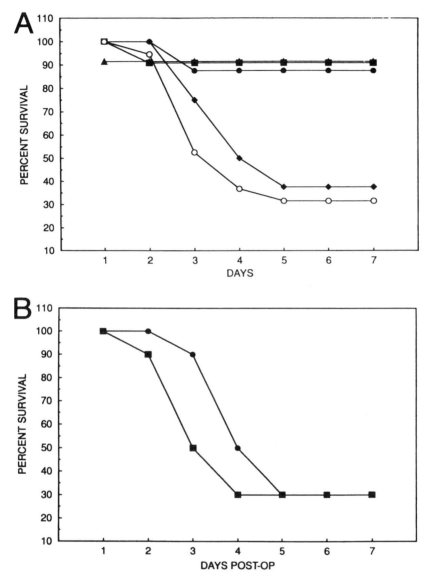

Fig 8–4.—A, Contrasting effects of route of nutrient administration on mortality of rats with 70% hepatectomy. Rats receiving total parenteral nutrition, the fat emulsion given as a bolus infusion (*open circles*) or continuously by incorporating it with the other nutrients (*closed diamonds*), had a much higher mortality than rats receiving the same nutrients at the same rates via the enteral route, TEN with fat emulsion given as a bolus (*closed squares*) and TEN with fat emulsion given continuously (*closed circles*) and rats eating rat chow ad libitum (*closed triangles*). **B,** Effect of isocaloric, isonitrogenous TPN with (*closed circles*) and without (*closed squares*) fat emulsion on mortality of rats with 70% hepatectomy. (Courtesy of Delany, HM, John J, Teh EL, et al: *Am J Surg* 167:135–144, 1994.)

the same nutrient solution was given enterally rather than parenterally. This study by Delany et al. is in contrast to the study by Fan and colleagues (2) that showed a reduction in major complications in patients undergoing major hepatic resection who received perioperative TPN. One difference between these 2 studies (other than 1 being done in rats and the other in patients) was that patients in the Fan study were allowed to consume some nutrients orally.—W.W. Souba, M.D., Sc.D.

References

1. Kudsk KA, Carpenter G, Peterson S et al: Effect of enteral and parenteral feeding in malnourished rats with E. coli-hemoglobin adjuvant peritonitis. *J Surg Res* 31:105–110, 1981.
2. Fan ST, Lo CM, Lai EC et al: Perioperative nutritional support in patients undergoing hepatectomy for hepatocellular carcinoma *N Engl J Med* 331:1547–1552, 1994.

Effect of Low and High Amounts of a Structured Lipid Containing Fish Oil on Protein Metabolism in Enterally Fed Burned Rats

Selleck KJ, Wan JM-F, Gollaher CJ, Babayan VK, Bistrian BR (Harvard Med School, Boston)
Am J Clin Nutr 60:216–222, 1994   140-95-8-9

Introduction.—The nutritional benefits of fat intake have been established in the treatment of burn injury. However, optimal fat intake has not been defined. The protein-sparing effects of a structured lipid (SL) were measured to determine optimal fat intake. The subsequent meta-

	Cumulative Nitrogen Balance	
Group	Preburn (days 1 + 2)	Postburn (days 3–6)
Control	209.4 ± 13.8	163.2 ± 12.9*
SL 10%	190.5 ± 12.7	162.3 ± 8.9*
LCT 10%	177.3 ± 10.1	145.7 ± 3.9*
SL 35%	153.3 ± 11.1† ‡	152.0 ± 10.9
LCT 35%	136.9 ± 13.2† ‡ §	137.1 ± 7.4

Abbreviations: SL, structured lipid; LCT, long-chain triglyceride
Note: Values are means ± SEM, no. = 7. Significance of diet effects, $P < .0001$ (two-way analysis of variance); significance of postburn vs. preburn, $P < .003$ (two-way analysis of variance).
* Significantly different from preburn, $P < .05$.
† Significantly different from control group, $P < .05$.
‡ Significantly different from LCT 10% group, $P < .05$.
§ Significantly different from SL 10% group, $P < .05$.
(Courtesy of Selleck KJ, Wan JM-F, Gollaher CJ, et al: *Am J Clin Nutr* 60:216–222, 1994.)

bolic responses were compared with those produced by similar amounts of long-chain triglyceride (LCT) in burned rats fed by gastrostomy.

Methods.—Male Sprague-Dawley rats were fed an enteral diet for 7 days and randomly placed in 1 of 5 groups. A control group received non-protein energy as dextrose. The remaining groups received 10% or 35% of nonprotein energy as SL or 10% or 35% of non-protein energy as LCT. Rats received a burn injury on day 3. Preburn, on day 2, indirect calorimetry and nitrogen balance were measured. The measurement was repeated postburn, on days 4 and 6.

Results.—The respiratory quotient was higher in rats fed the low-fat and control diets compared with those with high-fat diets. Total energy expenditure was significantly increased postburn, particularly with 35% LCT. A significant drop in nitrogen balance was found in the rats fed low-fat or no-fat diets postburn that was not seen in those fed 35% fat. The group fed 10% SL did significantly better than the groups fed 10% and 35% LCT (table).

Conclusion.—Results confirm the better protein-sparing effects of SLs compared with conventional LCT administration. Ten percent SL appears to be optimal for nutritional support in burn injury.

▶ Studies in both patients and animals suggest that both the quantity of lipid and the fatty acid composition of the lipid can significantly influence the metabolic responses associated with catabolic disease states. Structured lipids that contain a mixture of fish oils (first double bond after the third carbon, so-called ω-3 fatty acids) and medium-chain triglycerides appear to be superior to conventional lipids that contain longer-chain triglycerides (β-6 fatty acids). The study by Selleck et al. supports the authors' previous findings that SLs have unique protein-sparing properties that are not evident with conventional LCT administration. Structured lipids should be provided in low amounts (10% of total fat calories) to provide optimal nutritional support.—W.W. Souba, M.D., Sc.D.

Intraluminal Glutamine Refeeding Supports Mucosal Growth in Rat Jejunum
Wirén M, Skullman S, Wang F, Permert J, Larsson J (Univ of Linköping, Sweden)
Transplant Proc 26:1460–1463, 1994   140-95-8-10

Background.—Surgical patients often become malnourished and, as a result, may be at a higher risk of having surgical complications develop. Tissue levels of glutamine are reduced in this setting. Glutamine is metabolized by rapidly dividing cells and is very important to the integrity of the small bowel.

Objective.—The effects of refeeding glutamine on the proliferative activity of the small bowel mucosa were examined in malnourished rats

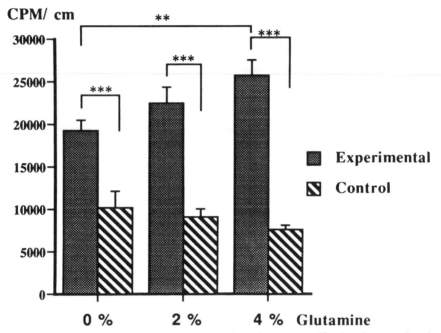

Fig 8–5.—Counts per minute (CPM)/cm mucosa 1 hour after injection of ³H-thymidine in study and control rats with different glutamine-containing diets. Values are means ± SEM. ** P < .01; *** P < .001. (Courtesy of Wirén M, Skullman S, Wang F, et al: *Transplant Proc* 26:1460–1463, 1994.)

after abdominal surgery. Study animals were starved for 3 days before undergoing laparotomy. After surgery they were re-fed for 3 days with a diet containing no glutamine, 2% glutamine, or 4% glutamine.

Results.—Their body weight decreased 12% during starvation and increased 10% during refeeding. The weight of the mucosa decreased in animals not re-fed glutamine. Both supplements increased the mucosal protein content, and the 4% supplement was associated with an increased DNA content. Thymidine incorporation, which took place mainly in the crypt cells, was increased in the 4% supplement group (Fig 8–5). Villous height was increased in this group and decreased in the nonsupplemented group.

Conclusion.—These results are consistent with a central role for glutamine in maintaining the integrity of the small bowel mucosa under conditions of starvation.

► Provision of glutamine in enteral diets provided to patients may stimulate mucosal turnover and maintain gut integrity. Enteral diets, in general, contain relatively small amounts of glutamine. This study is consistent with previous studies that have demonstrated the beneficial effects of glutamine on gut barrier function. The work also points out the need for carefully designed clinical studies that examine the potential salutory effects of luminal glutamine. Such studies have been much less common than investigations using glutamine-enriched parenteral nutrition.—W.W. Souba, M.D., Sc.D.

Triglyceride-Rich Lipoproteins Improve Survival When Given After Endotoxin in Rats

Read TE, Grunfeld C, Kumwenda Z, Calhoun MC, Kane JP, Feingold KR, Rapp JH (Univ of California, San Francisco; Veterans Affairs Med Ctr, San Francisco)

Surgery 117:62–67, 1995   140-95-8-11

Introduction.—Mobilization of triglyceride-rich lipoproteins is an early response to bacterial endotoxin. Animal studies have shown that triglyceride-rich chylomicrons administered before a lethal injection of endotoxin protect the animal from death by binding endotoxin and by accel-

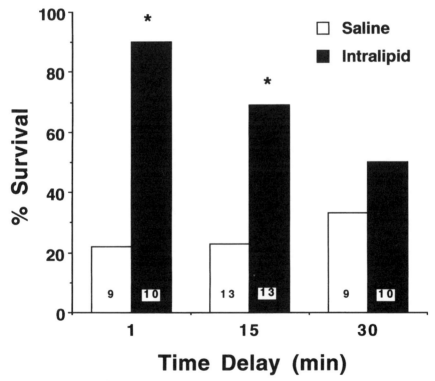

Fig 8–6.—Survival of rats after lethal dose of endotoxin, treated subsequently with either Intralipid or saline solution. Rats were given lethal dose of *Escherichia coli* endotoxin by IV infusion at time = 0, followed at various time intervals (1, 15, 30 minutes) by IV bolus infusion of either synthetic triglyceride-rich lipid emulsion Intralipid (1 g of Intralipid triglyceride/kg) or equal volume of normal saline solution. Survival was measured at 48 hours. Statistical significance was determined by χ^2 analysis, *$P < .05$. Number inside each bar represents total number of rats in that group. (Courtesy of Read TE, Grunfeld C, Kumwenda Z, et al: *Surgery* 117:62–67, 1995.)

erating endotoxin clearance. A study was undertaken to determine the protective effect of triglyceride-rich lipoprotein administration after endotoxin injection.

Methods.—Anesthetized rats were injected with a lethal dose of *Escherichia coli* endotoxin. At 1, 15, 30, 45, or 60 minutes after the endotoxin injection, they were given IV rat mesenteric lymph containing either nascent chylomicrons (1 g/kg) or normal saline solution. The number of surviving rats was determined at 48 hours. The experiment was repeated with half the dose of chylomicrons. The protocol was repeated in 2 more sets of experiments, with either a synthetic triglyceride-rich lipid emulsion, Intralipid, or chylomicron-deficient lymph substituting for lymph-containing chylomicrons. In another experiment, rats were given either chylomicrons or saline 1 minute after infusion of radio-iodinated endotoxin and were killed 15, 45, or 90 minutes later. The liver, spleen, heart, skeletal muscle, and blood were assayed for radio-iodine.

Results.—Survival was significantly improved with chylomicron infusion up to 30 minutes after endotoxin injection, with earlier administration predicting greater survival benefit. Survival was also significantly improved with Intralipid infusions up to 15 minutes after endotoxin injection (Fig 8–6). Survival was increased with both infusions in a dose-dependent manner. Radio-iodinated endotoxin distribution patterns demonstrated quicker clearance from blood and increased uptake by the liver with the chylomicron infusion.

Discussion.—Pretreatment with triglyceride-rich lipoproteins have a protective effect after endotoxins are already in the system for 15–30 minutes. The chylomicrons altered endotoxin metabolism, accelerating its plasma clearance, and increasing its uptake by the liver. Lipoproteins perform anti-inflammatory and anti-infectious functions.

▶ This is yet another study examining the effects of a specific nutrient on outcome after a catabolic insult. The early administration of triglyceride-rich lipoproteins (chylomicrons) had a protective effect against endotoxin by enhancing its plasma clearance and increasing its uptake by the liver. This translated into an improvement in survival after a lethal dose of endotoxin. Lipoproteins are generally thought of as playing a role in lipid transport—this study emphasizes that they also have important anti-inflammatory effects as well.—W.W. Souba, M.D., Sc.D.

Nutrition and Gut Function

Supplementation of an Elemental Enteral Diet With Alanyl-Glutamine Decreases Bacterial Translocation in Burned Mice

Tenenhaus M, Hansbrough JF, Zapata-Sirvent RL, Ohara M, Nyhan W (Univ of California, San Diego)
Burns 20:220–225, 1994   140-95-8–12

Percentage Translocation and Microbial Content of Nodes

Groups	Survivors (no.)	Translocation		Log$_{10}$ CFU/g MLN
		±	% +	
A Burn, Chow	29	9/20	31.0*	1.0 ± 0.3†
B Burn, Fast	42	27/15	64.3	2.5 ± 0.3
C Vivonex TEN	59	33/26	55.9	2.0 ± 0.25
D Vivonex TEN plus Ala-Gln	61	22/39	36.1†	1.17 ± 0.206†
E Normal Control	22	0/22	0.0	—

Abbreviations: CFU, colony-forming units; MLN, mesenteric lymph nodes.
* P = .0081 compared with burn fasted.
† P = .009 compared with burn fasted.
(Courtesy of Tenenhaus M, Hansbrough JF, Zapata-Sirvent RL, et al: Burns 20:220–225, 1994.)

Background.—Burn injury makes the bowel mucosa more permeable and enhances bacterial translocation (BT), the process whereby bacteria and their products, including endotoxin, escape the gut lumen to colonize the wound site and distant organs. A number of dietary elements such as glutamine (GLN) reportedly limit morbidity and mortality in stressed patients. Free glutamine, however, is not stable in solution.

Objective.—The value of alanyl-glutamine (ALA-GLN), a soluble form of GLN that remains stable in solution, was studied in mice subjected to a 32% full-thickness cutaneous burn injury.

Methods.—Group A of burn-injured mice was given standard rodent chow, group B was fasted for 24 hours and then fed chow, group C was fed Vivonex TEN, and group D was given Vivonex supplemented with ALA-GLN in a GLN equivalent of 14 g/L. A control group with no burn injury was fed rodent chow. Mesenteric lymph nodes were harvested 48 hours after burn injury, plated, and monitored for bacterial growth as evidence of BT.

Results.—No BT was observed in unburned control mice, but those that were injured and fasted had a 64% incidence. Burn-injured animals fed Vivonex TEN had a 56% rate of BT. Rodent chow provided the best protection against BT, with a 31% rate (table). Animals given Vivonex TEN had a 36% rate of BT when supplemental ALA-GLN was provided.

Conclusion.—An enteral supplement of ALA-GLN, given at an early stage of burn injury, may help pevent BT and the absorption of endotoxin.

Secretory Immunoglobulin A, Intestinal Mucin, and Mucosal Permeability in Nutritionally Induced Bacterial Translocation in Rats

Spaeth G, Gottwald T, Specian RD, Mainous MR, Berg RD, Deitch EA (Rheinische Friedrich-Wihelms-Univ, Bonn, Germany; Eberhard-Karls-Univ, Tuebingen, Germany; Univ of Medicine and Dentistry of New Jersey, Newark)
Ann Surg 220:798–808, 1994   140-95-8–13

Background.—An important and often under-appreciated function of the gut is bacterial translocation, i.e., acting as a barrier to prevent the spread of intraluminal bacteria and endotoxin to systemic organs and tissues. Several investigative groups have documented that parenteral and some enteral diets are associated with loss of intestinal barrier function. Certain therapeutic measures, including the provision of bulk-forming fibers, will limit or reverse diet-induced bacterial translocation. The mechanisms of this are unknown, but they could be hormonally mediated. The effects of nutritional modulation on intestinal permeability, mucin levels, and secretory immunoglobulin A in a model of nutritionally induced bacterial translocation were measured.

Methods.—In rats, intestinal mucin levels, mucosal protein content, immunoglobulin A, intestinal morphological structure, and permeability

Soluble Mucin Levels in Small Intestinal Washings

Soluble mucin

Group	n	Gut Length (ng/cm) Jejunum	Gut Length (ng/cm) Ileum	Mucosal Protein (ng/mg) Jejunum	Mucosal Protein (ng/mg) Ileum
IV-TPN	10	79.0 ± 64.6	93.5 ± 35.4	18.3 ± 17.5	28.2 ± 14.7
IV-TPN + fiber	8	27.8 ± 20.4	58.6 ± 35.7	6.6 ± 4.1	14.0 ± 8.8
p value		<0.05	<0.05	NS	<0.05
ORAL-TPN	9	62.0 ± 34.3	126.6 ± 56.3	9.3 ± 3.9	25.1 ± 9.2
ORAL-TPN + fiber	10	26.5 ± 16.4	78.7 ± 37.5	3.9 ± 2.0	16.5 ± 7.7
p value		<0.01	<0.05	<0.01	<0.05

(Courtesy of Spaeth G, Gottwald T, Specian RD, et al: *Ann Surg* 220:798–808, 1994.)

to horseradish peroxidase, bacterial translocation, and intestinal bacterial population levels were measured 7 days after they received total parenteral nutrition solution enterally or parenterally, and with or without enteral bulk fiber supplements. Control rats were fed chow.

Results.—In rats receiving total parenteral nutrition enterally and parenterally, the incidence of bacterial translocation was significantly reduced by the addition of fiber. Also in these rats, mucosal protein, immunoglobulin A, and insoluble mucin levels were decreased in the jejunum; mucosal protein levels were decreased to a greater extent than immunoglobulin A or mucin. In fiber-fed rats, similar decreases were observed, but the fiber was associated with consistent reduction in jejunal and ileal soluble mucin levels (table).

Conclusions.—The addition of bulk-forming fiber improves intestinal barrier function as measured by peroxidase permeability and bacterial translocation; however, mucosal protein content, mucin, or immunoglobulin A levels are not restored to normal. Bulk-forming fiber in fiber-free enteral diets may be clinically beneficial. The exact mechanism underlying the protective effect of fiber should be explored further.

Total Parenteral Nutrition, Bacterial Translocation, and Host Immune Function

Shou J, Lappin J, Minnard EA, Daly JM (The Univ of Pennsylvania, Philadelphia)
Am J Surg 167:145–150, 1994   140-95-8–14

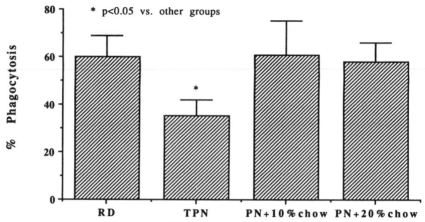

Fig 8–7.—Both parenteral nutrition (PN) and 10% chow and PN and 20% chow resulted in significantly increased mean peritoneal macrophage *Candida albicans* phagocytosis compared with the results in the total parenteral nutrition (TPN) group (P < .05). *Abbreviation: RD*, regular diet. (Courtesy of Shou J, Lappin J, Minnard EA, et al: *Am J Surg* 167:145–150, 1994.)

Introduction.—Infectious complications are significantly greater in perioperative and trauma patients receiving total parenteral nutrition (TPN) compared with those receiving enteral nutrition. The effects of TPN on splenocyte and peritoneal macrophage function and intestinal bacterial translocation were evaluated.

Study I.—Central vein cannulation was done on male Wistar rats. They received isocaloric feedings of a regular chow diet (RD) and were randomly allocated to also receive saline infusion or TPN for 7 days. Concanavalin A mitogenesis, superoxide production, and *Candida albicans* phagocytosis were analyzed upon harvesting splenocytes and peritoneal macrophages. In TPN-fed rats, 77% (10 of 13) had bacteria-positive mesenteric lymph nodes compared with a significantly lower 17% (2 of 12) in RD-fed rats. The RD group showed significantly lower incidence of splenocyte mitogenesis, peritoneal macrophage superoxide production and C. *albicans* phagocytosis.

Study II.—Thirty rats were randomly allocated to receive 7 days of RD, TPN, and parenteral nutrition (PN) with 10% or 20% of calories from oral chow (PN and 10% chow and PN and 20% chow). The TPN-induced suppression of C. *albicans* phagocytosis was reversed with PN and 10% chow. The combination of PN and 20% chow resulted in significant increase of splenocyte mitogenesis, peritoneal macrophage superoxide production, C. *Albicans* phagocytosis and killing, and a decreased incidence of bacteria-positive mesenteric lymph nodes (Fig 8–7).

Conclusion.—Administration of TPN is associated with bacterial translocation, which may have a significant role in TPN-associated immune dysfunction. Infectious complications of TPN may be reduced with the addition of a small amount of enteral feeding.

Role of Early Enteral Feeding and Acute Starvation on Postburn Bacterial Translocation and Host Defense: Prospective, Randomized Trials

Gianotti L, Alexander JW, Nelson JL, Fukushima R, Pyles T, Chalk CL (Univ of Cincinnati, Ohio; Shriners Burns Inst, Cincinnati, Ohio)
Crit Care Med 22:265–272, 1994   140-95-8-15

Background.—The amount of food intake, the route of administration, and the composition of the nutritional formula profoundly affect intestinal structure and function as well as systemic metabolic and immune responses. The effects of acute starvation in a preburn period and early nutritional support after thermal injury on the magnitude of microbial translocation from the intestine and the host's ability to kill translocating organisms were studied.

Methods.—Two prospective, randomized, experimental trials were performed. In the first, mice were starved for 0–24 hours before gavage with 10^{10} ^{14}C-labeled *Escherichia coli* and a 20% burn injury. In the second experiment, guinea pigs were burned over 40% of their bodies and randomly assigned to a complete enteral diet, 175 kcal/kg/day, or infusion of an equal volume of lactated Ringer's solution through a previously placed gastrostomy for 6, 24, or 48 hours. *Escherichia coli* were infused intragastrically after each feeding. All animals were killed 4 hours after gavage for examination.

Findings.—In the first experiment, 18 and 24 hours of preburn starvation increased translocation to the mesenteric lymph nodes only. It also increased bacterial killing in all tested tissues. In the second study, guinea pigs fed enterally for 6, 24, and 48 hours after burn injury had significantly lower bacterial translocation in all tissues compared with animals infused with lactated Ringer's solution. Also, the killing of translocating organisms was enhanced after 24 and 48 hours of feeding.

Conclusions.—Preburn starvation affects translocation and bacterial killing differently than postburn starvation. Postburn enteral nutrition reduces the load of viable bacteria in the tissues by the double mechanism of initial reduced translocation and subsequent improved ability to kill translocating bacteria.

Intestinal Microbial Translocation: Immunologic Consequences and Effects of Interleukin-4

Shou J, Motyka LE, Daly JM (Univ of Pennsylvania, Philadelphia)
Surgery 116:868–876, 1994   140-95-8-16

Introduction.—Bacterial translocation, a process by which intestinal bacteria cross the mucosal barrier and enter the lamina propria and then the mesenteric lymph nodes and other organs, increases in animals fed a chemically defined elemental diet (CDD). However, the impact of this

	Tissue Culture Results		
Tissues	RD	CDD	CDD + IL-4
Study 1			
Positive MLN (%)	0 (1/10)	70 (7/10)*	
Blood/liver spleen	0	0	
Study 2			
Positive MLN (%)			
Day 5	0 (0/10)	0 (0/10)	
Day 8	0 (0/16)	75 (12/16)†	25 (4/16)
CFU/MLN	0	151 ± 30†	63 ± 24‡
Blood/liver/ spleen	0	0	0

* $P < .01$ vs. regular diet (RD).
† $P < .05$ vs. RD.
‡ $P < .05$ vs. chemically defined elemental diet (CDD).
(Courtesy of Shou J, Motyka LE, Daly JM: *Surgery* 116:868–876, 1994.)

bacterial translocation on the lymph nodes and other organs has not been established. The effects of CDD-induced intestinal bacterial translocation and of interleukin-4 (IL-4) on mesenteric lymph node (MLN) lymphocyte, local peritoneal macrophage, and systemic Kuppfer cell (KC) function were studied in mice.

Methods.—Laboratory mice were randomly assigned to be fed either a regular diet, a CDD, or a CDD plus IL-4 for 14 days. The bacterial populations of MLNs and cecum were measured with cultures. Mesenteric lymph node lymphocytes were analyzed with immunoassays to determine mixed lymphocyte response and cytotoxic T-lymphocyte function. Peritoneal macrophages and hepatic KCs were harvested to assess production of tumor necrosis factor, fluorescent lipopolysaccharide binding to macrophages, and the ability of macrophages to phagocytose and kill *Candida albicans*. Kuppfer cells and hepatocytes were cocultured with tritiated leucine to determine the interaction of KCs with hepatocyte protein synthesis. The Ig-A levels in the terminal ileum were assayed.

Results.—Positive MLN bacterial cultures were found in 70% of the mice fed CDD and none of the control mice; the incidence was reduced to 25% in CDD-fed mice also receiving IL-4 (table). Chemically defined elemental diet feeding was associated with significant reductions in the mean mixed lymphocyte response and cytotoxic T-lymphocyte function in the MLN lymphocytes. Tumor necrosis factor production, macrophage binding with lipopolysaccharides, and C. *albicans* phagocytosis and killing were reduced in peritoneal macrophages in CDD-fed mice, but were similar in KCs in both groups. Lipopolysaccharide did not affect protein synthesis in hepatocyte cultures but did suppress protein synthesis in hepatocyte-KC cocultures similarly with both CDD and control groups. In CDD-fed animals given IL-4, peritoneal macrophage superoxide production and C. *albicans* phagocytosis and killing were significantly increased, as was the mean ileal tissue IgA level, compared with CDD-fed and control animals.

Conclusion.—Bacterial translocation induced by CDD feeding is associated with diminished cellular antimicrobial functions in MLN lymphocytes and peritoneal macrophages, but not hepatic KCs. Interleukin-4 administration improved peritoneal macrophage function and increased intestinal IgA, resulting in reduced bacterial translocation to the MLNs.

▶ Although the gut has traditionally been viewed as an organ of quiescence or inactivity, newer evidence has reshaped our thinking about the role of the gut in seriously ill patients. One key role of the gut relates to its function as a barrier to luminal bacteria and their toxins. Microbial translocation can be defined as the passage of both viable and nonviable microbes (bacteria, yeast, viruses) and microbial products (endotoxin) across an anatomically intact barrier. Factors that lead to translocation include: 1) direct injury to the enterocytes (chemotherapy, radiation therapy, inflammatory processes); 2) damage to intercellular tight junctions (endotoxin); 3) immunosuppressive drugs (steroids); 4) reduced intestinal blood flow (hemorrhage, sepsis); 5) an increase in the luminal microbial load (bacterial overgrowth, antibiotics); and 6) altered nutrition. Studies from numerous laboratories have demonstrated that bacterial translocation in animals, as evidenced by the presence of culture-positive mesenteric lymph nodes, is increased by; 1) hemorrhagic shock; 2) antibiotic therapy; 3) bowel obstruction; 4) steroid administration; 5) endotoxin treatment; 6) thermal injury; 7) TPN or feeding an elemental diet; 8) bowel irradiation; 9) administering chemotherapy; or 10) advanced malignant disease.

Studies in humans are not quite as clear-cut, but it has been shown that intestinal permeability is increased in burn patients, in patients receiving TPN, and in volunteers receiving endotoxin. Despite the lack of correlation between the development of septic complications (e.g., organ failure) and the detection of endotoxin and bacteria in the portal system, it does appear that the gut can become leaky under certain circumstances. Evidence for this event is compelling enough in some clinical circumstances that the gut has recently been described as the motor or driver of multiple organ failure in some critically ill patients. It is therefore prudent to use therapeutic measures to maintain gut barrier function. The best single way to maintain a healthy gut is to provide enteral nutrition to critically ill patients whenever feasible. Such feeding does not need to be full strength or at high rates. In fact, critically ill patients often do not tolerate high feeding rates. Even the slow delivery of enteral nutrition into the upper gastrointestinal (GI) tract is likely to be beneficial. Early feeding after burn injury has been shown to be beneficial in terms of reducing the hypermetabolic response, decreasing the incidence of translocation, and preserving intestinal morphology. Several studies of injured patients have demonstrated the superiority of enteral nutrition over PN (or no nutrition) in terms of reducing major complications.

Provision of growth factors (growth hormone, gut peptides) and specific nutrients (GLN, short chain fatty acids [SCFAs], nucleic acids) are 2 other methods that are likely to play a role in maintaining gut integrity. A number of growth factors may assist in preserving gut integrity in critically ill patients. Growth hormone works through the peptide IgF-1, which has been shown to improve barrier function. Besides GLN, other gut nutrients have also been investigated. The SCFAs acetate, butyrate, and proprionate are important fuels for the colon and have been shown to improve colonic function when given intraluminally of systemically. Also, RNA can stimulate intestinal epithelial turnover. None of these compounds is presently added to TPN solutions.—W.W. Souba, M.D., Sc.D.

Reversal by Short-Chain Fatty Acids of Colonic Fluid Secretion Induced by Enteral Feeding

Bowling TE, Raimundo AH, Grimble GK, Silk DBA (Central Middlesex Hosp Trust, London)
Lancet 342:1266–1268, 1993   140-95-8–17

Background.—Diarrhea is the most common complication of enteral feeding, affecting as many as 25% of patients. Research involving healthy subjects has shown that the ascending colon secretes salt and water in response to enteral feeding. The effects of short-chain fatty acids (SCFAs) on this secretory response were studied.

Methods.—Six healthy volunteers, mean age 25 years, were enrolled in the study. After baseline fasting colonic water and electrolyte movement was established, a standard polymeric enteral diet was infused into the stomach while the colon was perfused with a control electrolyte solution or test solution containing SCFA. The 2 perfusates were identical in electrolyte levels and osmolality.

Findings.—Water was absorbed throughout the colon in the fasting state. During the control infusion, water was secreted at a significant rate in the ascending colon, the median rate being 1 mL per minute. The secretion was significantly reversed during the SCFA infusion, resulting in a net absorption. Water absorption was significantly greater in the distal colon during the control infusion compared to the fasting one. During the test infusion, this absorption persisted. At all stages of the study, the movement of sodium, chloride, and potassium ions was similar to that of water. There was no significant change in bicarbonate movement at any stage.

Conclusions.—During enteral feeding, SCFA infusion directly into the cecum reverses the fluid secretion in the ascending colon. This finding may have implications for the treatment of diarrhea resulting from enteral feeding.

▶ The short-chain fatty acids are the C1-6 organic fatty acids. Acetate, propionate, and butyrate account for 83% of SCFAs, which are formed in the gastrointestinal tract of mammals by microbial fermentation of carbohydrates. The SCFAs are readily absorbed by intestinal mucosa, are relatively high in caloric content, and are readily metabolized by intestinal epithelium and liver. Supplementation of total parenteral nutrition (TPN) with SCFAs has been shown to reduce the small bowel mucosal atrophy seen with standard TPN. Similar effects on small bowel mucosa were seen with SCFA-supplemented TPN in rats with massive small bowel resection. The observation by Bowling et al. that infusion of SCFAs into the cecum reversed the fluid secretion seen in the ascending colon during enteral feeding is consistent with their role in salt and water absorption.—W.W. Souba, M.D., Sc.D.

Total Parenteral Nutrition: Basic and Clinical Research

Growth Retardation in Children Receiving Long-Term Total Parenteral Nutrition: Effects of Ornithine α-Ketoglutarate

Moukarzel AA, Goulet O, Salas JS, Marti-Henneberg C, Buchman AL, Cynober L, Rappaport R, Ricour C (Maimonides Med Ctr, Brooklyn, NY; Hôpital Necker Enfants Malades, Paris; Hôpital Saint Antoine, Paris; et al)
Am J Clin Nutr 60:408–413, 1994   140-95-8–18

Introduction.—Patients with impaired intestinal absorption may be dependent on long-term total parenteral nutrition (TPN). Although these children may have no signs of nutritional or endocrine deficiency, they may demonstrate growth retardation. Animal studies have shown that administration of ornithine α-ketoglutarate (OKG) has induced accelerated growth velocity. The effect of OKG supplementation on linear growth was studied in children dependent upon long-term TPN.

Methods.—Six prepubertal children, aged 9.5–16 years, who had received TPN for 5–10 years and had no known endocrinologic dysfunction, were studied during 2 consecutive 5-month periods. All patients were at least 1 SD below the 50th percentile for their expected height, although their heights had previously been at or above the age-appropriate 50th percentile. During the first study period, OKG was added to their otherwise unchanged parenteral solution. Ornithine α-ketoglutarate was not added to the solution during the second period. The patients were monitored with anthropometric measurements and blood analysis at baseline and monthly during the study.

Results.—During the OKG supplementation period, 5 of the 6 patients had increases in linear growth velocity of a median of 155%. During the second period, growth velocity decreased significantly in 3 children and continued to accelerate in 2 children. Growth velocity was unchanged in the sixth patient during both study periods. Overall, the median growth velocity increased from 3.8 cm/yr to 6.45 cm/yr during OKG supplementation and then decreased to 3.65 cm/yr during the second period. The median plasma insulin-like growth factor 1 (IGF1) increased significantly during OKG supplementation, except in the 1 patient who had no changes in growth velocity. The relative increases in IGF1 correlated positively with the relative increases in growth velocity. There were no other significant changes in blood parameters and no side effects of OKG.

Discussion.—Daily OKG supplementation may accelerate linear growth in children dependent on TPN. In addition, IGF1 synthesis increased in children responding with increasing growth velocity. However, more study is required with long-term follow-up of a larger group of patients to conclusively establish a relationship between OKG administration and improved growth velocity and to elucidate the mechanism involved.

▶ Recently, OKG has been proposed as a TPN additive that enhances protein economy. Its mechanism of action is unknown but may relate to its ability to stimulate insulin and growth hormone elaboration. α-Ketoglutarate is a key energy intermediate, and it may replenish tri-carboxylic acid-cycle intermediates during times of heightened metabolism. In this study, the authors demonstrated a beneficial effect on linear growth in children receiving long-term TPN. This clinical investigation, like others, has focused on a specific additive that may be added to standard TPN solutions to enhance their efficacy in promoting nitrogen economy. Children in particular experience growth retardation while on TPN, and supplemental OKG may be useful in promoting statural growth acceleration. The sample size in this study is small, and the authors acknowledge the need for a larger multicenter trial to confirm the results of this preliminary investigation.—W.W. Souba, M.D., Sc.D.

Factors Influencing Compensatory Feeding During Parenteral Nutrition in Rats
Beverly JL, Yang Z-J, Meguid MM (State Univ of New York-Health Science Ctr, Syracuse)
Am J Physiol 266:R1928–R1932, 1994   140-95-8–19

Background.—Animals given nutrients intravenously do not fully adjust their oral food intake to compensate for the infused calories. How efficiently nutrients are used depends on the timing of the infusion in relation to the diurnal cycle and also on the composition of the infusate. The more nutritionally complete an infusate, the better the compensation.

Objective.—The effects of both the diurnal timing of parenteral nutrition (PN) infusion and the composition of the available diet on compensatory feeding were examined in male rats given all their caloric needs as PN.

Observations.—When the timing of infused calories was more closely matched with the diurnal pattern of oral intake, with 75% of calories given during the dark phase and 25% in the light phase, compensation for infused calories increased from 70% to 80%. Comparable compensation occurred when the caloric distribution of the PN infusion had the same composition as the oral diet. With matching for both diurnal pattern and dietary composition, compensation for infused calories increased to 90%.

Conclusion.—The extent of compensatory feeding during infused nutrition is influenced by conditions that determine the metabolic use of the infused nutrients.

Parenteral Nutrition, Brain Glycogen, and Food Intake
Meguid MM, Beverly JL, Yang Z-J, Gleason JR, Meguid RA, Yue M-X (State Univ of New York Health Science Ctr, Syracuse; Syracuse Univ, NY)
Am J Physiol 265:R1387–R1391, 1993   140-95-8-20

Background.—When rats are given 100% of their daily energy requirements by IV parenteral nutrition (PN-100), they reduce their food intake about 80%. If PN-100 is stopped after several days of infusion, a delay in the return of food intake to control levels occurs. Whether whole brain glycogen content is changed during PN-100 and whether changes in brain glycogen may be causally related to alterations in food intake were studied.

Methods.—Male rats with jugular vein catheters were housed individually in metabolic cages, and their intake of food was measured daily. In experiment 1, the rats were randomly assigned to 1 of 2 treatment

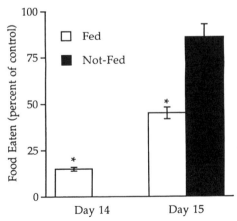

Fig 8–8.—Food intake of PN-100 rats during the last 24 hours of PN-100 infusion (day 14) and first 24 hours after PN-100 infusion was stopped (day 15). Rats were either allowed (Fed; experiment 1) or denied access to normal rat diet. (Not Fed; experiment 2) during 4-day PN-100 infusion period. The PN-100 solution provided 100% of daily caloric intake, determined during immediate 3-day preinfusion period. Values are means ± SE. *Intake different from control (P < .05). (Courtesy of Meguid MM, Beverly JL, Yang Z-J, et al: *Am J Physiol* 265-R1387–R1391, 1993.)

groups: the 45 rats in the control group received .9 N saline, and 45 rats received PN-100 via a jugular vein catheter for 4 days. All rats received .9 N saline infusions during the subsequent 4 days. Equal numbers of rats in each group were killed after 4 days of IV treatment and serially after the PN-100 was stopped. In experiment 2, the study design was similar, except that the 14 rats in the PN-100 group did not have access to food during the 4 days of PN-100.

Results.—In experiment 1, the PN-100 rats decreased their food intake to about 15% of control, but their total caloric intake (IV and eaten) was about 130% of control. The food intake of the PN-100 rats remained low for 3 to 4 days after the PN-100 was stopped. After 4 days of PN-100, the whole brain glycogen, plasma glucose, and plasma insulin values were higher in the PN-100 rats than in the controls. These values were similar to controls within 24 hours of stopping the PN-100. In experiment 2, in which the PN-100 group did not have access to food, these values were the same as the controls on the fourth day of PN-100. The food intake of the 2 groups of PN-100 rats was significantly different on the day after parenteral feeding was stopped (Fig 8–8).

Conclusions.—The increase in brain glycogen that occurs during PN is probably caused by hyperglycemia and hyperinsulinemia. Alterations in whole brain glycogen are apparently not causally related to the observed decrease in oral food intake by rats on PN.

▶ These 2 studies in animals receiving TPN have provided insight into the mechanisms that regulate oral (voluntary) food intake during IV feeding. It has not been established whether similar mechanisms occur in surgical patients fed parenterally. Although excess provision of calories via TPN increases brain glycogen content and delays the return of oral food intake after cessation of TPN, these 2 events are at least in part independent. Adjusting the diurnal timing of infused calories and the composition of the diet are 2 ways of increasing the compensation for intravenously infused calories.—W.W. Souba, M.D., Sc.D.

Perioperative Nutritional Support in Patients Undergoing Hepatectomy for Hepatocellular Carcinoma
Fan S-T, Lo C-M, Lai ECS, Chu K-M, Liu C-L, Wong J (Univ of Hong Kong; Queen Mary Hosp, Hong Kong)
N Engl J Med 331:1547–1552, 1994   140-95-8–21

Introduction.—Patients undergoing resection of hepatocellular carcinoma have high rates of morbidity and mortality, most commonly because of the loss of functioning liver mass and/or postoperative sepsis. Intensive nutritional therapy can reduce the catabolic response to surgery, increase protein synthesis, and enhance liver regeneration, which may reduce the risk of these common complications. Patients undergoing hepatectomy for hepatocellular carcinoma were prospectively stud-

Overall Postoperative Morbidity and
Hospital Mortality*

VARIABLE	PERIOPERATIVE NUTRITION (N = 64)	CONTROLS (N = 60)
Septic complications†		
Pulmonary infection	5 (1)	15
Wound infection	3	5
Subphrenic abscess	4	5 (4)
Urinary tract infection	0	2
Infected ascites	1	2
Biliary fistula	4	5
Central-catheter sepsis	1	0
Other complications		
Wound dehiscence	1	1
Myocardial infarction	0	3 (1)
Intraabdominal bleeding	4	1
Variceal bleeding	1	0
Peptic ulcer bleeding	1	2
Intestinal obstruction	1	0
Pleural effusion	9	12
Hepatic coma	4 (4)	4 (4)
Renal failure	2	1
Ascites requiring diuretic agent for control‡	16	30
Hospital mortality	5	9

* Some patients had more than 1 type of postoperative morbidity. Overall, postoperative morbidity occurred in 22 patients in the perioperative-nutrition group and 33 patients in the control group (34% vs. 55%, $\chi^2 = 5.29$, $P = .02$). Parentheses indicate the number of patients who died of the complication in the group shown.

† Septic complications occurred in 11 patients in the perioperative-nutrition group and 22 patients in the control group (17% vs. 37%, $\chi^2 = 5.97$, $P = .01$).

‡ Ascites requiring the use of diuretic agents occurred in 25% of the perioperative-nutrition group and 50% of the control group ($\chi^2 = 8.23$, $P = .004$).

(Courtesy of Fan S-T, Lo C-M, Lai ECS, et al: N Engl J Med 331:1547–1552, 1994.)

ied to determine the effect of perioperative nutritional support on postoperative morbidity and mortality.

Methods.—Patients with resectable hepatocellular carcinoma undergoing hepatectomy were randomly assigned to a control group (60 patients) or to receive perioperative nutritional support. Patients in the nutritional support group were given parenteral nutrition, consisting of 35% branched-chain amino acids, dextrose, and lipid emulsion for 30 kcal/kg/day, for 7 days preoperatively and 7 days postoperatively in addition to their usual oral diet preoperatively. The 2 groups were compared for hospital mortality, overall postoperative morbidity, anthropometric measurement changes, and liver and immunologic function.

Results.—Preoperatively, the 2 groups were comparable for age, sex, weight loss, the incidence of cirrhosis, and disease stage. Postoperative morbidity occurred in 34% of the nutrition group and 55% of the control group. The most significant differences were in the incidence of sepsis and the need for diuretics to control ascites. The hospital mortality rate was 8% in the nutrition group and 15% in the control group (table). Postoperatively, the nutrition group had higher levels of plasma glucose and serum urea, transferrin, prealbumin, and retinol-binding protein levels. They also lost less weight and had less hepatic function deterioration, as measured by indocyanine green clearance. The benefit of perioperative nutrition was more pronounced in the patients with underlying cirrhosis and in patients who underwent more extensive hepatectomy.

Discussion.—Perioperative nutritional support is beneficial in improving postoperative outcome in patients undergoing resection of hepatocellular carcinoma, particularly in patients with underlying chronic liver disease and those undergoing major hepatectomy. Solutions with branched-chain amino acids and medium-chain triglycerides may be particularly useful, because patients with cirrhosis often have glucose intolerance and insulin resistance.

▶ This study is important for several reasons. First, it is 1 of the few published randomized, controlled trials to demonstrate a significant reduction in hospital morbidity with parenteral nutrition in any patient group. Second, it strongly suggests that patients undergoing major hepatic resection for hepatoma should receive parenteral nutrition in the perioperative period. In addition, it demontrates a nutritional benefit in patients who were not malnourished. In contradistinction to the present study, the VA Cooperation trial (1) showed that only severely malnourished patients benefited from total parenteral nutrition. Although the Fan study did not report oral calorie intake, parenteral nutrition was associated with an improvement in hepatic function (better indocyanine green clearance) and a significant reduction in infectious complications. Of interest was that patients with preexisting cirrhosis had the greatest reduction in postoperative morbidity with parenteral nutrition.—W.W. Souba, M.D., Sc.D.

Reference

1. The Veterans Affairs Total Parenteral Nutrition Cooperative Study Group. Perioperative total parenteral nutrition in surgical patients. *N Engl J Med* 325:525–532, 1991.

A Prospective Randomized Trial of Total Parenteral Nutrition After Major Pancreatic Resection for Malignancy
Brennan MF, Pisters PWT, Posner M, Quesada O, Shike M (Mem Sloan-Kettering Cancer Ctr, NY)
Ann Surg 220:436–444, 1994   140-95-8–22

Morbidity in Patients Receiving TPN and Controls			
	TPN (n = 60)	**Control** (n = 57)	**p Value**
Major complications	27	13	0.02
Minor complications	32	24	0.30
Minor complications (excluding atelectasis)	23	13	0.11
Reoperation	6	3	0.18
Median length of stay (days)	16 (7–72)	14 (6–88)	

(Courtesy of Brennan MF, Pisters PWT, Posner M, et al: *Ann Surg* 220:436–444, 1994.)

Introduction.—Total parenteral nutrition (TPN) has been examined in many studies. Only 1 study has reported major positive results from use of TPN in perioperative management of patients with malignancies. No study exists in which a significant number of patients have had the same surgical procedure for malignancy while receiving TPN postoperatively.

Methods.—A prospective analysis was done to determine postoperative mortality and morbidity in 117 patients receiving TPN while undergoing major pancreatic resection for malignancy. Patients were randomly assigned on postoperative day 1 to receive or not receive TPN.

Results.—There were no significant benefits to receiving TPN in this group of patients. There was a significant increase in intra-abdominal abscess formation in the TPN group, as well as an increased incidence of peritonitis and intestinal obstruction. Postoperative mortality and length of stay showed no significant differences in either group (table).

Conclusion.—Routine use of TPN in patients undergoing major pancreatic resection for malignancy is not recommended. Further study is needed to determine why infectious complications are increased in patients receiving TPN.

▶ This provocative clinical study strongly suggests that the routine use of TPN after major pancreatic resection is not justifiable. In fact, the use of TPN was associated with a significantly higher incidence of major complications postoperatively. The authors compared patients receiving TPN with a group receiving standard 5% dextrose solutions—no enteral group was included. In the past, we have assumed that it is the absence of luminal nutrition that may be detrimental. It is well established that enteral feeding stimulates enterocyte proliferation and improves gut barrier function. This paper by Brennan and colleagues suggests that TPN in and of itself may be toxic inasmuch as the control group of patients in this study was treated with bowel rest and did not receive luminal nutrients. The principal questions raised by the work are; Why did the TPN group have an increase in major complications? Was the adrenal response to major surgery enhanced by TPN? Could the hyperglycemia associated with TPN have glycosylated IgG, preventing its binding to complement such that opsonization of bacteria was impaired? Did TPN induce some degree of cholestasis that could have impaired Kupffer cell clearance of bacteria in the liver? Although these questions were unanswered by this study, the work indicates that current TPN formulations should not be routinely used. Of interest is that feeding tubes were not placed in any of these patients—many surgeons would elect to use jejunal feedings after major pancreatectomy.—W.W. Souba, M.D., Sc.D.

Clinical Nutrition in Practice

Continuous Enteral Feeding Counteracts Preventive Measures for Gastric Colonization in Intensive Care Unit Patients
Bonten MJM, Gaillard CA, van Tiel FH, van der Geest S, Stobberingh EE
(Univ Hosp Maastricht, The Netherlands)
Crit Care Med 22:939–944, 1994   140-95-8–23

Background.—Gastric colonization by pathogens probably plays a causal role in the development of nosocomial pneumonia. A gastric pH of less than 3.5 is usually bactericidal. The effects of continuously administered enteral feedings on gastric pH and colonization were studied in a prospective, open trial of adult patients in 2 university hospital ICUs.

Methods.—Ninety-five patients with an ICU stay of 5 days or more were divided into 4 groups: group A1 included 9 patients who received gastric pH-increasing stress ulcer prophylaxis (antacids, ranitidine, or omeprazole); group A2 included 13 patients who received gastric pH-increasing stress ulcer prophylaxis and enteral feedings (Nutrison); group B1 comprised 12 patients who received topical antimicrobial prophylaxis (tobramycin, colistin, amphotericin B, sucralfate); group B2 comprised 9 patients who received topical antimicrobial prophylaxis and enteral feedings. Seven patients were studied twice. Gastric pH and colonization were measured on admission and at least twice weekly.

Results.—Gastric pH-increasing stress ulcer prophylaxis increased the risk of a gastric pH of more than 3.5 (odds ratio = 2.04). Enteral feeding ig,lex increased the risk of a gastric pH of more than 3.5 (odds ratio = 4.54) and the risk for gastric colonization by potentially pathogenic microorganisms (odds ratio = 4.52). Patients receiving gastric pH-increasing ulcer prophylaxis were colonized earlier than those who received both topical antimicrobial prophylaxis and sucralfate. In both groups A and B, patients receiving enteral feedings were colonized earlier than those without enteral feedings. The probability of remaining free of gastric colonization with potential pathogens in the 4 groups is shown in Figure 8–9.

Conclusions.—Gastric colonization by potential pathogenic organisms can be prevented in ICU patients by a combination of nonabsorbable antimicrobial agents and sucralfate unless continuous enteral feedings are given simultaneously. Further studies using intermittent vs. continuous enteral feedings, with continuous intragastric pH monitoring, are

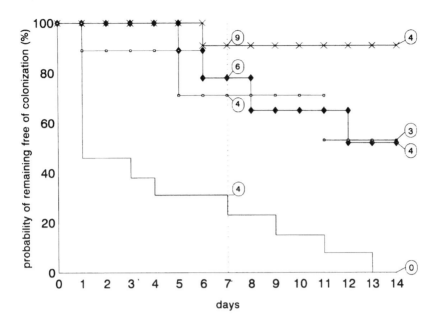

group A1 (n=9)   group A2 (n=13)   group B1 (n=12)   group B2 (n=9)

Fig 8–9.—Kaplan-Meier estimate of the probability of remaining free of colonization with potentially pathogenic microorganisms in the stomach in 4 groups of patients. All patients were free of colonization with potentially pathogenic microorganisms on day 0. Group A1, receiving gastric pH-increasing stress ulcer prophylaxis without enteral feeding; group A2, receiving gastric pH-increasing stress ulcer prophylaxis and enteral feeding; group B1, receiving topical antimicrobial prophylaxis without enteral feeding; group B2, receiving topical antimicrobial prophylaxis and enteral feeding. *Numerals within circles* refer to the numbers of patients free of colonization with potentially pathogenic microorganisms on days 7 and 14. Group B1 vs. B2, $P = .2194$; group B1 vs. A1, $P = .0222$; group B1 vs. A2, $P < .0001$; group B2 vs. A1, $P = .3505$, group B2 vs. A2, $P = .0014$; group A1 vs. A2, $P = .036$ (all by log-rank test). (Courtesy of Bonten MJM, Gaillard CA, van Tiel FH, et al: *Crit Care Med* 22:939–944, 1994.)

needed to learn if intermittent pH decreases will help prevent gastric colonization by potential pathogens.

▶ The methods used to prevent gastric colonization in patients in the ICU (which appears to be related to the development of nosocomial pneumonias) include the use of nonabsorbable topical antimicrobial agents, sucralfate, and enteral nutrition. In this study, the efficacy of antimicrobial prophylaxis was diminished when continuous enteral nutrition was simultaneously provided. The authors suggest that enteral feeding into the stomach should be administered intermittently because gastric pH may decrease when the feeding is stopped, thereby preventing gastric colonization. This hypothesis has been tested (1) and the results were equivocal.—W.W. Souba, M.D., Sc.D.

Reference

1. Lee B, Chang RWS, Jacobs S: Intermittent nosogastric feeding: A simple and effective method to reduce pneumonia among ventilated ICU patients. *Clin Intensive Care* 1:100–102, 1990.

Incidence and Recognition of Malnutrition in Hospital

McWhirter JP, Pennington CR (Ninewells Hosp and Medical School, Dundee, Scotland)
BMJ 308:945–948, 1994
140-95-8-24

Background.—A high incidence of protein energy malnutrition in hospital patients was first reported more than 15 years ago. Nutritional status affects recovery from injury or illness. The prevalence of malnutrition in patients admitted to the hospital, their nutritional status changes during hospitalization, and the effects of nutritional intervention were assessed.

Methods.—Five hundred consecutive admissions to 5 different services—100 each to general medicine, general surgery, orthopedic surgery, respiratory medicine, and geriatrics—in an acute care teaching hospital were studied prospectively. Nutritional status was determined from anthropometric data: body mass index, mid-arm circumference, mid-arm muscle circumference, triceps skinfold thickness, and weight loss before illness. Hospital records were reviewed for information about nutritional status. Patients who were hospitalized for more than 1 week were reassessed at the time of discharge.

Results.—At the time of admission, 40% of the patients were undernourished (body mass index < 20), and 34% were overweight (body mass index > 25) (table). The mean weight loss of the 112 patients who were reassessed at the time of discharge was 5.4%. The greatest weight loss was in those patients who were initially the most undernourished; 78% of these patients deteriorated nutritionally during hospitalization. The 10 patients who were referred for nutritional support had a mean

Nutritional Status of 500 Patients at Time of Admission to 1 of 5 Hospital Specialties

	Hospital specialty				
	General surgery (n=100)	General medicine (n=100)	Respiratory medicine (n=100)	Orthopaedic surgery (n=100)	Medicine for elderly (n=100)
Undernourished	27	46	45	39	43
Normal	25	30	17	30	27
Overweight	48	24	38	31	30

Note: Values are numbers of patients.
(Courtesy of McWhirter JP, Pennington CR: BMJ 308:945–948, 1994.)

weight increase of 7.9%. Only 96 of the 200 undernourished patients had any documentation of nutritional information in their records.

Conclusions.—There is a high incidence of protein energy malnutrition in hospital patients. Health and recovery from injury or illness are adversely affected by poor nutritional status. Malnutrition is often not recognized in hospitalized patients, suggesting that hospital staff should receive improved education about clinical nutrition.

▶ Nearly 20 years after the initial report (1) demonstrating a high incidence (50%) of malnutrition in hospitalized patients, the incidence remains unchanged. Since then, numerous studies have documented that poor nutritional status can adversely affect outcome. In surgical patients, poor nutritional status retards wound healing and predisposes the patient to a greater likelihood of complications. In this study by McWhirter, 40% of patients were undernourished on admission to the hospital and two thirds lost weight during their hospitalization. Although only a small number of these patients received nutritional support, those who did demonstrated an improvement in nutritional status. This continued lack of awareness of the importance of good nutrition emphasizes the need for aggressive educational programs.—W.W. Souba, M.D., Sc.D.

Reference

1. Bistrian BR, Blackburn GL, Vitale J, et al: Prevalence of malnutrition in general medical patients. *JAMA* 253:1567–1570, 1976.

Comparison of Specialized and Standard Enteral Formulas in Trauma Patients
Brown RO, Hunt H, Mowatt-Larssen CA, Wojtysiak SL, Henningfield MF, Kudsk KA (Univ of Tennesse, Memphis; Memphis State Univ, Tenn; Ross Laboratories, Columbus, Ohio)
Pharmacotherapy 14:314–320, 1994   140-95-8–25

Objective.—The values of a specialized enteral formula were compared with those of standard enteral treatment in a prospective series of 37 patients with major trauma who required enteral nutritional support.

Methods.—Nineteen patients were fed a specialized enteral formula containing supplements of arginine, linolenic acid, beta-carotene, and hydrolyzed protein for up to 10 days after admission to the trauma center. The 18 control patients received a standard enteral formula that contained intact caseinates and soy protein isolate and was supplemented by protein powder to provide a similar amount of nitrogen.

Results.—Ten of 18 control patients and only 3 of 19 fed the special enteral formula had infection develop (table). Nitrogen balance in the first 5 days was significantly more favorable in the special formula group, as was the change in serum C-reactive protein. The ratio of CD4 to CD8

Septic Morbidity at Study Entry and During Enteral Nutrition

	Specialized Diet (n=19)		Standard Diet (n=18)	
Infection	Entry	During Study	Entry	During Study
Pneumonia	9	1	8	7
Wound infection	1	0	1	1
Urinary tract infection	0	1	0	1
Sinus infection	0	0	1	1
Bacteremia	0	1	0	0
Totals	10	3	10	10*

* $P < .05$ between groups during enteral nutrition administration.
(Courtesy of Brown RO, Hunt H, Mowatt-Larssen CA, et al: *Pharmacotherapy* 14:314–320, 1994.)

lymphocytes increased more in the special formula group, but not significantly.

Conclusion.—A specially supplemented enteral formula containing hydrolyzed protein may lower the risk of infection after major trauma and enhance nitrogen balance and other indices of metabolic stress.

▶ This is yet another study that has evaluated the use of specific nutrients that, when delivered in high amounts, may have pharmacologic as well as nutritional effects. Besides the use of arginine and ω-3 fatty acids, other nutrients that are likely to be beneficial include glutamine, short chain fatty acids, and nucleic acids. It is unlikely that there is a single "magic bullet," and combination therapy using both nutrients and growth factors may be necessary to promote anabolism in critically ill patients.—W.W. Souba, M.D., Sc.D.

Can Morbidly Obese Patients Safely Lose Weight Preoperatively?
Martin LF, Tan T-L, Holmes PA, Becker DA, Horn J, Bixler EO (The Milton S Hershey Med Ctr, Hershey, Pa)
Am J Surg 169:245–253, 1995   140-95-8-26

Introduction.—There is increasing evidence suggesting that obese patients have increased perioperative mortality, prolonged hospital stays, and higher charges, compared with nonobese patients. Surgeons often advise obese patients to lose weight preoperatively, but there are questions about the amount of weight to be lost to reduce weight-related complications and about the possibility that perioperative weight loss might cause wound healing and other complications. The safety and feasibility of preoperative weight loss were examined in a prospective study.

Methods.—During a 4-year period, 100 severely obese patients scheduled to undergo gastric bypass surgery were asked to participate in a preoperative weight loss program; 70 agreed to participate. The patients dieted with a protein-sparing modified fast, consuming a liquid 420 Kcal,

TABLE 1.—Postoperative Medical Complications

	Dieters (n = 47)	Control (n = 53)
Death	1	0
Intra-abdominal abscess	1	0
Wound infection or seroma	7	7
Enterocolitis (*C. difficle*)	1	0
Empyema*	0	1
Pneumonia	0	1
Atelectasis	0	2
Wound dehiscence	1	2
Ventral hernia	3	3
Staple disruption	1	2
Adhesions/small bowel obstruction	2	1
Stricture of gastrojejunostomy	0	1
Revision of jejunojejunostomy	1	3
Deep venous thrombosis in calf	0	2
Venous thrombosis in bowel mesentery	0	1
Colon injury†	0	1
Pleural effusion†	1	0
Number of medical complications per patient		
None	33 (70%)	32 (60%)
One	9 (19%)	14 (26%)
Two	4 (9%)	5 (10%)
Three	1 (2%)	1 (2%)
Four	1 (2%)	

* Probable aftermath of community-acquired penumonia during 30 days postoperative.
† Result of intraoperative technical problems.
(Courtesy of Martin LF, Tan T-L, Holmes PA, et al: *Am J Surg* 169:245–253, 1995.)

70 g protein per day solution for 1–4 months. Perioperative accumulation of hydroxyproline in subcutaneously implanted polytetrafluoroethylene tubes was examined to study collagen formation in wound healing. Medical, psychological, and digestive status were monitored. Particular complications were specifically noted that were expected to increase (gallstone formation, hernia, and wound infection) or decrease (pulmonary, thrombotic, diabetic, and cardiovascular complications) after preoperative weight loss. The average follow-up was 42 months.

Results.—Of the 100 patients, 47 lost at least 7.5 kg before surgery and were termed dieters. The dieters were significantly more likely to be men, were initially significantly more obese, and had more psychopathology than the nondieters. Overall, 35% of the patients had at least 1 medical complication during the first 2 months postoperatively. The dieter and nondieter groups did not have significantly different types or numbers of medical complications (Table 1), including complications expected to be affected by acute weight loss (Table 2). The 2 groups also

TABLE 2.—Complications Influenced by Weight Loss

	Dieters (n = 47)	Non-Dieters (n = 53)
Might decrease		
Pulmonary	0	3
Thrombotic	0	3
Diabetic	0	0
Cardiovascular	0	0
Might increase		
Gallstone formation	10	11
Hernia	3	3
Wound infection or seroma	7	7

(Courtesy of Martin LF, Tan T-L, Holmes PA, et al: *Am J Surg* 169:245–253, 1995.)

did not differ significantly in the incidence and type of postoperative psychiatric or digestive complications. Collagen formation was not significantly different in the 2 groups.

Discussion.—Severely obese patients can safely lose up to 45 kg using a protein-sparing modified fast immediately before surgery without increasing the risk of postoperative complications. Randomized, prospective trials are required to evaluate a relationship between preoperative weight loss and improvements in patient outcome with various procedures.

▶ It may be intuitive that preoperative weight loss would be beneficial for obese patients requiring elective surgery. One might suspect a reduced incidence of cardiopulmonary and wound complications. However, some patients, such as those with malignancies, cannot delay their operation. In those who can wait, it will be expensive and will require a large multicenter trial to test the hypothesis. The best approach is to counsel patients to avoid weight gain so that if and when they do require surgery, they are not markedly obese.—W.W. Souba, M.D., Sc.D.

Gastroesophageal Reflux During Gastrostomy Feeding

Coben RM, Weintraub A, DiMarino AJ Jr, Cohen S (Univ of Pennsylvania, Philadelphia; Temple Univ, Philadelphia)
Gastroenterology 106:13–18, 1994   140-95-8-27

Objective.—Aspiration pneumonia is 1 of the most important complications in patients given gastrostomy tube feedings. How a gastrostomy tube affects the lower esophageal sphincter (LES) pressure was investigated prospectively.

Study Plan.—Five men and 5 women aged 67 to 93 years who were referred for endoscopic placement of a gastrostomy tube were included in the study. Eight of the patients had had a stroke and 2 were demented. The basal LES pressures were recorded before and after tube placement, and the pressure then was monitored at 15-minute intervals during the rapid infusion of 250 mL of an enteral feeding formula (Jevity) and 100 mL of water. After 2 hours, the formula was infused at a rate of 80 mL/hr. Five patients underwent scintigraphy during the infusion of formula labeled with ^{99}Tc-sulfur colloid.

Results.—The LES pressure did not change significantly after gastrostomy tube placement. Rapid infusion of the feeding formula lowered the pressure to incompetency levels. In contrast, the slow, continuous infusion of formula did not significantly reduce the LES pressure. The scintigraphic studies confirmed the occurrence of free gastroesophageal reflux up to the level of the sternal notch with rapid formula infusion. Free reflux did not occur during slow infusion of the formula.

Conclusion.—The finding that rapid, but not slow, infusion of a feeding formula via a gastrostomy tube promotes gastroesophageal reflux suggests obvious ways of avoiding aspiration pneumonia.

▶ This study indicates that, after gastrostomy tube placement, intragastric feeding be given slowly rather than in a bolus fashion. The authors suggest that the gastropexy associated with G-tube placement slightly increases LES pressure. The authors propose that bolus feeding into the stomach may be caused by gastric distention and relaxation of the LES, which could lead to gastroesophageal reflux. In elderly, debilitated patients with G-tubes, the incidence of aspiration pneumonia is as high as 20%.—W.W. Souba, M.D., Sc.D.

9 Growth Factors and Wound Healing

Introduction

Impaired wound healing contributes to hospital morbidity and mortality and increases the cost of health care markedly. Methods used to improve wound healing include the topical use of growth factors, the systemic administration of anabolic agents, the provision of nutritional support and specific nutrients, and the use of hyperbaric oxygen. None of these therapies are more important than meticulous wound care.

The ideal response to wounding has been lost almost entirely in phylogenetically advanced organisms, although the human fetus appears to heal with a scarless repair. The human liver also regenerates itself after partial removal, although the regenerated segment is not quite normal architecturally. Nonetheless, it seems to function quite well. In general, humans tend to heal with scar formation rather than regenerate lost organs or portions of tissue. Clinical wound problems, in general, become apparent when there is an abnormality in epithelialization, wound contracture, and/or collagen metabolism. Over the years, our understanding of these problems has progressed from the recognition of the importance of tissue perfusion to our current awareness of the role of peptides that modulate the normal healing process.

Although the biology of wound healing is complicated and incompletely understood, advances in our knowledge of the molecular biology of growth factors have enhanced our understanding of the regulation of normal and abnormal wound healing immensely. Studies on fetal wound healing and the cicatrization of hypertrophic scars have provided insights into the role of the supporting matrix proteins and the importance of angiogenesis and fibroblast proliferation. Each of these events can be altered or impaired and lead to a derangement in the final scar. Several known growth factors and their actions are shown in the table.

The hope is that these advances in the basic science of growth factors will have clinical applicability that will improve patient care and diminish morbidity and cost. Fibroblasts can now be transfected with vectors containing plasmids that encode for the biosynthesis of many of these growth factors. Such cells could be applied to nonhealing wounds and potentially enhance the healing process. Although optimism should be high, some caution is advised because of the relationship of these growth factors to the neoplastic process.

Wiley W. Souba, M.D., Sc.D.

Peptide Factors That Affect Wound Healing

Factor	Abbreviation	Source	Functions Regulated
Platelet-derived growth factor	PDGF	Platelets and macrophages	Fibroblast proliferation, chemotaxis, and collagenase production
Transforming growth factor β	TGF-β	Platelets, polymorphonuclear neutrophil leukocytes, T lymphocytes, and macrophages	Fibroblast proliferation, chemotaxis, collagen metabolism, and action of other growth factors
Transforming growth factor α	TGF-α	Activated macrophages and many tissues	Similar to EGF functions
Interleukin-1	IL-1	Macrophages	Fibroblast proliferation
Tumor necrosis factor	TNF	Macrophages, mast cells, and T lymphocytes	Fibroblast proliferation
Fibroblast growth factor	FGF	Brain, pituitary, macrophages, and many other tissues and cells	Fibroblast proliferation, stimulates collagen deposition and angiogenesis
Epidermal growth factor	EGF	Saliva, urine, milk, and plasma	Stimulates epithelial cell proliferation and granulation tissue formation
Insulin-like growth factor	IGF	Liver, plasma, and fibroblasts	Stimulates synthesis of sulfated proteoglycans, collagen, and cell proliferation
Human growth factor	HGF	Pituitary and thus plasma	Anabolism

(Courtesy of Cohen IK, Diegelmann: Wound healing, in Greenfield L (ed): *Surgery: Scientific Principles and Practice.* Philadelphia, JB Lippincott, 1993.)

Biology of Normal and Abnormal Wound Healing

Determination of Endogenous Cytokines in Chronic Wounds

Cooper DM, Yu EZ, Hennessey P, Ko F, Robson MC (Univ of Texas, Galveston)
Ann Surg 219:688–692, 1994   140-95-9–1

Background.—The ability to clone cytokines through recombinant DNA technology opens up the possibility of using these molecules to treat acute and chronic wounds, but it would be helpful to know the endogenous levels of particular cytokines in wounds.

Objective and Methods.—A method was developed for extracting minute amounts of cytokines from indolent, chronic wounds to characterize their microenvironment. Porous, inert hydrophilic dextranomer beads were examined for their ability to absorb or adsorb proteins and cytokines in vitro, using albumin alone; albumin combined with known amounts of cytokines; and clinical samples from chronic pressure ulcers. The amounts of platelet-derived growth factor (PDGF)-AB, basic fibroblast growth factor (bFGF), epidermal growth factor (EGF), and transforming growth factor-beta (TGF-β) extracted by the beads were estimated by enzyme-linked immunosorbent assay.

Findings.—From 88% to 98% of known amounts of albumin were recovered, as were 90% of admixed cytokines. Protein concentrations in 20 grade III/IV pressure ulcers were very similar, but endogenous levels of the growth factors varied widely. Concentrations of PDGF-AB ranged from 49 to 867 pg/mL; of bFGF from 47 to 697 pg/mL; and of EGF from undetectable levels to 247.5 pg/mL. No TGF-β was detected in 17 of the 20 pressure ulcers sampled.

Implications.—This appears to be a useful means of determining endogenous levels of cytokines. The amounts found in these chronic wounds were much lower than are reported for acute wounds. The markedly varying amounts of cytokines present in different chronic wounds may help explain the differences in wound healing reported from trials of exogenous cytokine treatment.

The Extracellular Matrix of the Fetal Wound: Hyaluronic Acid Controls Lymphocyte Adhesion

Dillon PW, Keefer K, Blackburn JH, Houghton PE, Krummel TM (The Pennsylvania State Univ, Hershey)
J Surg Res 57:170–173, 1994   140-95-9–2

Hypothesis.—The inflammatory response to tissue injury is determined to an important degree by adhesive interactions between lymphocytes and components of the extracellular matrix (ECM) in the environment of the wound. In fetal wounds, the ECM consists chiefly of hyaluronic acid and the inflammatory reaction to injury is minimal. The lack of inflammatory cell response in fetal wounds may reflect the inability of lymphocytes to adhere to hyaluronic acid.

Objective.—Tissues from 16-day gestational aged mouse fetuses were used to examine the ability of fetal lymphocytes to adhere to fibronectin, vitronectin, hyaluronic acid, and collagen types I, III, IV, and V.

Findings.—Lymphocytes from both the fetal spleen and the thymus bound to a significant degree to fibronectin, vitronectin, and collagen types I and III. They did not, however, bind to hyaluronic acid. Adhesive ability was unaffected by interleukin-1, interferon-γ, and phorbol dibutyrate.

Conclusion.—The inability of fetal lymphocytes to adhere to hyaluronic acid may help explain the relative lack of inflammation seen in fetal wounds. The result is tissue regeneration rather than inflammation and subsequent scar formation.

Fibronectin Gene Expression Differs in Normal and Abnormal Human Wound Healing

Sible JC, Eriksson E, Smith SP, Oliver N (Tufts Univ, Boston; Brigham and Women's Hosp, Boston)
Wound Rep Reg 2:3–19, 1994   140-95-9–3

Introduction.—Overproduction of fibronectin and type I collagen are seen in patients with hypertrophic scars and keloid formation. Extracel-

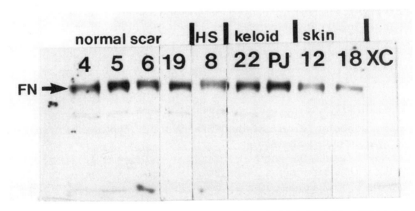

Fig 9–1.—Immunoprecipitation of fibronectin from cells pulse-labeled with Trans[³⁵S] label. Total fibronectin protein synthesized by fibroblasts derived from normal skin, normal scar, keloids, and a hypertrophic scar (*HS*). Patient numbers (or letters) are indicated at top. *FN* indicates the position at which fibronectin migrates. (Courtesy of Sible JC, Eriksson E, Smith SP, et al: *Wound Rep Reg* 2:3–19, 1994.)

lular matrix gene expression regarding differences in normal and abnormal scar formation is not well understood.

Methods.—The content of fibronectin messenger RNA (mRNA) and rates of fibronectin protein biosynthesis were analyzed in fibroblasts from keloid, hypertrophic scar, normal skin, and normal scar. Comparisons were made of normal and keloid tissues in the same patient to eliminate the problem of variation among individuals. To determine whether the expression of fibronectin protein correlated with mRNA levels in vitro, total fibronectin was specifically immunoprecipitated with cells pulse-labeled with Trans[^{35}S] label (Fig 9–1).

Results.—Three of 4 matched pairs of normal and keloid fibroblasts from the same patient exhibited higher rates of fibronectin production for the keloid sample. Fibronectin protein synthesized by fibroblasts showed that normal and abnormal wounds had higher fibronectin biosynthesis rates than fibroblasts from normal skin. Hypertrophic scar tissue showed a lower rate of fibronectin biosynthesis in fibroblasts than what was found in keloid and most normal scar tissue (see Fig 9–1).

Conclusion.—Differences in fibronectin gene expression can be observed in vivo and in vitro for both normal and keloid tissue. Although little difference is seen in fibronectin expression between keloid and normal scar formation, the rates of fibronectin biosynthesis and message levels in normal scars are more variable, suggesting that mature scars may be less homogeneous than keloid in matrix gene expression. These findings indicate that the fibronectin regulatory pathway in scar fibroblasts is influenced by the tissue environment.

Human Wound Healing Fibroblasts Have Greater Contractile Properties Than Dermal Fibroblasts

Germain L, Jean A, Auger FA, Garrel DR (Laval Univ, Québec; Hôpital l'Hôtel-Dieu, Montréal)
J Surg Res 57:268–273, 1994   140-95-9–4

Introduction.—Tissue contraction during wound healing can have important ramifications for posthealing structure and function. Its mechanism is not clear; however, both fibroblasts and myofibroblasts have been implicated in different theories. The physiologic events that cause contraction during healing were examined in an in vitro study.

Methods.—Wound fibroblasts were isolated from implants recovered after 12 days of subcutaneous implantation. Dermal fibroblasts were isolated from healthy skin. Some cells were cultured and plated in monolayers for immunofluorescence study. Other cells were cultured in a collagen solution, and the surface area of the collagen gels was measured daily to assess contractile properties.

Results.—Immunofluorescence studies demonstrated that less than 1% of the dermal fibroblasts and 30% to 40% of the wound fibroblasts

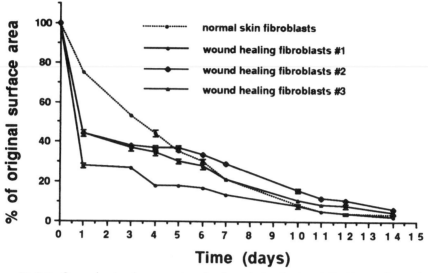

Fig 9–2.—Curves showing the contraction of collagen lattices by dermal fibroblasts and wound-healing fibroblasts. The extent of contraction is greater when wound-healing fibroblasts are used. Mean of duplicate ± standard deviation. (Courtesy of Germain L, Jean A, Auger FA, et al: *J Surg Res* 57:268–273, 1994.)

contained fiber networks of α-actin, a smooth-muscle cell marker. Compared with dermal fibroblasts, wound fibroblasts had significantly reduced surface areas of the collagen gels, indicating greater contractility (Fig 9–2).

Discussion.—These findings indicate the abundant presence of myofibroblasts in human granulation tissue 12 days after wounding but not in normal dermal tissue. In addition, granulating wound myofibroblasts demonstrate greater contractile capacity than do normal dermal fibroblasts in an in vitro environment. It is hypothesized that myofibroblasts induce wound closure by both individual and coordinated cellular contraction.

▶ The control of wound healing is of great interest to surgeons both as it relates to the clinical setting and to the laboratory. Wound healing advances are a good example of how a clinical observation has been taken to the bench and subsequent knowledge translated back to the bedside in the form of a biological therapy. For example, surgeons have long noted that certain wounds do not heal and have subsequently made important contributions to the biology of growth factors and their role in wound healing. The most important of these include EGF, bFGF, PDGF, and TGF. Cooper and colleagues (Abstract 140-95-9–1) demonstrated that the levels of these growth factors were much lower in chronic wounds than they were in acute wounds, suggesting a role for these compounds in modulating normal wound repair. Application of topical growth factors to certain wounds to promote healing is likely to have clinical relevance. Several studies have already demonstrated the ability of these agents to stimulate wound closure.

One of the most striking aspects of fetal wounds is the fact that they heal without an inflammatory response and generate a "scarless" repair hallmarked by an organized structural integrity rather than the disorganized scar matrix seen in adults. In adults, T lymphocytes play a crucial role in the disorganized collagen formation that characterizes the scar. Although fetal lymphocytes express the required receptors for binding to extracellular matrix glycoproteins, there is no intrinsic binding of these cells to hyaluronate (a pivotal matrix component). Without the ability to adhere to the interstitial matrix, fetal lymphocytes are unable to migrate into the zone of tissue injury and initiate an inflammatory response which can result in disorganized collagen formation. This is likely to be an important reason why fetal wounds exhibit a scarless repair.

Another important component of the altered wound healing seen in some adults is the excessive production of the matrix protein fibronectin. Overproduction of this protein, as well as type I collagen, is seen in patients with keloids and hypertrophic scarring. Fibroblasts harvested from keloids were noted to express elevated amounts of fibronectin compared with fibroblasts from normal skin. Related to this observation is the study by Germain et al. (Abstract 140-95-9–4) which demonstrated a marked increase in myofibroblasts in granulation tissue of the healing adult wound. Such cells possess a marked ability to contract as the wound heals and are not present in normal skin.

The significance of these findings collectively is that they add to our knowledge of the biology of normal and abnormal wound healing. With time, we will be able to block certain abnormal aspects of the reparative process such that wound healing will be enhanced and occur with less contraction and with more organized collagen. This kind of therapy will likely be used in surgical patients.—W.W. Souba, M.D., Sc.D.

Basic Research with Clinical Applicability

Modulation of Collagen Synthesis by Transforming Growth Factor-β in Keloid and Hypertrophic Scar Fibroblasts

Younai S, Nichter LS, Wellisz T, Reinisch J, Nimni ME, Tuan T-L (Univ of California, Davis–East Bay, Oakland; Univ of Southern California, Los Angeles)
Ann Plast Surg 33:148–151, 1994   140-95-9–5

Introduction.—Both keloid and hypertrophic scars can be characterized as benign fibrous growths that overproduce collagen. Transforming growth factor-β (TGF-β) has been found to promote excessive synthesis of matrix proteins, including collagen, in other similar biological models. The effects of TGF-β on collagen synthesis were studied in keloid fibroblasts (KFs), hypertrophic scar fibroblasts (HSFs), and normal skin fibroblasts (NSFs).

Methods.—Dermal fibroblasts obtained from biopsy specimens of keloids, hypertrophic scars, and normal skin were cultured in fibrin-gel ma-

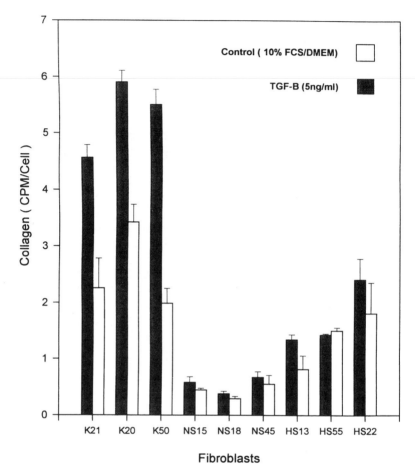

Fig 9–3.—Modulation of the rate of collagen synthesis by TGF-β. *Abbreviations:* K, keloid; HS, hypertrophic scar; NS, normal skin; CPM, counts per minute; FCS/DMEM, fetal calf serum/Dulbecco's modified Eagle's medium. (Courtesy of Younai S, Nichter LS, Wellisz T, et al: *Ann Plast Surg* 33:148–151, 1994.)

trices with or without TGF-β or an antibody against TGF-β. Collagen was labeled with ^{3}H-proline and measured after 48 hours.

Results.—Collagen secretion was highest in KFs; KFs secreted as much as 4 times more collagen than did the HSFs and as much as 12 times more collagen than did the NSFs. Exposure to TGF-β increased collagen secretion by the KFs by as much as 2.7 times, but such exposure did not affect collagen secretion in HSFs or NSFs. Similarly, collagen production was suppressed by 40% in KFs in the presence of anti–TGF-β antibody, but it was unaffected in HSFs and NSFs (Fig 9–3).

Discussion.—Although both KFs and HSFs overproduce collagen, only KFs demonstrate oversensitivity to TGF-β; the HSF response to

TGF-β is similar to that seen in NSFs. This suggests that hypertrophic scars are similar to normal fibroblasts and explains their frequent spontaneous regression, which does not occur with keloids. Further study of TGF-β receptors on keloids and of the intracellular signal transduction pathway of TGF-β may enable the development of treatment strategies for keloids and may elucidate the wound-healing process.

▶ One aspect of abnormal wound healing in which modulation of growth factor production may play a role is with regard to keloids and hypertrophic scars. Certain growth factors are likely to be overexpressed in these scars, and they may stimulate excessive collagen production, resulting in a nonpliable, painful, unsightly scar. Using specific monoclonal antibodies to these growth factors may be 1 method of diminishing collagen production. How, when, and how much antibody should be used has not yet been worked out in the clinical setting. Some of these growth factors also play a role in malignant transformation, and this must be kept in mind as well.—W.W. Souba, M.D., Sc.D.

Cytoprotection of Human Dermal Fibroblasts Against Silver Sulfadiazine Using Recombinant Growth Factors

McCauley RL, Li Y-Y, Chopra V, Herndon DN, Robson MC (Shriners Burns Inst, Galveston, Tex; Univ of Texas, Galveston)
J Surg Res 56:378–384, 1994   140-95-9–6

Background.—Rapid wound closure can significantly limit hospital morbidity and mortality in patients with large burn wounds, but topical antimicrobials such as silver sulfadiazine (SSD) and mafenide acetate (MA) have been associated with delayed wound healing. Both these agents have dose-related cytotoxic effects on human dermal fibroblasts.

Objective and Methods.—In vitro studies were carried out to determine the cellular responses of human dermal fibroblasts to SSD after exposure to 3 recombinant growth factors: epidermal growth factor (EGF), basic fibroblast growth factor (b-FGF), and platelet-derived growth factor (PDGF). Fresh human dermal fibroblasts isolated from normal skin were used in the studies. The cells were exposed to microsuspensions of .01%, .03%, and .05% SSD. Cell damage was assessed by phase-contrast microscopy, hemocytometer cell counts, and estimates of total cellular protein content (Fig 9–4).

Results.—Pre-exposure of human dermal fibroblasts to each of the growth factors resulted in cytoprotection against SSD in concentrations of .01% and .03%. At .05% SSD, the cells were destroyed but more slowly. Cytoprotection was most pronounced with b-FGF, whereas EGF was the least effective growth factor.

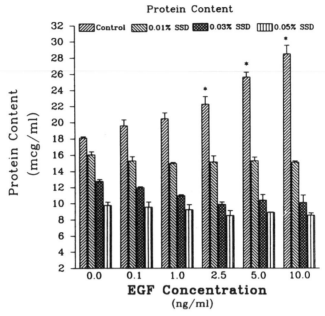

Fig 9–4.—Cytoprotection of fibroblasts against SSD with EGF. Comparison of hemocytometer cell counts with total protein assays with EGF. *P < .05 compared to PDGF controls by Scheffe's multiple comparison procedure. (Courtesy of McCauley RL, Li Y-Y, Chopra V, et al: *J Surg Res* 56:378–384, 1994.)

Conclusion.—Dermal fibroblasts activated by growth factors apparently either take up less antibiotic or are more resistant to its direct cytotoxic effects.

PDGF and TGF-α Act Synergistically to Improve Wound Healing in the Genetically Diabetic Mouse

Brown RL, Breeden MP, Greenhalgh DG (Shriners Burns Inst, Cincinnati, Ohio; Univ of Cincinnati, Ohio)
J Surg Res 56:562–570, 1994   140-95-9–7

Introduction.—Surgical patients with impaired wound healing experience significant morbidity and prolonged hospitalization. Previous studies with a murine model have demonstrated a synergistic effect of fibroblast mitogens, either BB homodimer of platelet-derived growth factor (PDGF-BB) or basic fibroblast growth factor (b-FGF), used together with insulin-like growth factor on wound healing in genetically diabetic mice with impaired wound healing. The effects on wound healing in genetically diabetic mice of 2 keratinocyte mitogens—epidermal growth factor (EGF) and transforming growth factor-α (TGF-α)—either alone

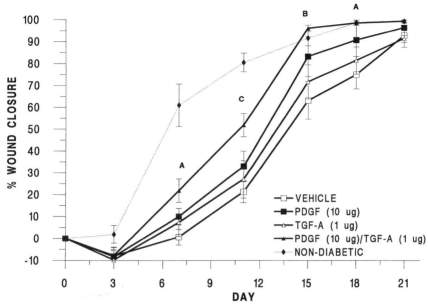

Fig 9–5.—Percentage of wound closure (mean ± standard error of mean) in genetically diabetic mice treated with vehicle (5% polyethylene glycol), PDGF-BB, TGF-α, or a combination of PDGF and TGF-α. The nondiabetic curve is included for comparison. A, $P < .05$ vs. vehicle; B, $P < .05$ vs. vehicle and TGF-α; and C, $P < .05$ vs. vehicle, TGF-α and PDGF-BB by analysis of variance and Duncan's multiple range test. (Courtesy of Brown RL, Breeden MP, Greenhalgh DG: *J Surg Res* 56:562–570, 1994.)

or in combination with a fibroblast mitogen, PDGF-BB, were investigated.

Methods.—Untreated, genetically diabetic mice were given full-thickness skin wounds on their backs. The wounds were treated topically with vehicle alone, PDGF-BB, EGF, or TGF-α, or with combinations of PDGF and either EGF or TGF-α for 5 days. Wound tracings were performed to monitor epithelial migration until either day 15 or 21, when the animal was sacrificed and the wound was examined histologically. The healing rates were compared with a representative healing curve for nondiabetic mice.

Results.—Compared with treatment with vehicle, wounds treated with EGF were not significantly affected, but treatment with PDGF-BB alone and TGF-α alone significantly enhanced wound healing. The combination of PDGF-BB and TGF-α induced a further increase in the wound healing rate comparable to the rate seen in nondiabetic mice (Fig 9–5). However, the addition of EGF did not increase the effects of PDGF-BB. The histologic analysis on day 15 revealed that cellular infiltration, formation of granulation tissue, vascularity, and re-epithelialization were all significantly advanced in the wounds treated with the combination of PDGF-BB and TGF-α, compared with the other wounds. By day 21, the differences were reduced as all the wounds approached complete healing.

Conclusion.—Both PDGF-BB and TGF-α had a synergistic effect on wound healing in genetically diabetic mice. However, EGF did not similarly increase the efficacy of PDGF-BB in promoting wound closure. Further studies should explore the possibility of increasing the synergy of PDGF-BB and TGF-α by adding a fibroblast progression factor.

Stimulation of All Epithelial Elements During Skin Regeneration by Keratinocyte Growth Factor

Pierce GF, Yanagihara D, Klopchin K, Danilenko DM, Hsu E, Kenney WC, Morris CF (Amgen Inc, Thousand Oaks, Calif)
J Exp Med 179:831–840, 1994   140-95-9-8

Introduction.—In several in vitro studies, keratinocyte growth factor (KGF), a fibroblast growth factor (FGF), has been shown to stimulate only epithelial cells that contain mesenchyme. Therefore, KGF has a much more specific target cell range than do basic or acidic FGFs. The influence of recombinant KGF (rKGF) on keratinocytes was studied in an in vivo model.

Methods.—A wound was created in rabbit ears by removing cartilage and the overlying skin. After its creation, the wound was treated with either various concentrations of rKGF or with vehicle alone and covered with Tegaderm occlusive dressing. One to 7 days later, the wound was harvested, bisected, and analyzed histologically and immunohistochemically.

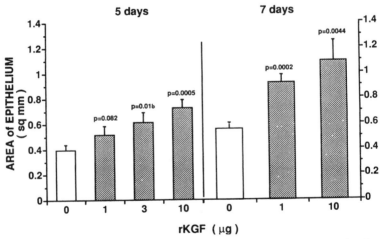

Fig 9–6.—Total area of regenerating epithelium at days 5 and 7 in rKGF-treated and control wounds. (Courtesy of Pierce GF, Yanagihara D, Klopchin K, et al: *J Exp Med* 179:831–840, 1994.)

Results.—Re-epithelialization was significantly enhanced with the application of 1–10 μg of rKGF, in a dose-dependent fashion (Fig 9–6). The histologic analysis revealed the migration of outer root sheath keratinocytes from within the underlying dermal wound bed as well as from the wound borders in rKGF-treated wounds, suggesting that rKGF stimulates adnexal elements. Treatment with rKGF did not affect the formation of granulation tissue, excluding an rKGF influence on platelet-derived growth factor or basic FGF. Immunostaining for cytokeratins 14 and 10 revealed that rKGF increased the expression of immature cytokeratin 14 but not the mature cytokeratin 10. The proliferating basal keratinocytes were localized at the wound margins after 30 hours in rKGF-treated wounds and in the suprabasal layer of the cytokeratin 14–positive neoepidermis by days 2 and 5. Treatment with rKGF also increased the number of hair follicles and proliferating follicular cells, as well as the number of hyperplastic sebaceous glands and proliferating sebocytes.

Discussion.—Treatment with rKGF, like treatment with epidermal growth factor or basic FGF, stimulates re-epithelialization. However, only rKGF also stimulates the proliferation and differentiation of adnexal structures. These findings suggest that rKGF directly stimulates both the progenitor cells within pilosebaceous units and the mature keratinocytes in the outer root sheath, and is, therefore, a significant paracrine stimulator functioning importantly in the skin regenerative process. Studying its effects may help elucidate the mechanisms of epithelial differentiation.

In Vivo Transfer and Expression of a Human Epidermal Growth Factor Gene Accelerates Wound Repair

Andree C, Swain WF, Page CP, Macklin MD, Slama J, Hatzis D, Eriksson E
(Brigham and Women's Hosp, Boston; Agracetus Inc, Middleton, Wis)
Proc Natl Acad Sci U S A 91:12188–12192, 1994   140-95-9–9

Introduction.—Epidermal growth factor (EGF) is present in platelets and may play an important role in regulating wound healing. Delivering exogenous EGF has therapeutic promise, but continuous delivery during the early stages of repair is problematic. The efficacy of particle-mediated gene transfer of an EGF expression plasmid was studied in a porcine wound model within an external chamber.

Methods.—Uniform partial-thickness excisional wounds were created on the dorsum of pigs. Expression plasmids containing the human EGF (hEGF) coding region and control plasmids containing the influenza virus hemagglutinin coding sequence were propagated. Gold particles were coated with the resulting DNA solution and were delivered with a particle-bombardment device. The porcine wounds were either not bombarded or were bombarded with uncoated gold particles, hEGF expression plasmid, or the control plasmid. Vinyl adhesive chambers were sealed to the surrounding skin and filled with normal saline, penicillin G, and streptomycin. Protein concentration, β-galactosidase activity, and hEGF concentration were monitored in wound fluid and biopsy samples.

Results.—There was β-galactosidase activity only in wounds bombarded with the control plasmid and not in unbombarded wounds or wounds bombarded with uncoated particles or EGF expression plasmid. Wounds bombarded with EGF expression plasmid had a mean 193-fold increase in EGF concentration within 24 hours; concentrations declined quickly during the first 5 days but remained detectable for at least 30 days. Protein concentrations indicated that re-epithelialization occurred in a mean of 8.2 days in EGF-bombarded wounds and in a mean of 10.3 days for all control wounds.

Discussion.—Particle-mediated in vivo gene transfer provides effective and persistent delivery of polypeptide growth factors to the wound bed. In addition, the wound chamber can provide protection of the wound and containment of the exogenous DNA, and permit both sampling of wound fluid and delivery to the wound. The transfer of hEGF to the wounds resulted in a 20% reduction in healing time.

▶ Because growth factors stimulate fibroblast proliferation, their application may enhance wound healing. In burn patients, the use of SSD is a key component of wound care because of its antimicrobial properties, but this agent delays wound healing by inhibiting the growth of fibroblasts. McCauley and associates (Abstract 140-95-9–6) demonstrated the protective effect of PDGF and bFGF on fibroblast integrity against SSD in vitro. The authors suggest that these agents may negate the inhibitory action of SSD on wound healing that is primarily influenced by fibroplasia and collagen deposition.

Consistent with these results is the work by Brown et al. (Abstract 140-95-9–7) which showed that growth factors can also act synergistically to accelerate wound healing in diabetic mice. Studies in patients have shown beneficial effects as well (1). These growth factors may work in an additive fashion because of preferential effects on various aspects of wound healing. For example, healing of the skin can be enhanced by KGF, a peptide similar to FGF. These kinds of studies have generally used topical application of synthetic growth factors, but optimal delivery of these compounds can be problematic.

One of the most exciting areas of growth factor research uses the technique of gene transfer to deliver growth factors. Such a technique promises localized and persistent delivery of growth factors to the healing wound. Andree and colleagues (Abstract 140-95-9–9) described the transfer of an hEGF expression plasmid to porcine partial-thickness wound keratinocytes by particle-mediated DNA transfer. Epidermal growth factor concentrations were increased almost 200-fold in the wound and healing was enhanced. This technique has promise because it overcomes the previous lack of a practical delivery system.—W.W. Souba, M.D., Sc.D.

Reference

1. Brown GL, Nanney LB, Griffen J, et al: Enhancement of wound healing by topical treatment with epidural growth factor. *N Engl J Med* 321:76–79, 1989.

Bombesin Improves Survival From Methotrexate-Induced Enterocolitis

Chu KU, Higashide S, Evers BM, Rajaraman S, Ishizuka J, Townsend CM Jr, Thompson JC (Univ of Texas, Galveston)
Ann Surg 220:570–577, 1994
140-95-9–10

Purpose.—Bombesin is a tetradecapeptide analogous to mammalian gastrin-releasing peptide. It stimulates the growth of numerous gastrointestinal tissues and may play a key role in the early development of the gastrointestinal tract. It may be clinically useful in maintaining the mucosal structure of the gut during periods of injury, such as trauma or chemotherapy. The ability of bombesin to improve survival from methotrexate-induced enterocolitis was examined in rats.

Methods.—Sixty rats were randomly allocated into 3 groups, all of which received an elemental diet as their only nutrition. This diet produces gut mucosal atrophy in rats. The animals received either saline or, beginning on either day 0 or day 14 of the study, bombesin in a dosage of 10 μg/kg subcutaneously 3 times a day. On day 14, all animals received methotrexate, 20 mg/kg intraperitoneally, which produces a lethal enterocolitis.

Results.—Bombesin prevented the ileal mucosal atrophy produced by the elemental diet, as evaluated by mucosal weight, DNA content, and total protein content (Fig 9–7). In addition, it significantly decreased mortality in rats given methotrexate. That was so whether bombesin was given as a pretreatment or at the same time as methotrexate.

Conclusion.—In this rat model of lethal methotrexate-induced enterocolitis, bombesin improved survival significantly, possibly through maintenance of gut mucosal structure. Clinically, bombesin may be useful in preventing enterocolitis in patients receiving toxic chemotherapy. Measures to reduce the side effects of chemotherapy can improve treatment tolerance and, thus, lead to more efficient therapy for cancer patients.

▶ The bowel is susceptible to injury in critically ill patients, and this is most apparent in cancer patients who receive chemotherapy. Antineoplastic drugs cause mucositis and intestinal epithelial damage which can manifest as mucosal erosions and/or a breakdown in gut barrier function. It is well known that a variety of gut-derived growth factors (gut peptides) act to stimulate mucosal cell proliferation and turnover. The production of these compounds—which act in part to maintain gut epithelial integrity—may be im-

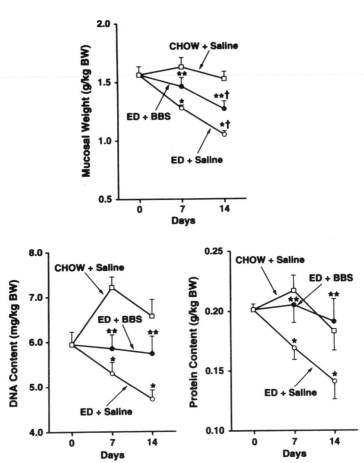

Fig 9–7.—Mucosal weight, DNA, and protein contents of ileal segment corrected for body weight (N indicates 6, mean ± SEM; *, P < 0.05 vs. CHOW + saline; **, P < 0.05 vs. elemental diet + saline; †, P < 0.05 vs. same group from Day 7). ED, elemental diet; BBS, bombesin. (Courtesy of Chu KU, Higashide S, Evers BM, et al: *Ann Surg* 220:570–577, 1994.)

paired during certain pathophysiologic states such as fasting or total parenteral nutrition.

In this study by Chu et al., exogenous bombesin stimulated mucosal growth and improved survival after methotrexate administration to rats. This observation is consistent with a role for bombesin in maintaining gut barrier function. Other growth factors, such as epidermal growth factor and basic fibroblast growth factor, have also been shown to stimulate mucosal proliferation. The safety and toxicity of these agents in the clinical setting have not yet been fully elucidated.—W.W. Souba, M.D., Sc.D.

The Effect of Insulinlike Growth Factor I on Wound Healing Variables and Macrophages in Rats

Mueller RV, Hunt TK, Tokunaga A, Spencer EM (Univ of California, San Francisco; Nippon Med School, Tokyo; California Pacific Hosp, San Francisco)
Arch Surg 129:262–265, 1994   140-95-9-11

Introduction.—Previous studies have demonstrated the importance of insulin-like growth factor I (IGF-I) in effective wound healing. The mechanisms of action of IGF-I in wounds have not been investigated in detail, however. Certain IGF-I deficiency states are also associated with deficits in wound healing and decreased wound macrophage concentrations. The effect of IGF-I depletion and restoration on the number of wound macrophages and wound healing variables was studied.

Methods.—Sham-operated and hypophysectomized healthy male Sprague-Dawley rats were used in a wound-healing model. The animals were randomly assigned to a 14-day infusion of IGF-I (10 μg per wound per day) or placebo infusion. Seventeen days after implantation, the animals were killed and the wound chambers removed for analysis. The concentration of wound macrophages was recorded, as were the wound healing variables of dry tissue weight, total protein, DNA, and hydroxyproline content.

Results.—The hypophysectomized rats had values of tissue dry weight, protein, DNA, and hydroxyproline that were, respectively, 73%, 42%, 39%, and 21% of sham-operated animals. Administration of IGF-I in-

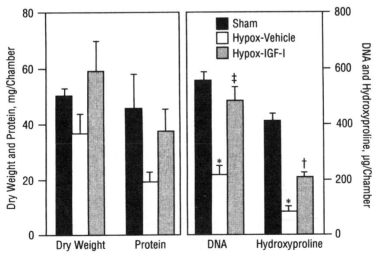

Fig 9–8.—Effect of hypophysectomy (*hypox*) and 14-day continuous local IGF-I infusion on dry tissue weight, protein, DNA, and hydroxyproline in wound chambers in 24 rats. Values are expressed as mean ± SEM. *Asterisks* indicate $P < .0001$ vs. sham; *dagger, $P < .01$; and *double dagger, $P < .0001$ vs. hypox-vehicle. (Courtesy of Mueller RV, Hunt TK, Tokunaga A, et al: *Arch Surg* 129:262–265, 1994.)

creased the values of tissue dry weight, protein, DNA, and hydroxypro-line to 118%, 82%, 87%, and 57% of sham, respectively (Fig 9–8). The number of wound macrophages showed a statistically significant decrease in hypophysectomized vs. sham-operated rats at all time points (days 3, 5, 7, and 11). In every instance, IGF-I infusion resulted in an increase in the number of wound macrophages. Although wound macrophage concentrations showed steady increases in sham-operated rats and in IGF-I–deficient rats receiving IGF-I infusions, IGF-I–deficient rats receiving the placebo infusion showed only a minimal increase.

Conclusion.—The effect of IGF-I infusions on the number of wound macrophages reinforces the principle that macrophages are key cells in wound healing. Macrophages are assumed to respond to various components of the wound environment, leading the intricate cascade of peptide signals that coordinate repair. There are likely to be additional effects of IGF-I on wound healing that are not mediated by macrophages.

▶ The beneficial effects of IGF-I on protein synthesis, gut barrier function, and cell growth attest to the anabolic effects of this naturally occurring peptide. Predictably, IGF-I stimulates wound healing in part by stimulating macrophage infiltration into healing wounds. While IGF-I is likely to modulate wound healing via mechanisms that do not involve macrophages, macrophages are thought to be necessary in the early stages of wound repair and are likely to orchestrate the various peptide signals that coordinate repair. The mechanism by which IGF-I controls wound macrophage concentration is unknown but could include a chemoattractant effect, diapedesis, and/or chemotaxis.—W.W. Souba, M.D., Sc.D.

Wound Healing in Clinical Practice

Comparison of Transcutaneous Oximetry and Laser Doppler Flowmetry as Noninvasive Predictors of Wound Healing After Excision of Extremity Soft-Tissue Sarcomas

Conlon KC, Sclafani L, DiResta GR, Brennan MF (Mem Sloan-Kettering Cancer Ctr, New York)
Surgery 115:335–340, 1994   140-95-9-12

Introduction.—Subjective methods of assessing wound healing in the early postoperative period are unreliable. Dependable methodology would be beneficial, particularly for patients with cancer for whom adjuvant therapy may be delayed until adequate wound healing has been achieved. Transcutaneous oximetry and laser Doppler flowmetry were investigated to determine whether they could identify the patient at risk for wound failure after limb-sparing surgery for soft tissue sarcoma of an extremity.

Methods.—On postoperative days 1, 4/5, 7, and 9, measurements of transcutaneous oxygen pressure ($tcPO_2$) were taken at breathing room air (BL) and 100% oxygen (rate $tcPO_2$). A perfusion index was calculated of

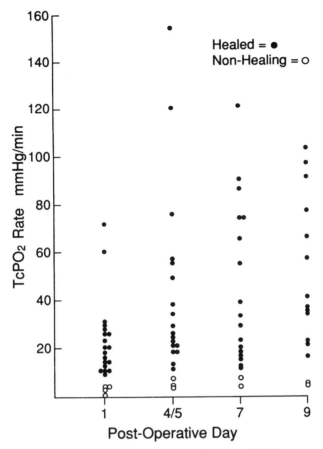

Fig 9–9.—Values of TcPo₂ rate change (air to 100% O₂) measured during postoperative period. Shown are individual measurements in healed (20 patients) and failed (4 patients) wounds. (Courtesy of Conlon KC, Sclafani L, DiResta GR, et al: *Surgery* 115:335–340, 1994.)

laser Doppler flowmetry measurements taken from multiple sites along the wound.

Results.—Four of 24 patients (17%) had nonhealing wounds. No significant differences between healed and nonhealing wounds were found in tcPO₂ (BL) values. On postoperative day 1, measurement of rate tcPO₂ was significantly lower in nonhealing than in healing wounds. Significant increases in rate tcPO₂ were seen in healing wounds from postoperative day 1 to postoperative days 7 and 9. This pattern was not observed in nonhealing wounds (Fig 9–9). Minimum rate tcPO₂ values were 9 mm Hg/min in healed wounds vs. maximum values of 7 mm Hg/min in nonhealing wounds. The laser Doppler flowmetry perfusion index failed throughout to differentiate between healing and nonhealing wounds.

Conclusion.—Measurement of tcPO$_2$ during oxygen inhalation therapy is a reliable predictor of wound healing in patients who have undergone excision of an extremity sarcoma.

▶ Clinical assessment of wound healing is often subjective and involves evaluation of color and capillary refill. Conlon and associates showed that the measurement of transcutaneous oxygen during oxygen inhalation can be used to differentiate viable from nonviable wounds in the early postoperative period after excision of an extremity sarcoma. The authors studied a group of patients in whom wound complications have been reported to be high and, thus, this simple, noninvasive technique is useful in these individuals. Patients with extremity sarcomas are frequently treated with brachytherapy in addition to surgery, and it would be interesting to evaluate the effect of iridium 192 seed placement into these wound beds on transcutaneous oxygen measurements.—W.W. Souba, M.D., Sc.D.

Reduction of Wound Infection in High-Risk Surgical Patients
Fonkalsrud EW, Buchmiller TL (Univ of California, Los Angeles)
Am Surg 59:838–841, 1993   140-95-9–13

Objective.—Two methods of wound management were compared in 183 consecutive patients who, over a 9-year period, underwent total colectomy and endorectal ileal pull-through. The indication was steroid-dependent ulcerative colitis in 156 cases, familial polyposis in 25, and Hirschsprung's disease in 2.

Management.—Ninety patients operated on between 1983 and 1987 had stapled skin closure and received IV antibiotics perioperatively. Ninety-three patients having surgery between 1988 and 1992 had their abdominal wounds probed daily for the first 5 postoperative days at 4 to 6 sites with a cotton swab moistened with 2% aqueous Mercurochrome solution. The ileostomy was closed about 4 months after primary surgery in 89 of the earlier patients and in 87 of those who underwent wound probing.

Results.—Among the patients not having ileostomy closure, 24% of those managed without wound probing and 4% of those having wound probing sustained wound infection. After ileostomy closure, the respective rates of wound infection were 3% and 1%. None of the patients who had their wounds probed required wound packing, and none were hospitalized for a prolonged period. Seventeen nonprobed patients who did not have ileostomy closure spent a mean of nearly 3 extra days in the hospital and required wound packing.

Conclusion.—Delayed wound healing and the need for open wound packing may be minimized in high-risk patients undergoing major colorectal surgery by probing the wound to evacuate clot or seroma for 5 days after surgery.

Colonic Anastomoses: Bursting Strength After Corticosteroid Treatment

Furst MB, Stromberg BV, Blatchford GJ, Christensen MA, Thorson AG
(Creighton Univ, Omaha, Neb)
Dis Colon Rectum 37:12–15, 1994   140-95-9–14

Introduction.—Leaking colonic anastomoses are responsible for numerous postoperative complications and a substantial number of deaths. Although corticosteroids are known to have an adverse effect on the healing of skin wounds, their influence on colonic anastomotic healing is unclear. The effect of corticosteroids on healing colonic anastomoses was studied.

Methods.—Male Sprague-Dawley rats were divided into 3 groups: 12 animals were unoperated and untreated, 48 were operated but untreated controls, and 48 were operated and treated. The bursting pressure was determined at time zero in the nonoperated, non–steroid-treated first group and in the operated groups after sacrifice at 4, 6, 8, and 20 days. All animals in the second and third groups underwent division and interrupted single-layer reanastomosis of the midtransverse colon. Each animal in the third group received 5 mg of cortisone acetate daily by IM injection into the thigh for 5 days preoperatively and daily until sacrifice.

Results.—Bursting pressure, recorded as the pressure at which leakage of air or gross rupture of the anastomosis was noted, was obtained

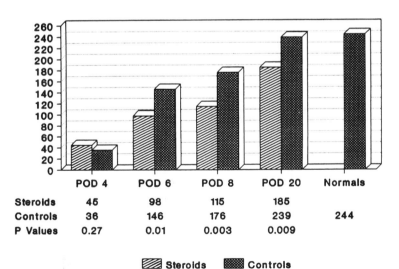

MEAN BURSTING PRESSURES

	POD 4	POD 6	POD 8	POD 20	Normals
Steroids	45	98	115	185	
Controls	36	146	176	239	244
P Values	0.27	0.01	0.003	0.009	

▨ Steroids   ▦ Controls

Fig 9–10.—Comparison of mean bursting pressures (mm Hg) with and without steroid treatment. (Courtesy of Furst MB, Stromberg BV, Blatchford GJ, et al: *Dis Colon Rectum* 37:12–15, 1994.)

within 5 minutes of sacrifice. The normal, unoperated animals had a mean bursting pressure of 244 mm Hg. At 4 days, there was no significant difference in mean bursting strength between treated animals and operated controls (45 vs. 37 mm Hg). Mean bursting pressures at 6, 8, and 20 days were, respectively, 145, 177, and 239 mm Hg for operated control animals and 98, 115, and 185 mm Hg, respectively, for steroid-treated animals (Fig 9–10). The differences at 6, 8, and 20 days were significant.

Conclusion.—In a rat model, corticosteroids significantly decreased the bursting strength of colonic anastomoses. This adverse effect continued even to the 20th postoperative day, when the bursting strength had returned to normal levels in untreated controls. The effect of corticosteroids is a factor that must be considered before colonic operation.

Impaired Wound Healing in Cushing's Syndrome: The Role of Heat Shock Proteins

Gordon CB, Li D-G, Stagg CA, Manson P, Udelsman R (Johns Hopkins Hosp, Baltimore, Md; Union Mem Hosp, Baltimore, Md)
Surgery 116:1082–1087, 1994   140-95-9-15

Introduction.—Glucocorticoids have been found to profoundly impair cellular responses to wounding. Heat shock proteins (HSP), induced in the adrenal cortex and in the vascular smooth muscle, play an important role in cellular repair during stress and have been found to help translocate the glucocorticoid receptor from cytosol to the nucleus. Heat shock proteins may also play an important role in wound healing, and HSP induction may be impaired in patients with Cushing's syndrome.

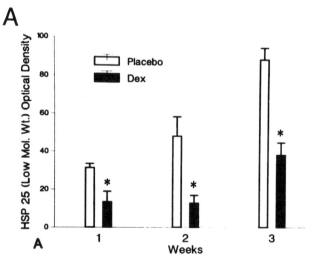

(continued)

Fig 9–11 (cont).

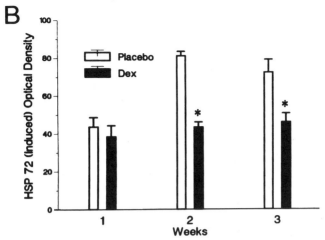

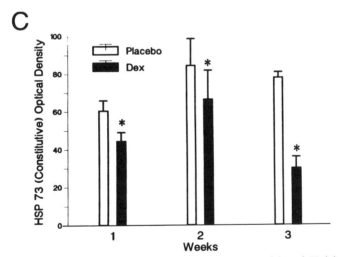

Fig 9–11.—Summary and graphic representation of HSP25 (**A**), 72 (**B**), and 73 (**C**) content of wound chamber tissue in rats treated with dexamethasone and placebo at 1, 2, and 3 weeks expressed as mean ± SEM optical density. *Sig. $F < .05$ by analysis of variance. (Courtesy of Gordon CB, Li D-G, Stagg CA, et al: *Surgery* 116:1082–1087, 1994.)

Methods.—Either 21-day release dexamethasone pellets or placebo pellets were implanted subcutaneously, and modified Hunt-Schilling wound chambers were inserted in each of 3 subcutaneous dorsal pockets in adult rats. One wound chamber was harvested weekly from each rat, and the adrenal gland was harvested at the third week. The wound tissue was analyzed with Western blot and immunohistochemistry for the presence of HSP 25, 72, and 73.

Results.—Whereas the control rats gained about 30 g each week, the animals treated with dexamethasone lost weight progressively, as is consistent with Cushing's syndrome. The mean combined adrenal weight was 47.9 mg in the placebo group and 22.8 mg in the dexamethasone group. The dexamethasone group had a total wet weight of wound tissue that was less than half of that of the control group, although the soluble protein fraction was similar in both groups. The HSP 25 and HSP 70 response increased progressively in the placebo group but was significantly attenuated in the dexamethasone group (Fig 9–11). Immunostaining for HSP 72 was intense in the collagen fibers of the fibroblasts, lymphocytes, macrophages, and vascular tissue in control wound tissue, but was much less intense in wound tissue from the dexamethasone group.

Discussion.—Heat shock proteins play a role in wound healing. However, although the total wound protein synthesis was unaffected by exogenous glucocorticoids, the insoluble protein fractions were qualitatively altered to diminish collagen content, and HSP expression was selectively attenuated. Further study is required to determine whether the wound HSP response can be manipulated in patients with Cushing's syndrome.

▶ Most of us have operated on patients receiving chronic steroid therapy and are familiar with the kinds of healing problems these patients can have. We tend to leave skin staples in longer, and we worry more about our bowel anastomoses. Glucocorticoids reduce collagen biosynthesis and decrease angiogenesis. These worries may be justifiable, as evidenced by the studies abstracted. Colonic anastomoses have a diminished bursting strength, although bursting strength is not necessarily an index of the potential for an anastomotic leak. The marked reduction in wound infection rates reported by Fonkalsrud (Abstract 140-95-9–13) using wound probing with 2% Mercurochrome, suggests that this technique may obviate the need for open wound packing in high-risk patients receiving steroids and undergoing total colectomy.

Steroids also selectively attenuate the expression of several HSPs. Heat shock proteins are highly conserved macromolecules, and they play a key role in the stress response and in the protein assembly, packaging, and repair. Some have referred to them as molecular chaperones. A glucocorticoid-mediated reduction in HSP expression in wounds may be 1 mechanism by which steroids impair wound healing in patients.—W.W. Souba, M.D., Sc.D.

Effects of Aging and Caloric Restriction on Extracellular Matrix Biosynthesis in a Model of Injury Repair in Rats
Reiser K, McGee C, Rucker R, McDonald R (Univ of California, Davis; State Univ of New York, Buffalo)
J Gerontol 50A:B40–B47, 1995   140-95-9–16

Introduction.—Previous animal studies have reported complex interactions between aging and caloric restriction affecting collagen cross-

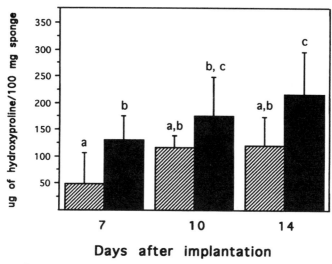

Days after implantation

Fig 9–12.—Effects of chronic caloric restriction and implantation time on accumulation of collagen. Values for hydroxyproline (means ± 1 SD) for rats, aged 10 months, that had been fed ad libitum or calorie restricted for 4 months are shown for sponges removed 7, 10, or 14 days after implantation. Hydroxyproline content was significantly influenced by both implantation time ($P < .02$) and caloric restriction ($P < .002$). Values sharing a common superscript are not significantly different from each other ($P < .05$). *Striped bars* = calorie restricted: *filled bars* = ad libitum fed. (Courtesy of Reiser K, McGee C, Rucker R, et al: *J Gerontol* 50A:B40–B47, 1995.)

linking. The effects of aging and caloric restriction on wound healing and repair were studied in rats, with analysis of both enzymatic cross-linking and nonenzymatic glycation in granulation tissue.

Methods.—After 2 weeks of ad libitum feeding, rats, aged 6 and 24 months, were assigned to either an ad libitum or a calorie-restricted group. Polyvinyl alcohol sponges were implanted either immediately before or after 4 months in the feeding assignment. The sponges were removed and analyzed for reducible and nonreducible enzymatic cross-links and hydroxyproline content at 7, 10, or 14 days after implantation.

Results.—Lysine hydroxylation in granulation tissue was not affected by either aging or caloric restriction. However, hydroxyproline accumulation was higher in younger animals and reached peak values with shorter implantation in younger than in older animals. Mean collagen accumulation was lower in chronically calorie-restricted animals with each implantation time than in animals fed ad libitum (Fig 9–12), although collagen accumulation was not affected by acute caloric restriction. Age significantly affected the collagen content of the reducible cross-links, difunctional dihydroxylysinonorleucine and hydroxylysinonorleucine, and the nonreducible cross-link, hydroxypyridinium, but caloric restriction had a significant interaction with age only on dihydroxylysinonorleucine.

Discussion.—Wound healing capacity is impaired by both aging and by chronic caloric restriction, as indicated by the amount of collagen deposited, the rate of healing response, collagen production, and collagen cross-linking.

▶ Most of us have made the clinical observation that wound healing is impaired in the elderly and in the malnourished patient. This study demonstrates that both aging and caloric restriction reduce wound healing and repair as manifested by a diminution in collagen accumulation and in cross-linking. The study did not include a group of older animals that were nutritionally replete to determine whether feeding could improve wound healing. The results, however, suggest that nutritional support of elderly patients may be 1 component of care that can improve wound healing.—W.W. Souba, M.D., Sc.D.

10 Gastrointestinal

Introduction

ESOPHAGUS AND STOMACH

The evolution of esophageal surgery began with therapies directed only to the cervical esophagus and included cervical esophagotomy for removal of foreign bodies. By the turn of the 20th century, malignant lesions of the cervical esophagus were amenable to surgical ablation, largely through the pioneering efforts of Czerny and Billroth.

The first phrenoesophageal diverticulum was resected in 1886 by Wheeler, and transabdominal procedures for relief of esophageal achalasia were performed in the early 1900s by von Mikulicz and Heller. In the United States, the first successful esophagogastrectomy for carcinoma was performed by Marshall at the Lahey Clinic in 1937. This was followed by rapid advances in thoracic surgery that were principally attained through progress in general anesthetic agents, blood replacement, and modifications in surgical technique which enhanced the probability of attaining acceptable morbidity and mortality rates.

Despite these extraordinary advances in the therapy of this organ, it was not until the post-World War II era that esophageal surgeons became acutely aware of the complexities of esophageal function and the disturbances created for this organ by intrinsic disease and surgical interventions. The contributions of Ingelfinger and colleagues and Code and associates in the 1950s advanced the knowledge base to enable understanding of the importance of physiology of this organ. As a result of these detailed physiologic advances, surgeons who were involved in care of the esophagus could properly document patients' diseases and provide a sound basis on which to select patients for operative approaches. This pioneering era encouraged the surgeon to emphasize function as well as technical approaches to the esophagus to enhance operative results.

Surgical therapy for carcinoma of the esophagus is often palliative and only rarely curative. Abstract 140-95-10-1 documents that residency training programs often emphasize a single technique for esophagectomy, because the safety and efficacy for teaching more than a single type of esophagectomy are poorly defined. Interestingly, transthoracic esophagectomy, transhiatal esophagectomy, and total thoracic esophagectomy that were performed within a single residency program were observed to have morbidity, mortality, and recurrence rates similar to those of other contemporary series. The report by Putnam and associates (Abstract 140-95-10–1) emphasizes the concept that a specific technique can be selected for individual patients who require esophagectomy for carcinoma. However, it is not the technique of esophagectomy that is used in training which determines outcome; rather, it is the stage of disease that is the determinant of survival and recurrence.

Despite recent advances in the therapy of esophageal carcinoma that apply adjuvant therapeutic principles with chemotherapeutics and irradiation, 50% to 60% of patients have incurable disease at the time they are seen. These patients require palliative therapy if possible, with the aim of relieving dysphagia because of a considerable reduction in the quality of life resulting from pain and obstruction related to the neoplasm.

The recent introduction of a new class of endoprostheses (see Abstract 140-95-10–2) promises a reduction in complications previously encountered with conventional plastic endoprostheses for the therapy of esophageal obstruction with inoperable disease. Although expandable metal stents are evolving, future developments will include a coating of the metal mesh with a membrane to prevent tumor ingrowth. Recent data (see Abstract 140-95-10–2) suggest that these metal stents are cost-effective and represent a safer alternative to conventional prostheses for palliation of malignant esophageal obstruction.

The growth in the application of molecular biology to various solid organs has been exponential over the past 5 years. The putative tumor suppressor gene p53 has been the most commonly implicated (60%) immunoreactive oncogene in mammalian neoplasms. Abstract 140-95-10–5 suggests that the mutated p53 gene with overexpression is possibly implicated in the pathogenesis of human esophageal cancers, specifically primary esophageal sarcoma and regional lymphatics. It is highly probable that this tumor suppressor gene and other oncogenes and gene products will be implicated in the neoplastic transformation of the organ. Furthermore, the application of molecular biological principles may enable surgeons to objectively evaluate prognosis and plan therapeutic interventions based on expression of these oncogenes, proto-oncogenes, growth factors, and tumor suppressor genes.

Step-sectioning techniques increasingly implicate the incidence and prevalence of synchronous esophageal carcinoma (see Abstract 140-95-10–7). The mechanisms of carcinogenesis and the evolution of molecular principles to establish an aggressive phenotype for various tumors of this organ are being identified and documented. Data suggest that significant prognostic indicators include a greater increase in the depth of invasion for those with multiple synchronous tumors of the esophagus. As a result, the entire esophagus can be considered a single all-encompassing entity for subsequent carcinogenesis, which supports the rationale that many surgeons apply for total esophagectomy in therapy for carcinoma.

Increasing recognition of esophageal adenocarcinoma in Western civilization raises increasing alarm as to the etiology of this neoplasm. Interestingly, Barrett's metaplasia usually always precedes esophageal adeno-carcinoma, is often recognized in specialized intestinal-type mucosa, and predominantly occurs in elderly white men who often have a history of heavy smoking. Abstract 140-95-10–9 confirms that adenocarcinomas located at the gastroesophageal junction were associated with Barrett's metaplasia in nearly one half the patients. The presence of high-grade dysplasia within this type of mucosa supports a Barrett's origin for one half of adenocarcinomas at this location. These data appear to lend credence to the tenet that patients with Barrett's metaplasia should be routinely placed in an aggressive endoscopic surveillance program.

This prospective approach should provide the clinician with the opportunity for early detection of adenocarcinoma that arises at the gastroesophageal junction in these short segments of specialized intestinal metaplasia. Early detection of such pathology, which is high grade and suggestive of in situ or invasive disease, warrants an esophagogastrectomy. The contributions of molecular biology to the identification of overexpression of oncogenes, proto-oncogenes, and mutated tumor suppressor genes may be of additional value to traditional pathologic approaches to identification of the high-risk patient.

The surgical literature currently emphasizes that identification of stage I and early stage II disease gives the patient a significantly enhanced probability of long-term survival with no nodal involvement. Esophagectomy remains the appropriate therapy in patients with nonmetastatic resectable carcinoma. It can now be done with low morbidity and mortality when it is performed by experienced surgeons (see Abstract 140-95-10–10).

The surgical literature embraces an increasing application of laparoscopic antireflux surgery for patients with documented gastroesophageal reflux disease. Although few studies document results similar to open techniques (see Abstract 140-95-10–14), the majority of reports show a significant reduction in the length of hospital stay, anesthetic requirements, complications, and esthetic sequelae. Emphasis must be placed on the size and tightness of the fundic wrap. The study by Peillon and associates (see Abstract 140-95-10–15) focuses on the role of the vagus nerves in initiating postoperative symptomatology. No advantage for exclusion of the vagi from the three quarter Nissen fundoplication wrap was evident for postoperative gastric emptying, and it did not appear to affect the outcome of reflux surgery. Because there is a high frequency of esophagogastroduodenoscopy reflux symptoms, health care cost containment issues have stimulated a re-evaluation of management for this disorder with expensive long-term medications. It is highly probable that we will see a resurgence of interest and progressive developments in the application of laparoscopic approaches for management of this esophageal disorder.

Consensus has developed with regard to the extraordinarily high prevalence rate of *Helicobacter pylori* colonization in duodenal ulcer patients; however, the relationship of this bacterial organism to peptic ulcer disease remains speculative. A recently conducted prospective randomized study by Walia and associates (see Abstract 140-95-10-17) determined that anterior lesser curve seromyotomy with posterior truncal vagotomy (ASPTV) is equivalent to proximal gastric vagotomy (PGV). Good-to-excellent results (Visick I & II) have been recorded for three quarters of patients in both groups. Although ASPTV is a good alternative to PGV for the treatment of chronic duodenal ulcer, both have recurrence rates that are high (14% for PGV, 12% ASPTV).

Since the introduction of the vagotomy as definitive therapy for duodenal ulcer by Dragstedt in 1945, antrectomy with truncal or selective vagotomy has emerged as the best operation because of its low recurrence rate (less than 2%). These alternatives include the most conservative approaches, which retain the stomach and duodenum and ensure a diminution in postgastrectomy symptoms that are much improved over those of lesser resection or drainage. Although PGV has been observed to have the lowest operative mortality and morbidity and the fewest postoperative sequelae, it is a demanding, technically exacting, and time-consuming procedure that is considered to be associated with a high rate of ulcer recurrence. As a consequence, the more simplistic ASPTV should now be considered a replacement for the PGV. Parietal cell vagotomy is the choice of many gastrointestinal surgeons for therapy of duodenal ulcer disease because of the occasional patient who is disabled by a selective vagotomy-antrectomy (see Abstract 140-95-10-18). However, selective vagotomy-antrectomy is preferable for patients with pyloric and prepyloric ulcers and for those with pyloric obstruction. Both procedures should be effective and safe when applied appropriately.

Kirby I. Bland, M.D.

Comparison of Three Techniques of Esophagectomy Within a Residency Training Program
Putnam JB Jr, Suell DM, McMurtrey MJ, Ryan MB, Walsh GL, Natarajan G, Roth JA (Univ of Texas MD Anderson Cancer Ctr, Houston)
Ann Thorac Surg 57:319–325, 1994   140-95-10-1

Background.—Residency training programs commonly teach a single technique of esophagectomy, because the safety and efficacy of teaching and performing more than a single type of this procedure have not been clarified. The results of teaching 3 techniques of esophagectomy for carcinoma of the intrathoracic esophagus were reviewed. Operation-specific and stage-specific survival, morbidity, mortality, and site of recurrence were assessed.

Patients and Methods.—Two hundred forty-eight patients underwent exploration for possible esophageal resection between 1986 and 1992. Of those, 221 were considered to be candidates for resection. Surgical indications included adenocarcinoma in 146, squamous cell carcinoma in 72, and other histologic findings in 3. Transthoracic esophagectomy was undertaken in 134, transhiatal esophagectomy in 42, and total thoracic esophagectomy in 45, with thoracic surgical residents or fellows performing the major components of all resections.

Results.—Complications were noted in 75% of the patients undergoing transthoracic, 69% undergoing transhiatal, and 80% undergoing total thoracic esophagectomy. The overall operative mortality rate was 6.8%. A higher leakage rate was observed in patients with a cervical anastomosis—at 13% compared with 6% for those with an intrathoracic anastomosis. The median survival was 22 months (19% 5-year survival), with no differences being observed with operation type or stage. None of the 27 patients with unresectable disease survived longer than 10 months. In patients with stage 3 or 2a adenocarcinoma, a trend toward improved survival was observed after transthoracic esophagectomy, despite comparable rates of local and distant recurrence.

Conclusion.—These 3 surgical techniques for esophagectomy performed within a residency training program had similar morbidity, mortality, and recurrence rates compared with those in other current series. Survival and sites of local or distant recurrence were independent of the technique used, although specific operations showed unique morbidity and mortality. These differences may help the surgeon with the selection of a surgical technique for individual patients.

▶ The interesting conclusions of this review support the assumption that the proper technique of site-specific disease is more important than the selection of technique for therapy of patients with carcinoma of the esophagus. Furthermore, the authors reiterated that survival and recurrence result from disease stage rather than from the technical approach selected by the surgeon.—K.I. Bland, M.D.

A Controlled Trial of an Expansile Metal Stent for Palliation of Esophageal Obstruction Due to Inoperable Cancer

Knyrim K, Wagner H-J, Bethge N, Keymling M, Vakil N (Städtische Kliniken, Kassel, Germany; Innere Abteilung IV, Krankenhaus Neukölln, Berlin, Germany; Kreiskrankenhaus, Bad Hersfeld, Germany; et al)
N Engl J Med 329:1302–1307, 1993   140-95-10–2

Introduction.—Dysphagia resulting from malignant esophageal obstruction usually can be palliated by endoscopic placement of a plastic prosthesis, but complications are frequent. An alternative is to insert a metal-mesh stent that collapses to 3 mm in diameter during placement but can then expand up to 16 mm.

Study Design.—This new type of endoprosthesis was evaluated in 39 adults who had dysphagia as a result of inoperable esophageal carcinoma and 3 others with extrinsic malignant obstruction of the esophagus. The

Complications and Recurrent Dysphagia

EVENT	PLASTIC PROSTHESIS (N = 21)	METAL STENT (N = 21)
	no. of patients (%)	
Complication	9 (43)	0*
Perforation	3 (14)	0
Aspiration pneumonia	1 (5)	0
Migration of device	5 (24)	0
Recurrent dysphagia	7	7†
Food-bolus impaction	1	3
Migration of device	5	0
Tumor ingrowth	0	3
Tumor overgrowth	0	2
Tracheoesophageal fistula	1	2

*P < 0.001 by Fisher's exact test for the comparison with the plastic-prosthesis group.
†Dysphagia recurred twice in three patients: one patient had food-bolus impaction and later had tumor ingrowth, one had tumor ingrowth and later had tracheoesophageal fistula, and one had food-bolus impaction and later had overgrowth at the distal end of the stent.
(Courtesy of Knyrim K, Wagner H-J, Bethge N, et al: N *Engl J Med* 329:1302–1307, 1993.)

patients were randomly assigned to receive either a plastic prosthesis 16 mm in diameter or an expansile metal-mesh stent and were followed at 6-week intervals for as long as they survived. If necessary, the stricture was dilated with a balloon catheter before stent placement. The 2 treatment groups were clinically comparable.

Results.—In all but 1 of the patients it was possible to place a prosthesis or stent. Mortality in the first month was 29% in patients who were given a plastic prosthesis and 14% in those who were given a metal-mesh stent. There were 3 placement-related deaths in the former group. Patients who were given a plastic prosthesis had significantly more complications from the placement or presence of the device. None of the metal-mesh stents migrated, but 5 plastic prostheses migrated, which led to recurrent dysphagia. In 3 patients with a metal-mesh stent, the ingrowth of tumor through the mesh led to recurrent dysphagia (table) and was treated by laser ablation. Two other patients in this group had a tracheoesophageal fistula and had a plastic prosthesis inserted through the stent.

Cost-Effectiveness.—Three patients died prematurely as a direct result of complications from the insertion of a plastic prosthesis. Metal stents cost $457 more per premature death avoided. Overall costs actually decreased when the time spent in the hospital for recovery and treating complications was taken into account.

Conclusion.—The metal-mesh esophageal stent is a relatively safe and cost-effective alternative to the conventional plastic prosthesis for palliation of patients with malignant esophageal obstruction.

▶ The application of expandable metallic stents is broadening its field from the biliary arena to inoperable gastrointestinal and rectal cancers. These applications are attractive because they should not dislodge nor require replacement. Long-term follow-up is warranted before widespread applicability can be ascertained.—V.E. Pricolo, M.D.

Impaired Healing of Cervical Oesophagogastrostomies Can Be Predicted by Estimation of Gastric Serosal Blood Perfusion by Laser Doppler Flowmetry

Pierie J-PEN, De Graff PW, Poen H, Van Der Tweel I, Obertop H (Univ Hosp, Utrecht, The Netherlands)
Eur J Surg 160:599–603, 1994   140-95-10–3

Objective.—Thirty patients who had cancer of the esophagus or esophagogastric junction underwent transhiatal esophagectomy with partial gastrectomy and had reconstruction with a gastric tube and cervical esophagogastrostomy. Perfusion of the stomach was monitored at 4 sites by laser Doppler flowmetry before and after construction of the gastric tube.

Results.—Perfusion was significantly lower at the most proximal part of the gastric tube than at more distal sites. An anastomotic stricture developed in half the 18 patients in whom perfusion of the proximal gastric tube was less than 70% of the preoperative value and in 1 of 12 patients (8%) who had greater baseline perfusion. Reduced perfusion of the gastric tube was not predictive of anastomotic leakage.

Conclusion.—In patients who have gastric tube reconstruction of the alimentary tract after resection of esophageal or esophagogastric cancer, preservation of perfusion to the proximal part of the gastric tube limits the risk of development of an anastomotic stricture.

▶ This prospective study involved 30 patients undergoing transhiatal esophagectomy and partial gastrectomy for cancer of the esophagus or esophagogastric junction with gastric tube reconstruction and cervical esophagogastrostomy. Operative measurement of gastric blood perfusion at 4 sites by laser Doppler flowmetry and perfusion of the same sites after construction of the gastric tube were expressed as percentages of preconstruction values.

These authors demonstrated that relative perfusion of the most proximal site of the gastric tube was significantly lower than at the more distal sites. Furthermore, 9 of 18 patients in whom the perfusion of the proximal gastric tube was less than 70% of the preconstruction values had an anastomotic stricture develop compared with only 1 of 12 patients with a relative perfusion of 70% or more. A reduction in perfusion of the gastric tube did not predict leakage. The majority of patients who did not develop a stricture had significantly higher relative blood perfusion than those who did.

Impaired anastomotic healing is unlikely if relative perfusion accounts for 70% or more of preconstruction values. However, perfusion of less than 70% partly predicts the occurrence of an anastomotic stricture, but leakage cannot be predicted. Because laser flow studies are relatively easy to perform in the operating room, this method would appear to be a useful adjunct in the attempt to predict whether blood flow to the gastric tube is adequate for a cervical esophagogastrostomy.—H.H. Simms, M.D.

The Value of Abrasive Cytology in the Early Detection of Oesophageal Carcinoma: A Pilot Survey in Ciskei

Lazarus C, Jaskiewicz K, Southall HA, Sumeruk RA, Nainkin J (Cecilia Makiwane Hosp, Mdantsane, Ciskei; South Africa Groote Univ of Cape Town; South Africa Rhodes Univ, Grahamstown, CP, South Africa)
S Afr Med J 84:488–490, 1994   140-95-10–4

Background.—In southern Africa, squamous cancer of the esophagus is the most common cancer among black men. Abrasive brush cytology has been used in China as a screening tool for esophageal cancer. The feasibility of brush cytology as a screening program for South Africans was examined.

Methods.—Over a 4-year period, villages in a district of Ciskei, South Africa, with a reported high prevalence of esophageal cancer were visited, and brush cytology screening was offered to the adults. A brush biopsy was performed by having the participants swallow a brush biopsy capsule that contained the brush attached to a long thread. After 10 minutes, the capsule dissolves, and the brush expands and is withdrawn with the thread. The cytologic material obtained is smeared onto a glass slide, fixed, stained, and examined.

Results.—Nine confirmed positive and 1 false positive cases were detected among the 1,336 adults (926 women and 410 men) screened. The predictive value of the brush cytology screening program was 90%. Because only 2 of the 9 positives underwent recommended treatment, the yield of the program was 2 cases or 688 people screened per case treated.

Conclusion.—The efficacy of brush cytology screening for esophageal cancer, as documented by Chinese studies, may be generalized to rural southern Africans. Further investigations are needed of the educational and economic implications of mass screening for esophageal cancer in southern Africa.

▶ These authors nicely demonstrated that a relatively benign technique using brush cytology with inexpensive brush biopsy capsules is an effective screening technique for the detection of early esophageal cancer. One thousand three hundred thirty-six research subjects underwent this procedure, and 9 true positive cases were identified, for a predictive value of 90%. In 7 of these 9 cases, the carcinoma was in an early stage, whereas in 2 it was advanced.

Although it was not possible to differentiate between sensitivity and specificity and therefore make distinctions between true and false negatives, this study has a high negative predictive value. This technique would appear to be of value for patients who are at high risk of esophageal carcinoma.—H.H. Simms, M.D.

---

p53 Immunoreactivity in Carcinosarcoma of the Esophagus
Casson AG, Kerkvliet N, O'Malley F, Inculet R, Troster M (Univ of Toronto; Mount Sinai Hosp, Toronto; Univ of Western Ontario, London, Canada)
J Surg Oncol 56:132–135, 1994   140-95-10-5

Background.—Mutations of the p53 tumor suppressor gene were recently reported in esophageal squamous cell cancers—primary esophageal adenocarcinomas—and associated premalignant Barrett's epithelium. A patient with a primary esophageal carcinosarcoma who was found to have p53 protein distribution in both the primary tumor and the regional lymph node metastases was studied.

Methods.—Distribution of the p53 protein in archival pathology specimens of the primary tumor, regional lymph nodes with and without metastases, and the normal esophagus was studied using a modified indirect immunoperoxidase technique.

Results.—The 57-year-old patient, a heavy cigarette smoker, had a 3-month history of fever, anterior chest wall pain, and a 10-kg weight loss. No history of dysphagia or any difficulty swallowing was obtained. Clubbing and hypertrophic pulmonary osteoarthropathy were revealed on an otherwise normal physical examination. The esophageal mass was biopsied at esophagoscopy, and a malignant stromal tumor was diagnosed. The patient underwent total esophagectomy, gastric interposition, and cervical esophagogastrostomy. No distant metastases were found. No immunoreactivity was seen in any negative control, in histologically normal esophagus from the patient's resection margin, or in nonmetastatic lymph nodes. Characteristic p53 protein nuclear staining with a heterogenous distribution of intensity was found in the sarcomatous component of the mass and in the lymph node metastases. Despite complete surgical resection and adjuvant chemoradiotherapy, the patient died 6 months after surgery with diffuse intrathoracic metastases.

Conclusion.—The p53 tumor suppressor gene was further implicated in the pathogenesis of human esophageal cancer.

▶ The tumor suppressor gene p53 mutation (overexpression) is recognized in approximately two thirds of mammalian neoplasms. The authors demonstrated the presence of diffuse p53 protein (mutation) distribution in a recently treated patient with primary esophageal carcinosarcoma. No immunoreactivity was seen in any negative control or histologically normal esophagus. In malignant specimens up to and including the resection margin, nuclear staining was characteristic for the p53 protein. A similar heterogeneous distribution was seen with regional lymph node metastases; nonmetastatic lymph nodes were immunonegative. These results further implicate the p53 tumor suppressor gene in the pathogenesis of human esophageal cancers.—H.H. Simms, M.D. and K.I. Bland, M.D.

Functioning of the Intrathoracic Stomach After Esophagectomy

Nishikawa M, Murakami T, Tangoku A, Hayashi H, Adachi J, Suzuki T (Yamaguchi Univ School of Medicine, Kogushi, Japan; Univ of Arkansas, Little Rock)
Arch Surg 129:837–841, 1994   140-95-10–6

Objective.—A case-control study was done to define the function of the intrathoracic stomach in terms of acid secretion and motility after esophagectomy.

Patients.—Twenty one patients were randomly selected from among 79 patients with esophageal cancer who had a subtotal esophagectomy and reconstruction with a 4-cm wide gastric tube, using the greater curvature of the stomach. The anastomoses were done in the neck in 17 patients and at the apex of the thorax in 4. All patients received either a digital pyloromyotomy or pyloroplasty. A control group of 14 healthy men was also studied.

Methods.—Acid secretion was monitored for at least 3 days after surgery and from 1 to 28 months after surgery using a newly developed pH probe placed in the intrathoracic stomach. The average pH value (average of all total monitoring values) and pH holding time (ratio of the period during which the pH value was 3 or higher, based on the entire continuous monitoring periods) were measured. Motility was measured by scintigraphy from 1 to 5 months after surgery.

Results.—The intrathoracic stomach remained at a pH of 3 or lower through postoperative day 3, with a temporal increase in pH in response to histamine-2 blockers. Follow-up measurements in the reconstructed gastric tube showed a 24-hour average pH value of 3.9 and a pH holding time of 52.2%, which was almost identical to that found in healthy controls. Scintigrams of the intrathoracic stomach showed no significant changes in gastric emptying. Almost all patients had a burst or slope type, indicating that the emptying of the intrathoracic stomach may not be static. Hemorrhagic ulcers developed after esophagectomy in 3 patients, but pH values did not differ significantly from those in patients who did not have hemorrhagic ulcers.

Conclusion.—These data indicate that acid secretion and motility of the intrathoracic stomach with truncal vagotomy may be unchanged after esophagectomy.

▶ This study investigated the function of the intrathoracic stomach after an esophagectomy in terms of acid secretion and motility. For acid secretion, a pH probe was placed in the intrathoracic stomach to measure the average pH value. For motility, digestive tract scintigraphy was performed using labeled indium-111.

The results demonstrate that there was no significant difference in pH values or pH holding time between patients and normal volunteers. The time activity curve of the intrathoracic stomach observed by scintigraphy underwent no change after surgery. Among 3 patients with hemorrhagic ulcers, 2 exhibited improvements after receiving a histamine block, whereas the other was not affected. These data demonstrate that the ability of acid secretion and motility of the intrathoracic stomach with truncal vagotomy are unchanged after esophagectomy.—H.H. Simms, M.D.

Prevalence and Clinicopathologic Features of Multiple Squamous Cell Carcinoma of the Esophagus
Pesko P, Rakic S, Milicevic M, Bulajic P, Gerzic Z (Univ Clinical Center, Belgrade, Yugoslavia)
Cancer 73:2687–2690, 1994   140-95-10–7

Introduction.—Independent synchronous esophageal carcinoma (SEC) can occur in grossly invasive esophageal cancer (GEC) patients. The clinicopathologic features of multiple primary esophageal carcinoma remain relatively unknown. The histology of GEC patients based on criteria for SEC was studied.

Methods.—Over a 4-year period, 54 squamous cell GEC patients had transthoracic esophagectomy and systemic lymphadenectomy. The esophagus was transected 3 cm from the pharyngoesophageal junction. The transected esophagus and lymph nodes were analyzed histologically. Tumors were classified as poorly, moderately, or well differentiated. To exclude secondary lesions, there had to be at least 1.5 cm of healthy tissue between the 2 lesions (Fig 10–1).

Results.—The SEC lesions, all of which were squamous cell carcinoma, were found in 31% of the patients. Second primary lesions all had a superficial or invasive carcinoma. There were no significant differences between patients with multiple or solitary cancer on the basis of sex, age, tumor site, differentiation, diameter, lymph involvement, or tumor stage.

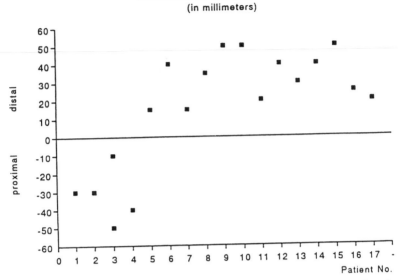

Fig 10–1.—Distance of SEC from GEC (in mm). *Abbreviations:* SEC, synchronous esophageal carcinoma; GEC, grossly invasive esophageal cancer. (Courtesy of Pesko P, Rakic S, Milicevic M, et al: *Cancer* 73:2687–2690, 1994.)

The depth of invasion for GEC was significantly deeper than SEC. Associated lesions did not influence tumor stage in multiple primary cancer patients.

Conclusion.—Invasive tumors were commonly found. Patients with advanced main tumor penetration should be expected to have a higher prevalence of multiple cancer sites. The whole esophagus can be considered to be a single entity.

▶ This study evaluated 54 surgical specimens from patients with grossly invasive esophageal cancer histopathologically, using step-sectioning techniques to determine the incidence and prevalence of SEC. Fifty-four patients with squamous cell GEC who underwent transthoracic esophagectomy were studied between 1987 and 1991. Lesions that were defined and classified as SEC were detected histologically in 17 of 54 patients (31%). All second primaries had a superficial carcinoma or invasive carcinoma. Significantly, the distance from the GEC to the SEC was 34 ± 12 mm.

The second lesion was significantly less invasive than the main tumor, and there was no significant difference in sex, age, main tumor site, tumor differentiation, tumor diameter lymph nodes, or tumor stage between patients with multiple cancer and patients with solitary cancer. The only significant prognostic indicator was a markedly greater increase in the depth of invasion in patients with multiple synchronous tumors. These results support the concept that the entire esophagus can be considered to be a single entity for subsequent carcinogenesis.—H.H. Simms, M.D.

Operative Procedures of Reconstruction After Resection of Esophageal Cancer and the Postoperative Quality of Life

Kuwano H, Ikebe M, Baba K, Kitamura K, Toh Y, Matsuda H, Sugimachi K (Kyushu Univ, Fukuoka, Japan)
World J Surg 17:773–776, 1993   140-95-10-8

Objective.—The influence of various reconstructive techniques on postoperative quality of life was examined in 50 patients who had resection of carcinoma from the thoracic esophagus. The patients had experienced no recurrence of cancer when they were interviewed.

Management.—Nine patients (group I) had reconstruction through the antethoracic route. The gastric tube was substituted for the esophagus in 8 patients and the colon in 1. Twenty-four patients (group II) had reconstruction through the retrosternal route by the use of the gastric tube. Seventeen patients (group III) had an intrathoracic anastomosis. The gastric tube was used in 16 of 17 group III patients; 1 patient in this group had colonic interposition.

Results.—Dysphagia developed postoperatively in 42% of group II patients, 22% of group I patients, and 6% of group III patients. It generally improved gradually over time. Dumping symptoms were similarly frequent in all groups and also tended to improve gradually. Hoarseness developed only in group II patients. Two group III patients had postoperative heartburn that was readily controlled medically. One third or more of patients in all groups lost more than 1 kg of body weight, but most patients had regained the weight after 3 years.

Conclusion.—Patients who remain free of recurrent esophageal cancer generally experience a gradual improvement in quality of life, regardless of the reconstructive method used.

▶ The influence of operative procedures for reconstruction after a resection of esophageal cancer on postoperative quality of life was investigated. The study included 3 groups of patients: Group I was composed of 9 patients who were reconstructed by the antethoracic route, group II included 24 patients who were reconstructed through the retrosternal route, and group III included 17 patients who were reconstructed through an intrathoracic anastomosis. The occurrence of postoperative dysphagia was far greater in those in group II compared with those in group I or group III, although this symptom improved over time.

There was no significant difference in the incidence of dumping between the 3 treatment groups. Performance data tended to improve after time, and the quality of life gradually improved in all patients as time elapsed postoperatively.—H.H. Simms, M.D.

Is Barrett's Metaplasia the Source of Adenocarcinomas of the Cardia?

Clark GWB, Smyrk TC, Burdiles P, Hoeft SF, Peters JH, Kiyabu M, Hinder RA, Bremner CG, DeMeester TR (Univ of Southern California, Los Angeles; Clarkson Memorial Hosp, Omaha, Neb; Creighton Univ, Omaha, Neb)
Arch Surg 129:609–614, 1994   140-95-10–9

Background.—Tumors located at the gastroesophageal junction have been hypothesized to be similar to esophageal adenocarcinomas, differing only because they arise from short segments of specialized intestinal metaplasia (Fig 10-2). The prevalence of Barrett's esophagus in patients with adenocarcinomas at the gastroesophageal junction was reported.

Methods.—One hundred patients with adenocarcinoma of the esophagus, cardia, or proximal stomach were included. All underwent esophagogastrectomy. In 42%, cardiac adenocarcinomas were associated with Barrett's esophagus.

Findings.—Specialized intestinal metaplasia was identified in the histologic sections from resected specimens in 42% of cardiac adenocarcinomas, 79% of esophageal adenocarcinomas, and only 5% of subcardiac adenocarcinomas (Fig 10-3). Preoperative endoscopic biopsy findings agreed with the final diagnosis of Barrett's esophagus in 33 of 38 esophageal tumors, in 6 of 13 cardiac tumors, and in the 1 subcardiac

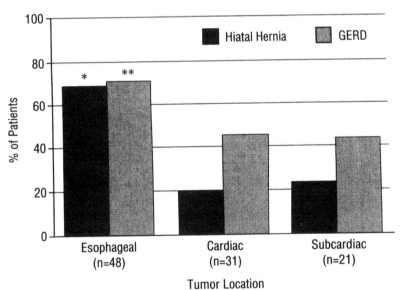

Fig 10–2.—Prevalence of hiatal hernia and history of gastroesophageal reflux symptoms, *GERD*, in patients with esophageal, cardiac, and subcardiac adenocarcinomas. *Abbreviations:* *, $P < 0.01$ vs cardiac and subcardiac tumors; **, $P < 0.05$ vs cardiac tumors and $P = 0.05$ vs subcardiac tumors (x^2). (Courtesy of Clark GWB, Smyrk TC, Burdiles P, et al: *Arch Surg* 129:609–614, 1994).

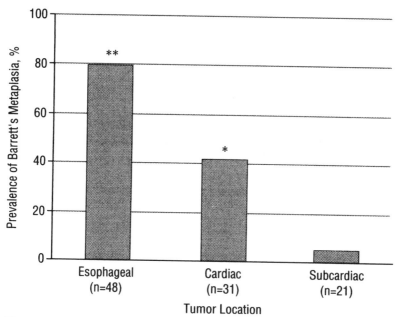

Fig 10–3.—Prevalence of specialized intestinal epithelium (Barrett's metaplasia) on histological examination of the surgical specimen in patients with esophageal, cardiac, and subcardiac adenocarcinomas. *Abbreviations:* *, P < 0.01 vs. cardiac and subcardiac tumors, **, P < 0.01 vs. cardiac and subcardiac tumors. (Courtesy of Clark GWB, Smyrk TC, Burdiles P, et al: *Arch Surg* 129:609–614, 1994.)

tumor. However, a preoperative endoscopic biopsy did not detect specialized intestinal metaplasia in 7 of 13 cardiac tumors. Compared with esophageal tumors, cardiac tumors were associated with shorter lengths of Barrett's mucosa. Barrett's metaplasia was dysplastic in 36 of 38 esophageal tumors, in 10 of 13 cardiac tumors, and in none of the subcardiac tumors.

Conclusion.—Adenocarcinomas at the gastroesophageal junction were associated with Barrett's metaplasia in almost half the patients. Because the length of the Barrett segment tends to be short, it can be missed on endoscopy. The finding of high-grade dysplasia in Barrett's mucosa supports a Barrett's origin for half the adenocarcinomas that arise at this location.

▶ This article examines the hypothesis that tumors located at the gastroesophageal junction are similar to esophageal adenocarcinomas and that they arise from short segments of specialized intestinal metaplasia. This hypothesis was tested in 100 patients who underwent an esophagogastrectomy for adenocarcinoma of the distal esophagus, cardia, or proximal stomach. Specialized intestinal metaplasia was identified in the histologic sections of approximately 42% of the cardiac adenocarcinomas and 70% of the esophageal adenocarcinomas but only 5% of subcardiac adenocarcinomas. Barrett's metaplasia was dysplastic in 36 of 38 esophageal tumors and 10 of 13 cardiac tumors.

This article supports the finding that adenocarcinomas located at the gastroesophageal junction are associated with Barrett's metaplasia in a large proportion of patients. Furthermore, the presence of high-grade metaplasia within Barrett's mucosa supports the Barrett's origin for half the adenocarcinomas that arise at this location. This article would appear to support the assertion that strong consideration should be given to esophagogastrectomy in patients with Barrett's metaplasia.—H.H. Simms, M.D.

Does Esophagectomy Cure a Resectable Esophageal Cancer?

Nakadi IE, Houben J-J, Gay F, Closset J, Gelin M, Lambilliotte J-P (Hôpital Erasme, Université Libre de Bruxelles, Brussels, Belgium)
World J Surg 17:760–765, 1993   140-95-10–10

Background.—Esophageal cancer is still difficult to treat. The role of surgery in patients with this disease needs to be more clearly defined. The value of esophagectomy in the cure of esophageal cancer was investigated.

Methods.—Four hundred one patients with esophageal cancer were assessed for curative resection between 1978 and 1990. One hundred eighty-seven patients, or 47%, underwent operation. Eleven patients with stage I, 24 with stage II, and 66 with stage III pathologic tumor node metastatis (TNM) who were followed up for at least 2 years were retrospectively studied. Esophagogastrectomy was done in 91% of the patients, and gastric transposition was achieved in 96%. The anastomoses were intrathoracic in 98%, and at the apex of the right thorax for tumors of the middle third of the esophagus. Staplers were used for three fourths of the sutures.

Findings.—Hospital mortality after surgery was 5.9%. Morbidity included strictures in 11%, esophagitis in 12%, and anastomotic leak in 2%. For patients with stages I, II, and III disease, respective actuarial 5-year survival rates were 90.9%, 52.3%, and 17.7%. The overall 5-year survival rate was 34.2%. This rate was 64.8% for patients with no nodal involvement a figure that declined to 17.7% when nodes were involved.

Conclusion.—Esophagectomy is the appropriate treatment for patients with nonmetastatic resectable carcinoma. The overall 5-year survival was 34.2%. If it is done in experienced medical centers, this procedure can be performed with low morbidity and mortality.

▶ This retrospective study involved 401 patients who underwent esophageal resection for cure. The significant findings were as follows: Actual 5-year survival was 90% in stage I, 52% in stage II, and 17% in stage III, with an overall 5-year survival rate of 34%, with a rate of 64.8% for those patients in whom no nodal involvement was detected. The overall operative mortality was 5.9%, but it increased to 15% in patients who were older than 70 years. Functional results were also satisfactory, because 77% of the patients remained symptom free and had only minor complaints.

This study supports the conclusion that esophagectomy is the appropriate treatment in patients who have nonmetastatic resectable esophageal carcinoma and that it can be accomplished with acceptable morbidity and mortality rates.—H.H. Simms, M.D.

Long-Term Results in Surgically Managed Esophageal Achalasia
Malthaner RA, Todd TR, Miller L, Pearson FG (Univ of Toronto)
Ann Thorac Surg 58:1343–1347, 1994   140-95-10–11

Background.—Achalasia, a motility disorder of the esophagus, can only be treated palliatively. Esophageal myotomy is the essential component of the surgical treatment of achalasia. Ten year follow-up data from a cohort of patients who had myotomy are provided.

Methods.—All patients who were operated on for achalasia from 1964 through 1983 at Toronto General Hospital were followed prospectively. Personal interviews were conducted with patients regarding post-myotomy symptoms and functional results, which were classified as excellent if the patients were asymptomatic; good if they experienced significant improvement with inconsequential ongoing symptoms; fair if they had definite improvement but with symptoms or endoscopic findings that required intermittent therapy; and poor if they had no improvement or worsening symptoms. The patients were divided into 2 groups: those whose first procedure was done at Toronto General Hospital and those who had undergone 1 or more previous operations elsewhere.

Results.—Complete, 10-year follow-up data were available for 35 patients. Of the 22 patients who had first been treated at Toronto General Hospital, good-to-excellent results were reported by 21 patients at 1 year postoperatively. The number reporting good-to-excellent results decreased to 17 of 22 at 5 years, 15 of 22 at 10 years, 11 of 16 at 15 years, and 6 of 9 at 20 or more years of follow-up. Of the 13 patients who were initially treated elsewhere, 3 had severe reflux damage that had to be treated with esophagectomy. All 10 of the remaining patients received conservative surgical management at the hospital. Of this group, 6 of 10 reported good-to-excellent results 1 year postoperatively; 6 of 10 at 5 years; 5 of 10 at 10 years; 2 of 6 at 15 years; and 1 of 2 at 20 years. When both groups were combined, 10 of 35 patients had poor results, and all were managed by esophagectomy.

Conclusion.—Long term follow-up of patients who had an esophagomyotomy and partial fundoplication for achalasia indicated that good-to-excellent results were obtained in most patients. Lifelong follow-up is warranted because of the steady deterioration of good results caused by the progressive and late complications of gastroesophageal reflux.

▶ This study identified the long-term results in patients who had undergone surgical treatment for achalasia with a minimum of 10 years of follow-up. Patients were divided into 2 groups: group A included patients who received surgical intervention only at the author's institution; group B included patients who had undergone 1 or more previous operations elsewhere. In group A excellent results were experienced by 95% of the patients at 1 year, 77% at 5 years, 68% at 10 years, 69% at 15 years, and 67% at 20 years or more. In group B there were 3 patients who required an immediate esophagectomy for chronic stricture secondary to reflux esophagitis. There were a total of 10 patients in both groups who underwent esophageal resection; 6 of the 10 esophagectomies were performed more than 10 years after the first operation.

Esophageal myotomy and partial fundoplication for achalasia showed good-to-excellent results in the majority of patients who were followed up long term. However, there was steady deterioration of good results because of the progressive and late complications of gastroesophageal reflux. Patients who are surgically treated for achalasia warrant lifelong follow-up to evaluate a late symptomatology.—H.H. Simms, M.D.

Outcome Effect of Adherence to Operative Principles of Nissen Fundoplication by Multiple Surgeons

Dunnington GL, De Meester TR, and the Department of Veterans Affairs Gastroesophageal Reflux Disease Study Group (Univ of Southern California, Los Angeles)
Am J Surg 166:654–658, 1993   140-95-10–12

Background.—Although surgical antireflux techniques can provide effective and long-lasting results in patients with complicated gastroesophageal reflux disease, gastroenterologists are hesitant to refer patients because reported results appear to be highly dependent on the surgeon. The outcomes of Nissen fundoplication, when performed for complicated disease by surgeons who had varied skill and experience but were in compliance with established principles of technique, were investigated.

Patients and Methods.—Fifty-eight patients with abnormal 24-hour pH studies and mucosal injury on endoscopy underwent Nissen fundoplication at 1 of 8 Veterans Administration hospitals. The mean patient age was 58 years. The participating surgeons met once to review 10 operative principles outlined by a surgeon who had extensive experience with the procedure. Surgery was performed by surgical residents under the supervision of surgical faculty; the results therefore reflected the efficacy of the surgical repair rather than the skill of any particular surgeon. Esophageal manometry, endoscopy, and 24-hour monitoring of esopha-

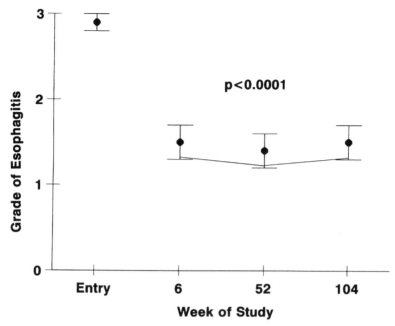

Fig 10–4.—Mean grade of esophagitis (range: 0 to 4) for patients at study entry, 6 weeks, 1 year, and 2 years postoperatively. (Courtesy of Dunnington GL, De Meester TR, VA Gastroesophageal Reflux Disease Study Group: *Am J Surg* 166:654–658, 1993.)

geal pH were done at 6 weeks postoperatively and repeated every 12 months. Symptom scoring was recorded at quarterly clinical examinations. Compliance with the 10 defined operative principles was assessed by a questionnaire.

Results.—Surgeon compliance was greater than 90% for 7 of the 10 operative principles. A significant improvement in symptomatic scores was noted at 52 and 104 weeks compared with preoperative scores (Fig 10-4). In addition, there was significant improvement in the total amount of time at a pH less than 4 at 52 weeks and 104 weeks. Significant improvement in the grade of esophagitis was also noted at 12 months.

Conclusion.—Ninety-three percent of the patients experienced symptom relief after surgery, and the rate of healing of esophagitis was 77%. Predictable and satisfactory results can be obtained after Nissen fundoplication when there is compliance with established technical principles. These findings should encourage the referral of patients with recurrent, progressive gastroesophageal reflux disease.

▶ This multi-institutional study reports the results of the adherence of numerous operators to standard (acceptable) technical principles rather than a specific technique. This review is particularly relevant in a time when the emphasis on technology (e.g., laparoscopy) should not make surgeons reluctant to accept time-honored and established operative principles of management.—K.I. Bland, M.D.

Laparoscopic Nissen Fundoplication

Jamieson GG, Watson DI, Britten-Jones R, Mitchell PC, Anvari M (Royal Adelaide Hospital, South Australia)
Ann Surg 220:137–145, 1994   140-95-10-13

Background.—Nissen fundoplication is a widely accepted surgical procedure for the management of gastroesophageal reflux disease. Nissen's original procedure did not divide the short gastric vessels; instead, the fundoplication was constructed using either the posterior or anterior stomach wall. An initial experience with laparoscopic Nissen fundoplication was reported.

Methods.—The experience included 155 patients over a 29-month period. All had symptomatic gastroesophageal reflux disease, as documented by endoscopy or esophageal manometry and ambulatory pH monitoring. Although 80 patients had hiatal hernias, they were longer than 5 cm in only 10 patients. The laparoscopic procedure involved 360-degree fundoplication, with the wrap secured by 3 or 4 sutures. Division of the short gastric vessels was not performed; the wrap was constructed using the anterior wall of the stomach, with a 52-French bougie positioned in the esophagus.

Results.—Failure to achieve an adequate wrap necessitated conversion to an open procedure in 19 patients. Median laparoscopic operating time was 120 minutes, decreasing to 90 minutes for the last 35 patients. Early in the experience, operating time was significantly reduced by the use of extracorporeal knot-tying. The median length of hospital stay for patients with completed laparoscopic procedures was 4 days. Readmission within the first month after surgery was required for 4 patients, all of whom had conversion to an open procedure. In 2 of these patients, a left pneumothorax resulted from a presumed pleural breach during mobilization of the esophagus. In 10 cases, open reoperation was necessary because of the poor outcome of the laparoscopic procedure—4 for severe dysphagia, 2 for recurrent reflux, 2 for acute paraesophageal hiatal hernia, and 1 for gastric obstruction. The remaining patient in this group died of mesenteric infarction. Another 7 patients were readmitted within days after discharge, 4 of whom had pulmonary emboli. Twenty-three patients had early, persistently troublesome dysphagia. Unexpectedly, postoperative barium and endoscopic studies showed that the wrap was fashioned from the body rather than the fundus of the stomach in 9 cases. Of 137 patients who were followed up for more than 3 months, 133 were well and without symptoms of reflux.

Conclusion.—The reported technique of laparoscopic Nissen fundoplication has many advantages in uncomplicated cases. Although it has yet to attain the overall usefulness of open fundoplication, laparoscopic fundoplication is likely to play an increasingly important role in the treatment of gastroesophageal reflux disease. A number of technical aspects facilitate the laparoscopic procedure, including placement of a tape around the esophagus to ease dissection of the posterior esophagus, dissection of a large window behind the esophagus to permit a tension-free fundoplication, and use of an endo-Babcock or other atraumatic grasping instrument to grasp the cardia and draw the esophagus into the abdomen.

▶ A large experience with laparoscopic Nissen fundoplication was provided. Although 12% of surgeries were not completed laparoscopically and 8% of patients required subsequent surgery, the results were excellent, given the early experience reported.

Three points made by the authors warrant discussion. First, they reduced the intra-abdominal pressure to 10 mm Hg based on 1 patient with mediastinal and subcutaneous CO_2 pressure that was also noted these findings; it did not cause a delay in discharge. These procedures are difficult to perform, especially early in the learning curve. A reduction in pressure to 10 mm Hg is an unnecessary maneuver that increases the difficulty of the procedure, especially in obese patients.

Second, a pneumothorax was noted in 2 patients, for which a chest tube was placed. In this regard, the authors provided a very conservative approach. Left pneumothorax arises during dissection of the hiatus when a closely applied left pleura is inadvertently opened; it was not the result of a pulmonary injury. Therefore, a tube is not needed. However, attention should be given to cardiopulmonary function because a tension pneumothorax can ensue that requires positive end-expiratory pressure or decompression.

Finally, the authors described a new complication of the anterior fundoplication: wrapping of the body of the stomach rather than the fundus, leading to a bilobed stomach. Although they suggest that this might be avoided by division of the short gastric vessels, they do not advocate that approach because the open experience is not associated with this complication, despite the short gastric vessels not having been divided. Although this might be avoided in open surgery, this complication can only be averted using the laparoscopic approach by division of the short gastric vessels.—J.F. Amaral, M.D.

Laparoscopic Antireflux Surgery: What Is Real Progress?
Collard JM, de Gheldere CA, De Kock M, Otte JB, Kestens PJ (Louvain Medical School, Brussels, Belgium)
Ann Surg 220:146–154, 1994   140-95-10–14

Background.—In theory, laparoscopic antireflux fundoplication is an attractive alternative to open surgery for patients with gastroesophageal reflux disease (GERD). However, there are no objective data to substantiate the claimed advantages of the laparoscopic approach, for example, lower complication rates, shorter hospital stays, and earlier rehabilitation. In an attempt to fill this void, a recent crude experience with laparoscopic and open antireflux surgery was reviewed.

Methods.—The analysis included 72 consecutive patients who underwent antireflux surgery. Fifty-six had disabling GERD that was refractory to medical therapy, 5 had a symptomatic hiatal hernia without GERD, and 11 had a previously unsuccessful antireflux surgery. Esophageal motility studies, which were performed in 70 patients, showed normal motility of the esophageal body in 67 patients, dysmotility in 2, and dyscontractility in 1. The lower esophageal sphincter resting pressure was less than 6 mm Hg in 37 patients, greater than 6 mm Hg in 30, and unevaluated in 3. All but 3 patients had abnormal results on esophageal pH monitoring. Patients were selected for transabdominal or transthoracic surgery based on the radiologic reproducibility of the gastroesophageal junction below the diaphragm. The decision to perform a laparoscopy or laparotomy was based on other surgical considerations, such as previous abdominal surgeries. The initial approach was laparoscopy in 39 patients, laparotomy in 28, and thoracotomy in 5. Sixty patients underwent subdiaphragmatic Nissen fundoplication, a procedure that involved division of the short gastric veins and posterior gastric vessels and construction of a tension-free wrap around the lower esophagus. Other operations included intrathoracic Nissen fundoplication in 3 patients with a short esophagus, subdiaphragmatic 240-degree fundoplication in 2 patients with severe motility disorders, a Lortat-Jacob repair in the 5 patients with hiatal hernia, and a duodenal diversion in 1 patient with delayed gastric emptying.

Results.—Pulmonary embolism occurred in 1 laparoscopy patient and 1 laparotomy patient, and hemothorax occurred in 1 thoracotomy patient. Patients undergoing laparoscopy had a mean hospital stay of 6.4 days compared with 7.8 days for laparotomy and 12.5 days for thoracotomy. The average postoperative morphine consumption, which was administered by patient-controlled analgesia, was 47 mg per 48 hours for laparoscopy and 46 mg per 48 hours for laparotomy with primary antireflux surgery. Ninety-three percent of laparoscopy patients returned to work within 3 weeks, although 92% of patients in the open surgery groups resumed their activities after more than 6 weeks. At follow-up evaluation, 88% of patients had no or only minimal symptoms, 10% had disabling side effects, and 3% had persistent or recurrent esophageal symptoms. Ninety-seven percent of the patients reported that they would undergo antireflux surgery again. Parietal herniations occurred in 4 patients: 1 incisional hernia and 1 recurrent hernia in the laparotomy group and 2 herniations of the wrap into the chest in the laparoscopy group; the latter complications probably resulted from a premature return to manual work. Scar esthetics were a complaint of 3 of the laparoscopy patients. Of the patients studied, 100% had normal lower esophageal sphincter pressure, and 95% had normal esophageal acid exposure.

Conclusion.—For appropriately selected patients, the laparoscopic approach to antireflux surgery is a viable one. Various antireflux procedures can be performed using the same steps as for conventional surgery. However, the laparoscopic approach does not significantly reduce the postoperative complication rate, postoperative discomfort, the length of hospital stay, or the risk of esthetic sequelae. For manual workers, an early return to work after laparoscopy may be inadvisable.

▶ The authors provide us with one of the few negative outcome studies of laparoscopic Nissen fundoplication. Notably, even though they conclude that laparoscopy is a good approach to the hiatal area for the management of GERD, they were unable to find any difference in the length of hospital stay, analgesic requirements, complications, or esthetic sequelae.

In large part, the lack of differences may be secondary to their methods. For example, the analgesic requirement was reported only for the first 48 hours not the entire hospital stay. Similarly, there was no mention of the esthetic result of the laparotomy or thoracotomy group, which makes the comment regarding the unsatisfactory esthetic result in 3 laparoscopic patients somewhat biased. Furthermore, would these 3 patients have been more satisfied with the esthetic result of a laparotomy or thoracotomy incision? Finally, the very long hospital stay reported for the laparoscopy group (6.4 days) in this study appears to be related more to the authors' reluctance to send patients home and to the use of nasogastric tubes than to an actual need to have them stay in the hospital.

Despite these problems, the authors' ultimate conclusion that laparoscopic Nissen fundoplication is not suitable for patients seems to be well founded and should be strongly considered in the evaluation of the patient with GERD.—J.F. Amaral, M.D.

Should the Vagus Nerves Be Isolated From the Fundoplication Wrap? A Prospective Study
Peillon C, Manouvrier J-L, Labreche J, Kaeffer N, Denis P, Testart J (Hôpital Charles Nicolle, Rouen, France)
Arch Surg 129:814–818, 1994   140-95-10–15

Purpose.—Patients undergoing fundoplication for gastroesophageal reflux (GER) sometimes have postoperative gastric emptying abnormalities. However, as many as 60% of patients with GER are found to have preoperative abnormalities of gastric emptying; most of the time, this problem goes unnoticed. An open, randomized, controlled trial was performed to examine whether careful dissection and isolation of the vagus nerves from a three quarter Nissen fundoplication wrap could reduce the incidence of postoperative gastric emptying abnormalities or otherwise affect postoperative outcomes.

Methods.—The study included 42 patients who were undergoing three quarter Nissen fundoplication for proven GER, a procedure that en-

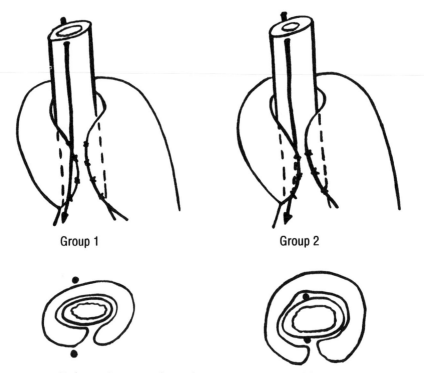

Group 1   Group 2

Fig 10–5.—Technique. In group 1, dissected vagus nerves were isolated from the wrap. In group 2, vagus nerves were included in the wrap. (Courtesy of Peillon C, Manouvrier J-L, Labreche J, et al: *Arch Surg* 129:814–818, 1994.)

tailed a periesophageal posterior gastric wrap with a circumference of 270 degrees. Half the patients were randomized to undergo dissection and exclusion of the vagus nerves from the wrap (Fig 10–5). Acid reflux and gastric emptying tests were performed before and 3 months after surgery (Fig 10–6).

Results.—Persistent dysphagia was present at follow-up in 2 patients with vs. 1 patient without isolation of the vagal nerves. On preoperative assessment, 30% of patients had below-average gastric emptying, according to the criteria of Bertrand and associates. Preoperatively and postoperatively, there was no significant difference in the mean number of radiopaque pellets remaining in the stomach 5 hours after ingestion. The number of pellets remaining at this time in the preoperative and postoperative studies was significantly and positively correlated.

Conclusion.—In patients with GER who are undergoing three quarter Nissen fundoplication, isolation of the vagus nerves from the fundoplication wrap does not appear to modify the risk of gastric emptying abnormalities nor to influence the surgical outcome. Preoperative and postoperative gastric emptying are positively correlated, suggesting a possible predisposition to postoperative gastric emptying disturbances. For pa-

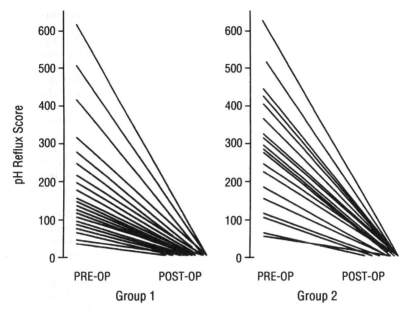

Fig 10–6.—Preoperative *(PRE-OP)* and postoperative *(POST-OP)* pH reflux test results. A normal pH reflux score is 0 to 90. (Courtesy of Peillon C, Manouvrier J-L, Labreche J, et al: *Arch Surg* 129:814–818, 1994.)

tients with delayed gastric emptying before surgery, there is no evidence that any modification of the fundoplication procedure improves gastric emptying.

▶ Patients with gastroesophageal reflux often have a set of preoperative symptoms replaced with a new set postoperatively. Considerable emphasis has been placed on the size and tightness of the wrap. This study focuses on the role the vagus nerves on postoperative symptoms. Although the study demonstrates no advantage to exclusion of the vagus nerves on postoperative gastric emptying, there were patients in both groups who had normal preoperative but delayed postoperative gastric emptying. Therefore, not all postoperative delayed gastric emptying existed preoperatively, which implicates some technical but unidentified event in the development of postoperative gastric emptying dysfunction.

In this regard, equal damage to the vagus nerves in both procedures cannot be excluded. However, to have an effect on gastric emptying, both vagal nerve fibers must be injured, a factor that makes this possibility less likely and raises questions about the effect of antireflux surgery on the intrinsic neuromuscular gastric activity. Nonetheless, it is important to remember that postoperative dyspeptic symptoms are not necessarily the result of too tight a wrap, but they may be the result of delayed gastric emptying. Furthermore, preoperative gastric emptying studies should be obtained to identify patients who are at risk for postoperative dyspepsia.—J.F. Amaral, M.D.

Gastroesophageal Leaks After Antireflux Operations

Urschel JD (Univ of Alberta, Edmonton, Canada)
Ann Thorac Surg 57:1229–1232, 1994   140-95-10–16

Introduction.—An unusual complication of antireflux operations is a postoperative gastroesophageal perforation. Although there has been some documentation of this complication, little about its incidence, predisposing factors, and treatment has appeared in the literature. Problems associated with this procedure were discussed.

Methods.—The charts of patients who underwent antireflux operations at 3 hospitals over a 10-year period were reviewed. After exclusion criteria were met (such as age and type of procedure) 1,005 operations were performed. Perforation was documented by contrast studies that showed leakage of the distal esophagus or proximal stomach.

Results.—The most common procedures were the modified (559 patients) or standard (363 patients) Nissen fundoplication and the operative mortality was less than 1%. Gastroesophageal leaks occurred in 12 patients (1.2%). Nine of these leaks occurred in patients who had the modified Nissen fundoplication. Significant predisposing factors included wrap quality (incomplete, intrathoracic, or excessive tension) and a previous hiatal operation. Postoperative fever was seen in 10 of the 12 patients between postoperative days 1 and 5. Hypotension, respiratory distress, and ileus were also seen postoperatively. Diagnosis of the perforation was made at a median of 8 days after surgery. The leak was thought to be caused by sutures that had cut the esophageal wall. Six of the perforations were well contained and responded to conservative treatment. Two of the other 6 were treated conservatively. One had late empyema and 1 died. The other 4 were treated surgically and 1 died, for a mortality rate of 17% in patients with a perforation.

Conclusion.—Most of the leaks were present in the first week after surgery. Contained peritoneal leaks respond to conservative treatment. Uncontained leaks require aggressive surgical intervention.

▶ Health care cost containment has stimulated a reevaluation of the management of gastroesophageal reflux disorders with expensive long-term medications. This has led to a resurgence of interest in the surgical management of gastroesophageal reflux disease in general and to the development of a laparoscopic approach to the management of the disorder.

The author has concisely identified 4 strong associations with gastroesophageal leakage after open reflux surgery: previous hiatal surgery; incomplete fundal wrap; intrathoracic wrap; and too much tension on the wrap. Many surgeons who perform laparoscopic fundoplications have adopted an approach in which either the short gastric vessels are not divided and/or the wrap is not made completely.

This study raises significant questions about these laparoscopic approaches. In addition, one cannot help but wonder whether similar successful results (12 leaks in 1,005 operations) would be achieved with a laparoscopic approach.—J.F. Amaral, M.D.

Anterior Lesser Curve Seromyotomy With Posterior Truncal Vagotomy Versus Proximal Gastric Vagotomy: Results of a Prospective Randomized Trial 3–8 Years After Surgery
Walia HS, El-Karim HA (Al-Amiri Hosp, Kuwait)
World J Surg 18:758–763, 1994   140-95-10–17

Purpose.—Proximal gastric vagotomy (PGV) has long been recognized as being a beneficial procedure for patients who have duodenal ulcer, and a number of innovative modifications have been proposed to offset the technical difficulty and high recurrence rate of the initial procedure. After it became apparent that only 1 vagal nerve was needed for normal gastric emptying, the procedure of anterior lesser curve seromyotomy and posterior truncal vagotomy (ASPTV) was introduced. A prospective, randomized trial of these 2 procedures, with 3 to 8 years of follow-up, was conducted.

Methods.—The study included 100 patients with a history of chronic duodenal ulcer that was refractory to standard medical therapy. It was performed at a Kuwait hospital; most of the patients were young men with ASA physical status I risk; 80% were expatriates. The research subjects were randomized to undergo PGV according to the technique of Rossi and Braasch or ASPTV using the method of Taylor and associates. The results were evaluated 3 to 8 years after surgery.

Results.—The mean operative time was 109 minutes for PGV vs. 76 minutes for ASPTV. When assessed soon after surgery, those in both groups had a mean reduction of 85% in basal acid output and of 88% in insulin-stimulated peak acid output. At 1 year, basal acid output remained at 70% of its preoperative level and insulin-stimulated peak acid output was 60% of its preoperative level. Seventy-six percent of patients in both groups had good-to-excellent results using Visick I or II classifications. Ulcers recurred in 14% of the PGV group and in 12% of the ASPTV group.

Conclusion.—For patients who have refractory duodenal ulcer, ASPTV is a safe and simple procedure. Like PGV, it effectively reduces acid secretion, morbidity, mortality, and ulcer recurrence. Therefore, ASPTV appears to be a viable alternative to PGV for the surgical treatment of chronic duodenal ulcer.

▶ The so-called Taylor procedure has been modified and simplified to include an anterior lesser curve seromotomy with a posterior truncal vagotomy. This technical variation has gained notoriety and popularity since the introduction of laparoscopic approaches for the therapy of duodenal ulcer disease. This series confirms the clinical applicability of this procedure, which compares very favorably with the formal, highly selective vagotomy.—V.E. Pricolo, M.D.

Twenty Years After Parietal Cell Vagotomy or Selective Vagotomy Antrectomy for Treatment of Duodenal Ulcer: Final Report
Jordan PH Jr, Thornby J (Baylor College of Medicine, Houston; VA Hosp, Houston)
Ann Surg 220:283–296, 1994   140-95-10–18

Purpose.—Patients who undergo operative treatment for duodenal ulcer are at risk of surgical mortality as well as mechanical and metabolic morbidity. In recent years, surgeons have made progress in the development of operations that have low morbidity and mortality. At the same time, the need for such operations has declined, partly because of dramatic improvements in medical therapy. Surgical therapy still plays an important role in the treatment of duodenal ulcer, particularly in certain socioeconomic environments. In such a setting, a prospective, randomized trial of parietal cell vagotomy (PCV) and selective vagotomy-antrectomy (SV-A) was performed.

Methods.—Thirty-five consecutive patients who had duodenal, pyloric, or prepyloric ulcers participated in a pilot study of PCV, which was initiated in 1972. Thereafter, 200 patients were randomized to undergo either PCV or SV-A. A single surgeon was responsible for all operations and follow-up studies. The latter included an annual in-hospital evaluation if possible. Each of these visits included gastric analyses if the patients consented. Suspected recurrences were evaluated by endoscopy. The clinical results were evaluated using a modified Visick grading scale.

Results.—There were no operative deaths. Many patients had minor complaints during the early postoperative period; in some cases, these symptoms resolved by the next visit. Dumping was significantly more frequent after SV-A than after PCV, particularly for the first 10 years. There was no significant difference in the frequency of diarrhea, nor was there a significant difference in the percentage of patients with Visick grade I or II results for the 2 operations; however, significantly more patients who underwent PCV had Visick grade I results. Patients who underwent SV-A had a lower recurrence rate-by-life table analysis than those who underwent PCV.

Conclusion.—This long-term experience shows that both SV-A and PCV are effective and safe operations. For patients who have pyloric and prepyloric ulcers and pyloric obstruction, SV-A is preferred. Because patients occasionally become disabled after SV-A, the authors recommend PCV for patients who have duodenal ulcers.

▶ Dr. Jordan clearly deserves credit having been willing for many years to perform an operation that originated in Europe. Most American surgeons initially approached it with a great deal of reluctance and skepticism. Over the years, Dr. Jordan has consistently published updates and longer follow-ups on his extensive experience. He has carefully presented data and proved that careful patient selection, meticulous attention to technical detail during the operation, and prolonged follow-up are all necessary to the success of this operation.

This operation can be performed in many patients with minimal side effects. The recent emphasis placed on *Helicobacter pylori* as a pathogen commonly associated with duodenal ulcer, as well as several other benign and malignant gastroduodenal conditions, certainly raises questions regarding the therapeutic approach that should be used with these patients as well as a possible causal relationship between the pathogen and recurrences. To a large extent, the broader applicability of highly selective vagotomy for duodenal ulcer disease is going to be based on the individual surgeon's familiarity with this technique.—V.E. Pricolo, M.D.

Long-Term Follow-Up of Patients with Roux-en-Y Gastrojejunostomy for Gastric Disease
McAlhany JC, Hanover TM, Taylor SM, Sticca RP, Ashmore JD Jr (Greenville Hospital System, SC)
Ann Surg 219:451–457, 1994   140-95-10–19

Introduction.—Reports of postoperative chronic abdominal pain, nausea, vomiting, or bezoar formation (Roux stasis syndrome) have caused concern about the use of a Roux-en-Y gastrojejunostomy to treat or prevent bile reflux gastritis. Long-term results were evaluated in patients who had a Roux-en-Y gastrojejunostomy (Fig 10–7 and 10–8).

Methods.—Twenty-four consecutive patients (12 men) with a mean age of 50 (range, 26–76 years) had a Roux-en-Y gastrojejunostomy between 1976 and 1981. Indications for surgery included bile reflux gastritis in 12 patients, peptic ulcer disease in 6, and revisional operative therapy in 6. Long-term follow-up (mean, 12 years; range, .5 to 16.5 years) was accomplished by reviewing medical records, interviewing, and performing an upper gastrointestinal series on symptomatic patients.

Results.—Of 22 evaluable patients, the clinical condition that prompted surgery was corrected in 21 (table). A Roux-en-Y gastrojejunostomy succeeded in preventing or treating bile reflux gastritis in all 22. Despite this success, clinical failure (Visick scale III or IV) occurred in 8 patients (36%); 7 of the 8 had clinical failure within 6 months of operation, including Roux stasis syndrome in 6.

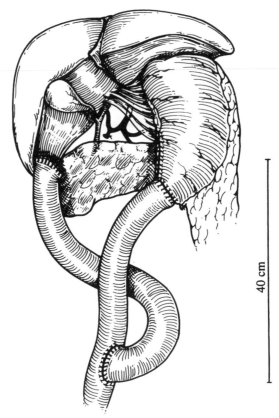

40 cm

Fig 10–7.—Roux-en-Y gastrojejunostomy after gastrectomy. (Courtesy of McAlhany JC, Hanover TM, Taylor SM, et al: *Ann Surg* 219:451–457, 1994.)

Conclusion.—Although a Roux-en-Y gastrojejunostomy is safe and often successful, unsatisfactory long-term results suggest caution in using this procedure for primary or remedial gastrointestinal disease.

▶ The issues of reflux gastritis and indications for a Roux-en-Y gastrojejunostomy are seldom addressed in the literature nowadays, with the increased incidence of gastric operations. Interestingly, the results of this series were not as satisfactory as those usually reported.—V.E. Pricolo, M.D.

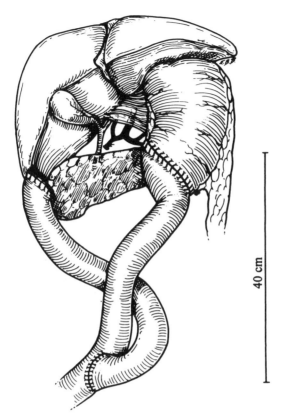

Fig 10–8.—Roux-en-Y gastrojejunostomy after revision of loop gastrojejunostomy. (Courtesy of McAlhany JC, Hanover TM, Taylor SM, et al: *Ann Surg* 219:451–457, 1994.)

Clinical Response of Roux-en-Y Gastrojejunostomy in 22 Patients		
	Visick I-II	**Visick III-IV**
Bile reflux gastritis	5	5
Peptic ulcer disease	5	1
Revisional operative therapy	4	2
Total	14 (64%)	8 (36%)

(Courtesy of McAlhany JC, Hanover TM, Taylor SM, et al: *Ann Surg* 219:451–457, 1994.)

Gastric Cancer Risk After Vagotomy

G Lundegårdh, Ekbom A, McLaughlin JK, Nyrén O (Univ Hosp, Uppsala, Sweden; National Cancer Inst, Bethesda, Md)
Gut 35:946–949, 1994   140-95-10–20

Introduction.—Vagotomy has replaced gastric resection as the preferred surgery for peptic ulcer in Sweden. However, diminished gastric acid secretion might increase the risk of gastic cancer. The risk of gastric cancer after vagotomy was studied.

Methods.—A Swedish registry provided information on 7,198 patients who had a vagotomy for benign gastric or duodenal disease between 1971 and 1979. Patients were followed up until 1988.

Results.—The average patient age at surgery was 49 years. Excluding the first year of follow-up, 34 cases of gastric cancer developed in the patients who had undergone vagotomy. This figure was not significantly different than the 26 cases that were expected. The duration of follow-up, sex, age at surgery, underlying diagnosis, and surgical procedures did not affect risk for gastric cancer.

Conclusion.—Decreased gastric secretion after vagotomy does not increase the risk of gastric cancer for as long as 18 years after the procedure. A longer follow-up is necessary to exclude the possibility of excess risk.

▶ With the increasing trend toward preservation of the gastric antrum for ulcer disease of the stomach and duodenum, a significant number of patients are available nowadays for long-term follow-up. This interesting study comes from Sweden, one of the European countries that embraced the philosophy of highly selective vagotomies much earlier than the United States.

A concern of any gastric-reducing procedure is that the change in the pH environment of the stomach might possibly lead to increased cancer rates, as shown by intestinal metaplasia findings over time. This very large study with significant follow-up offers reassurance, at least for the first 10 years after surgery.—V.E. Pricolo, M.D.

Factors Predisposing to Further Hemorrhage and Mortality After Peptic Ulcer Bleeding

Mueller X, Rothenbuehler J-M, Amery A, Harder F (Basel-Univ, Basel, Switzerland; Frimley Park Hosp Natl Health Service Trust, Surrey, England)
J Am Coll Surg 179:457–461, 1994   140-95-10–21

Background.—Mortality associated with peptic ulcer hemorrhage has remained unchanged, mainly because of rebleeding in an increasingly aging population. The early identification of patients who are at high risk of rebleeding and subsequent prompt treatment may decrease rebleeding and death rates. The value of clinical and endoscopic findings in predicting further bleeding or death in patients who are admitted with peptic ulcer bleeding was studied.

Methods and Findings.—The patients included 157 individuals who were admitted during a 2-year period with bleeding from a peptic ulcer. Nineteen patients died, 37 had further bleeding, and 31 had early surgery. The variable that best predicted additional bleeding was shock. A transfusion requirement of more than 4 units of blood in the first 48 hours and endoscopic stigmata of recent hemorrhage were other significant factors. The fatality rate and the number of coexisting illnesses per patient correlated strongly. Other predictors of increased mortality were steroid use, onset of bleeding during hospitalization, alcohol use, further bleeding, and the need for more than 4 units of blood in the first 48 hours.

Conclusion.—Shock continues to be the most valuable predictor of further bleeding. It is superior to endoscopic stigmata. The close correlation between mortality and coexisting illness demonstrates that most deaths in this patient population are caused by nonpeptic ulcer disease.

▶ One hundred fifty-seven patients who were admitted over a 2-year period with bleeding from peptic ulcer were reviewed retrospectively. The predictive value of individual risk factors in identifying patients who are at risk of further bleeding or dying was determined by the chi-square test with a Yates correction. A period of shock was the factor that best predicted further bleeding.

Transfusion requirements of more than 4 units of blood during the first 48 hours and endoscopic stigmata of recent hemorrhage also significantly predicted further hemorrhagic episodes. The number of coexisting illnesses per patient was strongly related to the mortality rate. Other factors that indicated increased hospital mortality rate were steroid usage, the onset of bleeding during the period of hospitalization, alcohol use, and the transfusion of 4 units of blood during the first 48 hours.

These data would strongly suggest that shock remains the most valuable sign of predicting further bleeding and is superior to endoscopic stigmata. This close relationship between the mortality rate and coexisting illness emphasizes that most deaths result from nonpeptic ulcer disease in patients who have had peptic ulcer bleeding.—H.H. Simms, M.D.

Ten-Year Follow-Up of a Prospective, Randomized Trial of Selective Proximal Vagotomy With Ulcer Excision and Partial Gastrectomy With Gastroduodenostomy for Treating Corporeal Gastric Ulcer
Emås S, Grupcev G, Eriksson B (Karolinska Hosp, Stockholm)
Am J Surg 167:596–600, 1994   140-95-10–22

Background.—Partial gastrectomy with gastroduodenostomy is the established procedure for elective surgical treatment of type I corporeal

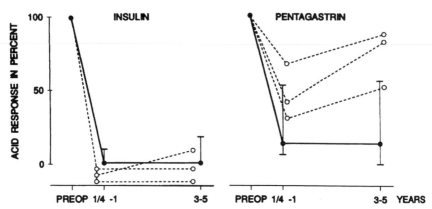

Fig 10–9.—Median gastric acid responses and ranges 3 months to 5 years after selective proximal vagotomy for type I gastric ulcer, expressed in percent of the preoperative response of 11 patients without recurrent ulcer (*filled circles*) and 3 patients with recurrent ulcer (*open circles*). Responses to insulin hypoglycemia (**left**) and pentagastrin (**right**) are shown. Median preoperative responses and ranges in mmoL are given in the Results section. (Courtesy of Emås S, Grupcev G, Eriksson B: *Am J Surg* 167:596–600, 1994.)

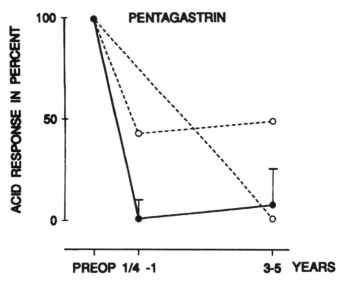

Fig 10–10.—Median gastric acid responses to pentagastrin and ranges 3 months to 5 years after partial gastrectomy for type I gastric ulcer, expressed in percent of the preoperative response of seven patients without recurrent ulcer (*filled circles*) and two patients with recurrent ulcer (*open circles*). Median preoperative response and range in mmoL are given in the Results section. (Courtesy of Emås S, Grupcev G, Eriksson B: *Am J Surg* 167:596–600, 1994.)

gastric ulcer. In the hope of minimizing side effects, various types of vagotomies have replaced gastric resection for treatment of duodenal ulcer. Ten-year follow-up data were presented to reliably evaluate results after the 2 operations.

Methods.—Patients with a preoperative diagnosis of recurrent or slow-healing benign type I corporeal gastric ulcer located at or proximal to the angulus were randomly assigned to undergo selective proximal vagotomy with ulcer excision or partial gastrectomy with gastroduodenostomy. Before surgery, basal gastric acid secretion and maximal acid response to regular insulin and pentagastrin were determined. The pentagastrin and insulin tests were repeated between 3 months and 1 year postoperatively and then at intervals up to 5 years (Fig 10-9).

Results.—Thirty patients participated; 16 underwent selective proximal vagotomy and 14 had a partial gastrectomy. The median time for follow-up was 10.1 years (range, 1.7–15.3 years) for both groups. Three patients in the selective proximal vagotomy group had a recurrence of ulcer, 1 each at 4, 4.5, and 10 years postoperatively. Two patients in the partial gastrectomy group had ulcers recur, 1 each at 4 and 10 years. Graded according to a modified Visick scale, the results overall were very good to good for 73% of the patients who had a selective proximal vagotomy and 71% after a partial gastrectomy. After 10 years, nutritional status was comparable between the 2 groups. The vagotomy reduced the median acid response to insulin hypoglycemia by 100% and to pentagastrin by 80% 3–12 months after surgery. That reduction remained unchanged 3–5 years after surgery. Partial gastrectomy reduced the median acid response to pentagastrin by 99% at 3–12 months and 97% at 3–5 years (Fig 10-10).

Conclusion.—For the surgical treatment of type I gastric ulcer, selective proximal vagotomy with ulcer excision is an alternative to partial gastrectomy. Five treatment failures during 10 years among 30 surgically treated patients is as important a finding as the comparison of 2 equally useful operations.

▶ Over a 10-year period, this study evaluated 30 patients with a type I corporeal gastric ulcer who had been randomly allocated to undergo either selective proximal vagotomy with ulcer excision or a partial gastrectomy with gastroduodenostomy. The median time for follow-up was 10.1 years. Ulcers recurred in 3 patients at 4, 4.5, and 10 years after selective proximal vagotomy and in 2 patients at 4 and 10 years after partial gastrectomy. The overall results, as assessed using the modified Visick scale, were assessed as being very good and good for 73% of the patients after selective proximal vagotomy and 71% after partial gastrectomy. Selective proximal vagotomy reduced the median acid response to insulin hypoglycemia by 100% and to pentagastrin by 80% for at least 3–5 years. Partial gastrectomy reduced the median acid response to pentagastrin by 97%. These results suggest that selective proximal vagotomy and ulcer excision are viable alternatives to partial gastrectomy for treating type I gastric ulcers.—H.H. Simms, M.D.

11 Biliary Tract and Gallbladder

Introduction

Assessment of the biliary tract by state-of-the-art imaging is increasingly used both preoperatively and intraoperatively. Evaluation of the biliary tree for strictures, neoplasms, and stone disease can be accomplished with endoscopic retrograde cholangiopancreatography (ERCP), percutaneous transhepatic cholangiography (PTC), ultrasonography, or CT.

The important articles by the hepatobiliary and liver transplantation units in London and Bristol (Abstracts 140-95-11-1 and 140-95-11-2) confirm that radiologic imaging ineffectively produces a definitive diagnosis for the etiology of biliary strictures. Direct tissue procurement using a needle biopsy is often difficult; as a result many clinics are encouraging the use of biliary cytology with direct examination of bile samples and/or brushings (brush cytology). The availability of these techniques may enhance the establishment of the etiology for biliary strictures. Techniques to establish an effective methodology for procurement of tissue with brush methods may be more sensitive than traditional measures that use bile cytology.

Notably, few studies have been devoted to examination of the diameter of the cystic duct; instead, the majority of these analyses have used indirect assessment methodology. The report from Nice, France, at the Hôpital Universitaire de Cimiez (Abstract 140-95-11-4) evaluates the role of the diameter of the cystic duct in the natural history of gallstones to confirm that maximal and minimal cystic duct diameters possess a statistical relationship that increased with a greater level of disease, from stone-free patients to those with cholelithiasis and from the latter to those with choledocholithiasis.

The continuing concern regarding concomitant procedures at the time of indicated colectomy was reviewed by the Division of Colon and Rectal Surgery at the Mayo Clinic. Unless clear contraindications exist, patients with asymptomatic gallstones who are undergoing colorectal surgery should have a concomitant cholecystectomy (Abstract 140-95-11-15). Additionally, the prophylactic administration of parenteral antibiotics remains of interest for patients who undergo elective open biliary tract surgery. Included in these reviews is an original prospective trial from a Canadian university hospital experience that compares cefotetan with cefoxitin. The pharmacodynamic properties of these cephalosporins to reduce the incidence of infection is evident (Abstract 140-95-11-6). Interventional approaches to the hepatobiliary tree require periprocedural coverage with prophylactic antibiotics.

The report from Brussels, Belgium, confirms the advantages of endoscopic placement of metal mesh self-expandable stents for chronic pancreatitis (Abstract 140-95-11-7). This suggests a satisfactory, low morbidity alternative to biliary tract diversion that provides effective long-term biliary drainage.

The increasing applications of laparoscopic cholecystectomy and the potential consequences for both litigious as well as therapeutic misadventures are documented in Abstracts (140-95-11-8 through 140-95-11-10). In addition, laparoscopic approaches to the gallbladder have introduced 2 potential intraoperative complications that are not encountered with open surgery: biliary spillage and intra-abdominal stone loss. The review by Johnston and associates (Abstract 140-95-11-8) affirms that the combination of gallstones in the peritoneal cavity with bile is associated with an enhanced risk of intra-abdominal adhesions and abscess formation. At laparoscopic cholecystectomy, the operating surgeon should make every attempt to retrieve stones that are lost during the procedure.

Kirby I. Bland, M.D.

A Prospective Study of Biliary Cytology in 100 Patients With Bile Duct Strictures

Kurzawinski TR, Deery A, Dooley JS, Dick R, Hobbs KEF, Davidson BR (Royal Free Hosp, London)
Hepatology 18:1399–1403, 1993   140-95-11–1

Background.—Depending on the tissue diagnosis, balloon dilation, stenting, surgical resection, and even liver transplantation may all be appropriate treatments for biliary strictures. The diagnostic value of exfoli-

| | Group 2: Results by Sampling Method | | | |
| | ERCP | | PTC | |
Parameters	Bile	Brush	Bile	Brush
Sensitivity	33% (10/30)	71% (17/24)	0% (0/9)	67% (10/15)
Specificity	100% (7/7)	100% (7/7)	NA	NA
Accuracy	46% (17/37)	77% (24/31)	0% (0/9)	67% (10/15)

NA, not applicable: no benign strictures in this group.
(Courtesy of Kurzawinski TR, Deery A, Dooley JS, et al: *Hepatology* 18:1399–1403, 1993.)

Moving?

I'd like to receive my *Year Book of Surgery* without interruption.
Please note the following change of address, effective:

Name: _____

New Address: _____

_____

City: _____ State: _____ Zip: _____

Old Address: _____

_____

City: _____ State: _____ Zip: _____

Reservation Card

Yes, I would like my own copy of *Year Book of Surgery*. Please begin my subscription with the current edition according to the terms described below.* I understand that I will have 30 days to examine each annual edition. If satisfied, I will pay just $67.95 plus sales tax, postage and handling (price subject to change without notice).

Name: _____

Address: _____

City: _____ State: _____ Zip: _____

Method of Payment
○ Visa   ○ Mastercard   ○ AmEx   ○ Bill me   ○ Check (in US dollars, payable to Mosby, Inc.)

Card number: _____ Exp date: _____

Signature: _____

LS-0908

*Your *Year Book* Service Guarantee:

When you subscribe to the *Year Book*, we'll send you an advance notice of future volumes about two months before they publish. This automatic notice system is designed to take up as little of your time as possible. If you do not want the *Year Book*, the advance notice makes it quick and easy for you to let us know your decision, and you will always have at least 20 days to decide. If we don't hear from you, we'll send you the new volume as soon as it's available. And, of course, the *Year Book* is yours to examine free of charge for 30 days (postage, handling and applicable sales tax are added to each shipment.).

BUSINESS REPLY MAIL

FIRST CLASS MAIL   PERMIT No. 762   CHICAGO, IL

POSTAGE WILL BE PAID BY ADDRESSEE

Chris Hughes
Mosby-Year Book, Inc.
200 N. LaSalle Street
Suite 2600
Chicago, IL 60601-9981

BUSINESS REPLY MAIL

FIRST CLASS MAIL   PERMIT No. 762   CHICAGO, IL

POSTAGE WILL BE PAID BY ADDRESSEE

Chris Hughes
Mosby-Year Book, Inc.
200 N. LaSalle Street
Suite 2600
Chicago, IL 60601-9981

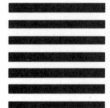

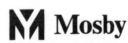

Mosby

Dedicated to publishing excellence

ative bile and brush cytology methods in establishing the nature of biliary strictures was analyzed.

Methods.—During a 2-year period, 100 consecutive patients with biliary tract strictures who were given a diagnosis using endoscopic retrograde cholangiopancreatography (69 of 93 patients) or percutaneous transhepatic cholangiography (36 of 93 patients) were followed. Group 1, which consisted of the first 47 patients, was assessed using bile cytology alone. Group 2, which consisted of the next 46 patients, was assessed using bile and brush cytology methods. Seven patients were excluded because of inadequate follow-up.

Results.—Eighty-one patients had confirmed malignant strictures, whereas benign strictures were confirmed in 12 patients. Malignant lesions were correctly identified in 16 of 42 patients in whom bile cytology alone was used (sensitivity, 33%). Results were not significantly different for samples that were taken endoscopically and percutaneously (table). The specificity of bile cytology in this group was 100%. Diagnostic accuracy was 40% overall and it did not differ for patients using samples that were taken endoscopically or percutaneously. Malignant lesions were correctly identified in 27 of 39 patients (sensitivity, 69%) in whom bile and brushing cytology was combined, demonstrating significantly greater sensitivity of the combined cytologies. Results were not significantly different for samples that were taken endoscopically and percutaneously. As in the bile cytology only group, the specificity was 100%. The diagnostic accuracy of bile and brush cytology combined was 74%, which was also significantly better than bile alone. No complications associated with the procedures occurred.

Conclusion.—Brush methods are more sensitive than bile cytology and should be done routinely in cases of biliary stricture. In this study, about 25% of the patients remained without a tissue diagnosis. Better results may be achieved by combining brush cytology with fine-needle aspiration cytology.

▶ These authors compared 100 patients who underwent 2 forms of bile cytologic investigation. Group 1 included 47 patients who were studied using bile cytology alone, and group 2 comprised 46 patients who were studied using bile and brush cytologic techniques. Combined bile and brush cytology was more sensitive than bile cytology alone for malignant disease—69 vs. 33% for the diagnosis of malignant strictures. In addition, for patients in group 2 who received both bile and brush cytology the cytologic study of brushings was more sensitive—69 vs. 26%. No false positive results were obtained in either group, and it would seem that bile cytology is an effective way of obtaining a tissue diagnosis with brush methods that are more sensitive than bile cytology. It would appear that both techniques should be performed to increase the overall sensitivity in patients who have biliary strictures of unknown etiology.—H.H. Simms, M.D.

Assessment of the Common Bile Duct Before Cholecystectomy Using Ultrasound and Biochemical Measurements: Validation Based on Follow-Up

Watkin DS, Haworth JM, Leaper DJ, Thompson MH (Southmead Hosp, Bristol, England)

Ann R Coll Surg Engl 76:317–319, 1994   140-95-11-2

Objective.—Even before the introduction of laparoscopic cholecystectomy (LC), there was debate about the need for routine operative cholangiography. Some more selective approach might be appropriate. A combination of biochemical measurements and ultrasound was studied as a means of assessing the common bile duct before LC.

Methods.—Two hundred fifty-three patients were studied before undergoing LC. Those who had known bile duct stones were excluded from the study, whereas those with a history of jaundice, pancreatitis, or abnormal liver function tests were included. On the day before the operation, all patients underwent measurement of serum bilirubin, alkaline phosphatase, and alanine aminotransferase levels along with ultrasound measurement of the bile duct diameter. If the results of these studies were normal, direct-contrast cholangiography was not performed.

Results.—Biochemical and ultrasound testing yielded abnormal results in 47 patients. Of these, only 6 patients were found to have bile duct stones on cholangiography. Follow-up was available on all 253 patients, including 93 who had repeat biochemical and ultrasound testing after 12 months. Only 2 patients showed evidence of missed stones of the common bile duct, and both of these stones passed spontaneously. No cases of bile duct injury occurred.

Conclusion.—For patients who are to undergo LC, the combination of ultrasound and liver function testing can safely obviate the need for routine operative cholangiography. With the use of selective cholangiography for patients who have abnormal results, there is no increase in postoperative morbidity resulting from missed stones or bile duct injuries.

▶ A resurgence of interest in the role of cholangiography at the time of cholecystectomy was noted, because all American surgeons are not properly trained and competent in the technique of intraoperative laparoscopic cholangiography. Nonetheless, the natural history of choledocholithiasis has not been modified by the introduction of new technology. Although the proponents of routine cholangiography will detect unsuspected common duct stones in a certain percentage of patients, they must realize that intraoperative cholangiography is not technically possible in all patients. The proponents of a selective approach possibly will fail to identify a small percentage of stones that may or may not be clinically relevant.—V.E. Pricolo, M.D.

Surgical Management of Choledochal Cysts

Scudamore CH, Hemming AW, Teare JP, Fache JS, Erb SR, Watkinson AF
(Univ of British Columbia, Vancouver, Canada)
Am J Surg 167:497–500, 1994   140-95-11–3

Introduction.—Although choledochal cysts are an uncommon cause of biliary obstruction, they are being detected more frequently with improved biliary imaging techniques. Eighty-five percent of these cysts are reportedly of type 1—that is, fusiform dilatations of the common bile duct—that are managed by complete surgical excision. However, type IVa cysts, in which cystic dilatation extends up into the intrahepatic biliary tree, can pose a surgical challenge. An experience with choledochal cysts, including 14 patients with type IVa cysts, was evaluated.

Patients.—Twenty-three consecutive patients with choledochal cysts were treated during a 5-year period. There were 18 women and 5 men, with a mean age of 36 years; abdominal pain, jaundice, and fever were the most common symptoms. The cysts were type I in 8 patients, type III in 1, and type IVa in 14. The patients with type I cysts underwent complete excision plus a hepaticojejunostomy and a modified Hutson loop formation. Thirteen of the 14 patients with type IVa cysts had complete excision of the cyst plus a hepaticojejunostomy and cystojejunostomy and a modified Hutson loop formation. Hepatic lobectomy was required in the remaining patient in this gruop. Differences in outcome were examined using Fisher's exact test.

Outcomes.—None of the patients with type I cysts had cholangitis or evidence of anastomotic stricture at a mean follow-up of 36 months. By contrast, 4 of the 14 patients with type IVa cysts had some evidence of recurrent cholangitis at a mean follow-up of 33 months. In 3 of these 4, the Hutson loop was used to achieve access to the biliary tree. Three of the patients had anastomotic strictures that were treated nonoperatively.

Conclusion.—Patients undergoing resection of type IVa choledochal cysts have a high incidence of recurrent cholangitis and anastomotic stricture. The construction of a Hutson loop at the time of primary resection for both biliary tract surveillance and as a route for intervention was recommended. The high incidence of type IV cysts in this study may reflect the tertiary referral nature of the study unit.

▶ This series of choledochal cysts is atypical, because the majority (14 of 23) had type IVa cysts. In other reports, the frequency was greatest for type I variants. The authors convincingly document the surgical approaches and conclude that the management of the more complex variant with intra- and extrahepatic dilation of the biliary duct (type IVa) includes extrahepatic cyst excision. Reconstruction with a Roux-en-Y to the intrahepatic portion of the cyst as a hepaticojejunostomy in the liver hilum is essential. These authors further recommend construction of the modified Hutson loop to enhance attempts at subsequent reintervention when necessary.—K.I. Bland, M.D.

Relationship Between Cystic Duct Diameter and the Presence of Cholelithiasis

Castelain M, Grimaldi C, Harris AG, Caroli-Bosc FX, Hastier P, Dumas R, Delmont JP (Hôpital Universitaire de Cimiez, Nice, France)
Dig Dis Sci 38:2220–2224, 1993   140-95-11–4

Introduction.—The diameter of the cystic duct was measured in patients with cholelithiasis or choledocholithiasis and in patients without biliary calculi.

Methods.—The cystic ducts of 168 patients were visualized using endoscopic retrograde cholangiopancreatography (ERCP). Based on ERCP findings, patients were placed in 1 of 3 groups: group I, no calculi in the gallbladder or common bile duct, 57 patients; group II, stones found in the gallbladder but absent from the common bile duct, 27 patients; and group III, stones present in the common bile duct with or without gallbladder stones, 34 patients. Cystic duct diameter was measured at the widest and narrowest dimensions.

Results.—The largest diameters were found in group III patients, and the smallest diameters were found in group I patients. Diameter sizes increased with the severity of disease and were significantly different in all 3 groups.

Conclusion.—The increase in cystic duct size with greater severity of disease may facilitate the migration of gallstone fragments after lithotripsy as well as the instrumentation of the cystic duct during ERCP and laparoscopic cholecystectomy.

▶ More and more attention is now being devoted to the ability to predict choledocholithiasis at the time of laparoscopic cholecystectomy. In addition to the traditionally analyzed variables (e.g., age, liver function tests, the presence of multiple stones and common bile duct diameter, and a history of pancreatitis), cystic duct diameter is assuming an interesting role. The presence of larger cystic ducts would probably make transcystic choledochoscopy and stone extraction possible.—V.E. Pricolo, M.D.

Incidental Cholecystectomy During Colorectal Surgery

Juhasz ES, Wolff BG, Meagher AP, Kluiber RM, Weaver AL, van Heerden JA (Mayo Clinic, Rochester, Minn)
Ann Surg 219:467–474, 1994   140-95-11–5

Introduction.—Incidental, asymptomatic gallstones are often found during colorectal surgery. The value of incidental cholecystectomy during colorectal surgery was assessed retrospectively.

Methods.—All patients who had asymptomatic cholelithiasis noted during surgery over a 5-year period were studied. Charts were reviewed, and the patients received questionnaires.

Results.—Three hundred five patients had asymptomatic cholelithiasis, of whom 195 (64%) had an incidental cholecystectomy and 110 (36%) did not. The groups were similar in terms of sex, age, and primary and associated medical conditions. Operative morbidity, long-term risk for small bowel obstruction, and survival curves were similar for both groups. Patients who did not have cholecystectomy had a 12% probability of needing this procedure 2 years later and a 22% probability 5 years later.

Conclusion.—Incidental cholecystectomy was not associated with increased postoperative morbidity. There was a substantial long-term risk of asymptomatic gallstones becoming symptomatic. Unless clearly contraindicated, patients who are found to have asymptomatic gallstones during abdominal surgery should have a concomitant cholecystectomy.

▶ The benefits of an incidental cholecystectomy during abdominal operations for unrelated problems (e.g., aortic aneurysmectomy) have been proven to outweigh its risks. Therefore, similar conclusions could be drawn for procedures in which concurrent contamination is evident.—V.E. Pricolo, M.D.

Comparison of Single-Dose Cefotetan and Multidose Cefoxitin as Intravenous Prophylaxis in Elective, Open Biliary Tract Surgery: A Multicentre, Double-Blind, Randomized Study
Lapointe RW, Roy AF, Turgeon PL, Lewis RT, Dagenais MH, Joly JR, Scudamore CH, Roy PD, Conly JM, Syrotuik J (St-Luc Hosp, Montreal; Queen Elizabeth Hosp, Montreal; Hôpital du Saint-Sacrement, Université Laval, Quebec, PQ, Canada; et al)
Can J Surg 37:314–318, 1994   140-95-11–6

Background.—Cefotetan is a new IV cephamycin antibiotic that has in vitro microbiological activity similar to that of cefoxitin. Because of this similarity, any pharmacokinetic difference should be considered in deciding which of these 2 agents is preferable, assuming that their efficacy and side effects are similar. The overall elimination half-life of cefotetan is 3.5 hours, substantially longer than that of cefoxitin (.8 hours).

Study Design.—The safety and prophylactic effectiveness of single-dose cefotetan compared with a standard prophylactic regimen of cefoxitin in elective, open biliary tract surgery were evaluated in a multicenter, double-blind, randomized study. Preoperatively, 76 of 111 patients who were undergoing elective, open biliary tract surgery were assigned to receive a 2-g IV dose of cefotetan, and 35 were assigned to receive cefoxitin 2 g in 3 doses.

Outcome.—Overall, 2 (1.8%) incisional wound infections were reported; both occurred in patients who received cefotetan. The mean duration of hospitalization was similar in both treatment groups. Similarly, there were no significant differences in the frequency of adverse events in the cefotetan group (12.6%) and the cefoxitin (10.4%) group. None of the 16 adverse events in the cefotetan group or the 5 events in the cefoxitin group were severe or serious. Several abnormal postoperative changes in hematologic and biochemical indicators were mainly attributed to surgery. In particular, abnormal postoperative prothrombin times and increased bleeding did not differ significantly between the 2 treatment groups.

Conclusion.—Cefotetan is safe and effective to use in reducing postoperative infections after elective, open biliary tract surgery. Because a single dose of cefotetan is equally as effective as 3 dose of cefoxitin, it appears to be a cost-saving substitute for prophylaxis in elective biliary tract surgery.

▶ This study compared the safety, tolerance, and prophylactic effectiveness of a single 2-g IV dose of cefotetan with a standard prophylactic regimen of cefoxitin in reducing the incidence of postoperative infections after elective, open biliary tract surgery. One hundred eleven patients were entered in a multicenter, double-blind randomized comparative study with a 4-week follow-up period. Patients were randomized to receive either cefotetan or cefoxitin at a ratio of 2:1; therefore, 76 patients received cefotetan and 35 received cefoxitin.

Two incisional wound infections were reported by the patients in the cefotetan group, for an overall infection rate of 1.8% (2 of 111). No significant differences were found in the failure rate nor in any other indicator of efficacy. The incidence of adverse events for cefotetan (12.6%) was not statistically different from that for cefoxitin (10.4%). Several hematologic biochemical parameters were found to be normal preoperatively and abnormal postoperatively, but no relationship was found between these variations and the study drugs. It would appear that cefotetan is as effective and comparable to cefoxitin both in terms of safety and in reducing the incidence of infection after elective, open biliary tract surgery.—H.H. Simms, M.D.

Influence of Compression Stockings on Lower-Limb Venous Haemodynamics During Laparoscopic Cholecystectomy
Wilson YG, Allen PE, Skidmore R, Baker AR (Frenchay Hospital, Bristol, England)
Br J Surg 81:841–844, 1994   140-95-11–7

Introduction.—Although laparoscopic cholecystectomy has the advantages of allowing more rapid recovery and reducing postoperative pain, the prolonged pneumoperitoneum required for some procedures may cause significant alterations in lower limb venous return. This can increase the risk of thromboembolism. The effects of pneumoperitoneum on lower limb venous return were studied in a prospective, randomized trial.

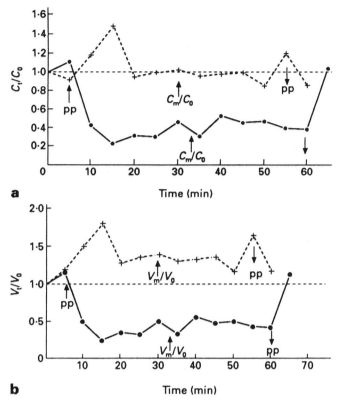

Fig 11–1.—**a** Standardized venous capacitance ratio (C_t/C_o) plotted against time; **b** standardized venous outflow ratio (V_t/V_o) plotted against time. *Dotted line,* with compression stockings; *solid line,* no stockings. *Abbreviations: pp,* pneumoperitoneum; C_m/C_o and V_m/V_o, standardized venous capacitance and outflow rations at mid-operation. (Courtesy of Wilson YG, Allen PE, Skidmore R, et al: *Br J Surg* 81:841–844, 1994.)

Methods.—Forty patients without an increased risk of a thromboembolic disorder who underwent elective laparoscopic cholecystectomy were randomly assigned to surgery with or without compression stockings. All patients were positioned in a 20-degree reverse Trendelenburg tilt with the right side up. They wore pressure cuffs on both calves and both thighs to monitor venous blood flow. The venous capacitance and outflow values were calculated as fractions of baseline values.

Results.—Capacitance and outflow ratios fell during the procedure and returned to normal after the release of pneumoperitoneum in 65% of the patients without stockings. By contrast, capacitance and outflow ratios either remained consistent or increased during the procedure, returning to baseline after the release of pneumoperitoneum (Fig 11–1). At the midpoint of the procedure, the median capacitance ratios were .89 in the group without stockings and 1.48 in the group with stockings, and the median outflow ratios were .89 in the group without stockings and

1.71 in the group with stockings. The ratios for both values were consistently but nonsignificantly lower in left legs than in right legs.

Discussion.—These data suggest that a resistance to venous return occurs in the lower limbs during pneumoperitoneum and that this occurrence can be controlled by the use of graded compression stockings. Capacitance and outflow may be reduced by blood pooling caused by pneumoperitoneum, and this pooling can be prevented by the stockings. Blood pooling affects stasis and can induce endothelial injury. Graded rather than uniform compresssion has been shown to increase venous flow velocity, thereby reducing stasis and endothelial injury. The trend toward lower capacitance values for left legs than for right legs may be caused by compression of the left iliac vein by the right common iliac artery. Because at least 2 of the 3 components of Virchow's triad are affected by pneumoperitoneum, it is recommended that both graduated compression stockings and subcutaneous heparin be used to prevent thromboembolic complications during laparoscopic surgery.

▶ Wilson and colleagues have provided us with an excellent and timely study on venous outflow from the legs during laparoscopic surgery. They documented a clear and marked reduction in venous outflow from the legs with pneumoperitoneum, which is abolished by the use of graded venous compression stockings. Although they were unable to comment on the incidence of thromboembolic phenomena during laparoscopic procedures, their study strongly argues for the use of graded compression stockings in laparoscopic surgery.

At least 2 elements of Virchow's trial are activated by pneumoperitoneum: stasis and endothelial injury. Theoretically, this can lead to potential thromboembolic complications. Furthermore, the reduction in venous flow is associated with important hemodynamic changes that were not evaluated in their study. These changes may also have important consequences, particularly in the patient with preexisting cardiopulmonary disease.

We currently use graded venous compression stockings in all our laparoscopic surgeries and agree with the authors' conclusion.—J.F. Amaral, M.D.

The Need to Retrieve the Dropped Stone During Laparoscopic Cholecystectomy
Johnston S, O'Malley K, McEntee G, Grace P, Smyth E, Bouchier-Hayes D
(Beaumont Hospital, Dublin, Ireland)
Am J Surg 167:608–610, 1994   140-95-11–8

Objective.—Bile leakage, which is sometimes accompanied by loss of gallstones, can occur during laparoscopic cholecystectomy. One recent series of 60 laparoscopic cholecystectomies reported a bile leakage rate of 13%. The effects of bile, alone and in combination with gallstones, on the peritoneal cavity were evaluated in rats.

Methods.—Ninety Sprague-Dawley rats were randomized to 6 equal groups. Respectively, those in groups 1–3 had 2 mL of saline, sterile bile, or infected bile intraperitoneally injected. After a 3- to 5-mm lower midline abdominal incision, the animals in groups 4 and 5 had a single gallstone less than 3 mm in diameter placed in the right upper quadrant. After the wound was closed, group 4 rats were injected with sterile bile and group 5 rats with infected bile. Laparotomy was followed by sterile saline injection only in group 6 animals. All rats were killed and examined after 4 weeks.

Results.—Seventy-three percent of rats in group 4 and 67% of those in group 5 had intra-abdominal adhesions compared with none in groups 1–3. Two of the group 4 animals had 2 intra-abdominal abscesses. There were no intra-abdominal lesions in the group 6 rats.

Conclusion.—In small amounts, intraperitoneal bile leakage appears to be relatively harmless. However, bile leakage combined with gallstones can significantly increase the risk of postoperative adhesions and intra-abdominal abscesses. If "lost" gallstones are associated with intra-abdominal abscess formation, the increased incidence of this complication should soon become apparent. By contrast, the associated risk of adhesions may take longer to define and its clinical significance longer still. In this study, it was possible that the lesions in groups 4 and 5 were related to infected gallstones.

▶ Laparoscopic cholecystectomy has introduced 2 potential intraoperative complications that are not applicable to open surgery: bile spillage and stone loss. Although these events occur with open cholecystectomy, they are easily managed. Bile spillage occurs in 9% to 15% and stone loss occurs in 1% to 2% of laparoscopic cholecystectomies. Early clinical studies on laparoscopic cholecystectomy indicated that these events did not matter and that no special management was needed.

The authors provide us with strong evidence that bile spillage alone, whether infected or not, is not likely to lead to any postoperative problem. However, bile and stones are likely to lead to a high incidence of adhesions and a low incidence of abscess. Given these findings, one can be comfortable there will be no untoward sequelae after irrigation and aspiration of bile, but what about dropped stones?

Clearly, every effort should be made to remove any dropped stones and prevent any further stone spillage by closing holes in the gallbladder and placing it in a specimen bag as soon as possible. However, conversion to open surgery seems to be a drastic step in managing lost stones, because the morbidity of a right upper quadrant incision is much greater than any potential stone-related complications. A right upper quadrant incision has almost a 100% adhesion rate, a definite incidence of significant wound infection and hernia formation, and no guarantee that all the stones will be retrieved. Furthermore, clinical experience after 4 years has not confirmed this experimental study, with only a few isolated case reports of abscess in the literature. Finally, right upper quadrant adhesions are rarely the cause of bowel obstruction. Therefore, until further evidence has been accumulated, a "wait and see" policy appears to be most prudent.—J.F. Amaral, M.D.

Preoperative Transdermal Scopolamine Does Not Reduce the Level of Nausea and Frequency of Vomiting After Laparoscopic Cholecystectomy

Sohi HS, Heipel J, Inman KJ, Chinnick B, Cunningham DG, Holliday RL, Girotti MJ (Victoria Hosp, London, Ont, Canada)
Can J Surg 37:307–312, 1994   140-95-11–9

Introduction.—Nausea and vomiting cause significant morbidity after laparoscopic cholecystectomy. Several studies have focused on the use of transdermal scopolamine to reduce the degree of postoperative nausea and the frequency of postoperative vomiting, but the results have been contradictory. To investigate further, a homogeneous group of patients scheduled for laparoscopic surgery were studied to determine whether preoperative transdermal scopolamine could reduce the degree of nausea and the frequency of postoperative vomiting by 30%.

Study Design.—In a randomized, double-blind, placebo-controlled study, 125 men and women aged 20–60 years who were scheduled to undergo elective laparoscopic cholecystectomy were studied. The patients applied a skin patch that contained either scopolamine or placebo

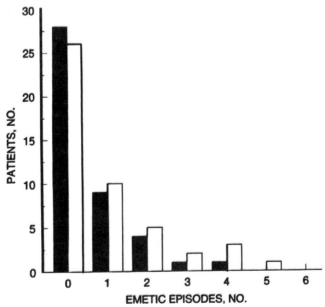

Fig 11–2.—Mean frequency of emetic episodes in treatment (*black bars*) and control (*white bars*) groups 6 hours after laparoscopic cholecystectomy. (Courtesy of Sohi HS, Heipel J, Inman KJ, et al: *Can J Surg* 37:307–312, 1994.)

Mean (SEM) Preoperative and Postoperative Levels of Nausea on the Visual Analogue
Scale in the Treatment and Control Groups

	Nausea level, mm		
Time	Treatment	Control	*p* value
Preoperatively	2.9 (9.4)	3.8 (11.0)	0.695
6 h postoperatively	25.5 (34.5)	23.9 (35.6)	0.827
12 h postoperatively	14.3 (26.8)	20.9 (31.4)	0.289
24 h postoperatively	3.3 (9.4)	5.9 (15.2)	0.328

(Courtesy of Sohi HS, Heipel J, Inman KJ, et al: *Can J Surg* 37:307–312, 1994.)

behind the right ear on the evening before surgery and wore it for at least 24 hours postoperatively. Anesthetic procedures and postoperative care, including analgesia, were standardized. Postoperative nausea was assessed using a visual analogue scale, and the frequency of vomiting and the use of antiemetics were monitored during the first 24 hours postoperatively (Fig 11–2).

Outcome.—There were no significant differences in the level of nausea, frequency of emesis, and the use of antiemetics between the treatment and control groups (table). Similarly, there were no significant differences in the overall frequency of side effects, although there was a definite trend toward increased visual blurring in the treatment group. Heavier patients and women had higher levels of postoperative nausea than their counterparts. In addition, there was a definite trend for patients with a history of travel sickness to require additional antiemetics in both groups.

Conclusion.—Transdermal scopolamine before laparoscopic cholecystectomy does not reduce the frequency or level of nausea and vomiting postoperatively. The use of transdermal scopolamine in patients undergoing laparoscopic cholecystectomy is not recommended, because of the drug's lack of efficacy as well as the potential for deleterious side effects and related health care costs.

▶ Postoperative nausea and vomiting are the most common complaints after laparoscopic surgery and among the most common if not the most common reasons for admission. In a randomized, prospective trial, the authors have evaluated the preoperative use of transdermal scopolamine. Unfortunately, not only was there no difference in postoperative nausea and vomiting between placebo and scopolamine groups, there was a trend toward more side effects in the scopolamine group.

This type of study is important as we continue to search for ways to reduce health care costs while improving quality. It is hoped that more efforts will be made to eliminate postoperative nausea and vomiting after these procedures.—J.F. Amaral, M.D.

Management of Common Bile Duct Stricture Caused by Chronic Pancreatitis With Metal Mesh Self Expandable Stents

Deviere J, Cremer M, Baize M, Love J, Sugai B, Vandermeeren A (Hôpital Erasme, Université Libre de Bruxelles, Brussels, Belgium)

Gut 35:122–126, 1994   140-95-11-10

Background.—The use of self-expandable metal mesh stents in malignant bile duct strictures provides immediate drainage and prevents the early complications associated with plastic stents. However, long-term results are marred by tumoral ingrowth and more commonly ingrowth through the metallic mesh into the stent. Ingrowth and subsequent reocclusion appear to be tumor related. A new treatment method was investigated in patients who had severe chronic pancreatitis (CP) and benign symptomatic biliary stricture.

Patients and Methods.—Self-expandable metal mesh stents were placed in 20 patients who had CP and signs of biliary obstruction. Persistent cholestasis was noted in all patients; 7 patients also had jaundice, and 3 had overt cholangitis. Plastic endoprostheses had been used previously in 11 patients. The mean follow-up was 33 months, and it included clinical assessment, ultrasonography, and endoscopic retrograde cholangiopancreatography (ERCP).

Results.—Endoscopic stent placement was successful in all patients and led to rapid resolution of cholestasis, jaundice, and cholangitis. No early clinical complications were observed. In 18 patients, successive ERCPs and cholangioscopies showed that the metal mesh was initially embedded in the bile duct wall. By 3 months, the mesh was covered with a continuous tissue. Epithelial hyperplasia developed within the stent in 2 patients, resulting in recurrent biliary obstruction at 3 months and 6 months after placement. Treatment consisted of endoscopic placement of standard plastic stents, and 1 of the 2 patients ultimately required surgical drainage. In all other patients, the stent lumen remained patent and functional during the follow-up period. Subsequent obstruction was not observed in any patient who was free of clinical or radiologic signs of epithelial hyperplasia after 6 months.

Conclusion.—This new treatment may be an effective, low-morbidity alternative to surgical biliary diversion. Additional controlled follow-up studies are needed to confirm these initial findings.

▶ The application of expandable metal stents to nonmalignant diseases may find a particularly favorable arena in chronic pancreatitis, where surgeons may be particularly reluctant to reoperate and perform biliary enteric anastomosis, especially in the absence of the gallbladder.—V.E. Pricolo, M.D.

Medicolegal Analysis of Bile Duct Injury During Open Cholecystectomy and Abdominal Surgery

Kern KA (Hartford Hospital, Conn; Univ of Connecticut School of Medicine, Hartford)

Am J Surg 168:217–222, 1994   140-95-11–11

Background.—Numerous series of open cholecystectomies have reported bile duct injury and bile leakage in .1% to .5% of patients. A recent review of more than 40,000 open operations documented bile duct injury in .2% of cases. Such injuries can lead to stricture formation, chronic illness, or death. A recent textbook on malpractice litigation indicates that biliary fistula formation complicating routine gallbladder surgery is the most common meritorious reason for negligence actions. Bile duct injuries have become more prevalent since the advent of laparoscopic cholecystectomy.

Objective.—The medicolegal ramifications of bile duct injuries were studied by analyzing 68 patients who were injured in the course of open cholecystectomy and abdominal surgery. These cases were litigated between 1970 and 1991.

Findings.—Cholecystectomy performed for cholelithiasis accounted for 72% of injuries. Five patients underwent common bile duct exploration and 7 had other abdominal operations. The delay in recognizing the injury averaged 16 days but could be as long as 6 weeks. Twelve patients (18%) died. The average out-of-court settlement was $250,000, but the median jury award in successfully litigated cases was $500,000.

Discussion.—Bile duct injuries incurred at open cholecystectomy or other abdominal operations carry a high mortality rate if they are not detected promptly. The most prevalent injury is division and dissection of the common bile duct or common hepatic duct when it is mistaken for the cystic duct. It is often believed that a biliary anomaly such as a duct of Luschka or a supernumerary bile duct is present. Deaths related to biliary complications of elective cholecystectomy are a major source of negligence litigation. The likelihood of an award being made depends more on expert judgment that accepted standards of care were not followed than on the severity of injury.

▶ This timely article discusses the medicolegal issues associated with an uncommon but potentially disastrous complication—bile duct injury. Three points are worthy of note. Although anomalies do occur (15% to 20%), they rarely are responsible for injury. Therefore, when an anomaly is suspected, the surgeon must exercise extreme caution and document the anomaly with cholangiography.

Second, most cases of bile duct transection occur when the surgeon mistakenly identifies the common duct as the cystic duct. Therefore, no tubular structure should ever be divided before its junction with the gallbladder has been confirmed. Furthermore, any large tubular structure (larger than 5 mm) requires confirmation by cholangiography that it is the cystic duct and not the common duct.

Third, early recognition is of paramount importance in reducing the long-term morbidity and mortality of the injury. Finally, the author also argues that not all litigated cases result in a jury verdict in favor of the plaintiff.

The most important reason for documentation is to show that the injury was not a deviation from accepted standards of care. In this era of laparoscopic cholecystectomy, the rate of injury to the common duct and the severity of injury itself appear to be greater. Adherence to the points made in this article is likely to reduce injuries as well as verdicts in favor of the plaintiff.—J.F. Amaral, M.D.

Helium Pneumoperitoneum for Laparoscopic Cholecystectomy: Ventilatory and Blood Gas Changes

McMahon AJ, Baxter JN, Murray W, Imrie CW, Kenny G, O'Dwyer PJ (Western Infirmary, Glasgow, Scotland; Royal Infirmary, Glasgow, Scotland)
Br J Surg 81:1033–1036, 1994   140-95-11–12

Introduction.—Pneumoperitoneum in laparoscopic surgery is usually achieved with carbon dioxide. However, concerns about respiratory acidosis and increased ventilation have led to investigations of an alternative gas for abdominal insufflation. Helium has been found to be suitable in animal studies. The effects of helium and carbon dioxide pneumoperitoneum on ventilatory and arterial blood gas changes were compared during laparoscopic cholecystectomy.

Methods.—Laparoscopic cholecystectomy was performed on 60 consecutive patients, using helium for pneumoperitoneum in 30 patients and carbon dioxide in 30 patients. Minute ventilation, peak airway pressure, end-tidal carbon dioxide and oxygen tension, and arterial carbon dioxide and oxygen tension were monitored. The alveolar-arterial oxygen gradient was calculated.

Results.—The patients who were insufflated with either gas had comparable preoperative characteristics. Minute ventilation increased significantly with carbon dioxide but not with helium. Peak airway pressure rose significantly with both gases. Arterial carbon dioxide and hydrogen ion concentrations increased significantly with carbon dioxide pneumoperitoneum. Significant increases in the alveolar-arterial oxygen gradient and the ratio of arterial to end-tidal carbon dioxide tension were seen with helium pneumoperitoneum. Four patients in the helium group had accidental insufflation into the abdominal wall, resulting in surgical emphysema that lasted 3 to 5 days.

Discussion.—Ideally, the gas used for pneumoperitoneum would be chemically, physiologically, and pharmacologically inert; would not support combustion; and would be highly water soluble and able to dissolve in the bloodstream if a gas embolism occurred. Carbon dioxide, although it increases the ventilatory requirements, is highly water soluble. Nitrous oxide does not induce changes in arterial blood gases, but it supports combustion, which excludes it from use in laparoscopic procedures that require diathermy. The usefulness of helium is limited only by its poor water solubility, which can result in surgical emphysema and indicate less safety than carbon dioxide if a gas embolism occurs.

▶ The authors have provided us with a detailed, nonrandomized comparison of carbon dioxide and helium pneumoperitoneum. As expected, changes caused by absorption of carbon dioxide (increased arterial P_{CO_2} and decreased pH) were not seen in the helium pneumoperitoneum patients. However, helium pneumoperitoneum did induce respiratory changes in peak airway pressure, the alveolar-arterial oxygen gradient, and the alveolar arterial CO_2 gradient. Furthermore, helium is not as soluble as carbon dioxide, resulting in a prolonged time for resolution of subcutaneous emphysema.

The latter may be the most important finding because it raises serious concerns about helium emboli during surgery. Because carbon dioxide pneumoperitoneum can be easily controlled by careful monitoring and adjustment of respiratory function during surgery, it is rapidly reversed by relieving the pneumoperitoneum. Because it has a very low risk of embolism, there appears to be no need to change to helium.—J.F. Amaral, M.D.

12 Oncology

Introduction

As in previous years, this year has been replete with significant studies in both basic surgical science and clinical literature. However, of particular note has been the significant movement toward molecular and biological markers and the study of molecular events in carcinogenesis and metastasis. In the event that one is left with the impression that clinical studies are not important, there have also been a number of significant findings in the evaluation of patients with malignant disease.

Technical advances in the diagnosis of breast disease have been made through more thorough pathologic evaluation of smaller amounts of tissue. This has been done using immunohistochemistry and improved DNA analysis. In addition, advances are underway to use MRI and positron emission tomography scanning for radiographic evaluation of the breast. Studies that will yield a more in depth appreciation of the molecular events as well as the prediction of metastasis are currently underway. Clinical studies, such as sentinel lymph node biopsy and the limitations of breast-conserving surgery, will help define the future surgical management of breast cancer.

Extensive studies have been published regarding the molecular genetics of colorectal cancers. Vogelstein and others have made significant advances in defining the stepwise progression of benign to malignant transformation as well as local to disseminated disease progression. This has practical applicability in the management of colorectal cancer, and it forms a model for the study of benign to malignant transformation that may be applicable to other malignant diseases as well. Significant clinical studies with preoperative radiation therapy and/or postoperative adjuvant therapies have also been performed. New surgical techniques of coloanal anastomosis with resection of low-lying carcinoma of the rectum are being perfected and studied thoroughly.

Advances are being introduced in the management of soft tissue sarcoma through the development of better prognostic indicators and use of brachytherapy as well as a better definition of the indications for adjuvant radiation therapy. Unfortunately, the treatment of soft tissue sarcoma is still limited by the poor results of adjuvant chemotherapy; however, trials of neoadjuvant chemotherapy are currently underway and will probably be the subject of future YEAR BOOK citations.

Gastric cancer remains a disease with poor prognosis unless it is diagnosed early. Again, neoadjuvant therapy will probably play a major role in future clinical trials. The extent of resection, selection of patients, and adjuvant immunochemotherapy have been studied over the past year.

In summary, this year has resulted in numerous detailed molecular studies that have led to a better understanding of the pathogenesis of various malignant processes. In addition, the utilization of randomized prospective trials and prospective databases have better defined clinical parameters that will significantly enhance the treatment of patients with malignant disease.

Timothy J. Eberlein, M.D.

Carcinoma of the Breast

New Horizons in the Diagnosis and Treatment of Breast Cancer Using Magnetic Resonance Imaging
Cross MJ, Harms SE, Cheek JH, Peters GN, Jones RC (Baylor Univ Med Ctr, Dallas)
Am J Surg 166:749–755, 1993   140-95-12–1

Objective.—Rotating delivery of excitation off-resonance (RODEO) is a new steady–state, fat–suppressed MRI sequence designed to achieve optimal image contrast for breast imaging with a T1-weighted, 3-dimensional image. It is hoped that the RODEO method will aid surgeons in the diagnosis and treatment of breast cancer, particularly in achieving clear tumor margins. The potential role of the RODEO method in surgical decision making was assessed in a prospective, nonrandomized study.

Methods.—The study sample comprised 100 women with a high suspicion of breast cancer. All had palpable or nonpalpable breast masses that were demonstrated by conventional imaging modalities. Physical examination and mammography were performed in every case, and some form of biopsy was performed in most cases. Forty–one patients underwent preoperative RODEO MRI followed by mastectomy and serial sectioning of the surgical specimens.

Results.—Eighty-five pathologically confirmed lesions were detected by RODEO; 64 proved to be malignant. The sensitivity of RODEO was 95% with 3 false negatives compared with 58% and 27 false negatives for conventional imaging. The RODEO method detected 21 cancers that were not seen on mammography and sonography, most of which were multifocal in nature. The specificity of RODEO MRI was 37% compared with 85% for conventional imaging. Accuracy was 76% for RODEO MRI and 66% for conventional imaging. In some cases, RODEO MRI found lesions that were initially missed on pathologic examination.

Conclusion.—The RODEO MRI method is a highly sensitive technique that aids in locating possible multicentric breast cancer and evaluating patients for conservative surgery. It may also be used clinically to assess the response to chemotherapy or to evaluate women who have normal mammograms but with high-risk markers for future breast cancer. Further studies are needed to identify the distinguishing MRI features that are suspicious for malignancy.

▶ This very nice prospective study of 100 patients documents the improved sensitivity of RODEO MRI techniques over standard mammography in detecting occult malignancies. There is no doubt that this technology is more sensitive, but there are 2 issues surrounding it: its expense in this cost-consciousness health environment and its ability to determine benign lesions from occult malignant lesions. The latter can only be addressed with continued experience and by larger numbers of patients entered into prospective trials.—T.J. Eberlein, M.D.

Difficulties in Diagnosis of Carcinoma of the Breast in Patients Less Than Fifty Years of Age

Lannin DR, Harris RP, Swanson FH, Edwards MS, Swanson MS, Pories WJ (East Carolina Univ School of Medicine, Greenville, NC; Univ of North Carolina, Chapel Hill)
Surg Gynecol Obstet 177:457–462, 1993   140-95-12–2

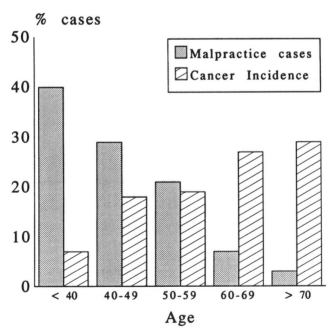

Fig 12–1.—Age distribution for malpractice suits from the Physicians Insurers Association of America Breast Cancer Study compared with the age distribution for carcinoma of the breast from the North Carolina State Tumor Registry. (Courtesy of Lannin DR, Harris RP, Swanson FH, et al: *Surg Gynecol Obstet* 177:457–462, 1993.)

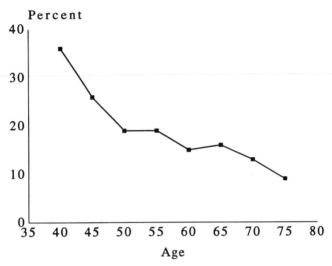

Fig 12–2.—Percent of carcinomas not detected by mammography or physical examination (interval carcinomas) in the Breast Cancer Detection Demonstration Project. (Courtesy of Lannin DR, Harris RP, Swanson FH, et al: *Surg Gynecol Obstet* 177:457–462, 1993.)

Introduction.—One of the most common causes of medical malpractice suits in the United States is delay in the diagnosis of breast carcinoma, particularly in women younger than 50 years of age, even though the incidence of breast carcinoma is considerably lower in this age group than in women older than 50 years of age (Fig 12–1). Diagnostic data from several sources were analyzed to determine whether medical fac-

Two Estimates of Cost per Diagnosed Carcinoma of the Breast		
Age, yrs.	20 to 49	≥50
ECU		
Clinic visits at $40	41 $ 1,640	8 $ 320
Mammograms at $90	16 $ 1,440	5 $ 450
Biopies at $1,000	7.5 $ 7,500	1.9 $1,900
Total cost per carcinoma	$10,580	$2,670
BCBS of North Carolina		
Biopsies per 10,000 women	64.21	103.95
Biopsies per carcinoma	5.7	2.6
Cost per biopsy	$ 1,885	$2,051
Cost per carcinoma	$10,744	$5,333

Abbreviations: ECU, East Carolina University; *BCBS,* Blue Cross Blue Shield.

Note: The ECU estimate takes into account clinic visits and mammograms for patients referred to the Breast Clinic, but not for all patients with presumably normal findings who were not referred. The BCBS data are more accurate and are state-wide, but only consider biopsy cost.

(Courtesy of Lannin DR, Harris RP, Swanson FH, et al: *Surg Gynecol Obstet* 177:457–462, 1993.)

tors make diagnosis more difficult in women younger than 50 years of age.

Methods.—Records were reviewed of all patients who went to a university breast clinic during a 2½ year period without a previous diagnosis of carcinoma of the breast. Data were also derived from Blue Cross and Blue Shield and from published reports of the Breast Cancer Detection Demonstration Project.

Results.—Nearly twice as many women younger than 50 years of age went to the university breast clinic than women older than 50 years. There were no significant age–related differences in the performance of fine-needle aspiration or open biopsy, which were performed if there were abnormal findings with either the physical examination or mammography. Both mammography and physical examination were significantly less sensitive in women younger than 50 years of age. An abnormal mammogram had a positive predictive value of 28% in women younger than 50 years of age and 53% in women older than 50 years of age and respective sensitivities of 68% vs. 91%. An abnormal physical examination had a positive predictive value of 11% in women younger than 50 years of age and 57% in women older than 50 years of age and respective sensitivities of 74% vs. 77%. In addition, nonpalpable tumors were much larger in the younger women than in the older women, either because of the background density of the breast or the diffuse growth of the tumors. The data from the Breast Cancer Detection Demonstration Project confirmed that mammography and physical examination are less sensitive and less predictive in women younger than 50 years of age than in older women (Fig 12-2). Cost comparisons of diagnosis at the breast clinic and from Blue Cross Blue Shield indicated that diagnosis of breast carcinoma costs at least twice as much in women younger than 50 years of age than in older women (table).

Discussion.—The biological factors involved in tumor development cause more diagnostic difficulties than physician error. Diagnosis is more difficult in women younger than 50 years of age because both mammography and physical examination are much less accurate in these women than in women older than 50 years of age.

▶ This article objectively documents what we all recognize: It is much more difficult to detect a cancer in young women, because of the very dense stroma of the surrounding normal breast tissue. The dense stroma results in a much less sensitive mammography in the young women, and somewhat surprisingly it accounts for why palpable cancers in young women are often much larger. The use of positron emission tomographic scanning and MRI may help to identify cancers in dense stroma earlier; however, experience and improved interpretation of these new modalities will be needed before they are more useful in large populations of young women.—T.J. Eberlein, M.D.

Occurrence and Prognosis of Contralateral Carcinoma of the Breast

Singletary SE, Taylor SH, Guinee VF, Whitworth PW Jr (Univ of Texas MD Anderson Cancer Ctr, Houston; Sarah Cannon Surgical Group, Nashville, Tenn)
J Am Coll Surg 178:390–396, 1994   140-95-12-3

Background.—In women with breast cancer, the risk of a second carcinoma developing in the contralateral breast concerns both the patient and physician. Morbidity and mortality rates associated with a second contralateral breast carcinoma have not yet been determined. Therefore, some women may undergo mastectomy in a contralateral breast to prevent development of a second carcinoma. Whether a prophylactic mastectomy is an appropriate option in patients who are treated for breast carcinoma was studied.

Patients and Methods.—The medical records of 142 consecutive patients who were given a diagnosis of and surgically treated for breast carcinoma between 1965 and 1988 were retrospectively reviewed. Of these, 55 had a previous carcinoma of the breast (metachronous) (Fig 12–3), and 87 had a contralateral carcinoma of the breast that was detected within 4 months of enrollment (synchronous) (Table 1).

Results.—At 3.1%, a low occurrence of bilateral breast carcinoma was noted. The frequency of metachronous breast carcinoma was relatively constant over time (Table 2). The nodal status of the second breast carcinoma was associated with the method of discovery rather that the stage of the first carcinoma. Second carcinoma survival rates were similar for metachronous and synchronous disease.

Conclusion.—In breast cancer patients, the contralateral breast should be carefully evaluated at initial diagnosis and during follow-up examinations. The likelihood of early identification of a second carcinoma is high, with good subsequent survival rate. Therefore, candidates for a prophylactic mastectomy should be selected on the basis of their emotional needs.

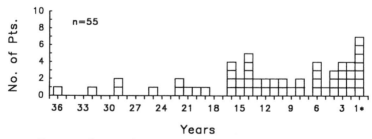

Fig 12–3.—Time interval in years between the diagnosis of first and second metachronous carcinoma of the breast. Asterisk indicates time interval of 5–12 months between diagnosis before registration at The University of Texas M.D. Anderson Cancer Center, Houston. (Courtesy of Singletary SE, Taylor SH, Guinee VF, et al: *J Am Coll Surg* 178:390–396, 1994.)

TABLE 1.—Method of Discovery of Synchronous and Metachronous Carcinomas of the Breast

Method of discovery	Synchronous		Metachronous	
	—First, n=87—	—Second, n=87—	—First, n=55—	—Second, n=55—
Breast self-examination	65 (74)	14 (16)	24 (43)	27 (49)
Physician examination	10 (12)	25 (29)	3 (6)	12 (22)
Screening mammography	10 (12)	38 (44)	—	14 (25)
Prophylactic mastectomy	—	7 (8)	—	1 (2)
Blind biopsy	—	3 (3)	1 (2)	—
Unknown	2 (2)	0 —	27 (49)	1 (2)

*Numbers in parentheses are percentages.
(Courtesy of Singletary SE, Taylor SH, Guinee VF, et al: *J Am Coll Surg* 178:390–396, 1994.)

TABLE 2.—Correlation of Axillary Nodal Status Between First and Second Metachronous Carcinomas of the Breast*

Histologic nodal status, first carcinoma	Histologic nodal status, second carcinoma			
	Negative	Positive	Unknown	Total
Negative	12	6	0	18 (33)
Positive	6	4	1	11 (20)
Unknown	18	7	1	26 (47)
Total	36 (65)	17 (31)	2 (4)	55 (100)

*Numbers in parentheses are percentages.
(Courtesy of Singletary SE, Taylor SH, Guinee VF, et al: J Am Coll Surg 178:390–396, 1994.)

▶ In this paper the authors document the risk of contralateral breast cancer that is diagnosed simultaneously as quite small; therefore, opposite breast biopsy procedures can be avoided unless they are directed by physical examination or mammography. The need for long-term follow-up is also emphasized because the risk of contralateral breast cancer is linearly increased with time. This approach will minimize the procedures performed on contralateral breasts.—T.J. Eberlein, M.D.

Long-Term Risk of Breast Cancer in Women With Fibroadenoma

Dupont WD, Page DL, Parl FF, Vnencak-Jones CL, Plummer WD Jr, Rados MS, Schuyler PA (Vanderbilt Univ, Nashville, Tenn)
N Engl J Med 331:10–15, 1994   140-95-12–4

Background.—Fibroadenomas usually occur in young women, and they were previously considered to be unrelated to a risk of breast cancer. However, recent studies have found a relationship between these benign breast tumors and subsequent invasive breast cancer. The correlation between the histologic features of fibroadenomas and the long-term risk of breast cancer was examined in a retrospective cohort study.

Methods.—Patients who were eligible for the study were diagnosed as having fibroadenomas between 1950 and 1968 and did not have breast cancer before or within 6 months after their study entry biopsy. There were 2 control groups, the first consisting of the patients' sisters-in-law and the second of women listed in the Connecticut Tumor Registry. Histologic slides of all patients were reviewed and classified. Follow-up data on the rate of subsequent breast cancer, which were available for 1,835 patients (90%), were compared with the rates in the 2 control groups.

Results.—Complex fibroadenomas, (those with cysts greater than 3 mm in diameter) sclerosing adenosis, epithelial calcifications, or papillary apocrine changes were identified in 22.7% of 2,458 consecutive biopsy specimens. Proliferative disease was more common adjacent to complex fibroadenomas than to noncomplex lesions. The risk of invasive breast cancer was 2.17 times higher among the women with fibroadenomas than among their sisters-in-law and 1.61 times higher relative to the control women from the Connecticut Tumor Registry. This difference was consistent, because the sisters-in-law had lower observed risks for breast cancer than the women in the tumor registry. Among patients with complex fibroadenomas, the relative risk increased to 3.1 and remained elevated for decades after diagnosis. Risk was also increased by the presence of benign proliferative disease adjacent to the fibroadenoma and by a family history of breast cancer in conjunction with complex fibroadenoma.

Conclusion.—Fibroadenomas are a long-term risk factor for breast cancer, although the histologic features of the tumor, the presence or absence of proliferative disease, and the patient's family history influence this risk. If these additional factors are present, regular mammographic surveillance at 35 or 40 years of age and testing for mutations in the *BRCAI* gene may be appropriate. Women with neither a complex lesion nor a family history can be assured that a fibroadenoma does not appreciably influence their risk of breast cancer.

▶ This article further extends the authors' observations that benign proliferative disease in the breast increases the risk of breast cancer. Regardless of whether this proliferation is intraductal hyperplasia, intraductal hyperplasia with atypia, or lobular carcinoma *in situ*, each increases the subsequent risk of carcinoma. This risk is further increased by family history.

This study looks specifically at fibroadenoma and the surrounding breast tissue. Again, proliferation and family history increase risk. This is particularly true with complex fibroadenomas, which obviously indicate an increase in proliferative activity. The good news is that in women without a family history of breast cancer and without a complex proliferative lesion in the fibroadenoma, the risk of subsequent breast cancer is not appreciably influenced.—T.J. Eberlein, M.D.

Lymphatic Mapping and Sentinel Lymphadenectomy for Breast Cancer

Giuliano AE, Kirgan DM, Guenther JM, Morton DL (Saint John's Hosp, Santa Monica, Calif)
Ann Surg 220:391–401, 1994   140-95-12–5

Purpose.—The value of axillary lymph node dissection (ALND) for staging and prognostic purposes in breast cancer is widely accepted. However, the debate continues about the optimal extent of dissection. Some nodal metastases may be missed by blind sampling or level I dissection; on the other hand, ALND may result in lymphadema. Studies in patients with melanoma have shown intraoperative lymph node mapping with sentinel lymphadenectomy to be an effective and minimally invasive technique for detecting lymph node metastases. The feasibility and accuracy of this technique in breast cancer patients was evaluated.

Methods.—The research subjects were 172 women with potentially curable breast carcinoma who were undergoing ALND as part of their therapy. All had intraoperative lymphatic mapping and sentinel lymphadenectomy immediately before modified radical mastectomy or breast-conserving surgery. Two women had synchronous bilateral primary tumors, so a total of 174 procedures were performed. The mapping procedure was performed with an injection of isosulfan blue vital dye at the primary breast cancer site. The surgeons then identified the axillary lymphatics and followed them to the first or "sentinel" node, which was selectively excised before ALND.

Results.—Nearly two thirds of the procedures led to the identification of sentinel nodes, which accurately predicted the axillary nodal status in 96% of cases. The surgeon's rate of sentinel node detection increased with experience (Fig 12–4). There was a 95.7% false negative rate, but all

Blue Nodes
Identified (%)

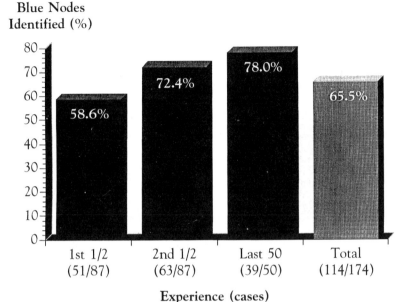

Fig 12–4.—The incidence of blue node detection according to the surgeon's experience with lymphatic mapping and sentinal lymphadenectomy. (Courtesy of Giuliano AE, Kirgan DM, Guenther JM, et al: *Ann Surg* 220:391–401, 1994.)

these cases occurred in the first part of the study (Fig 12–5). For the last 87 procedures, the sentinel nodes were 100% predictive. Dye uptake by an involved node was highly unlikely to occur by chance alone. In 38% of patients with clinically negative but pathologically positive axillary nodal status, the sentinel node was the only positive lymph node identified. In the last 54 procedures, the anatomical location of the sentinel node was assessed. Ten of these patients had metastases in only level II nodes, which might have been missed by sampling or level I axillary dissection.

Conclusion.—In some women with breast cancer, the use of intraoperative lymphatic mapping can lead to accurate identification of the sentinel axillary lymph node, which is the most likely to contain metastases. With the use of this technique, the surgeon can ensure accurate staging of node-negative patients without the morbidity that attends formal dissection. Lymphatic mapping and sentinel lymphadenectomy have the potential to enhance the accuracy of staging for breast cancer; with further experience, this technique may even alter the role of ALND.

▶ This is a novel technique that uses vital dye and then sentinel lymph node biopsy is based on the substantiated data in melanoma. The problem in breast cancer is that the lymphatic drainage is less predictable, which accounts for why sentinel nodes were identified in only 65% of the patients in this study. The second issue is that whereas sentinel lymph node biopsy may

False-Negative (%)

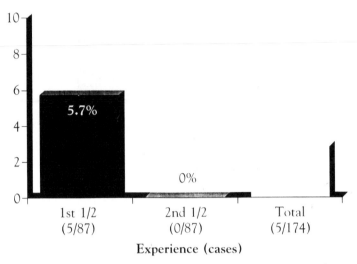

Fig 12–5.—The incidence of false negative sentinel nodes according to the surgeon's experience with lymphatic mapping and sentinel lymphadenectomy. (Courtesy of Giuliano AE, Kirgan DM, Guenther JM, et al: *Ann Surg* 220:391–401, 1994.)

be predictive of disease in the axilla, this biopsy alone cannot accurately stage the axilla. This is an issue in many medical centers, because the number of positive lymph nodes is important in selecting patients for various adjuvant protocols. However, it may well be very useful in identifying node-negative patients and thereby avoiding axillary dissection. A learning curve is obligatory with this technique.—T.J. Eberlein, M.D.

Axillary Lymph Node Dissection for T1a Breast Carcinoma: Is It Indicated?
Silverstein MJ, Gierson ED, Waisman JR, Senofsky GM, Colburn WJ, Gamagami P (The Breast Ctr, Van Nuys, Calif)
Cancer 73:664–667, 1994   140-95-12–6

Introduction.—Despite the current trend toward breast conservation and a more limited dissection of the axilla in breast cancer, there is agreement regarding the need for some form of axillary dissection in all patients with invasive disease. However, routine node dissection has recently been eliminated for intraductal carcinoma. Whether node dissection could be eliminated for T1a carcinomas as well was determined.

Patients and Methods.—From 1979 through 1992, 1,128 node dissections were performed on patients with breast cancer. The patients were classified according to T category and axillary node positivity. Disease-

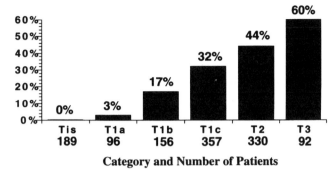

Category and Number of Patients

Fig 12–6.—Axillary node positivity by T category. There is no significant difference between Tis (DCIS) and T1a lesions. There is a significant difference between T1a lesions and all larger T categories. (Courtesy of Silverstein MJ, Gierson ED, Waisman JR, et al: *Cancer* 73:664-667, 1994.)

free survival (DFS) and breast cancer–specific survival were determined for 6 subgroups: Tis (ductal carcinoma in situ, DCIS), T1a T1b, T1c, T2, and T3. Those with T4 lesions or lobular carcinoma in situ were excluded. Treatment evolved during the study period. All patients with invasive carcinomas underwent axillary node dissection (levels 1 and 2).

Results.—Nodal positivity was 0% for DCIS and 3% for T1a lesions. There was a large increase in nodal positivity in lesions larger than 5 mm: 17% for T1b, 32% for T1c, 44% for T2, and 60% for T3 (Fig 12–6, table). Seven-year DFS ranged from 91% in the DCIS category to 48% in T3 tumors. Seven-year breast cancer–specific survival rates decreased from 99% in DCIS patients to 59% in T3 patients.

Conclusion.—Axillary dissection was long thought to be both prognostic and therapeutic. More recent studies suggest that the procedure is only prognostic and that survival is unchanged whether or not axillary node dissection is performed. It is clear that axillary node positivity in-

Nodal Positivity for Various T Categories			
Category	No. of patients	No. of positive dissections (%)	P value
Tis (DCIS)	189	0 (0)	0.015
T1a	96	3 (3)	0.0007
T1b	156	27 (17)	0.0006
T1c	357	115 (32)	0.0015
T2	330	145 (44)	0.0014
T3	92	55 (60)	

Rate of nodal positivity was statistically different as each T category was compared with the next more advanced T category.
(Courtesy of Silverstein MJ, Gierson ED, Waisman JR, et al: *Cancer* 73:664-667, 1994.)

creases as the size of the invasive component becomes larger. Both DFS and breast cancer–specific survival decrease with every increment in T value. Elimination of axillary node dissection should be considered for T1a lesions that are without numerous poor prognostic signs. The procedure continues to be indicated for T1b and larger lesions, and axillary lymph node status remains the most important single prognostic indicator.

▶ This selected retrospective study indicates that patients with DCIS or tumors of less than 5 mm may be spared axillary lymph node dissection, based on the statistical likelihood of having a positive lymph node. As emphasized by the authors, this also depends on the pathologic features. In patients who have estrogen receptor negative tumors and lymphatic vessel invasion, one may certainly want to alter this conclusion.

Similarly, in patients with DCIS the size of the primary lesion is also an indicator for axillary dissection. If a mastectomy is performed, sampling of the lymph nodes is easy and convenient. If breast conservation is performed, axillary lymph node dissection should be considered for DCIS lesions larger than 2 cm.—T.J. Eberlein, M.D.

Determinants of Receiving Breast-Conserving Surgery: The Surveillance, Epidemiology, and End Results Program, 1983–1986

Samet JM, Hunt WC, Farrow DC (Univ of New Mexico School of Medicine, Albuquerque; Univ of Washington, Seattle)

Cancer 73:2344–2351, 1994   140-95-12-7

TABLE 1.—Numbers and Treatment of Local-Stage Breast Cancers in Non-Hispanic Whites by SEER Area, 1983–1986

SEER participant	n	Any surgery (%)	Breast-conserving surgery (%)
San Francisco	3443	99.1	35.2
Connecticut	3414	97.7	30.0
Detroit	3095	99.7	27.3
Hawaii	276	98.6	31.6
Iowa	3115	99.7	14.8
New Mexico	775	97.4	23.7
Seattle	3055	99.7	36.7
Utah	1022	99.0	25.2
Atlanta	1466	99.5	18.2
All SEER areas	19661	99.1	27.8

(Courtesy of Samet JM, Hunt WC, Farrow DC: *Cancer* 73:2344–2351, 1984.)

TABLE 2.—Odds Ratio With 95% Confidence Intervals for Receipt of
Breast-Conserving Surgery for SEER Area and Other Predictors in a
Multivariate Model

Variable	Category	OR	95% CI
SEER area	San Francisco/Oakland	1.27	(1.15, 1.40)
	Connecticut	1.14	(1.04, 1.25)
	Detroit	0.98	(0.87, 1.11)
	Hawaii	1.32	(1.04, 1.69)
	Iowa	0.57	(0.50, 0.64)
	New Mexico	1.03	(0.87, 1.23)
	Seattle	1.39	(1.25, 1.54)
	Utah	1.05	(0.91, 1.21)
	Atlanta	0.62	(0.54, 0.71)
Age at diagnosis (yr)	Younger than 55	1.00	—
	55–64	0.77	(0.71, 0.84)
	65–74	0.66	(0.60, 0.72)
	75–84	0.74	(0.67, 0.82)
	85 or older	1.88	(1.63, 2.18)
Physicians per 10,000	Fewer than 16.5	1.00	—
	16.5–26.3	0.96	(0.84, 1.10)
	26.3 or more	1.01	(0.87, 1.16)
Percent of county with	Less than 16.5	1.00	—
college education	16.5–24.0	1.05	(0.92, 1.21)
	24.0 or more	1.40	(1.20, 1.63)
Percent of county	Less than 6.1	1.00	—
below poverty level	6.1–8.6	0.94	(0.84, 1.05)
	8.6 or more	0.84	(0.75, 0.94)
Cancer center in	No	1.00	—
county	Yes	1.15	(1.01, 1.30)
City of 100,000 or	No	1.00	—
more in county	Yes	1.13	(1.03, 1.25)

Abbreviations: SEER, surveillance, epidemiology, and end results; *OR*, odds ratios; *CI*, confidence
intervals.
(Courtesy of Samet JM, Hunt WC, Farrow DC: *Cancer* 73:2344-2351, 1994.)

Background.—Although breast-conserving surgery was used with increasing frequency during the 1980s, most women still have a mastectomy. A marked variation in the proportion of women undergoing breast-conserving surgery across regions of the United States has been documented. Characteristics of the county of residence as predictors of the receipt of breast-conserving surgery were examined. Whether regional variations persisted after these variables were considered was also determined.

Methods.—Data were obtained from all 19,661 non-Hispanic caucasian women with localized breast cancer who were diagnosed from 1983 through 1986 in the 9 regions covered by the Surveillance, Epidemiology and End Results (SEER) Program (Table 1). Data on county characteristics were acquired from standard sources and merged with the SEER data.

Findings.—Age was a strong predictor of type of surgery performed. After adjusting for age, county characteristics that significantly predicted the use of breast-conserving surgery were physician-to-population ratio, education and income levels, the presence of a cancer center, and residence in a city of at least 100,000 (Table 2). Marked regional variations persisted after these factors were controlled in a multiple logistic regression analysis.

Conclusion.—Patient age and county characteristics do not explain the regional variation in the treatment of localized breast cancer across the SEER regions. Further research is needed to explore the decision making of individual patients and their physicians regarding type of surgery.

▶ This manuscript utilizes data from almost 20,000 women in the surveillance, epidemiology, and End Results Program. It clearly documents that there is a striking variation in the rate of breast conservation; However, this regional variation is not explained simply by patient age or the county characteristics of the patient's domicile. It would seem logical that the patient's education concerning breast cancer and the influence of her physician may play a major role. Obviously, better education regarding the randomized prospective trials on breast conservation for both the patients and their treating physicians is necessary.—T.J. Eberlein, M.D.

Conservation Approaches for the Management of Stage I/II Carcinoma of the Breast: Milan Cancer Institute Trials
Veronesi U, Luini A, Galimberti V, Zurrida S (Istituto Nazionale per lo Studio e la Cura dei Tumori, Milan, Italy)
World J Surg 18:70–75, 1994   140-95-12–8

Background.—In 1981, the Milan Cancer Institute demonstrated good results with a conservative technique, known as the QUART method, for the management of breast cancer. This method, which consists of quadrantectomy, high-energy radiation therapy to the mammary level, complete axillary dissection, and the elimination of radiation therapy to the regional lymph nodes remains in use today, with some variations. The results of the 3 major Milan Cancer Institute trials of breast conservation therapy for patients with stage I or II breast carcinoma were reanalyzed.

Milan I Study.—In the first study, beginning in 1973, 701 patients were randomized to receive a Halsted mastectomy or QUART. On the most recent analysis, the survival curves of the 2 groups were superimposable, and patients with positive axillary lymph nodes had a trend toward better survival with QUART than with mastectomy (Fig 12–7).

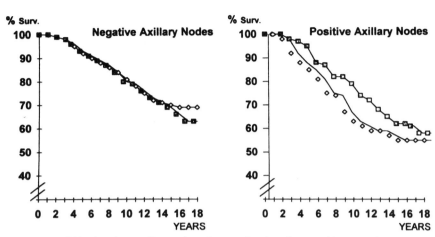

Fig 12–7.—Milan I study: overall survival in relation to lymph node status. (Courtesy of Veronesi U, Luini A, Galimberti V, et al: *World J Surg* 18:70-75, 1994.)

Local recurrences occurred in 8 patients in the mastectomy group and in 17 of the QUART group. However, most of the latter recurrences had little effect on prognosis. Radiation therapy appeared to have no onco-genic effect.

Milan II Study.—In the second study, initiated in 1985, 705 patients were randomized to receive QUART or tumorectomy, axillary dissec-tion, and radiation therapy (TART). Local relapses and new carcinomas occurred in 5.3% of the QUART group and in 13.3% of the TART group, but the 7-year survival was nearly identical. In the QUART group but not the TART group, the number of local recurrences increased pro-gressively with greater tumor size. The risk of local recurrence was in-creased with both treatments in patients with an extensive intraductal component (EIC)—9% in the QUART group vs. 28% in the TART group (Fig 12–8). In the TART group, the local recurrence rate was high, even in patients with negative resection margins.

Milan III Study.—Finally, in the third study, 567 patients were ran-domized to QUART or quadrantectomy plus axillary dissection without radiation therapy (QUAD). In the QUAD group, radiation therapy was given only for recurrences. The local recurrence rates were .3% in the QUART group vs. 8.8% in the QUAD group. The local recurrence rate was low in patients older than age 55 years, regardless of treatment. (Fig 12–9). Again, EIC predicted local recurrence. The survival of the 2 groups was similar. (Fig 12–10).

Conclusion.—An analysis of these 3 studies suggests that quadrantec-tomy plus radiation therapy is a safe treatment for stage I or II breast carcinoma. At up to 19 years of follow-up, survival was no different from

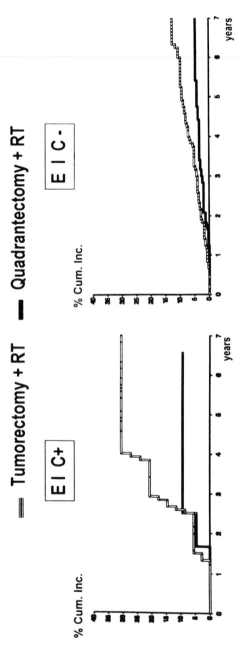

Fig 12-8.—Milan II study: incidence of local recurrence in relation to the presence of an EIC. (Courtesy of Veronesi U, Luini A, Galimberti, et al: *World J Surg* 18:70–75, 1994.)

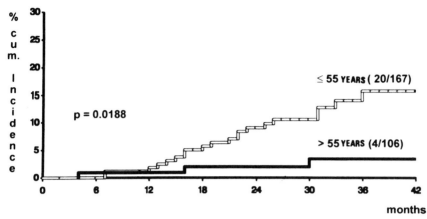

Fig 12–9.—Milan III study: incidence of local recurrence in relation to patient age. (Courtesy of Veronesi U, Luini A, Galimberti V, et al: *World J Surg* 18:70-75, 1994.)

that in women treated by Halsted mastectomy. Minimizing the extent of resection from quadrantectomy to lumpectomy carries a 3-fold increase in the risk of local recurrence, as does withholding radiation therapy, although quadrantectomy alone may be effective in postmenopausal women. A young age and the presence of EIC are the main risk factors for local recurrence.

▶ This study looks at 3 specific Milan trials. The first was a randomization between a Halsted mastectomy or breast conservation; the second was a trial in which both arms of the randomization received breast conservation and documented the increased risk of local recurrence with either treatment in patients who had an extensive intraductal component (EIC). In the third trial, patients were randomized to breast conservation with or without radiation therapy. As could be predicted, local recurrence increased with EIC, but the survival of the 2 groups was comparable.

These researchers have been among the leading pioneers in breast conservation. In these 3 trials they are trying to identify the size of the tumor excision and whether radiation therapy is necessary. Simple excision of the tumor resulted in a higher recurrence rate, but radiation therapy could be eliminated in small tumors in older women.—T.J. Eberlein, M.D.

▶↓ I have included 3 successive manuscripts that look at the risk of cancer recurrence in the breast and help define selection criteria for inclusion of patients in breast conservation.—T.J. Eberlein, M.D.

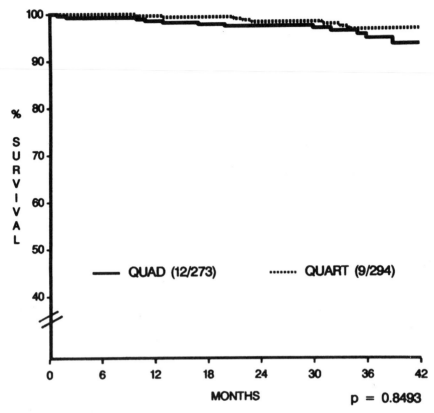

Fig 12–10.—Milan III study: overall survival of the 2 treatment arms. (Courtesy of Veronesi U, Luini A, Galimberti V, et al: *World J Surg* 18:70-75, 1994.)

Risk Factors in Breast-Conservation Therapy

Borger J, Kemperman H, Hart A, Peterse H, van Dongen J, Bartelink H (Netherlands Cancer Inst/Antoni van Leeuwenhoek Huis, Amsterdam)

J Clin Oncol 12:653–660, 1994   140-95-12-9

Background.—Reported series of breast-conservation therapy (BCT) have yielded 5-year breast recurrence rates of 1% to 13%. However, recurrence rates are much higher in certain patient subgroups that are defined by such factors as young age, extensive intraductal component, margin involvement, and vascular invasion. However, there is debate about the signficance of these factors. The clinical and pathologic factors associated with an increased risk of local recurrence after BCT were examined.

Methods.—A series of 1,026 patients with stage I or II breast cancer who were treated at a Dutch cancer center from 1979 to 1988 was ana-

TABLE 1.—Summarized Results of Proportional Hazards Analysis for Local Recurrence Counting All Breast Failures (First Analysis)

Variable	No. Assessable	Step 0	Step 1	Step 2	Step 3
Age	1,026	.036	.0049	.0058	<u>.0058</u>
Nonlinearity		.088	.043	.058	.058
Residual tumor reexcision	1,026	.0069	.032	.050	.16
Estrogen receptor	743	.051	.030	.042	.18
Nonlinearity		.32	.57	.063	.076
Histologic type	969	.046	.086	.50	.55
CIS component	885	.025	.41	.26	.29
Vascular invasion	805	.0001	.0006	.0006	<u>.0027</u>
Margin involvement	723	.0001	<u>.0001</u>	<u>.022</u>	<u>.033</u>
Clinic of surgery	1,026	.28	.025	.046	.086
Whole-breast dose	1,026	.041	.071	.23	.34
Nonlinearity		.19	.22	.17	.11

Notes: Only variables from Table 3 with a *P* value ≤ .05 in at least 1 step are listed. Underlined are variables controlled for. Including nonlinearity.
(Courtesy of Borger J, Kemperman H, Hart A, et al: *J Clin Oncol* 12:653–660, 1994.)

lyzed. Management was with BCT, consisting of local excision and axillary lymph node dissection, followed by irradiation—up to 50 Gy to the whole breast and 15–25 Gy of boost irradiation. The median follow-up was 66 months.

TABLE 2.—Actuarial 5-Year Results According to Risk Groups (Univariantly Displayed)

| | Local Recurrence Rate | | | | Disease-Specific Survival | |
| | All Recurrences | | First Failure | | | |
	%	No.	%	No.	%	No.
All	4	45/1,026	2	38/1,026	91	928/1,026
Microscopic incomplete	16	10/94	8	7/94*	78	78/94
Vascular invasion	11	16/151	8	11/151	80	119/151
Age < 40 years	8	18/187	6	14/187	85	159/187
No risk factors	1	5/409	1	5/409	93	383/409

*Nonsignificant in multivariate analysis.
(Courtesy of Borger J, Kemperman H, Hart A, et al: J Clin Oncol 12:653–660, 1994.)

Findings.—On univariate analysis the significant risk factors of local recurrence were age, residual tumor at re-excision, histologic tumor type, any carcinoma in situ component, vascular invasion, microscopic margin involvement, and whole breast radiation dose. On proportional hazard regression analysis, the independent risk factors were age, margin involvement, and vascular invasion (Table 1). A second analysis, which included only recurrences occurring before regional or distant failure, found only young age and vascular invasion to be significant predictors. In a third analysis to predict the necessity of local salvage, the same 2 predictors remained significant (Table 2). For patients without these risk factors, 5-year breast recurrence rates were only 1% compared with 6% for those younger than 40 years old and 8% for those with vascular invasion.

Conclusion.—Three independent predictors were identified for local recurrence after BCT: incomplete excision, vascular invasion, and age younger than 40 years. Marginal involvement is less important when analyzing only breast recurrences as the first site of failure. On their own, the other 2 risk factors are not strong enough to affect patient selection for BCT.

The Relationship Between Microscopic Margins of Resection and the Risk of Local Recurrence in Patients With Breast Cancer Treated With Breast-Conserving Surgery and Radiation Therapy

Schnitt SJ, Abner A, Gelman R, Connolly JL, Recht A, Duda RB, Eberlein TJ, Mayzel K, Silver B, Harris JR (Harvard Med School, Boston; Dana-Farber Cancer Inst, Boston; Faulkner Hosp, Jamaica Plain, Mass)
Cancer 74:1746–1751, 1994   140-95-12–10

Purpose.—In patients treated with conservative surgery and radiation therapy for early-stage breast cancer, microscopic involvement of the resection margins and the presence of an extensive intraductal component (EIC) are significantly related to the likelihood of local recurrence. However, these relationships have not been adequately defined. The local recurrence rate was related to microscopic margin involvement and the presence or absence of EIC in 181 patients with stage I or II infiltrating ductal carcinoma and at least 3 years of follow-up.

Results.—All patients received a radiation dose to the surgical site of 60 Gy or more and had evaluable final microscopic margins of resection. The patients were followed up for a median of 86 months. The presence of tumor at the linked margin of resection was defined as a positive margin; tumor within 1mm of the inked margin was defined as a close margin, and no tumor within this distance was defined as a negative margin. The presence of tumor at the margin in 3 or less low-power fields was defined as a focally positive margin. The presence or absence of EIC was evaluable in 157 of the patients.

Results.—A recurrence at or near the primary site—that is, true recurrence/marginal miss (TR/MM)—developed within 5 years in 7% of patients. The 5-year TR/MM rate was 0% in patients with negative margins, 4% in those with close margins, 6% in those with focally positive

TABLE 1.—Sites of First Recurrence in Relation to Microscopic Margin Involvement (Crude 5-Year Rates)

Margin status	No. of patients	NED	D < 5 yr	Site of first recurrence			
				Breast, TR/MM (%)	Breast, other*	Regional nodes	Distant metastases
Negative	70	52 (74)	5 (7)	0 (0)	2 (3)	1 (1)	10 (14)
Close	25	19 (76)	3 (12)	1 (4)	0 (0)	0 (0)	2 (8)
Positive	86	45 (52)	3 (3)	11 (13)	2 (2)	1 (1)	24 (28)
Focally positive	48	29 (60)	2 (4)	3 (6)	2 (4)	0 (0)	12 (25)
> Focally positive	38	16 (42)	1 (3)	8 (21)	0 (0)	1 (3)	12 (32)

Values are No. (%).
Abbreviations: NED, no evidence of disease; D < 5 yr, dead with less than 5 years of follow-up.
*Recurrence elsewhere in breast, in skin of breast, or unclassifiable breast recurrence.
(Courtesy of Schnitt SJ, Abner A, Gelman R, et al: *Cancer* 74:1746–1751, 1994.)

TABLE 2.—Final Model Assessing Factors Associated With TR/MM or Other Recurrences Vs. Having NED

	TR/MM versus NED		Other recurrences versus NED	
	RR	P	*RR*	P
> Focally positive margins	14.9	0.0001	2.7	0.03
T stage (I versus II)	3.7	0.11	6.1	0.003
1–3 positive nodes	0.3	0.16	0.3	0.01
Node status unknown	1.0	0.94	1.5	0.39
Size > 3 cm	0.2	0.06	0.5	0.14

Abbreviations: NED, no evidence of disease; RR, relative risk.
(Courtesy of Schnitt SJ, Abner A, Gelman R, et al: *Cancer* 74:1746–1751, 1994.)

margins, and 21% in those with more than focally positive margins (Table 1). Respective 5-year rates of distant failure were 14%, 8%, 25%, and 32%. Axillary lymph nodes were positive in 59% of patients with positive margins vs. 38% of those with negative or close margins. The 5-year TR/MM rate was 20% for patients with an EIC vs. 7% for those without. For the 127 patients without an EIC, the 5-year TR/MM rate was less than 10%, regardless of margin status. Among the 30 patients with an EIC, the 5-year TR/MM rate was 0% for those with negative or close margins vs. 50% for those whose margins were more than focally positive. The presence of more than focally positive margins was the most significant predictor of TR/MM recurrence (Table 2).

Conclusions.—Breast-conserving surgery and radiation therapy appear to be an appropriate treatment for early-stage breast cancer patients with uninvolved margins. This is true regardless of the presence or absence of EIC. Breast-conserving therapy and radiation therapy, including a radiation boost to the primary site, may also be a reasonable treatment choice for selected patients with an EIC-negative tumor and only focal marginal involvement. Longer follow-up in more patients is needed to confirm these relationships.

Ipsilateral Breast Tumor Recurrence Postlumpectomy Is Predictive of Subsequent Mortality: Results From a Randomized Trial
Whelan T, Clark R, Roberts R, Levine M, Foster G, and Investigators of the Ontario Clinical Oncology Group (McMaster Univ, Ont, Canada; Hamilton Civic Hosps Research Ctr, Ont, Canada; Ontario Cancer Inst/Princess Margaret Hosp, Toronto)
Int J Radiat Oncol Biol Phys 30:11–16, 1994   140-95-12–11

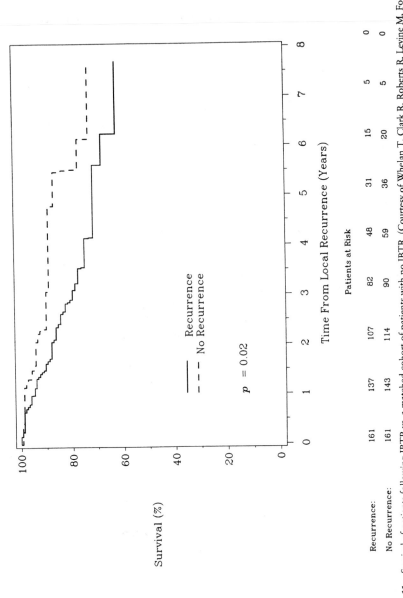

Fig 12–11.—Survival of patients following IBTR vs. a matched cohort of patients with no IBTR. (Courtesy of Whelan T, Clark R, Roberts R, Levine M, Foster G, and Investigators of the Ontario Clinical Oncology Group: *Int J Radiat Oncol Biol Phys* 30:11–16, 1994.)

Background.—Isolated local-regional recurrence after mastectomy usually carries a poor prognosis. As the use of breast conservation treatment increases so does the significance of local breast recurrence. The relationship between ipsilateral breast tumor recurrence (IBTR) after lumpectomy and the subsequent outcome in a cohort with node-negative breast cancer was investigated.

Methods.—Eight hundred thirty-seven women with node-negative disease were studied in a randomized trial conducted between 1984 and 1989 in Ontario. All the study participants had undergone a lumpectomy and axillary dissection and were randomly assigned to postoperative radiation or no further treatment. Radiation was delivered in a dosage of 40 Gy in 16 fractions to the whole breast, followed by a boost of 12.5 Gy in 5 fractions to the primary site. Patients were followed up for a median of 66 months.

Findings.—Complete data were available for 799 patients. At 5 years, the cumulative rate of IBTR was significantly greater for the patients who received no further treatment than for those who received radiation. The respective rates were 30% and 8%. Overall survival in the 2 groups did not differ. Factors significantly and independently predictive of mortality were nuclear grade and tumor size. A high tumor grade carried a relative risk of 2.28, and a tumor size of 2 cm or more, 1.64. Increased mortality was also predicted by IBTR (Fig 12–11). The results for distant relapse were comparable. An IBTR within 1 year of operation correlated with a greater risk of distant relapse and mortality.

Conclusion.—Ipsilateral breast tumor recurrence independently predicts distant failure and mortality. Therefore, the association of local breast recurrence and distant relapse for node-negative breast cancer appears to be real rather than merely a result of measurement bias.

▶ In Abstract 140-95-12–9 higher recurrence rates in young patients were documented. This could be the result of there being more patients with breast-conserving treatment in the younger age group. Through their analysis, these authors concluded that tumor vascular invasion predicted recurrence, although in a hazard regression analysis, margin involvement was also important.

This issue regarding margin involvement is better addressed in Abstract 140-95-12–10 in which groups were analyzed on the basis of negative margins, close margins, focally positive margins, or more than focally positive margins. All groups had satisfactory recurrence rates, except for the group that had more than focally positive margins; this group also had a higher rate of distant failure. However, even in EIC-positive patients whose margins were negative or close, recurrence rates were acceptable. As a result, breast conservation and radiation therapy seemed to be a reasonable treatment choice if the margins were uninvolved, even if the tumor was EIC-positive. However, more than focally positive margins should either undergo another excision or be considered for mastectomy.

In Abstract 140-95-12–11, which reports on a randomized treatment of women undergoing breast conservation with or without radiation therapy, overall survival between the 2 treatment groups was no different. However, IBTR predicted increased mortality, especially if it occurred within 1 year of surgery. This is somewhat contrary to the NSABP B06 trial, which showed a higher rate of recurrence in women who were not treated with radiation, but it did not change overall survival. In this study, IBTR may be a marker for more aggressive disease, the cause of a poor outcome, or a combination of both. Further analysis of ongoing trials will help to resolve this dilemma.—T.J. Eberlein, M.D.

▶↓ I have grouped the next 4 articles together because they examine specific pathologic features in an attempt to develop prognostic markers in the treatment of breast cancer.—T.J. Eberlein, M.D.

Tumor Microvessel Density, p53 Expression, Tumor Size, and Peritumoral Lymphatic Vessel Invasion Are Relevant Prognostic Markers in Node-Negative Breast Carcinoma

Gasparini G, Weidner N, Bevilacqua P, Maluta S, Palma PD, Caffo O, Barbareschi M, Boracchi P, Marubini E, Pozza F (St Bortolo Regional Med Ctr, Vicenza, Italy; St Chiara Regional Med Ctr, Trento, Italy; Univ of Milan, Italy; et al)
J Clin Oncol 12:454–466, 1994   140-95-12–12

Objective.—The value of both conventional and alternative prognostic factors was examined in a series of 254 consecutive patients with node-negative breast carcinoma (NNBC), who were followed up for a median period of 62 months.

Methods.—In addition to the usual prognostic features, intratumoral microvessel density (MVD) was determined by immunostaining with anti-CD31 antibody. Peritumoral lymph vessel invasion (PLVI) was related to relapse-free survival (RFS) and overall survival (OS). The expression of p53 and c-*erb*B-2 proteins was determined immunocytochemically.

Observations.—Overall RFS after approximately 5 years of follow-up was 82%, and for OS it was 89%. Twenty of the 30 deaths were caused by breast cancer. The MVD significantly predicted both RFS and OS on univariate analysis, and it was the strongest independent predictor of RFS on multivariate analysis. Patients whose tumors were highly vascularized were nearly 6 times more likely to relapse than those with less vascular tumors. The PLVI was the next most prominent prognostic factor, followed by the overexpression of p53 and then tumor size. For OS, tumor size was the most significant independent variable. Bivariate analysis indicated that MVD was a factor in relapse in both p53-positive and negative tumors. The MVD was the most significant prognostic factor for all types of metastasis. Tumor size predicted visceral metastasis, and both PLVI and the expression of p53 protein predicted bone recurrence.

Conclusion.—In addition to the usual prognostic features, MVD, PLVI, and the expression of p53 are helpful in selecting high-risk patients with NNBC who may be eligible for adjuvant treatment. Quantifying MVD may be useful not only as a prognostic factor but for predicting the response to drugs that inhibit angiogenesis.

---

p53 Gene Mutations and Steroid Receptor Status in Breast Cancer: Clinicopathologic Correlations and Prognostic Assessment
Caleffi M, Teague MW, Jensen RA, Vnencak-Jones CL, Dupont WD, Parl FF (Vanderbilt Univ, Nashville, Tenn)
Cancer 73:2147–2156, 1994   140-95-12–13

Introduction.—A number of different genetic changes that occur in sporadic breast cancer may be involved in the pathogenesis of malignant transformations and progression. The tumor suppressor gene p53 is the most commonly mutated gene that is identified in human cancers. The frequency of p53 gene mutations in primary breast cancer was assessed, including their correlation with steroid receptor status and other established clinicopathologic parameters.

Methods.—The study material consisted of genomic DNA samples from 192 primary breast cancers. Exons 5–9 were analyzed by denaturant gradient gel electrophoresis in all tumors to identify mutations. A biochemical steroid hormone binding assay and an estrogen receptor (ER) immunohistochemical assay were performed as well. In 20 of the

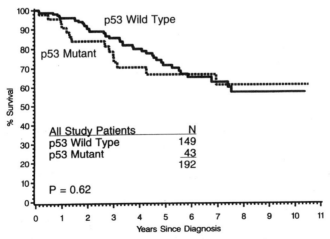

Fig 12–12.—p53 status and survival time for all patients. (Courtesy of Caleffi M, Teague MW, Jensen RA, et al: *Cancer* 73:2147–2156, 1994.)

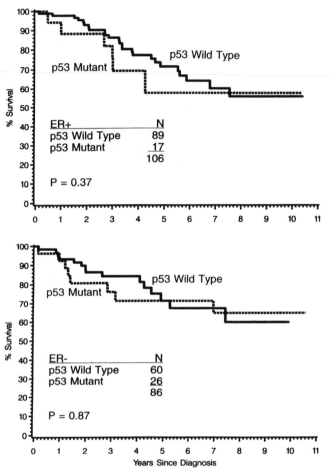

Fig 12–13.—A, p53 status and survival time for patients with ER-positive cancers. **B,** p53 status and survival time for patients with ER-negative cancers. (Courtesy of Caleffi M, Teague MW, Jensen RA, et al: *Cancer* 73:2147–2156, 1994.)

tumors, the precise nature of the p53 mutations was assessed by DNA sequencing.

Results.—Twenty-two percent of the tumors showed p53 gene alterations, most of which were localized in exons 5 and 6. Most of these alterations were found on DNA sequencing to be missense mutations resulting from G or C substitutions. Younger women, black women, and tumors lacking an ER and/or progesterone receptor were more likely to have p53 mutations. The presence of p53 mutations was unrelated to family history, tumor size, histologic grade or type, nodal status, or disease stage. Survival was no different for patients with mutant vs. wild-type p53 tumors (Fig 12–12); this was also true when the comparison was limited to node-negative patients or to those with ER-positive or ER-negative tumors (Fig 12–13). There were also no survival differences between patients with mutations in exons 5 and 6 vs. those with mutations in exons 7–9.

Conclusion.—As in previous studies, a consistent relationship was found between ER-positive breast cancers and wild-type p53 and between ER-negative tumors and p53 mutations. However, p53 does not appear to play any significant prognostic role in predicting survival. Mutations of p53 appear to be more common in younger women and in black women.

Overexpression of p53 and HER-2/neu Proteins as Prognostic Markers in Early Stage Breast Cancer
Marks JR, Humphrey PA, Wu K, Berry D, Bandarenko N, Kerns B-JM, Iglehart JD (Duke Univ, Durham NC; Washington Univ, St Louis, Mo)
Ann Surg 219:332–341, 1994   140-95-12–14

Background.—The most common genetic abnormalities associated with breast cancer are p53 and HER-2/*neu* oncogene overexpression. Patients with tumors containing p53 or HER-2/*neu* have shorter survival times. A cohort of patients with early stage breast cancers were analyzed retrospectively for both oncogenes to relate overexpression to clinico-pathologic parameters and survival.

Methods and Findings.—Immunostaining for p53 and HER-2/*neu* was performed on 230 paraffin-embedded specimens of stage I and II breast cancers. Twenty-four percent of the cohort was positive for p53, 17% for HER-2/*neu*, and 4% for both. Immunostaining of p53 correlated significantly with increasing tumor size, stage, and low estrogen and progesterone receptor contents. In a univariate analysis, p53 and HER-2/*neu* were found to indicate overall and failure-free survival. Patients with both oncogene abnormalities had an additive effect on survival. In a multivariate analysis, nodal status, HER-2/*neu*, and p53 all had independent prognostic values (Fig 12–14, table).

Conclusion.—Although proven, the prognostic value of the p53 and HER-2/*neu* oncogenes is limited. An approach that combines several molecular genetic markers with established pathologic criteria may help clinicians more accurately predict prognosis in patients with early stage breast cancer.

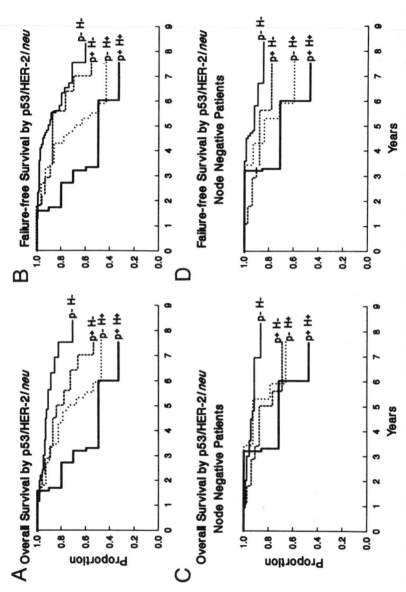

Fig 12–14.—Kaplan-Meier survival curves separated by staining for both p53 and HER-2/*neu*. **A,** overall survival and **B,** failure-free survival for all stage I and II patients (n = 230). **C,** overall and **D,** failure-free survival for node-negative patients (n = 147). Each curve represents a nonoverlapping subset of patients. (Courtesy of Marks JR, Humphrey PA, Wu K, et al: *Ann Surg* 219:332–341, 1994.)

Independent Prognostic Variables by Multivariate Analysis

Prognostic Variable	Relative Risk	P Value
Overall Survival		
HER-2/neu	3.4	0.0001
Nodal status	2.6	0.002
p53	2.4	0.005
Failure-free Survival		
Nodal status	3.7	0.0001
HER-2/neu	3.2	0.0001
p53	1.8	0.04

(Courtesy of Marks JR, Humphrey PA, Wu K, et al: *Ann Surg* 219:332–341, 1994.)

Frequent *p*53 Gene Mutations and Novel Alleles in Familial Breast Cancer

Glebov OK, McKenzie KE, White CA, Sukumar S (Salk Inst for Biological Studies, La Jolla, Calif; Scripps Mem Hosp Oncology Research Program, Encinitas, Calif)
Cancer Res 54:3703–3709, 1994   140-95-12–15

Introduction.—Evidence suggests that the p53 protein is a transcriptional regulator that delays growth, allowing damaged DNA to be repaired before replication. The frequency of p53 gene mutation varies in breast tumors. It was hypothesized that patients with a family history of breast cancer (FHBC) would evidence a greater frequency of p53 gene mutations and greater genomic instability than patients with sporadic breast cancer (SBC).

Methods.—A DNA sample was extracted from surgical breast tumor specimens, adjacent normal breast tissue, and the peripheral blood of 75 SBC patients and 29 FHBC patients. Sequence and allele analysis followed polymerase chain reaction (PCR) and cloning. Allelic loci were analyzed by comparing tumor cell DNA with normal cell DNA in the same patient.

Results.—There was a highly significant difference in the frequency of p53 mutation between the 2 groups of patients. Eleven of the 75 SBC tumors and 17 of the 29 FHBC tumors contained DNA with a mutation in the p53 exons 5–9. Most of the FHBC mutations were on exon 5, and 7 of the 16 with this mutation had a G to C transversion at codon 156. More FHBC patients than SBC patients had alleles of altered length in breast tumor DNA, and the patterns of allelic loss in chromosome 17 were different. Allele losses occurred more frequently in the q arm and more often involved multiple loci in FHBC patients, whereas allele losses occurred more frequently in the p arm and more frequently involved a single locus in SBC patients. In FHBC patients p53 mutations were closely associated with loss of TP53 alleles, whereas these were independent occurrences in SBC patients.

Discussion.—The DNA in breast tumors found in FHBC patients differs from that found in SBC patients in the frequency of p53 mutations, the mutation sequence, the frequency of altered-length alleles, and the loci of allelic losses on chromosome 17. These findings support the hypothesis that patients with a family history of breast cancer have a higher incidence of p53 gene mutations, and the multiple-loci allele losses indicated increased genomic instability. However, it is unclear whether the genomic instability was caused directly by the p53 mutations or by defects in a repair gene that result in p53 mutations.

▶ The first article (Abstract 140-95-12–12) showed that PLVI and intratumoral MVD are associated with a much higher relapse rate than less vascular tumors. Tumor size was also an important prognostic factor, especially for overall survival. This verifies work initially begun by Weidner and Folkman, which documented a poor prognosis in patients with increased vascularity.

In Abstract 140-95-12–13, an association between wild-type p53 and better prognosis tumors (ER-positive). Mutations of p53 are more frequently associated with ER-negative tumors, but in this study p53 did not predict for overall survival.

In Abstract 140-95-12–14, p53 was combined with the HER2/*neu* protein. Once again, p53 was associated with ER-negative tumors and tumors of a larger size as well as a more advanced stage. However, when p53 was combined with HER2/*neu* expression, the prognosis was improved for predicting overall and failure-free survival. Another major advantage was that with better immunostaining techniques we are able to obtain the kind of specific genetic information on very small tumor samples needed to improve our ability to predict survival and select patients who can be treated with minimally invasive biopsy procedures.

The final article (Abstract 140-95-12–15) documents that patients with a FHBC have more frequent p53 mutations. Once again these genetic markers are not predictive in every patient with breast cancer, but by combining family history and/or multiple genetic markers, prediction of survival can be enhanced using p53, HER2/*neu* expression and MVD in and around primary tumors.—T.J. Eberlein, M.D.

Colorectal Cancer

▶↓ The next 6 articles address genetic and biological markers in colorectal cancers. These are not necessarily definitive studies, nor will these markers be used definitively in the diagnosis or treatment of colorectal cancer; instead, these articles were selected to acquaint the reader with some of the cutting-edge studies that will assist us in the earlier diagnosis and novel treatment of colorectal cancer.—T.J. Eberlein, M.D.

High Frequency of Allelic Deletion on Chromosome 17p in Advanced Colorectal Cancer

Khine K, Smith DR, Goh H-S (Singapore Gen Hosp; Howard Hughes Med Inst, Ann Arbor, Mich; Imperial Cancer Research Fund Laboratories, London; et al)

Cancer 73:28–35, 1994   140-95-12–16

Objective.—Theoretically, both 5q and 17p alleles must be deleted or mutated to inactivate a tumor suppressor gene. Most studies of allelic deletions have been done in Western populations. The connection between chromosome 5q and 17p deletions and the development of colorectal cancer in a predominantly Chinese population was studied in Singapore, where the incidence of colorectal cancer is rapidly increasing.

TABLE 1.—Relation of Chromosome 5q and 17p Deletion to Dukes Stage

Location	Dukes' stage	No. of cases examined	No. of informative cases	Deletion/ informative cases (%)	P value*
5q	A	25	18	7/18 (39)	NS
	B	25	21	4/21 (19)	
	C	30	25	8/25 (32)	
	D	22	15	7/15 (47)	
17p	A	25	25	17/25 (68)	0.006
	B	25	24	14/24 (58)	
	C	29	29	18/29 (62)	
	D	21	18	17/18 (94)	

* Fisher exact test; not significant if $P > .05$.
Abbreviation: NS, not significant.
(Courtesy of: Khine K, Smith DR, Goh H-S: *Cancer* 73:28–35, 1994.)

TABLE 2.—Relation of Chromosome 5q and 17p Deletion to Metastasis

Location	Metastasis	No. of cases examined	No. of informative cases	Deletion/ informative cases (%)	P value*
5q	Distant metastasis				
	Positive	16	8	2/8 (25)	NS
	Negative	86	71	24/71 (34)	
	Lymph node metastasis				
	Positive	43	33	13/33 (39)	NS
	Negative	59	46	13/46 (28)	
17p	Distant metastasis				
	Positive	15	14	13/14 (93)	0.028
	Negative	85	82	53/82 (65)	
	Lymph node metastasis				
	Positive	41	39	29/39 (74)	NS
	Negative	59	57	37/57 (65)	

* Fisher exact test; not significant if P > .05.
Abbreviation: NS, not significant.
(Courtesy of: Khine K, Smith DR, Goh H-S: *Cancer* 73:28–35, 1994.)

Methods.—Chromosomal deletions in tumors from 102 patients with colorectal cancer (age ranges, 23–84 years) were examined using the restriction fragment length polymorphism method. Genomic DNA was analyzed for allelic loss using a CS-9000 scanner. A 50% reduction in signal intensity was considered to indicate a deletion.

Results.—There were 22 proximal and 80 distal tumors. There were 25 Dukes' A, 25 Dukes' B, 30 Dukes' C, and 22 Dukes' D tumors. Sixteen patients had distant metastasis, and 43 had lymph node involvement. The chromosome 5q allele was seen in 33% of informative cases and was deleted in 26 patients; chromosome 17p was found in 69% of informative cases and was deleted in 66 patients; in 19 patients, both alleles were lost. There was a significantly higher incidence of 17p deletion in patients with Dukes' D tumors and distant metastasis. (Table 1). No association was found between Dukes' stage and 5q deletion. There was a significant association and perhaps a causal relation, between 17p deletion and liver metastasis. This association with distant metastasis but not with lymph node metastasis suggests that bloodborne spread arises from a different genetic origin than lymphatic spread and therefore should be investigated further. Although mutation of the p53 gene is related to transformation of adenoma to adenocarcinoma in colorectal cancer, it does not appear to be involved in metastasis (Table 2).

Conclusion.—The loss of chromosome 17p allele may be useful as a prognostic indicator of distant metastasis.

▶ The first of the 6 articles is Abstract 140-95-12–16. The ongoing genetic model suggests that *ras* gene mutations as well as allelic deletion of chromosome 5q are early changes in the development of colorectal tumors. On the other hand, chromosome 17p and 18q deletions are late changes in colorectal tumorigenesis. The 17p and 18q deletions are associated with an increased tendency toward metastasis.

This study involves a predominantly Chinese population from Singapore. In essence, these authors found that in their own population p53 is not involved in the metastatic process but rather that deletion of 17p is associated with distant metastasis and not lymph node metastasis. Of course, this is very interesting and suggests a hematologic spread rather than a spread through the lymphatics. The 5q deletion has no such tendency toward metastasis, which confirms its position in the genetic model.—T.J. Eberlein, M.D.

Multifactorial Analysis of Local Recurrences in Rectal Cancer, Including DNA Ploidy Studies: A Predictive Model

Moran MR, Rothenberger DA, Gallo RA, Goldberg SM, James EC (Univ of North Dakota, Grand Forks; Univ of Minnesota, Minneapolis)

World J Surg 17:801–805, 1993   140-95-12–17

TABLE 1.—Local Recurrences vs. > 3 Positive Nodes[*]

| >3 positive nodes | Local recurrences | |
	No[*]	Yes
No[†]	97	11 (11.2%)
Yes	14	11 (44.0%)
Total	111	22 (16.5%)

[*]$P = .0001$.
[†]"No" also includes patients with positive nodes.
(Courtesy of Moran MR, Rothenberger DA, Gallo RA, et al: *World J Surg* 17:801–805, 1993.)

Objective.—Although 16% to 18% of patients who have undergone colorectal cancer resections will have a recurrence, there is no accurate method for predicting local recurrences. A better predictive model would enable physicians to select appropriate treatments and tests. The predictive capabilities of DNA ploidy patterns and of Dukes' staging in the same patients were compared.

Methods.—A total of 138 patients aged 23–90 years who had abdominal resections for rectal cancer and had been followed-up for at least 3.5 years or until death were categorized according to the type of first recurrence—local, distant, or none. There were 29 stage A, 56 stage B, and 53 stage C patients; 64 patients died. Cellular DNA content was measured, DNA variables were analyzed, and 37 other variables were also examined.

Results.—The significant risk factors identified were 3 positive lymph nodes, macroscopic local invasion of the tumor, and DNA ploidy (Tables 1–3). Using these factors, discriminant values (DV) for each type of patient were calculated. Patients with DVs less than $-.6$; are predicted not to have a local recurrence. In the 3 subgroups of patients, there were 56 very low-risk patients with DVs less than -1.9; there were only 2 recurrences in this group. There were 55 moderate risk patients with DVs between -1.9 and $-.6$; there were 9 recurrences in this group. There were 27 high-risk patients with DVs greater than $-.6$; there were 14 patients in this group.

TABLE 2.—Local Recurrences vs. Transmural Invasion[a]

| Local invasion | Local recurrences | |
	No	Yes
No	105	8 (6.5%)
Yes	17	7 (29.2%)
Total	122	15 (10.9%)

[a]$P = .0016$.
(Courtesy of Moran MR, Rothenberger DA, Gallo RA, et al: *World J Surg* 17:801–805, 1993.)

TABLE 3.—Local Recurrences vs. DNA*

Local recurrences

DNA diploid	No	Yes
No	65	9 (12.2%)
Yes	48	16 (25.0%)
Total	113	25 (18.1%)

*$P = .05$.
(Courtesy of Moran MR, Rothenberger DA, Gallo RA, et al: *World J Surg* 17:801–805, 1993.)

Conclusion.—Use of DNA ploidy to predict local recurrence produced significantly better results than Dukes' staging. Assigning patients to risk groups would seem to be a better way to evaluate therapeutic treatment methods.

▶ This article was included because it represents large series of patients. It relied on DNA ploidy to predict the local recurrence of rectal cancers. A very intriguing model was set up by analyzing various risk factors for recurrence, such as positive nodes, microscopic local invasion of the tumor, and DNA ploidy. The authors then showed a direct correlation between the risk factors and local recurrence.

Although other articles have documented DNA analysis in rectal cancer, this is the first time that it has been used in a predictive model for local recurrence. Obviously, this might be extremely beneficial in selecting patients for preoperative chemotherapy or radiation therapy, and it can be done on a relatively small tumor biopsy sample.—T.J. Eberlein, M.D.

Prognostic Factors of Colorectal Cancer: K-ras Mutation, Overexpression of the p53 Protein, and Cell Proliferative Activity

Tanaka M, Omura K, Watanabe Y, Oda Y, Nakanishi I (Kanazawa Univ, Japan)
J Surg Oncol 57:57–64, 1994   140-95-12–18

Objective.—As colon carcinogenesis develops, tumor characteristics evolve that are prognostic of the course of the disease. The value of 2 molecular assays in predicting and evaluating the progress of the disease was compared.

Methods.—Eighteen adenomas, 5 intramucosal carcinomas, and 39 invasive carcinomas, 1 from each of 62 patients, were examined histopathologically. Point mutations in K-*ras* 12, 13, and 61 codons were identified. Nuclear localizations of p53 protein and peripheral cell nuclear antigen (PCNA) were determined.

TABLE 1.—Colorectal Cancer: Multivariate P-Values for the
Relationship of Various Clinicopathologic Markers and
K-ras Mutation*†

Variable	Coefficient	Odds ratio	P-value
Age	1.408	1.25	NS
Sex	0.753	1.04	NS
Tumor differentiation	0.143	0.20	NS
Depth of invasion	1.704	1.53	NS
Infiltrative growth at periphery of the tumor	−0.076	0.08	NS
Lymphatic invasion	0.641	0.91	NS
Vascular invasion	2.491	2.63	<0.01
Lymph node metastasis	0.251	0.31	NS
Stage	0.711	0.98	NS
Hematogenous recurrence	2.841	2.38	0.02
Hematogenous metastasis	2.491	2.63	<0.01
Overexpression of the p53 protein	−1.098	1.99	NS
PCNA activity	1.358	1.67	NS

* *Abbreviation:* NS, not significant.
† Stage grouping according to TNM classification for cancer of the colon and rectum; infiltrative growth at periphery of the tumor, classification according to Japanese Research Society for gastric cancer, expanding, intermediate, or infiltrating.
(Courtesy of Tanaka M, Omura K, Watanabe Y, et al: *J Surg Oncol* 57:57–64, 1994.)

Results.—Ten tumors had mutations at codon 12 and 5 at codon 13; none had mutations at codon 61 of the K-*ras* gene. The frequency of mutation increased as the malignancy progressed from an adenoma to a carcinoma. Overexpression of p53 protein was found in 2 of 13 adenomas. The frequency of overexpression in carcinomas was 64%, and the reactivity was higher than with either adenomas or normal mucosa. The PCNA immunoreactivity levels were higher in carcinomas than in adenomas, although the difference was not significant. K-*ras* mutation correlated significantly with vascular invasion, distant recurrence, and distant metastasis. There was no correlation between K-*ras* mutation and either overexpression of p53 or PCNA activity. The PCNA labeling index correlated significantly with clinicopathologic variables of adenocarcinomas (Tables 1 and 2).

Conclusion.—The extent of lymph node metastasis, tumor node metastasis stage, lymphatic invasion, and K-*ras* mutation are significant predictors of survival.

▶ This article is a relatively small study of only 39 invasive carcinomas, but it confirmed that the K-*ras* mutation was significantly associated with vascular invasion and distant metastasis. The correlation with previous findings that

TABLE 2.—Prognostic Factors of Survival Time Using the Cox
Proportional Hazard Model

Prognostic factors	Coefficient	Relative risk	P-value
Lymph node metastatis	1.951	7.27	<0.01
Stage	2.192	5.37	0.02
Lymphatic invasion	1.480	4.48	0.04
K-ras mutation	2.219	3.69	0.05
Depth of invasion	1.959	3.57	0.07
Tumor differentiation	0.915	3.15	0.08
Hematogenous metastasis	1.731	3.00	0.09
Peritoneal seeding	1.554	1.80	0.19
Size of tumor	0.201	1.61	0.21
p53 protein overexpression	−1.462	1.60	0.21
Age	0.017	0.13	0.72
Infiltrative growth at periphery	0.186	0.06	0.80
Sex	0.047	0.00	0.96
PCNA	0.029	0.00	0.98

Abbreviation: PCNA, peripheral cell nuclear antigen.
(Courtesy of Tanaka M, Omura K, Watanabe Y, et al: *J Surg Oncol* 57:57–64, 1994.)

there is no relationship between p53 and survival grade of differentiation for Dukes' stage in colorectal cancer was also significant.—T.J. Eberlein, M.D.

Allelic Loss of Chromosome 18q and Prognosis in Colorectal Cancer

Jen J, Kim H, Piantadosi S, Liu Z-F, Levitt RC, Sistonen P, Kinzler KW, Vogelstein B, Hamilton SR (Johns Hopkins Univ, Baltimore, Md; Finnish Red Cross Blood Transfusion Service, Helsinki)
N Engl J Med 331:213–221, 1994   140-95-12–19

Background.—Determining the prognosis and selecting patients with colorectal cancer for postoperative adjuvant treatment currently depend on pathologic and clinical staging. Chromosome 18q loss is a genetic event that has been associated with tumor progression. The value of 18q allelic loss as a prognostic marker for colorectal cancer was studied.

Methods.—One hundred forty-five consecutively resected stage II or III colorectal carcinomas, which were formalin fixed and paraffin embedded, were studied. The status of chromosome 18q was examined using microsatellite markers and DNA from the tumors.

Findings.—Patients with stage II cancer and no evidence of allelic loss of chromosome 18q had a 5-year survival rate of 93% compared with 54% of patients with stage II disease and allelic loss. Among patients with stage III disease, the respective survival rate was 38% and 52% in those with and without allelic loss. In a univariate analysis, patients with

Estimated Hazard Ratios for Selected Individual Prognostic
Factors in All 145 Patients Studied

FACTOR	CATEGORY	HAZARD RATIO	95% CONFIDENCE INTERVAL	P VALUE*
Chromosome 18q	Loss vs. no loss	2.83	1.32–6.08	0.008
TNM stage	III vs. II	2.33	1.27–4.28	0.006
Vein invasion	Yes vs. no	3.29	1.83–5.91	<0.001
Perineural invasion	Yes vs. no	3.08	1.73–5.48	<0.001
Tumor differentiation	Moderate vs. well	2.43	0.57–10.3	0.24
	Poor vs. well	4.28	0.94–19.4	0.06
Race	White vs. other†	0.61	0.34–1.10	0.10
Sex	Male vs. female	1.30	0.74–2.29	0.36
Tumor side‡	Left vs. right	1.63	0.87–3.05	0.13
Tumor site	Colon vs. rectum	0.83	0.41–1.66	0.59
Adjuvant therapy	Yes vs. no	0.74	0.40–1.38	0.34

* P values result from a test of the hypothesis that the hazard ratio equals 1.0.
† The "other" category contained 40 black patients, 1 Asian patient, and 1 Hispanic patient.
‡ The tumor side was based on the position of the tumor relative to the splenic flexure.
(Courtesy of Jen J, Kim H, Piantadosi S, et al: N Engl J Med 331:213–221, 1994.)

chromosome 18q allelic loss had a 2.83 overall estimated hazard ratio for death (table). Chromosome 18q allelic loss remained a strong predictor after adjustments for tumor differentiation, vein invasion, and tumor node metastasis (Fig 12–15).

Conclusion.—In patients with stage II colorectal cancer, the status of chromosome 18q has strong prognostic value. Patients with stage II disease and allelic loss have a prognosis similar to that of patients with stage III cancer, who may benefit from adjuvant treatment. Patients with stage II disease and no chromosome 18q allelic loss have a survival rate comparable to that of patients with stage I disease and may not require additional treatment.

▶ Deletion of chromosome 18q has been noted as being a genetic event associated with progression of tumor in colorectal cancer. In this article, the author shows that by including chromosome 18q, deletion is a prognostic factor and that a stage II patient has the prognosis of the stage III patient. This would have obvious implications in the selection of patients for appropriate adjuvant therapy; however, a small note of caution is warranted: The prognosis of patients with stage III disease was unchanged by knowledge of the status of chromosome 18q. Therefore, in the future 18q would have to be combined with other genetic and biochemical assays to improve the prognosis of all patients with colorectal cancers.—T.J. Eberlein, M.D.

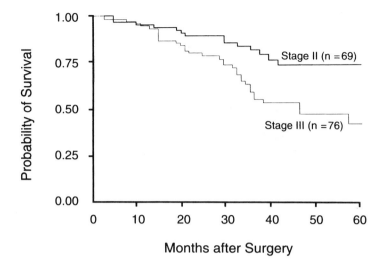

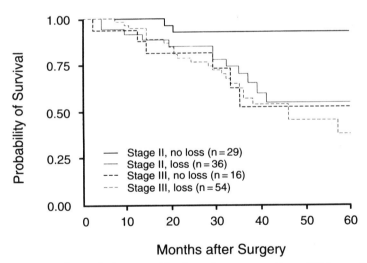

Fig 12–15.—Overall survival of patients with colorectal cancer, according to TNM stage alone (**A**) and both TNM stage and chromosome 18q allelic loss (**B**). The survival rate of patients with stage II disease was significantly better than that of patients with stage III disease ($P = 0.006$). However, when the patients were subclassified according to their status for chromosome 18q, the survival rate of patients with stage II disease whose tumor had chromosome 18q allelic loss was similar to that of patients with stage III disease, whereas patients with stage II disease whose tumor retained both alleles of chromosome 18q had a significantly better outcome. (Courtesy of Jen J, Kim H, Piantadosi S, et al: *N Engl J Med* 331:213–221, 1994.)

c-*myc* mRNA Overexpression Is Associated With Lymph Node Metastasis in Colorectal Cancer

Sato K, Miyahara M, Saito T, Kobayashi M (Oita Med Univ, Japan)
Eur J Cancer 30A:1113–1117, 1994   140-95-12–20

Introduction.—Recent studies have suggested that evidence of oncogene overexpression in patients with colorectal cancer may be a useful prognostic indicator. However, others have found no correlation between oncogene expression and the malignant potential of colorectal cancer. The relationship between these oncogene overexpressions and the clinicopathologic features in patients with colorectal cancer was examined.

Relationship Between c-*myc* Overexpression and Pathologic Findings

	Overexpression (%)	
	Positive	Negative
Differentiation		
Well	5 (20)	5 (50)
Moderately	18 (72)	5 (50)
Poorly	2 (8)	0 (0)
Depth of penetration		
< pm	5 (20)	5 (50)
ss,a1	11 (44)	3 (30)
>s,a2	9 (36)	2 (20)
Lymphatic vessel invasion		
Positive	20 (80)	3 (30)*
Negative	5 (20)	7 (70)
Vessel invasion		
Positive	8 (32)	1 (10)
Negative	17 (68)	9 (90)
Lymph node metastasis		
Positive	17 (68)	2 (20)*
Negative	8 (36)	8 (80)
Liver metastasis		
Positive	4 (16)	0 (0)
Negative	21 (84)	10 (100)
Dukes' classification		
A,B	8 (32)	8 (80)*
C,D	17 (68)	2 (20)

Abbreviations; pm, cancer confined to the proper muscular layer; ss and a1, cancer that has invaded the serosa or adventitia to some extent; s and a2, cancer that has invaded the serosa or adventitia extensively.
* Significant difference ($P < .05$).
(Courtesy of Sato K, Miyahara M, Saito T, et al: *Eur J Cancer* 30A:1113–1117, 1994.)

Patients.—The level of expression of c–*myc*, c–*fos*, and c-Ki-*ras* genes was examined in 35 Japanese patients with nonhereditary colorectal cancer. The 18 men and 17 women were aged 42–89 years. Thirty-one underwent curative resection of the primary lesion with lymphadenectomy, and 4 with liver metastasis had noncurative resection. Northern blot hybridization was performed on fresh resected specimens of colorectal tumors and their corresponding normal mucosa.

Results.— Overexpression of the c–*myc* gene was detected in 25 patients (71%), overexpression of the c–*fos* gene was detected in 16 (46%), and overexpression of the c-Ki-*ras* gene was detected in 18 (51%). The pathologic findings of the c–*myc* overexpression-positive group and the negative group are shown in the table. Lymphatic invasion was present in 20 of the 25 patients (80%) with c–*myc* gene overexpression but in only 3 of 10 (30%) without it. Lymph node metastases were found in 17 patients (68%) with c–*myc* gene overexpression but in only 2 (20%) of those without it. The depth of tumor penetration did not significantly differ between positive and negative expression of the c–*myc* gene. The survival rate tended to be poorer in patients with c–*myc* overexpression than in those without it, but the difference did not reach statistical significance. No significant relationship was found between the clinicopathologic features and overexpression of the c–*fos* gene or the c-Ki-*ras* gene.

Conclusion.—The detection of c–*myc* overexpression by northern blot hybridization is a useful indicator for determining the malignant potential of colorectal cancer.

▶ In the article, c-*myc* expression was associated with lymphatic invasion and lymph node metastasis. Probably as a result of the relatively small sample, the presence of c-ki-*ras* and c-*fos* overexpression did not correlate with any clinical features.—T.J. Eberlein, M.D.

Study of c-erbB-2 Protein and Epidermal Growth Factor Receptor Expression and DNA Ploidy Pattern in Colorectal Carcinoma
Nakae S, Shimada E, Urakawa T (Kobe Rosai Hosp of the Labour Welfare Corp, Japan)
J Surg Oncol 54:246–251, 1993   140-95-12–21

Background.—The excessive expression of oncoproteins that possess receptor-type tyrosine kinase activity, epidermal growth factor receptor (EGFR), and c-*erb*B-2 oncogene product helps predict the outcome in several human cancers, including breast and esophageal tumors. Several lines of evidence have confirmed the involvement of the c-*erb*B-2 oncogene product in the development of human malignant neoplasms (e.g.,

TABLE 1.—Colorectal Carcinoma: Relationship Between Clinicopathologic Findings and c-erbB-2 Staining

Variable	n	c-erbB-2 staining		
		Negative	Positive	
Tumor size				
≤5cm	18	7	11	
>5cm	26	12	14	N.S.*
Histological type				
Well differentiated	34	15	19	
Moderately differentiated	7	3	4	
Poorly differentiated	2	1	1	
Mucinous	1	0	1	N.S.
Subserosal invasion				
Negative (m, sm, pm)	5	3	2	
Positive (ss, a_1, s, a_2, si, ai)	39	16	23	N.S.
Lymph node metastasis				
Negative	26	10	16	N.S.
Positive	18	9	9	N.S.

gastric carcinoma). The behavior of colorectal cancer has been closely related to its DNA ploidy.

Objective.—The expression of these products was examined using immunohistochemical techniques and monoclonal antibodies against c-*erb*B-2 protein and EGFR in 31 cases of colonic and 13 cases of rectal carcinoma. All the patients had both the primary tumor and lymph nodes resected. In addition, the DNA ploidy pattern was studied by estimating the DNA volume of tumor-cell nuclei.

Lymphatic vessel invasion						
Negative	8		6		2	P <0.1
Positive	36		13		23	
Venous invasion						
Negative	17		8		9	N.S.
Positive	27		11		16	
Dukes classification						
A	4	}34	3	}18	1	}16
B	19		7		12	P <0.05
C	11		8		3	
D	10		1		9	

* *Abbreviation:* N.S., not statistical.
(Courtesy of Nakae S, Shimada E, Urakawa T: *J Surg Oncol* 54:246–251, 1993.)

Results.—Expression of c-*erb*B-2 protein was identified in 56.8% of the 44 cases and of EGFR in 53.7% of the cases. No significant association could be found between the expression of c-*erb*B-2 protein and tumor size, the histologic type of tumor, nodal metastasis, or venous invasion. More tumors with subserosal invasion and more with lymph vessel invasion stained positively (Table 1). Significantly more Dukes' D tumors stained positively for c-*erb*B-2 protein. Aneuploidy of DNA was found in 63.6% of well-differentiated adenocarcinomas and in all 7 moderately

TABLE 2.—Colorectal Carcinoma Relationship Between Clinicopathologic Findings and DNA Ploidy Pattern

Variable	n	DNA ploidy pattern		
		Diploidy	Aneuploidy	
Tumor size				N.S.*
5cm	17	6	11	
>5cm	25	8	17	
Histological type				$P < 0.1$
Well differentiated	33	12	21	
Moderately differentiated	7	0	7	
Poorly differentiated	1	1	0	
Mucinous	1	1	0	
Serosal invasion				$P < 0.1$
Negative (m, sm, pm, ss, a_1)	15	8	7	
Positive (s, a_2, si, ai)	27	6	21	
Lymph node metastasis				$P < 0.01$
Negative	25	13	12	
Positive	17	1	16	

differentiated neoplasms; it correlated significantly with the presence of Dukes' C or D changes (Table 2).

Conclusion.—The overexpression of c-erbB-2 protein or EGFR might be a useful marker of distant disease in patients who have colorectal cancer. At the same time, the pattern of DNA ploidy might help predict nodal metastasis.

Lymphatic vessel invasion				
Negative	8	1	7	N.S.
Positive	34	13	21	
Venous invasion				
Negative	16	5	11	N.S.
Positive	26	9	17	
Dukes classification				
A	4 }22	1 }11	3 }11	
B	18	10	8	
C	10 }20	0 }3	10 }17	P <0.05
D	10	3	7	

* Abbreviation: N.S., not statistical.
(Courtesy of Nakae S, Shimada E, Urakawa T: *J Surg Oncol* 54:246–251, 1993.)

▶ This is a relatively small study in which C-*erb*B-2 expression was associated with the Dukes' D tumor. In aneuploid tumors, DNA content was more often associated with lymph node metastasis.

We are beginning to assimilate a model of tumorigenesis in colorectal cancer that suggests early genetic changes as well as later genetic changes are more often associated with either lymph node or hematogenous spread. However, as is true of many of these studies, they are relatively small and in general represent only select patient populations. Only through large prospective studies that examine all these genetic markers will it be possible to more definitively construct a model to form the basis for patient selection for future adjuvant trials.—T.J. Eberlein, M.D.

Pathologic Determinants of Survival Associated With Colorectal Cancer With Lymph Node Metastases: A Multivariate Analysis of 579 Patients

Newland RC, Dent OF, Lyttle MNB, Chapuis PH, Bokey EL (Concord Hosp, Australia; Australian Natl Univ, Australia; University of Sydney, Australia)
Cancer 73:2076–2082, 1994   140-95-12–22

Introduction.—For patients who have undergone surgery for colorectal cancer and have known residual tumor, the presence or absence of lymph node metastases is a major determinant of survival. Although this is a large and prognostically diverse group of patients, few studies have evaluated the independent prognostic significance of the major pathologic variables. Such a study was done using multivariate analysis.

Methods.—Prospectively collected data on 579 patients who were treated at 1 institution over a 21.5-year period were used. They represented 31% of all patients whose primary tumor was treated by bowel resection during that time. Pathologic documentation was standardized, and all patients were followed up for at least 6 months. All had known residual tumor and regional lymph node metastases that were demonstrated in the surgical specimen. A Kaplan-Meier survival analysis was performed, with Cox proportional hazards regression used to examine the multivariate models.

Multivariate Survival Analysis

Variable	Estimated coefficient	Hazard ratio	*P*
Aged ≥ 75 yr	0.685	1.98	< 0.001
Apical node involved	0.584	1.79	< 0.001
Spread involving free serosal surface	0.535	1.71	< 0.001
Spread beyond muscularis propria	0.516	1.68	0.029
Rectum	0.423	1.53	< 0.001
Venous invasion	0.399	1.49	< 0.001
High-grade carcinoma	0.392	1.48	< 0.001
Male	0.237	1.27	0.046

(Courtesy of Newland RC, Dent OF, Lyttle MNB, et al: *Cancer* 73:2076–2082, 1994.)

Results.—Eight variables were found to be significantly associated with survival on univariate analysis. Multivariate analysis found that 6 of the variables had significant independent effects on survival; the most important of these was apical lymph node involvement, followed in order by spread involving a free serosal surface, invasion beyond the muscularis propria, rectal location, venous invasion, and higher tumor grade. Age older than 75 years and male sex were also associated with poorer survival (table). The number of involved nodes had no independent effect on survival.

Conclusion.—Six pathologic variables were identified as having independent prognostic effects on survival for patients with colorectal cancer and lymph node metastases. The most powerful predictor is apical lymph node involvement, which is used in the subclassification of Dukes' stage C tumors. Direct spread beyond the muscularis propria is used in the Astler-Coller subclassification. Approaches to stratification of this large and prognostically diverse patient group should include all 6 independent variables.

Variables Related to Risk of Recurrence in Rectal Cancer Without Lymph Node Metastasis
Ogiwara H, Nakamura T, Baba S (Hamamatsu Univ School of Medicine, Japan)
Ann Surg Oncol 1:99–104, 1994   140-95-12-23

Purpose.—More surgeons are using local excision of rectal cancer or selective preservation of the pelvic autonomic nerves in an attempt to reduce the incidence of urinary and sexual dysfunction. However, because local excision does not remove areas involved in lymphatic spread, the decision to use this procedure must be carefully considered. It is particularly important to identify patients who are at risk of failure after resection and who might benefit from postoperative adjuvant therapy. Prognostic factors for recurrence were investigated in a retrospective study of patients undergoing radical resection for rectal carcinoma without lymph node metastasis.

Methods.—The analysis included 142 patients undergoing radical resection of Dukes A or B rectal carcinoma—a tumor confined to the rectal wall without nodal involvement—during a 9-year period. The patients were 75 men and 67 women, with a median age of 62 years. Possible predictors of recurrence that were evaluated included macroscopic and microscopic pathologic characteristics, immunohistochemical staining for p53, and the DNA ploidy pattern of the primary tumor.

Results.—Five-year disease-free survival was 87%, and overall survival was 91%. Rates of local control and freedom from distant metastases were both 93%. Depth of tumor invasion, vascular or lymphatic involvement, tumor differentiation, and tumor size were all significantly related

Survival Data for Patients Undergoing Radical Operation for Rectal Cancer Without Lymph Node Metastases

	No. of patients	Five-year disease-free survival (%)	Local control (%)	Freedom from distant metastases (%)	Overall survival (%)
Overall	142	87	93	93	91
Depth of invasion					
sm, pm	52	98*†	100†‡	100	100†‡
ss(a$_1$), s(a$_2$)	90	81	89	90	87
Vascular/lymphatic vessel involvement					
Absent	82	90	91	97†	94
Present	60	84	94	89	90
Differentiation					
Well	123	87	93	93	93†
Moderately	15	79	90	87	77
Others	4	87	93	93	93
Tumor size (cm)					
<2.0	8	100	100	100	100
2.0–5.0	57	89§	96	93	90§
5.0–8.0	63	84¶	90§	92§	90
≥8.0	14	83§	90	92	92

* $P < .001$ (Kaplan-Meier).
† $P < .05$ (generalized Wilcoxon).
‡ $P < .01$ (Kaplan-Meier).
§ $P < .05$ vs. tumor size (< 2.0) (Kaplan-Meier).
¶ $P < .01$ vs. tumor size (< 2.0) (Kaplan-Meier).
(Courtesy of Ogiwara H, Nakamura T, Baba S: *Ann Surg Oncol* 1:99–104, 1994.)

to recurrence and prognosis (table). The p53 staining and DNA ploidy pattern were not significant predictors.

Conclusion.—Among patients with rectal cancer, those with tumors confined to the rectal wall and no lymph node metastases generally have an excellent prognosis after radical resection. A number of features suggest consideration of adjunctive radiotherapy and chemotherapy, including serosal tumor invasion, vascular or lymphatic involvement, moderately differentiated adenocarcinoma, and lesions larger than 2 cm. Patients with these characteristics should not be treated with local excision, regardless of the absence of lymph node metastases.

Selection Factors for Local Excision or Abdominoperineal Resection of Early Stage Rectal Cancer
Willett CG, Compton CC, Shellito PC, Efird JT (Harvard Med School, Boston)
Cancer 73:2716–2720, 1994   140-95-12–24

Introduction.—Patients with distal rectal carcinoma whose tumors are low, small, completely excisable, and exhibit favorable histologic features can achieve good rates of local control and survival with conservative surgical techniques. However, no randomized trial has compared outcome after local excision procedures and abdominoperineal resection in such a patient population. A review of patients with early stage rectal cancer who were managed by local excision or abdominoperineal resection focused on selection factors for conservative techniques.

Methods.—From 1962 to 1991, 56 patients with T1 and T2 tumors underwent local excision, whereas 69 were managed with abdominoperineal resection. Tumors in both groups were limited to the submucosa and muscularis propria. Thirty patients in the local excision group received postoperative radiation therapy. Since 1986, patients treated with local excision have received IV 5-fluorouracil for 3 consecutive days during the first and last week of radiation treatment. The outcome was analyzed by stage, treatment modality, and pathologic features of tumor grade, as well as by vessel involvement.

Results.—Five-year actuarial recurrence-free survival was 72% in the local excision group and 87% in the abdominoperineal resection group. In both groups, rates of recurrence-free survival and local control were better in patients whose tumors demonstrated favorable histologic features than in those whose tumors exhibited unfavorable histologic features. Venous/lymph vessel involvement was also associated with lower rates of local control and recurrence-free survival, both in the local excision group (Table 1) and the abdominoperineal resection group (Table 2).

Conclusion.—Patients with early stage rectal cancer without poorly differentiated histologic features or venous/lymph vessel involvement can achieve excellent rates of survival and local. control with local exci-

TABLE 1.—Five-Year Actuarial Results for Patients Undergoing Local Excision of Rectal Cancer Based on Histological Features

	No. of patients	5-year actuarial (%)		
		RFS	LC	FDM
Depth of invasion				
Submucosa	34 (12)	76	83	91
Muscularis propria	22 (7)	66	80	79
Tumor grade				
Well/moderately well differentiated	40 (14)	77	88*	88
Poorly differentiated	16 (5)	55	64	80
Venous/lymph vessel invasion (one patient not evaluable)				
Absent	34 (15)	85*	97*	88
Present	21 (4)	47	54	82
Histologic features				
Favorable	28 (11)	87*	96*	90
Unfavorable	28 (8)	57	68	81

Abbreviations: RFS, recurrence-free survival; LC, local control; FDM, freedom from distant metastases.
Values in parentheses indicate number of patients at risk at 5 years.
* $P < .05$.
(Courtesy of Willett CG, Compton CC, Shellito PC, et al: *Cancer* 73:2716–2720, 1994.)

sion. The outcome is significantly less favorable if one or both of these tumor characteristics are present. Abdominoperineal resection yields better results, but patients with high-risk T1 and T2 rectal cancers may benefit from radical resection combined with pelvic irradiation and 5-fluorouracil-based chemotherapy.

▶ Abstracts 140-95-12–22, 140-95-12–23, and 140-95-12–24 were grouped together because of their relationship to recurrence and survival.

Abstract 140-95-12–22 examines 579 patients from a single institution. The drawback of this study is that it spans more than 2 decades. Using statistical methodology and multivariate analysis, the authors found that the most important independent effect on survival was apical lymph node involvement. I would not necessarily agree with the authors that the tumor node metastases staging system should be changed to include these variables; how-

TABLE 2.—Five-Year Actuarial Results for Patients Undergoing Abdominoperineal Resection Based on Histologic Features

	No. of patients	5-year actuarial (%)		
		RFS	LC	FDM
Depth of invasion				
Submucosa	11 (6)	100	100	100
Muscularis propria	58 (34)	85	89	89
Tumor grade				
Well/moderately well differentiated	58 (35)	91*	92	92
Poorly differentiated	11 (5)	70	80	80
Venous/lymph vessel invasion				
Absent	58 (37)	91†	92†	92
Present	11 (3)	73	80	82
Histologic features				
Favorable	49 (32)	91*	91	93
Unfavorable	20 (8)	79	89	84

Abbreviations: RFS, recurrence-free survival; LC, local control; FDM, freedom from distant metastases.
Values in parentheses indicate number of patients at risk at 5 years.
* P between .05 and .10.
† P < .05.
(Courtesy of Willett CG, Compton CC, Shellito PC, et al: *Cancer* 73:2716–2720, 1994.)

ever, it does seem that apical lymph node involvement, the spread of a tumor involving a free serosal surface, and some of the other features that these authors identified would certainly be important in patient selection for adjuvant trials that involve radiation and chemotherapy in the rectum or chemotherapy in colon tumors.

The study by Ogiwara and associates (Abstract 140-95-12–23) explores the variables related to the risk of recurrence of rectal carcinoma. All these patients did not have lymph node involvement, and whereas survival was excellent, serosal tumor invasion as well as lymphatic vessel invasion by large size tumors were associated with a higher risk of recurrence. As a result, these local tumor features may be important in treating patients with adjuvant chemotherapy/radiation. The authors have shown that *ras, myc,* and DNA ploidy are more useful in patients with Dukes' C rectal carcinoma. Ideally, large tumors with poor risk features would not be treated with local excision but would better be treated with more radical surgery.

Similar conclusions are put forth in the article by Willett and co-workers (Abstract 140-95-12–24), who conclude that well-differentiated tumors that are confined to the muscularis propria which did not have venous or lymphatic involvement were potential candidates for local excision with or without postoperative radiation therapy. Obviously, size is an important consideration, as is comorbid disease.—T.J. Eberlein, M.D.

▶↓ The next 3 articles (Abstracts 140-95-12–25, 140-95-12–26, and 140-95-12–27) deal with a new technique that spares the sphincter in low-lying rectal cancers.—T.J. Eberlein, M.D.

Treatment of Rectal Cancer by Low Anterior Resection With Colo-anal Anastomosis
Paty PB, Enker WE, Cohen AM, Lauwers GY (Mem Sloan-Kettering Cancer Ctr, New York)
Ann Surg 219:365–373, 1994   140-95-12–25

Introduction.—Coloanal anastomosis in combination with low anterior resection (LAR/CAA) has been used to treat rectal cancer at the study institution for nearly 2 decades. All patients treated between 1977 and 1990 were studied retrospectively to determine the results of cancer treatment, identify risk factors for pelvic recurrence, and assess the long-term success of sphincter preservation.

Patients and Methods.—The study group consisted of 90 men and 44 women with a median age of 59 years. The median tumor diameter was 4 cm, and the median distance from the anal verge to the lowest edge of the tumor was 6.5 cm; all but 3 tumors were mobile. Transection at the distal margin of the specimen was performed from the abdominopelvic approach in 64% of patients and from the transanal approach in 36% of patients. Either the sigmoid colon or the descending colon was used for reconstruction. Anastomosis was end-to-end in 131 cases; colonic J pouches were used in 3 cases. All pathologic slides were reviewed. In all but 6 cases, a distal resection margin was measured and recorded. Sixty-five patients received adjuvant pelvic radiation. The median follow-up was 4 years.

Results.—Twenty–nine of the 134 patients have died of rectal cancer—25 with recurrence and 4 with persistent liver metastases. The median time to cancer death was 3.8 years. The overall actuarial survival for 5 years was 73%. Stratified by stage, actuarial survival at 5 years was 100% for stage A, 79% for stage B1, 70% for stage B2, 58% for stage C, and 13% for stage D. Most recurrences (64%) occurred at distant sites only. Pelvic disease was controlled by LAR/CAA for 121 of 134 patients, with or without radiation therapy. An increased risk of pelvic recurrence (Table 1) was associated with mesenteric implants, a positive micro-

TABLE 1.—Univariate Analysis of Risk Factors for
Pelvic Recurrence

Feature	Group	No. of Recurrences/ N (%)	p
Patient factors			
Gender	Male	10/90 (11%)	0.33
	Female	3/44 (7%)	
Age	<60 yr	6/69 (9%)	0.56
	≥60 yr	7/65 (11%)	
Tumor factors			
Mesenteric implants	Present	6/7 (86%)	0.000003
	Absent	7/127 (6%)	
Perineural invasion	Present	2/4 (50%)	0.0004
	Absent	11/127 (9%)	
T stage	T1-2	2/64 (3%)	0.008
	T3	11/67 (16%)	
Blood vessel invasion	Present	3/8 (38%)	0.005
	Absent	10/123 (8%)	
Grade	G1-2	9/118 (8%)	0.01
	G3	4/13 (31%)	
Lymphatic invasion	Present	4/18 (22%)	0.06
	Absent	9/113 (8%)	
Mucinous	Present	2/11 (18%)	0.28
	Absent	11/120 (9%)	
Size	<4 cm	7/77 (9%)	0.54
	≥4 cm	6/54 (11%)	
N stage	N0	7/84 (8%)	0.42
	N1-2-3	6/47 (13%)	
Above anal verge	<6 cm	5/48 (10%)	0.76
	≥6 cm	8/86 (9%)	
Treatment factors			
Microscopic margins	Positive	2/2 (100%)	0.000003
	Negative	11/132 (8%)	
Anastomosis	EEA	3/47 (6%)	0.26
	Handsewn	10/87 (11%)	
Adjuvant chemotherapy	Any	1/19 (5%)	0.66
	None	12/115 (10%)	
Radiation therapy	≥45 Gy	5/36 (14%)	0.80
	None	8/69 (12%)	
Surgical distal margin	<2 cm	3/48 (6%)	0.42
	≥2 cm	9/80 (11%)	

(Courtesy of Paty PB, Enker WE, Cohen AM, et al: *Ann Surg* 219:365–373, 1994.)

TABLE 2.—Comparison of Patients With Short and Long Distal
Resection Margins: Distribution of Tumor Stages and Doses of
Pelvic Radiation Therapy

	Patients with Distal Margin < 2 cm N (%)	Patients with Distal Margin > 2 cm N (%)	p
Tumor stage			
T12N0	20 (42%)	30 (38%)	0.42
T3N0	9 (19%)	23 (29%)	
T12N123	7 (15%)	6 (8%)	
T3N123	12 (25%)	21 (26%)	
Adjuvant pelvic radiation			
None	28 (58%)	39 (49%)	0.56
15–30 Gy	10 (21%)	19 (24%)	
≥45 Gy	10 (21%)	22 (28%)	

(Courtesy of Paty PB, Enker WE, Cohen AM, et al: *Ann Surg* 219:365–373, 1994.)

scopic resection margin, a T3 tumor, perineural invasion, blood vessel invasion, and a high tumor grade. Eight of the 13 patients with pelvic recurrence ultimately required a permanent colostomy. Patients with short and long distal margins had similar distributions of tumor stage and received adjuvant pelvic radiation with similar frequencies and schedules (Table 2). Therefore, the favorable outcome with short distal margins was unlikely to be related to a selection bias.

Conclusion.—Treatment with LAR/CAA was effective for a large proportion of patients with mid-rectal cancers and some distal cancers. Overall, more than 90% of patients avoided a permanent colostomy with control of pelvic tumor. Pelvic recurrence was associated with the presence of histopathologic markers of aggressive disease in the primary tumor but not with short distal resection margins. Postoperative radiation, when used in combination with LAR/CAA, has significant risks and adverse effects; its routine use for all T3 or N1 tumors may be unwarranted.

Long-Term Functional Results of Coloanal Anastomosis for Rectal Cancer

Paty PB, Enker WE, Cohen AM, Minsky BD, Friedlander-Klar H (Mem Sloan-Kettering Cancer Ctr, New York)
Am J Surg 167:90–95, 1994   140-95-12–26

Objective.—In a small number of rectal cancer patients who are eligible for coloanal anastomosis (CAA) with low anterior resection (LAR),

Clinical Characteristics of Patients	
Age at operation (y) (median)	59
Range (y)	23–90
Gender (M/F)	51: 30
Duke's stage (Duke test)	39A: 26B: 20C: 3D
Tumor location above AV (cm) (median)	Median: 6
Range (cm)	3–11
Distal margin of resection (cm)	2.0
Range (cm)	0.1–6.0
Anastomotic technique	52 handsewn: 29 stapled
Anastomotic location	31 high (apex): 50 low (dentate)
Temporary diversion	73 yes: 8 no
Adjuvant pelvic radiation	40 yes: 41 no

Abbreviation: AV, anal verge
(Courtesy of Paty PB, Enker WE, Cohen AM, et al: *Am J Surg* 167:90-95, 1994.)

the goal is to preserve anorectal function. To assess the long-term results of such surgery, a survey was performed.

Methods.—A total of 81 primary rectal cancer patients, who had LAR/CAA for an average of 4.3 years but without a colostomy, responded to the survey (table).

Results.—The median stool frequency was 2 per day with 22% of patients having 4 or more movements daily (Fig 12–16). More than half

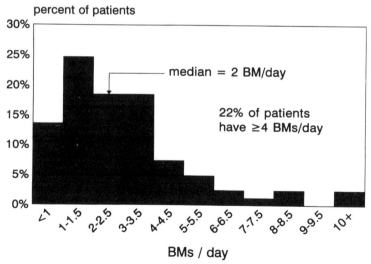

Fig 12–16.—The distribution of patients according to the number of bowel movements (BM) experienced in a typical day. (Courtesy of Paty PB, Enker WE, Cohen AM, et al: *Am J Surg* 167:90-95, 1994.)

the patients reported complete fecal continence, 21% reported gas incontinence, 23% occasional staining, and 5% a significant leak. Thirty-two percent wore a pad at least part time. Urgency was present in 19% of patients, whereas 32% had difficulty with evacuation. A functional score (FS) was developed based on continence, frequency, and evacuation that ranged from 1 (excellent) to 4 (poor). Functional scores were good or excellent in 56% of patients, fair in 32%, and poor in 12%. The most common problem was stool frequency. Lifestyle changes included avoidance of certain foods by 56%, avoidance of certain activities by 17%, and medication dependence by 37%. Almost three quarters of the patients said they were pleased or satisfied. There was no correlation between surgical procedure and either continence or urgency. Stool frequency improvement correlated significantly with time since surgery, age at surgery, and stapled anastomosis. Multiple evacuation correlated significantly with male sex and receipt of adjuvant radiotherapy and marginally with pelvic lymph node dissection.

Conclusion.—Low anterior resection/coloanal anastomosis can be used in only a small number of rectal cancer patients. It is a satisfactory option in the majority of patients who are not eligible for intrapelvic anastomosis. In 10% of patients with poor bowel function, additional studies of surgical technique and adjuvant therapy is desirable.

▶ The first 2 articles (Abstracts 140-95-12–25 and 140-95-12–26) are from the Memorial Sloan-Kettering Cancer Center, where Drs. Enker and Cohen have been pioneers in the technique of sparing the sphincter in the treatment of low-lying rectal cancers. Colostomy was avoided in more than 90% of the patients. It should be emphasized that careful selection, as well as perfection of the surgical technique, is necessary to attain these results. Recurrence is associated with lymphatic vessel invasion and high tumor grade.

The article by Paty (Abstract 140-95-12–26) presents a subset of the Memorial Sloan-Kettering's experience with CAA. In this study, 81 patients are presented, including 23% with occasional staining and 5% with a significant leak; almost one third of the patients wore a pad at least part of the time. These functional abnormalities were more significant in males, especially those who received adjuvant radiation therapy or more extensive lymph node dissection.

This article underscores the importance of meticulous technique as well as the learning curve involved in perfecting this procedure. However, CAA/LAR of a rectal cancer may well be an increasingly utilized method of treatment, especially in young patients.—T.J. Eberlein, M.D.

New Perspective in the Treatment of Low Rectal Cancer: Total Rectal Resection and Coloendoanal Anastomosis

Leo E, Belli F, Baldini MT, Vitellaro M, Mascheroni L, Andreola S, Bellomi M,

Zucali R (Nazionale per lo Studio e la Cura dei Tumori, Milan, Italy)
Dis Colon Rectum 37:S62–S68, 1994   140-95-12-27

Objective.—Patients with lower rectal cancer who have abdominoperineal resection receive a permanent colostomy. The more conservative technique of total rectal resection (TRR) with coloendoanal anastomosis (CEAA), which preserves the sphincter, produces good results and a better quality of life for the patient.

Methods.—A total of 55 patients aged 30 to 79 years with primary or recurring lower rectal cancers within 7 cm of the anal verge received TRR with CEAA in which the sigmoid colon was divided proximally and the rectum was sectioned. The rest of the sigmoid colon was used to prepare a colic J-shaped pouch. A hand-sewn pouch–endoanal anastomosis with the external sphincter was done. The patients received temporary colostomies.

Results.—After 7–14 months, 7 patients had recurrent invasive lesions, and 3 had reoperations. Five patients had distant metastases. In 9 patients colostomies could not be closed. No patients experienced incontinence, but 9 patients had occasional minor urine leakage. After colostomies were closed, 74% of patients had 1 or 2 bowel movements a day, and 12% had 3 or 4 bowel movements a day (table). Patients having CEAA should be selected carefully. Meticulous resection of perirectal tissue is the most important consideration in lowering the frequency of local and pelvic recurrence.

Conclusion.—This combination of procedures is a suitable alternative to traditional surgery for lower rectal cancer.

▶ In this article, a small series of patients was presented. Nearly three quarters of these patients had good functional results, although nearly 15% had recurrent lesions. This emphasizes that patients must be carefully selected for this procedure, because recurrence is directly related to the extent of re-

Postoperative Functional Results in 45 Patients After
Colostomy Closure

Bowel movements	
1 or 2/day	34 (74%)
3 or more/day	12 (26%)
Continence	
1 Perfect	36 (78%)
2 Incontinent to gas	0
3 Occasional minor leak	10 (22%)
4 Frequent major soiling	0

(Courtesy of Leo E, Belli F, Baldini MT, et al: *Dis Colon Rectum*
37:S62–S68, 1994.)

section of perirectal tissue, however, this may diminish the functional results. Another difference between this series and the Memorial Sloan-Kettering series is that these patients underwent J-pouch reconstruction utilizing the sigmoid colon, whereas the majority of the Memorial Sloan-Kettering patients had straight coloanal anastomosis.—T.J. Eberlein, M.D.

▶↓ The next 2 papers (Abstracts 140-95-12-28 and 140-95-12-29) deal with either preoperative or postoperative radiation therapy for carcinoma of the rectum.—T.J. Eberlein, M.D.

Downstaging of Advanced Rectal Cancer Following Combined Preoperative Chemotherapy and High Dose Radiation

Chen E-T, Mohiuddin M, Brodovsky H, Fishbein G, Marks G (Thomas Jefferson Univ Hosp, Philadelphia)
Int J Radiat Oncol Biol Phys 30:169–175, 1994   140-95-12-28

Background.— Tumor fixation in rectal cancer has been recognized as the single most important pretreatment factor for predicting the achievement of a curative resection, as well as predicting overall and disease-free survival. Preoperative radiation and chemotherapy treatment in locally advanced rectal carcinoma is an appropriate consideration in improving these outcomes. The results of treating patients with advanced rectal cancer with preoperative adjuvant treatments were analyzed.

Methods.— Patients with primary low rectal cancers were examined for preoperative treatment, undergoing complete physical examinations, blood work, proctosigmoidoscopy with biopsy, colonoscopy, and radiographic studies. Patients were selected for treatment if they had clinical and radiographic evidence of tumors with full-thickness involvement of the bowel wall. The extent of tumor fixation was graded as partially

TABLE 1.—Clinical Downstaging

Postchemoradiation stage

PrechemoRT stage	Mobile	Partially fixed	Fixed	% Downstaging
Partially fixed (n = 3)	2	1	—	67
Fixed (n = 24)	11 (46%)	6 (25%)	7	71
Adv fixation (n = 4)	2 (50%)	—	2 (50%)	100

Abbreviation: RT, radiation.
(Courtesy of Chen E-T, Mohiuddin M, Brodovsky H, et al: *Int J Radiat Oncol Biol Phys* 30:169–175, 1994.)

TABLE 2.—Patterns of Failure by Clinical Stage

Clinical stage	Local	Local + distant	Distant
Partially fixed (*n* = 3)	—	—	—
Fixed (*n* = 24)	1 (4%)	4 (17%)*	3 (13%)[†]
Adv fixation (*n* = 4)	—	—	—
Total (*n* = 31)	1 (3%)	4 (13%)	3 (10%)

* Includes 2 patients with node-positive disease.
† Includes 2 patients with liver metastases at surgery.
(Courtesy of Chen E-T, Mohiuddin M, Brodovsky H, et al: *Int J Radiat Oncol Biol Phys* 30:169–175, 1994.)

fixed, fixed, and advanced fixation. Patients were treated with high-dose preoperative radiation using a 4-field pelvis technique with shaped alloys. All fields were treated daily using megavoltage beams, with a median dose to the whole pelvis of 45 Gy. This was followed by a boost field that encompassed the tumor and presacral region using opposed high-energy lateral fields for an additional 10.8 Gy, with a resultant total median dose of 55.8 Gy. Concurrent with the start of radiation, infusional 5-fluorouracil was begun in either low-dosage continuous infusions (200–300 mg/m²/day) or 2 cycles of short-course 5-fluorouracil infusions at the same dosage over 5 days. All patients then underwent surgical resection at a median of 7.5 weeks after the preoperative treatment course.

Results.— Thirty-one patients—24 with fixed, 3 with partially fixed, and 4 with advanced fixed tumors—underwent treatment. After preoperative therapy, 23 (74%) were clinically downstaged (Table 1). Surgical resection was completed with negative margins in 29 patients (94%). The 3-year actuarial survival was 68%, and sites of failure included local, distant, and combined local and distant metastases in 8 patients (Table 2). The treatment was generally well tolerated.

Conclusion.—Combined high-dose preoperative radiation and chemotherapy for advanced rectal cancers resulted in significant clinical downstaging and improved surgical and survival outcomes. Preoperative combined modality therapy should be selectively considered for patients with fixed rectal cancers.

▶ The authors confirm previous studies that showed preoperative radiation therapy for carcinoma of the rectum results in significant downstaging. All patients in this study had at least partially fixed tumors; therefore, preoperative treatment also resulted in easier surgical resection. A survival benefit was also demonstrated; however, it has not been uniformly identified in other series of patients undergoing preoperative radiation therapy. This may be related to the relatively poor prognosis of patients with fixed tumors, but it also may be related to the dose of radiation therapy.—T.J. Eberlein, M.D.

The Importance of Patient Selection for Adjunctive Postoperative Radiation Therapy for Cancer of the Rectum: Patient Selection in Adjunctive Therapy

Lingareddy V, Mohiuddin M, Marks G (Thomas Jefferson Univ Hosp, Philadelphia, Pa)

Cancer 73:1805–1810, 1994   140-95-12–29

Objective.—The success of adjuvant radiation treatment of patients with rectal cancer depends on their careful selection.; however, criteria have not been defined. Clinical selection features of the disease with treatment outcome after adjuvant postoperative radiotherapy were evaluated.

Methods.—A total of 120 clinically favorable patients with resectable rectal adenocarcinomas were divided into 3 groups. All patients received 5 Gy preoperatively and were followed for at least 5 years. Group 1 consisted of 32 patients with stage A or B1 cancers who received no further treatment; group 2, 54 patients with Stage B2, C1, or C2 cancers, received 45 Gy of postoperative radiotherapy; group 3, 53 stage B2 and C patients, received 45 Gy of postoperative radiotherapy and had the worst prognosis.

Results.—No group 1 patients had severe radiation complications. Two group 2 patients and 3 group 3 patients had serious small bowel complications that required surgery. Group 1 had the highest rate of local recurrence, with 21% of stage B2, 50% of stage C1, and 40% of stage C2 carcinomas recurring. Group 3 had the highest rate of distant metastases, with 50% for stage C1 and 52% for stage C2 tumors. The respective 10-year actuarial survival rates for groups 1, 2, and 3 were 38%, 62%, and 28%. Group 3 patients had the most clinically unfavorable factors, older age, more males, distal tumor location, more abdominoperineal resections, and more stage C2 tumors. The 5-year survival rate of 41% is consistent with the results shown in other studies.

Conclusion.—The 5- and 10-year survival of patients with rectal carcinoma who were treated with preoperative low-dose and postoperative high-dose radiotherapy was excellent and better than postoperative radiotherapy alone in poorly selected patients. It was also better than for patients who were treated without postoperative radiotherapy.

▶ The next article shows that low-dose preoperative radiation therapy combined with high-dose postoperative radiation therapy is well tolerated. Again, whereas the results of using a small amount of preoperative radiation therapy in this series appear to be beneficial, a comparison was made with other historic series. Therefore, selection bias and the excellent quality of the surgical technique used by these authors may have played a role in the overall outcome. Final determination of the role of preoperative radiation therapy can be obtained only through randomized prospective trials that are carefully designed to specifically address the role of preoperative radiation therapy.—T.J. Eberlein, M.D.

Prospective Comparison of Laparoscopic and Conventional Anterior Resection

Tate JJT, Kwok S, Dawson JW, Lau WY, Li AKC (The Chinese Univ of Hong Kong; Prince of Wales Hosp, Shatin, New Territories, Hong Kong)
Br J Surg 80:1396–1398, 1993   140-95-12-30

Objective.—The results of conventional and laparoscopically assisted anterior resection were compared in 25 patients with cancer of the sigmoid colon or upper rectum. Patients older than age 65 and those with a fixed mass were excluded from the study. The patients were not randomized; instead, age and the presence of metastases dictated the type of surgery performed.

Methods.—Laparoscopic surgery was performed in 11 patients by a team of 4 surgeons using a subumbilical incision and 4 accessory cannulas. The tumor was mobilized laparoscopically, the necessary arteries divided, the bowel divided proximal and distal to the tumor, and an anastomosis carried out. Six of the 11 patients required only a muscle-splitting incision. Fourteen other patients had conventional anterior resection. In both groups the inferior mesenteric artery was ligated as far as possible proximally to maximize the clearance of lymph nodes.

Results.—Laparoscopically assisted surgery required a mean of 205 minutes compared with 123 minutes for conventional surgery. A normal diet was resumed about a day earlier in the laparoscopy group. These patients required fewer doses of pethidene than those who were managed conventionally. Their hospital stay averaged 12 days compared with 14 days after conventional surgery (Table 1). Resection specimens were

TABLE 1.—Details of Patient Recovery After Operation

	Laparoscopic ($n=11$)	Conventional ($n=14$)	P
Time to restart diet (days)	2·5(0·2)	3·6(0·3)	0·008*
Total analgesia (doses of intramuscular pethidine)	2·6(0·4)	7·4(2·1)	0·011†
Length of hospital stay (days)	12·3(3)	14·3(6)	0·079*

Note: Values are mean (s.d.).
* Mantel-Cox test
† Mann-Whitney U test
(Courtesy of Tate JJT, Kwok S, Dawson JW, et al: *Br J Surg* 80:1396–1398, 1993.)

TABLE 2.—Details of Resection Specimens

	Laparoscopic ($n=11$)	Conventional ($n=14$)
Dukes' stage		
A	1	0
B	4	9
C	5	4
Carcinoid	1	0
No. of nodes resected*	10 (2–14)	13 (2–18)
Length of bowel resected (cm)*	14 (11–21)	15 (7–25)
Distal resection margin (cm)*†	2·0 (0·5–5)	2·5 (2–5)

* Values are median (range).
† Does not include 'doughnut' resected by staple gun. There were no significant differences between the 2 groups.
(Courtesy of Tate JJT, Kwok S, Dawson JW, et al: *Br J Surg* 80:1396–1398, 1993.)

comparable in the 2 groups, and major complications were similarly frequent.

Conclusion.—Laparoscopic anterior resection is a technically feasible approach to cancers of the sigmoid colon and upper rectum (Table 2). Patients recover more rapidly than after the conventional open operation.

▶ This article was selected because of the extensive discussions that surround laparoscopic surgery. In this small series, patients were not randomized but instead were selected by age or clinical diagnosis of the tumor. Despite this, the length of surgery was longer in the laparoscopic patients, and their hospital stay was slightly less. Cooperative group trials are now in progress that are examining randomized patient populations, especially those with right colon cancers that compare laparoscopic and conventional surgery. The results of these trials will be forthcoming in the next few years.—T.J. Eberlein, M.D.

Recurrent Squamous Cell Carcinoma of the Anal Canal: Predictors of Initial Treatment Failure and Results of Salvage Therapy

Longo WE, Vernava AM III, Wade TP, Coplin MA, Virgo KS, Johnson FE (St Louis Univ, Mo; John Cochran VA Med Ctr, St Louis, Mo)
Ann Surg 220:40–49, 1994   140-95-12–31

Introduction.—Squamous cell carcinoma of the anal canal is a rare clinical occurrence. The current primary therapy of choice is combined chemotherapy and radiation therapy. Abdominoperineal resection is used to treat patients with recurrent cancer after primary therapy fails. In patients with squamous cell carcinoma of the anal canal, various factors

Outcome of Primary Treatment of 164 Evaluable Patients With
Squamous Cell Carcinoma of the Anal Canal, By Stage*

Stage	Treatment	Percent Alive
Stage I (N = 78)	Local excision only (N = 9)	6/9 (67%)
	Local excision plus RT (N = 5)	5/5 (100%)
	Multimodality therapy (N = 59)	48/59 (81%)
	APR plus RT (N = 1)	1/1 (100%)
	APR plus chemotherapy and RT (N = 4)	3/4 (75%)
Stage II (N = 59)	Local excision only (N = 3)	0/3 (0%)
	Local excision plus chemotherapy (n = 2)	1/2 (50%)
	Local excision plus RT (N = 1)	0/1 (100%)
	Multimodality therapy (N = 37)	26/37 (70%)
	APR only (N = 5)	5/5 (100%)
	APR plus RT (N = 4)	1/4 (25%)
	APR plus chemotherapy and RT (N = 7)	4/7 (57%)
Stage III (N = 12)	Local excision only (N = 1)	1/1 (100%)
	Multimodality therapy (N = 6)	3/6 (50%)
	APR only (N = 1)	1/1 (100%)
	APR plus RT (N = 1)	0/1 (0%)
	APR plus chemotherapy and RT (N = 3)	2/3 (6%)
Stage IV (N = 15)	Local excision only (N = 2)	0/2 (0%)
	Multimodality therapy (N = 12)	1/12 (8%)
	APR plus RT and chemotherapy (N = 1)	0/1 (0%)

* Multimodality = local excision followed by chemotherapy and RT.
(Courtesy of Longo WE, Vernava AM III, Wade TP, et al: *Ann Surg* 220:40–49, 1994.)

were assessed as predictors of therapeutic failure, and outcomes after various forms of therapy were compared.

Methods.—Data on 221 patients were derived from the database of all hospitals of the Department of Veterans Affairs for a 5-year period and from local tumor registrars. Pathology reports were analyzed to determine tumor staging. Other data collected included demographic information, diagnostic and surgical procedures, use and toxicity of chemotherapy and radiation therapy, metastatic status, development and management of recurrent disease, and survival. Logistic regression analysis determined the variables that predicted therapeutic failure.

Results.—Most of the patients were treated with local excision plus postoperative chemotherapy and radiation therapy; these patients had a higher survival rate than those treated with any of those 3 strategies alone. However, postoperative chemotherapy and radiation therapy did not enhance survival of the patients who underwent abdominoperineal resection. Overall survival was higher in patients who underwent local excision with adjuvant chemotherapy and radiation therapy than in patients who underwent abdominoperineal resection (table). However, in patients with disease recurrence, salvage abdominoperineal resection enhanced survival compared with salvage chemotherapy with or without radiation therapy. Only treatment modality and tumor stage predicted the probability of survival.

Discussion.—These outcome data indicate that multimodality therapy is the most effective treatment strategy for primary disease. Recurrent disease, which is significantly predicted by tumor stage, can best be treated with abdominoperineal resection, which enhanced survival in more than half the affected patients in this cohort.

▶↓ This manuscript emphasizes the importance of a multimodality approach to the treatment of squamous cell carcinoma of the anal canal. Since the publications of Nigro and colleagues from Wayne State, this is not unusual; however, proper treatment of patients with recurrent squamous cell carcinoma of the anal canal is still controversial. This series demonstrated that abdominoperineal resection results in enhanced survival in more than half the patients. Failure of primary treatment was related to stage at diagnosis; as a result, a multimodality approach to primary tumors of squamous origin in the anal canal has been verified in this large group of VA patients.—T.J. Eberlein, M.D.

Sarcoma

▶↓ The next 4 articles deal with soft tissue sarcoma. They address 4 specific issues that are important in the management of this malignancy, specifically, prognosis in retroperitoneal soft tissue sarcoma, prognostic factors and extremity sarcoma, brachytherapy, and adjuvant chemotherapy. Whereas none of these manuscripts is by any means definitive, each sheds light on important aspects in the management of soft tissue sarcoma.—T.J. Eberlein, M.D.

Outcome and Prognosis in Retroperitoneal Soft Tissue Sarcoma
Catton CN, O'Sullivan B, Kotwall C, Cummings B, Hao Y, Fornasier V (Princess Margaret Hosp, Toronto; St Michael's Hosp, Toronto)
Int J Radiat Oncol Biol Phys 29:1005–1010, 1994   140-95-12-32

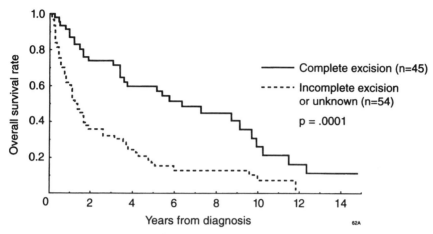

Fig 12–17.—Uncorrected survival for 45 patients who underwent complete excision compared to 59 patients who did not. (Courtesy of Catton CN, O'Sullivan B, Kotwall C, et al: *Int J Radiat Oncol Biol Phys* 29:1005–1010, 1994.)

Objective.—Because retroperitoneal soft tissue sarcomas (RSTSs) are usually not diagnosed until late in the course of the disease, the 5-year survival rate is poor. Although there have been some trials to assess the benefit of postsurgical radiotherapy for treatment of RSTS, the studies have been small. The effects of radiotherapy on patient outcome were assessed retrospectively in 104 patients whose average age at diagnosis was 62 years.

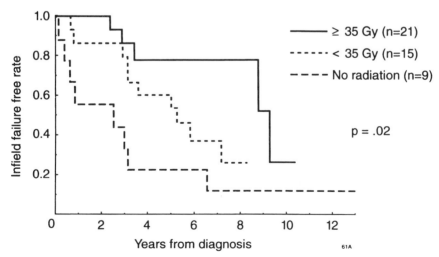

Fig 12–18.—Forty-five patients treated with complete excision. The effect of adjuvant irradiation dose on the infield failure free rate. (Courtesy of Catton CN, O'Sullivan B, Kotwall C, et al: *Int J Radiat Oncol Biol Phys* 29:1005–1010, 1994.)

Methods.—Treatment consisted of complete excision and postoperative irradiation using a dose of 20 Gy per 20 fractions per 4 weeks to 50 Gy per 25 fractions per 5 weeks delivered by a 20-megaelectron volt linear accelerator. Some patients also received adjuvant chemotherapy.

Results.—Localized disease was present in 74 patients; 20 patients had a recurrence. There were 35 high- and 36 low-grade tumors; 33 were not graded. There were 42 liposarcomas, 22 leiomyosarcomas, 19 malignant fibrous histiocytomas, 7 fibrosarcomas, and 14 with other histologic results. Forty-five patients had complete tumor excisions. Treatment consisted of adjuvant irradiation in 36 patients, with 16 also receiving chemotherapy. Respective 5- and 10-year survival rates were 36% and 14%. Both locoregional and distant relapse free rates (RFR) significantly increased for patients whose tumors were completely excised (Fig 12–17). Patients who were treated with higher dose adjuvant radiation benefitted significantly when infield relapse rates alone were considered (Fig 12–18). Time to relapse approached significance for these patients.

Conclusion.—Failure to excise the tumor completely was the main cause of recurrence in patients with RSTS. Postoperative radiation therapy at higher doses delayed but did not prevent recurrence.

▶ This article looked at 104 patients with RSTS. Although almost one third of the patients in this series had adjuvant radiation therapy and a number also received chemotherapy, the most important issue in the prevention of recurrence was complete excision. Radiation therapy, especially at high doses, may delay recurrence, but it does not prevent it. Our own series show that radiation therapy can be associated with significant morbidity. Until better systemic treatment and/or radiation sensitizers are developed, complete excision will remain the only rational attempt at curative treatment for this malignancy.—T.J. Eberlein, M.D.

Prognostic Factors Predictive of Survival and Local Recurrence for Extremity Soft Tissue Sarcoma
Singer S, Corson JM, Gonin R, Labow B, Eberlein TJ (Harvard Med School, Boston; Harvard School of Public Health/Dana Farber Cancer Inst, Boston)
Ann Surg 219:165–173, 1994   140-95-12–33

Background.—Although standard surgical management of soft tissue sarcoma has been evolving, there is debate about the required size of resections and when adjuvant therapy is indicated. It has been difficult to identify patients who can benefit from adjuvant radiation or chemotherapy. In a retrospective study of 182 patients with soft tissue sarcomas of the extremities, prognostic factors as well as the size and grade of the tumor were sought, and patients who might benefit from adjuvant or neoadjuvant chemotherapy were identified.

| | Predictors of Survival | | | |
Variable	Parameter Estimate	Standard Error	p value	Risk Ratio
Grade				
High *vs.* low	1.56	0.655	0.018	4.76
Size				
> 10 cm *vs.* < 5 cm	1.22	0.442	0.006	3.40
Histology				
Angio, synovial,				
Ewing's *vs.* lipo,				
fibro, peripheral				
nerve	2.54	0.505	0.0001	12.67
Age at diagnosis	0.028	0.012	0.015	1.03
Mean mitotic activity				
(mitoses/10 hpf)	0.055	0.020	0.005	1.06

Abbreviation: hpf, high-power field
(Courtesy of Singer S, Corson JM, Gonin R, et al: *Ann Surg* 219:165-173, 1994.)

Methods.—Data collected prospectively from the 182 patients aged 16-80 years who had soft tissue sarcomas of the extremities were analyzed for factors governing survival and local recurrence. Patients were assessed according to the characteristics of the primary tumor, the type of treatment, and their disease status and survival.

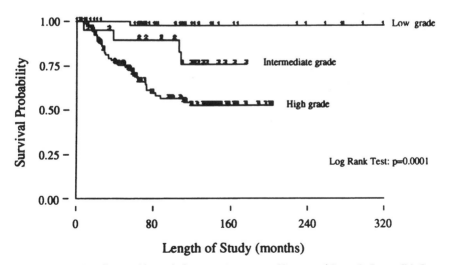

Fig 12–19.—Overall survival by grade for extremity sarcoma. (Courtesy of Singer S, Corson JM, Gonin R, et al: *Ann Surg* 219:165-173, 1994.)

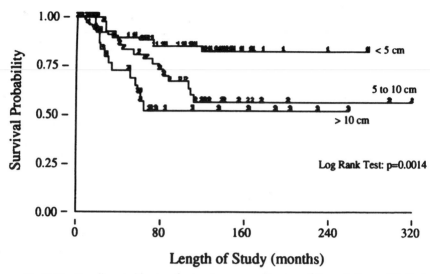

Fig 12–20.—Overall survival by size of extremity sarcoma. (Courtesy of Singer S, Corson JM, Gonin R, et al: *Ann Surg* 219:165–173, 1994.)

Results.—There was a 13-fold increased risk of death associated with a histologic diagnosis of Ewing's sarcoma, synovial sarcoma, and angiosarcoma, compared with a diagnosis of liposarcoma, fibrosarcoma, or malignant peripheral nerve sheath tumor. Important prognostic factors for survival are shown in the table. They include high-grade sarcomas (Fig

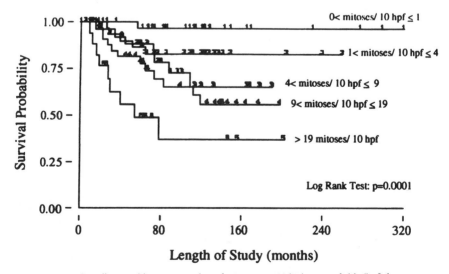

Fig 12–21.—Overall survival by mean number of mitoses per 10 high-power fields (hpf) for sarcoma of an extremity. (Courtesy of Singer S, Corson JM, Gonin R, et al: *Ann Surg* 219:165–173, 1994.)

12–19), sarcomas larger than 10 cm (Fig 12–20), and patient age at diagnosis; these factors were not important for local recurrence. The mean mitotic activity of the tumor was shown to have prognostic value after adjusting for other prognostic factors (Fig 12–21). Locally recurrent disease or microscopically positive margins were the only prognostic factors for local recurrence. There was no difference in the overall survival of patients who did or did not receive adjuvant chemotherapy.

Conclusion.—Grade, size, mitotic activity, and histologic type are prognostic factors for survival in soft tissue sarcomas of the extremities. The mean mitotic activity can be helpful in selecting patients for future adjuvant or neoadjuvant trials and primary therapy. Future chemotherapy trials should include patients with large, high-grade tumors that have high mitotic activity.

▶ The authors studied a series of 182 patients with extremity soft tissue sarcoma. As previously reported, grade and size were associated with survival; however, an objective correlation between mitotic activity and survival was introduced in this article. Therefore, histology and mean mitotic activity may be helpful in selecting patients for an adjuvant protocol. Complete excision of low-grade sarcomas and complete excision with adjuvant radiation therapy for high-grade sarcomas continue to be the treatments of choice.—T.J. Eberlein, M.D.

A Prospective Randomized Trial of Adjuvant Brachytherapy in the Management of Low-Grade Soft Tissue Sarcomas of the Extremity and Superficial Trunk

Pisters PWT, Harrison LB, Woodruff JM, Gaynor JJ, Brennan MF (Mem Sloan-Kettering Cancer Ctr, New York)
J Clin Oncol 12:1150–1155, 1994   140-95-12–34

Introduction.—Adjuvant radiotherapy delivered by the brachytherapy (BRT) technique was found in a previous trial to improve local control of resected soft tissue sarcomas of the extremity and superficial trunk. However, disease-specific survival was not affected, perhaps because only 29 of 126 patients who were enrolled in the study had histologic low-grade sarcomas. In this trial, which was designed to evaluate the impact of adjuvant BRT, all 45 patients had localized, low-grade tumors.

Patients and Methods.—Eligible patients had been admitted to the study institution between July 1982 and June 1992. All had localized extremity lesions that could be completely resected by a limb-sparing procedure or completely resected localized superficial trunk sarcomas. After resection of all gross disease, 22 patients were randomized to BRT and 23 to no adjuvant BRT. The 2 groups were similar in age and sex distribution, tumor characteristics (site, size, and depth), number with primary vs. recurrent sarcomas, and microscopic tumor margins (positive vs. neg-

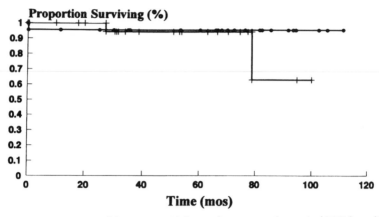

Fig 12–22.—Overall survival for patients with low-grade sarcomas who received BRT (—·—) vs. no BRT (+). (Courtesy of Pisters PWT, Harrison LB, Woodruff JM, et al: *J Clin Oncol* 12:1150–1155, 1994.)

ative). Those in the BRT arm received iridium-192 (45 Gy) that was delivered to the tumor bed for 4–6 days.

Results.—As of January 1, 1993, the overall median follow-up among survivors was 67 months. The predominant histopathologic diagnosis was liposarcoma in both BRT (59%) and no-BRT (61%) groups. There were 6 local recurrences in the BRT group and 5 in the no-BRT group. One patient from the BRT group died of systemic disease, but the remaining patients were treated successfully with additional therapy and are alive with no evidence of disease. As a result, adjuvant therapy had no impact on survival (Fig 12–22). There was no relationship between microscopic tumor margin status and local recurrence in either study arm.

Conclusion.—Local recurrence rates after resection of low-grade soft tissue sarcomas of the extremity and superficial trunk are not lowered by adjuvant radiation in the form of BRT. These patients with low-grade tumors had a very low rate of distant failure and responded well to additional therapy when local recurrences developed. Although BRT yields results similar to those of external beam therapy in patients with high-grade sarcomas, the latter method may be required to prevent local recurrence in low-grade tumors.

▶ In this article from Memorial Sloan-Kettering, adjuvant BRT in the management of low-grade soft tissue sarcomas was explored. No reduction in local recurrence resulting from BRT was reported; however, this most likely was because all the tumors were low-grade and were adequately treated with surgical excision. Brachytherapy is still extremely useful in patients with high-grade sarcoma, especially near joints and where external beam radiation therapy may result in significant morbidity.—T.J. Eberlein, M.D.

Adjuvant CYVADIC Chemotherapy for Adult Soft Tissue Sarcoma— Reduced Local Recurrence But No Improvement in Survival: A Study of the European Organization for Research and Treatment of Cancer Soft Tissue and Bone Sarcoma Group

Bramwell V, Rouesse J, Steward W, Santoro A, Schraffordt-Koops H, Buesa J, Ruka W, Priario J, Wagener T, Burgers M, Van Unnik J, Contesso G, Thomas D, van Glabbeke M, Markham D, Pinedo H (London Regional Cancer Centre, Canada; Institut Gustave-Roussy, Villejuif, France; Christie Hosp, Manchester, England et al)

J Clin Oncol 12:1137–1149, 1994   140-95-12-35

Introduction.—Soft tissue sarcomas exhibit a high rate of metastasis, despite good local control through surgery and adjuvant therapy. Trials of chemotherapy regimens have had mixed results, perhaps because of the variability of patient populations. The effects of adjuvant chemotherapy in adult patients with soft tissue sarcomas were evaluated.

Methods.—Eligible patients had no evidence of metastasis and were able to start chemotherapy no later than 13 weeks after the first resection of the primary tumor or local recurrence; radiotherapy was not among the exclusion criteria. Of 468 patients who met eligibility requirements, 317 were entered into analysis, with 145 randomized to the cyclophosphamide, vincristine, doxorubicin, and dacarbazine (CYVADIC) regimen and the rest serving as controls. On day 1, patients received IV boluses of cyclophosphamide (500 mg/m²), vincristine (1.4 mg/m²), and doxorubicin (50 mg/m²); dacarbazine (400 mg/m² by 1-hour infusion)

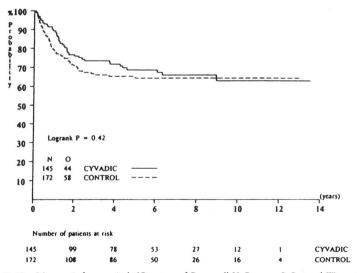

Fig 12–23.—Metastasis-free survival. (Courtesy of Bramwell V, Rouesse J, Steward W, et al: *J Clin Oncol* 12:1137-1149, 1994.)

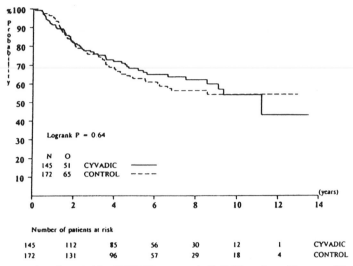

Fig 12–24.—Overall survival for CYVADIC vs. control, all eligible patients. (Courtesy of Bramwell V, Rouesse J, Steward W, et al: *J Clin Oncol* 12:1137–1149, 1994.)

was given on days 1 to 3. Cycles were repeated every 28 days for 8 courses.

Results.—The CYVADIC and control groups were well balanced in terms of sex, age, surgical procedure and margins, and tumor size. The limbs were the site of 68% of sarcomas; 42% of patients received postoperative irradiation. Only 52% of patients completed the full 8 courses of chemotherapy, usually because of side effects or toxicity. One toxic death occurred after the first course of chemotherapy. With a median follow-up of 80 months, the respective rates of relapse-free survival were significantly higher and the local recurrence significantly lower for the CYVADIC group than for the control group (56% vs. 43% and 17% vs. 31%). The 2 groups did not differ significantly in distant metastases (Fig 12–23) or in overall survival (Fig 12–24). The overall reduction in local recurrence was achieved by the effects of chemotherapy in patients with head, neck, and trunk sarcomas; those in the group with limb tumors did not experience this benefit.

Conclusion.—Treatment with adjuvant CYVADIC did not significantly lower the incidence of distant metastases or extend overall survival in these adult patients with soft tissue sarcomas. Based upon these results, the European Organization for the Research and Treatment of Cancer does not recommend adjuvant chemotherapy with CYVADIC outside the context of a clinical trial.

▶ This article reports on a large cooperative trial of the European Organization for Research and Treatment of Cancer. In this study, 317 eligible patients were evaluated. From numerous previous studies, the authors concluded that in extremity soft tissue sarcoma adjuvant chemotherapy does not improve overall survival. Because of a reduction in local recurrence, they are studying neoadjuvant chemotherapy. Outside a clinical trial setting, adjuvant chemotherapy for soft tissue sarcoma is generally not indicated; surgery with or without radiation therapy remains the primary treatment.—T.J. Eberlein, M.D.

Gastric Cancer

▶↓ The following 4 articles address specific issues related to the management of gastric cancer, including prognostic factors, the extent of surgery, and the results of adjuvant therapy.—T.J. Eberlein, M.D.

---

erbB-2 Expression in Well-Differentiated Adenocarcinoma of the Stomach Predicts Shorter Survival After Curative Resection
Motojima K, Furui J, Kohara N, Izawa K, Kanematsu T, Shiku H (Nagasaki Univ School of Medicine, Japan)
Surgery 115:349–354, 1994   140-95-12–36

Objective.—Amplification of the c-*erbB*-2 oncogene has been shown in adenocarcinomas and is associated with increased c-*erbB*-2 messenger RNA (mRNA). The tyrosine kinase oncogene is similar in structure to the epidermal growth factor receptor. Histochemical analysis on 120 gastric carcinomas showed a correlation between *erbB*-2 expression and mortality for patients with well-differentiated gastric adenocarcinomas but not for patients with poorly differentiated gastric adenocarcinomas.

Methods.—Tissue samples were stained and the bound antibody was determined.

Results.—The *erbB*-2 protein was detected in 33 specimens, most of which exhibited heterogeneous expression of the oncogene within the same sample. The presence of the *erbB*-2 protein was detected in 8 of 46 poorly differentiated carcinomas. The positivity of *erbB*-2 increased

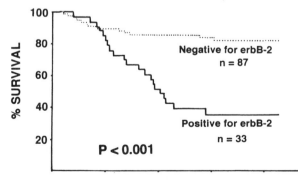

Fig 12–25.—Survival of patients with gastric carcinoma after curative resection. Cumulative survival rates of 120 patients with erbB-2-positive or negative gastric carcinomas. (Courtesy of Motojima K, Furui J, Kohara N, et al: *Surgery* 115:349–354, 1994.)

TABLE 1.—Relationship Between erbB-2 Expression and Clinicopathologic
Characteristics in 120 Patients With
Gastric Carcinomas

Variables	No. of patients	No. of patients positive for erbB–2 (%)	Significance
Age of patients			
<65 yr	48	13 (29)	
≥65 yr	72	20 (28)	NS
Gender of patients			
Male	79	20 (27)	
Female	41	13 (32)	NS
Surgical resection			
Proximal	5	2 (40)	
Total	32	10 (31)	
Distal	83	21 (25)	NS
Tumor location			
Cardia	19	8 (42)	
Middle	61	12 (24)	
Antrum	40	13 (35)	NS
Tumor size			
<5 cm	66	12 (18)	
≥5 cm	54	21 (39)	$p < 0.01$
Serosal invasion			
Negative	96	21 (22)	
Positive	24	12 (50)	$p < 0.01$
Nodal involvement			
Negative	65	8 (12)	
Positive	55	25 (45)	$p < 0.01$
Histologic subtype			
Well differentiated	74	25 (34)	
Poorly differentiated	46	8 (17)	NS

Abbreviation: NS, not significant
(Courtesy of Motojima K, Furui J, Kohara N, et al: *Surgery* 115:349–354, 1994.)

with tumor stage, becoming significant between stages I and II or III. Invading cancers had significantly higher *erbB*-2 expression than superficial carcinomas. Thirty-six patients died of recurrent disease. The 5-year survival rate was 70%. Patients with *erbB*-2 positive tumors had significantly lower survival rates than patients with *erbB*-2 negative tumors (Fig 12–25). There was no correlation between *erbB*-2 positivity and the mortality of patients with poorly differentiated adenocarcinomas. Expression of *erbB*-2 correlated significantly with tumor size, serosal invasion, and nodal involvement (Table 1). In patients with well-

TABLE 2.—Multivariate Analysis of Clinicopathologic Variables and *erb*B-2 Expression for Predicting Recurrent Disease in 120 Patients

Variables	Unfavorable component	Hazard ratio	p Value
Nodal involvement	Positive	3.8	0.0003
*erb*B-2 expression	Positive	2.9	0.0051

(Courtesy of Motojima K, Furui J, Kohara N, et al: *Surgery* 115:349–354, 1994.)

differentiated tumors, nodal involvement was predictive of recurrent disease. (Table 2).

Conclusion.—The expression of *erb*B-2 is predictive of metastatic disease in patients with well-differentiated gastric adenocarcinomas. Such expression is seldom found in poorly differentiated tumors, which carry a worse prognosis but probably involve a different oncogenic progression mechanism.

▶ This article shows that *erb*B-2 expression correlated with a poor prognosis in well-differentiated gastric adenocarcinomas; however, it was not shown to correlate in poorly differentiated carcinomas, which may indicate that either a different oncogene mechanism is involved in poorly differentiated carcinomas or that a poorly differentiated carcinoma has such a bad prognosis it overcomes the influence of *erb*B-2 expression.

As more groups study molecular and genetic markers in gastric and other malignancies, a better understanding of the mechanism of carcinogenesis will be identified. It is hoped that this will then result in more optimal patient selection for adjuvant trials.—T.J. Eberlein, M.D.

Significant Prognostic Factors by Multivariate Analysis of 3926 Gastric Cancer Patients
Kim J-P, Kim Y-W, Yang H-K, Noh D-Y (Seoul National Univ College of Medicine, Korea)
World J Surg 18:872–878, 1994   140-95-12–37

Background.—Early detection and management of gastric cancer, the leading cause of cancer death, are primary goals. Significant prognostic factors, including sex, age, location of the primary tumor, gross type, histologic type, depth of invasion, number of lymph node metastases, and type of treatment were analyzed for their effects on 5-year survival.

Patients and Methods.—Medical records and pathologic reports of 3,926 selected patients with gastric cancer who were treated between 1981 and 1991 were retrospectively reviewed. The UICC TNM staging system was used. Prognostic factors were evaluated using univariate and

Prognostic Factors for Gastric Cancer and Ratio of Relative Risk by
Multivariate Analysis

Prognostic factor	p Value	Relative risk	95% Confidence interval
Depth of invasion	< 0.001*	3.969	2.338–6.739
Lymph node metastasis	< 0.001*	3.105	2.595–3.715
Gross type	0.003*	1.810	1.230–2.663
Location	0.041*	1.564	1.018–2.402
Histologic differentiation	0.002*	1.453	1.152–1.833
Age	0.506	1.116	0.8076–1.542
Sex	0.554	0.9659	0.8610–1.084

* Statistically significant.
(Courtesy of Kim J-P, Kim Y-W, Yang H-K, et al: *World J Surg* 18:872–878, 1994.)

multivariate analyses (table). In addition, immunochemosurgery, postoperative chemotherapy, and surgery alone were assessed for their effects on survival in stage III patients.

Results.—The overall 5-year survival rate of patients with operable gastric cancer was 46.8%. The 5-year survival rates, based on UICC clinical staging, were 90.7% for stage I, 64.5% for stage II, 33.4% for stage III, and 4.9% for stage IV. After analyzing the 5-year cumulative survival for each prognostic factor, univariate analysis showed some significance for age, depth of invasion, lymph node metastasis, location of primary tumor, histologic differentiation, and gross type. Multivariate analysis identified depth of invasion and lymph node metastasis as being the most powerful prognostic factors. Additional significant factors included gross type, location, and histologic differentiation. With respect to postoperative treatment, significantly better survival rates were noted in stage III patients who were treated with immunochemosurgery compared with postoperative chemotherapy and surgery alone.

Conclusion.—The depth of invasion and the number of lymph node metastases are significant prognostic factors in gastric cancer. In patients with advanced gastric cancer, immunochemosurgery may prove beneficial after curative gastric resection.

▶ The article from Seoul, Korea, analyzes almost 4,000 gastric cancer patients. Dr. Kim has invested a lifetime studying this disease, and as one of the international leaders he documents the depth of invasion in lymph node metastasis as being an indicator of a poor prognosis. Immunochemosurgery, that is, a combination of approaches, early postoperative immunotherapy followed by chemotherapy, is introduced. This particular retrospective analysis did not show an appreciable difference between immunochemotherapy or postoperative chemotherapy; however, the author has previously shown that immunochemotherapy was more effective than postoperative chemotherapy in a randomized prospective trial.—T.J. Eberlein, M.D.

A Prospective Randomized Trial Comparing R₁ Subtotal Gastrectomy With R₃ Total Gastrectomy for Antral Cancer

Robertson CS, Chung SCS, Woods SDS, Griffin SM, Raimes SA, Lau JTF, Li AKC (Chinese Univ of Hong Kong, Shatin)

Ann Surg 220:176–182, 1994   140-95-12-38

Introduction.—Survival rates for patients with localized gastric cancer are higher in Japan, where radical surgery with extended lymph node dissection is the common treatment, than in the United States. To determine the contribution of total gastrectomy to survival, subtotal gastrectomy and total gastrectomy were compared prospectively and randomly.

Methods.—Patients with localized gastric adenocarcinoma were randomly assigned to have either the subtotal gastrectomy (25 patients), involving tumor excision and omental resection, or the total gastrectomy (30 patients), involving total omental excision, splenectomy, distal pancreatectomy, lymphatic clearance of the celiac axis, and skeletonization of the porta hepatis vessels. The patients were followed up every 3 months.

Results.—There was only 1 perioperative death—a patient who underwent total gastrectomy and died of intra-abdominal sepsis. The patients who underwent total gastrectomy had longer operations, lost more blood, required more blood transfusions, and had longer hospital stays (Table 1). These patients also had significantly more postoperative complications, including left subphrenic abscess, some of which required relaparotomies, and an esophagojejunal anastomotic leak (Table 2). None of the patients who underwent subtotal gastrectomy experienced

TABLE 1.—Operative Details

	R₁	**R₃**	
Median operation time (min)*	140	260	$p < 0.05$
(range)	(100–300)	(140–375)	
Median blood loss (mL)*	300	600	$p < 0.05$
(range)	(150–1070)	(250–2300)	
No. of patients transfused*	7	23	$p < 0.05$
Median no. of units transfused*	0	2	$p < 0.05$
(range)	(0–6)	(0–6)	
Median postoperative stay (days)	8	16	$p < 0.05$
(range)	(6–17)	(7–97)	

Note: Mann-Whitney U-test.
* Relates to primary procedure only.
(Courtesy of Robertson CS, Chung SCS, Woods SDS, et al: *Ann Surg* 220:176–182, 1994.)

TABLE 2.—Major Morbidity

No. of Patients	Complications	Comments
14	Left subphrenic abscess	5 patients had 6 open drainage operations 4 patients had 7 percutaneous aspirations 4 patients managed conservatively 1 died of sepsis
7	Relaparotomies	5 patients had 6 open drainage operations for L subphrenic abscess 2 patients had 3 secondary haemorrhages (all related to L subphrenic abscess)
3	Oesophagojejunal anastomotic leak	

(Courtesy of Robertson CS, Chung SCS, Woods SDS, et al: *Ann Surg* 220:176–182, 1994.)

major complications or required reoperation. Survival was significantly greater in the subtotal gastrectomy group than in the total gastrectomy group (Fig 12–26).

Discussion.—These findings suggest that the routine performance of total gastrectomy is not responsible for the increased survival of patients

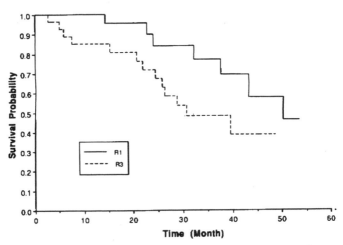

Fig 12–26.—The overall survival curves for the R_1 and R_3 groups. (Courtesy of Robertson CS, Chung SCS, Woods SDS, et al: *Ann Surg* 220:176–182, 1994.)

with gastric carcinoma in Japan. Total gastrectomy resulted in lower survival and higher morbidity than subtotal gastrectomy.

▶ Although this is a small randomized and prospective series, one of the major issues in the management of gastric cancer is addressed. The extent of surgical excision in general in the Pacific Basin series results in higher survival than in the United States. However, in this randomized series total gastrectomy was associated with reduced survival and increased morbidity. In addition to total gastrectomy, the patients also underwent splenectomy and distal pancreatectomy as well as extensive lymph node dissection. This may well have accounted for the increased morbidity.—T.J. Eberlein, M.D.

The Second British Stomach Cancer Group Trial of Adjuvant Radiotherapy or Chemotherapy in Resectable Gastric Cancer: Five-Year Follow-Up
Hallissey MT for the British Stomach Cancer Group (Queen Elizabeth Hosp, Birmingham, England; Epsom Gen Hosp, England)
Lancet 343:1309–1312, 1994   140-95-12-39

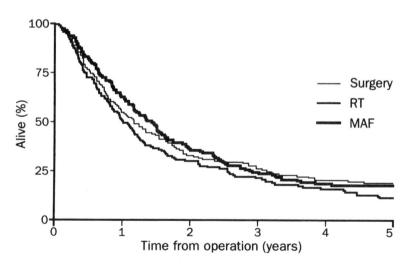

Treatment		No at risk			
S	145	81	49	40	31	29
RT	153	79	47	34	26	18
MAF	138	88	50	35	27	26

Fig 12–27.—Survival by treatment. (Courtesy of Hallissey MT, for the British Stomach Cancer Group: *Lancet* 343:1309–1312, 1994.)

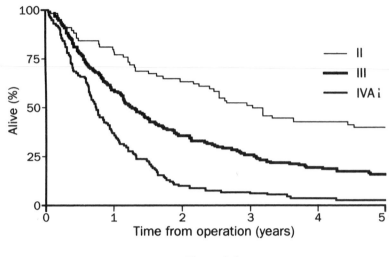

Fig 12–28.—Survival by BSCG-II stage. (Courtesy of Hallissey MT, for the British Stomach Cancer Group: *Lancet* 343:1309–1312, 1994.)

Introduction.—Survival in patients undergoing surgery alone was compared with that of patients who received adjuvant radiotherapy (RT) or chemotherapy, consisting of mitomycin, doxorubicin, and fluorouracil (MAF). Results of this trial were reported with minimum follow-up of 5 years.

Patients and Methods.—Eligible patients, who were recruited from 10 centers in the United Kingdom, had undergone resection for histologically proven adenocarcinoma of the stomach. They were entered into the trial within 4 weeks of surgery, because results of an earlier trial had shown adjuvant treatment to be most effective when started early. A total of 436 patients entered the trial between June 1981 and July 1986; 145 were randomized to surgery alone, 153 to surgery plus RT, and 138 to surgery plus MAF. Of the patients allocated to chemotherapy, 23 were not treated and 39 required dose modifications. The protocol-defined RT dose was given to 102 of 117 patients.

Results.—After at least 5 years 372 patients had died, including 327 from recurrent cancer. The median duration of survival for the group as a whole was 14 months; the longest duration of survival was 9.8 years. The 3 treatment groups did not differ significantly in survival rates (Fig 12–27). Five–year survival was 20% for surgery alone, 12% for surgery plus RT, and 19% for surgery plus MAF. The final clinicopathologic stage influenced both 5-year survival and the median duration of survival (Fig 12–28). Patients with stage II cancer had a 5-year survival rate of 39% and a median survival of 38 months; the corresponding figures for stage IVA were 5% and 9 months.

Conclusion.—The addition of chemotherapy or radiotherapy to surgical resection did not yield a survival advantage for patients with gastric cancer. Overall survival remains low for this malignancy, indicating a need for increased early diagnosis and more effective chemotherapy regimens. The use of adjuvant treatment should be limited to controlled trials.

▶ The final article in this series is from the British Stomach Cancer Group, which reports on a series of 436 patients with minimum 5-year follow-up. Adjuvant therapy of either kind did not prolong survival, emphasizing the need for earlier diagnosis. Neoadjuvant trials are currently underway, and whereas they have been associated with increased morbidity, they may demonstrate a survival benefit in selected patients.—T.J. Eberlein, M.D.

Pancreatic Cancer

A Comparison of Long Term Results of the Standard Whipple Procedure and the Pylorus Preserving Pancreatoduodenectomy

Kozuschek W, Reith HB, Waleczek H, Haarmann W, Edelmann M, Sonntag D (Ruhr Univ Bochum, Germany)
J Am Coll Surg 178:443–458, 1994   140-95-12–40

Background.—Patients undergoing the standard Whipple procedure experience intestinal disturbances such as dumping, diarrhea, dyspepsia, and ulcers at the gastroenterostomy. In one study, a postoperative, usually persistent weight loss of 10–40 kg was observed. Some authors have suggested that preserving the stomach, pylorus, and small portions of the duodenum might prevent complications that arise from the loss of gastric reservoir function, thereby improving postoperative malnutrition. To date, no studies have compared the long-term results of the standard vs. the pylorus-preserving Whipple procedure in terms of digestive and endocrine function. A recent experience with these 2 procedures was reviewed, focusing on the postoperative complications and nutritional status.

Patients.—The nonrandomized study included 68 patients who were operated on for malignant disease between 1985 and 1992. Forty-three patients had the pylorus-preserving Whipple procedure, or pancreatoduodenectomy (PPPD), and 25 had the standard Whipple procedure. On average, 3 cm of the duodenum was preserved in the former group. The

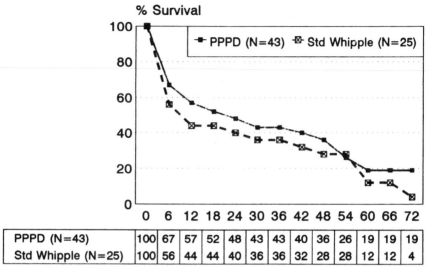

	0	6	12	18	24	30	36	42	48	54	60	66	72
PPPD (N=43)	100	67	57	52	48	43	43	40	36	26	19	19	19
Std Whipple (N=25)	100	56	44	44	40	36	36	32	28	28	12	12	4

Time in months

Fig 12–29.—For patients with periampullary carcinoma, the survival time in months was similar for the pylorus preserving modified Whipple procedure (PPPD) vs. the standard Whipple group. The average survival time was 43.2 (PPPD) vs. 36.3 months. (Courtesy of Kozuschek W, Reith HB, Waleczek H, et al: *J Am Coll Surg* 178:443–458, 1994.)

constitution and postoperative results of the 2 groups were compared, including nutritional status and weight behavior as well as extensive functional tests, such as orocecal transit time, blood glucose daily profile, oral and IV glucose tolerance tests, and maximal beta-cell stimulation.

Findings.—For patients with carcinoma, survival was 57% at 1 year and 19% at 5 years (Fig 12-29). The PPPD group had a significantly better capacity for food uptake and development of body weight: Eighty-six percent reached their preoperative weight within 1 year compared with 43% of the standard Whipple group (Fig 12-30). Gastric or jejunal ulcers only occurred in the standard Whipple group. The PPPD group showed no clinical signs of digestive disorders, such as dumping syndrome (table). Preserving the opening mechanism of the pylorus did not impede nutrition or digestion. Transit time was preserved in the PPPD group, but it was significantly increased in the standard Whipple group. Postoperative exocrine function was only slightly decreased by PPPD. Postoperative glucose metabolism was only slightly affected in the PPPD group, but it was depressed in the standard Whipple group.

Conclusion.—The pylorus-preserving Whipple procedure has some important long-term advantages over the standard Whipple procedure. The restricted organ loss of the PPPD leaves the secretory and functional capacity of the upper gastrointestinal tract almost unaltered. Patients are therefore better able to regain their preoperative weight without gastric

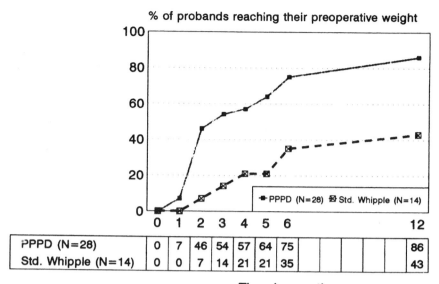

% of probands reaching their preoperative weight

	0	1	2	3	4	5	6				12
PPPD (N=28)	0	7	46	54	57	64	75				86
Std. Whipple (N=14)	0	0	7	14	21	21	35				43

Time in months

Fig 12–30.—More patients were able to gain their preoperative weight in the PPPD group as compared to the standard Whipple group. The difference was significant ($P < .05$), 6 and 12 months postoperatively. (Courtesy of Kozuschek W, Reith HB, Waleczek H, et al: *J Am Coll Surg* 178:443–458, 1994.)

or jejunal ulcers and without clinical signs of digestive disorders. There was no difference in survival between the 2 operations.

▶ This article reports on a nonrandomized study; therefore, selection bias is possible. Whereas no survival disadvantage to pyloric-sparing Whipple procedures was shown, this study did show a somewhat better functional result. Pyloric-sparing Whipples are somewhat easier to perform and have generally

Digestion After PPPD and Standard Whipple Procedure, One Year After Operation

Digestion	*PPPD, n=28*	*Whipple, n=19*
Normal	24 (86)	8 (43)
50 to 90 percent of normal . .	4 (14)	11 (57)
Dumping syndrome	0	2
Emesis	0	1 (5)
Peptic ulcer	0	2 (11)
Enzyme supplement required .	2 (7)	6 (32)

Numbers in parentheses are percentages.
(Courtesy of Kozuschek W, Reith HB, Waleczek H, et al: *J Am Coll Surg* 178:443–458, 1994.)

not been associated with reduced survival. Although careful selection is necessary, especially when there is a large tumor and/or involvement in the wall of the duodenum, pyloric-preserving Whipple procedures are particularly attractive in the treatment of nonmalignant disease.—T.J. Eberlein, M.D.

Factors Influencing Survival After Resection of Pancreatic Cancer: A DNA Analysis and a Histomorphologic Study

Böttger TC, Störkel S, Wellek S, Stöckle M, Junginger T (Johannes Gutenberg Univ, Mainz, Germany)
Cancer 73:63–73, 1994   140-95-12–41

Objective.—The prognosis for patients with pancreatic cancer is poor. Resection results in a mean survival time of 16 months and carries a 5% to 10% mortality. Factors influencing survival have not been well established, but the DNA content of tumor cells could be predictive. The prognostic potential of DNA contents and that of histologic variables were compared.

Methods.—Paraffin-embedded tumor sections from 41 patients were stained, graded from 1 to 4 using the tumor-metastasis node classification of the International Union Against Cancer and analyzed for DNA content using the Leytas method. Patients were followed up at 3-month intervals, and all died by the end of the study.

Results.—The DNA histogram showed 1 hypotriploid, 7 triploid, 21 hypertriploid, and 12 tetraploid patterns. About half the patients with

Multivariate Analysis for Prognostic Relevant Factors in Pancreatic Cancer*

Independent variable	Regression coefficient	Standard error	*P*-value	Partial correlation ratio† (r^2 par)
R0 vs R1/R2				
resection	0.9211	0.2825	0.0025	0.2382
Tetraploid	0.7469	0.2394	0.0037	0.2226
Nuclear grading	−0.1589	0.3966	0.6911	0.0047
Grade of				
differentiation	−0.2544	0.3991	0.5282	0.0119
Tumor stage	−0.1958	0.2234	0.3869	0.0222
Tumor size 2 cm	−0.0868	0.2097	0.6816	0.0051

* Multiple linear regression with log-normally distributed errors.
† Relative reduction of the error sum of squares attained by incorporating the respective variable as an additional regressor.
Abbreviations: RO, no residual tumor; R1, microscopic residual tumor; R2, macroscopic residual tumor.
(Courtesy of Böttger TC, Störkel S, Wellek S, et al: *Cancer* 73:63–73, 1994.)

tumors less than 2 cm and 12.5% of patients with tumors larger than 2 cm survived 18 months. About 45% of patients with no lymph node metastasis and 18% of patients with lymph node metastasis survived 18 months. About 70% of patients with tumor stage 1A but no patients with tumor stage 1B survived 18 months. Although the differences were not significant, about 36% of patients with grade 1 and 2 tumors survived 18 months, whereas only 16% of patients with grade 3 and 4 tumors survived that long. In patients who had tumors with a nuclear grade of 1 or 2, 61% survived 18 months, whereas only 11% of patients who had tumors with a nuclear grade of 3 or 4 survived that long. No patients with residual tumors survived 18 months, whereas 32% of patients without residual tumors survived that long. The DNA content was not associated with tumor size or stage, grade of differentiation, or nuclear grade.

Conclusion.—The DNA histogram type was the strongest prognostic indicator of survival (table). Additional studies on more patients should be done to establish the clinical suitability of these criteria.

▶ Survival of pancreatic cancer remains poor. In this study, despite the radical nature of the operative procedure, DNA content had the strongest influence on the prognosis. Until more effective systemic treatments are introduced, biological and genetic markers associated with pancreatic cancer may lead to biological or immunotherapeutic treatments.—T.J. Eberlein, M.D.

Liver

Liver Transplantation for Hepatocellular Carcinoma
Chung SW, Toth JL, Rezieg M, Cameron R, Taylor BR, Greig PD, Levy GA, Langer B (Univ of Toronto, Canada)
Am J Surg 167:317–321, 1994   140-95-12–42

Background.—Hepatocellular carcinoma (HCC) has traditionally been treated by surgical resection, with high tumor recurrence rates depending on the stage of the lesion. Orthotopic liver transplantation (OLT) has been performed in patients with locally unresectable HCC or with unifocal or multifocal tumors in a cirrhotic liver. The value of this treatment has been questioned because a high incidence of early tumor recurrence in the transplanted liver has been reported. An experience with OLT in 29 patients with HCC was reported.

Patients.—The patients were 22 men and 7 women, with an average age of 53 years. All were carefully screened before OLT to select only those whose tumors had favorable morphologic features confined to the liver and were not associated with major complications of either the tumor or liver disease. Twenty-five patients had cirrhosis, and 19 of them had known or suspected HCC before OLT. Hepatitis B surface antigen (HBsAG) testing was positive in 19 patients. Immunotherapy or adjuvant chemotherapy was not given before or after OLT. The patients were followed up for a mean of 33 months.

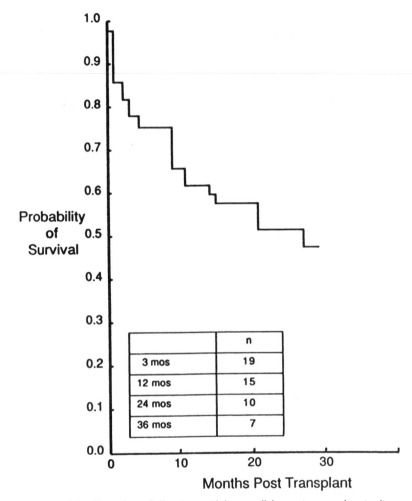

Fig 12–31.—Life-table analysis of all patients with hepatocellular carcinoma undergoing liver transplantation. (Courtesy of Chung SW, Toth JL, Rezieg M, et al: *Am J Surg* 167:317–321, 1994.)

Outcomes.—Overall actuarial survival after OLT was 75% at 3 months, 61% at 1 year, and 46% at 3 years (Fig 12–31). Survival was significantly better in HBsAg-negative than in HBsAg-positive patients at 69% vs. 18% at 3 years (Fig 12–32). The 2 survivors in the HBsAg-positive group had recurrent and aggressive hepatitis B viral infection.

Conclusion.—For carefully selected patients with otherwise unresectable HCC, OLT is associated with a low recurrence rate. However, mortality is high among patients who are HBsAg positive, suggesting that they are poor candidates for OLT. Further gains in survival may be possible with adjuvant chemotherapy.

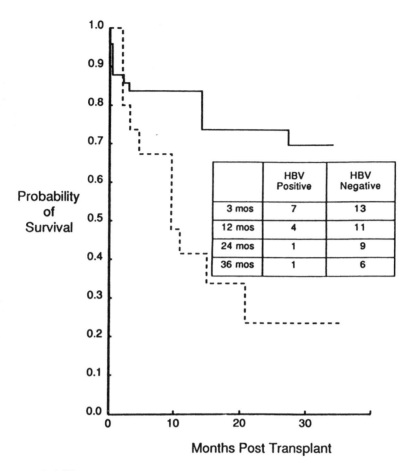

	HBV Positive	HBV Negative
3 mos	7	13
12 mos	4	11
24 mos	1	9
36 mos	1	6

Months Post Transplant

p = 0.045

Fig 12–32.—Life-table analysis comparing patients with hepatocellular carcinoma who were either hepatitis B virus (*HBV*) positive or HBV negative undergoing liver transplantation. *Solid line,* HBV negative; *dotted line,* HBV positive. (Courtesy of Chung SW, Toth JL, Rezieg M, et al: *Am J Surg* 167:317–321, 1994.)

▶ Liver transplantation can result in significant survival. In this series, patients who were HBsAG negative had a significantly improved survival over patients who were HBsAG positive. Because HCC is associated with hepatitis infection, improved screening and earlier diagnosis might result in patients being treated with surgery; OLT could then be avoided.—T.J. Eberlein, M.D.

Surgical Management of Regional Lymph Nodes in Patients With Melanoma

Slingluff CL Jr, Stidham KR, Ricci WM, Stanley WE, Seigler HF (Univ of Virginia Health Sciences Ctr, Charlottesville; Duke Univ Med Ctr, Durham, NC)
Ann Surg 219:120–130, 1994   140-95-12–43

Purpose.—There is retrospective evidence that elective lymph node dissection may improve prognosis for patients with melanomas of intermediate thickness. However, this contention has not held up in 2 prospective, randomized trials. To obtain a clearer understanding of the behavior and appropriate management of draining lymph nodes and reassess the clinical value of elective lymph node dissections (ELNDs), a large series of patients with cutaneous melanoma who had or were at risk of lymph node metastases were evaluated.

Methods.—The retrospective study included 4,682 patients who were treated at a single institution for localized or regional melanomas. The site of the primary lesion was carefully recorded and grouped according to regions, based on expected drainage patterns. The patients were followed for a median of 5 years, with 314 patients being followed for more than 10 years.

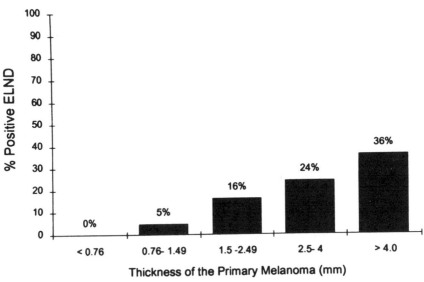

Thickness of the Primary Melanoma (mm)

Fig 12–33.—The results of ELND. For melanomas < 0.76-mm thick, 0 of 43 ELND performed in 43 patients were positive. For melanomas 0.76 to 1.49 mm in thickness, 14 of 298 ELND performed in 295 patients were positive. For melanomas 1.5 to 2.49 mm in thickness, 47 of 291 ELND performed in 284 patients were positive. For melanomas 2.5 to 4.0-mm thick, 45 of 186 ELND performed in 182 patients were positive. For melanomas > 4-mm thick, 40 of 111 ELND performed in 107 patients were positive. The total results were 146 of 929 ELND (16%) performed in 911 patients were positive. (Courtesy of Slingluff CL Jr, Stidham KR, Ricci WM, et al: *Ann Surg* 219:120–130, 1994.)

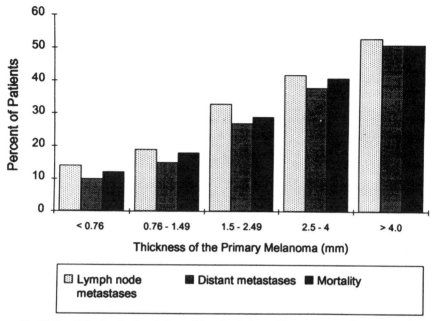

Fig 12–34.—Risk of regional and distant failure by thickness. The percentage of patients in whom lymph node metastases developed during the follow-up period is shown for each of 5 thickness ranges. These closely match the percentage of patients with distant metastases and the mortality rate. For the 5 thickness ranges (< 0.76, 0.76 to 1.49, 1.5 to 2.49, 2.5 to 4, and > 4mm, respectively), the numbers of patients were 769, 1612, 1091, 676, and 534, and the median follow-up periods were 5.0, 5.4, 4.8, 3.8, and 3.2 years. (Courtesy of Slingluff CL Jr, Stidham KR, Ricci WM, et al: *Ann Surg* 219:120–130, 1994.)

Findings.—Ten percent of patients with nodal metastases had them in contralateral nodes, with 6% in nodal basins that would not have been predicted by the classic models of lymph node drainage. Thirteen percent of patients with metastases and 3% of patients overall had nodal metastases to more than 1 nodal basin. For all thicknesses, nodal and distant metastases were comparable in incidence. At baseline, 3,550 patients had clinically negative regional nodal basins: 26% of them underwent ELND. The percentage of patients with positive nodes ranged from 0% in patients with melanoma thicknesses less than .76 mm to 36% of those with thicknesses greater than 4 mm (Fig 12–33). Nodal metastases occurred in 23% of patients who underwent ELND: 143 at the time of the operation and 71 later. In the latter group, 44% had metastases in a previously dissected basin and 56% in a previously undissected basin. Patients with clinically negative nodes who were treated with and without ELND, stratified for thickness and primary site, showed no significant difference in survival (Fig 12–34, table).

Conclusion.—The findings cast doubt on the value of ELND in patients with melanoma. In patients with intermediate-thickness melanomas, the risk of nodal metastases is no more common than the risk of

Survival With Or Without Elective Lymph Node Dissection			
Thickness	No LND (n)	ELND (n)	p Value
	5-year survival estimates*		
Extremity			
<0.76 mm	90% (233)	100% (28)	0.048
0.76–1.5 mm	90% (363)	91% (139)	0.234
1.5–2.5 mm	81% (168)	88% (131)	0.053
2.5–4.0 mm	68% (74)	66% (87)	0.695
>4.0 mm	62% (63)	59% (48)	0.274
Trunk			
<0.76 mm	94% (260)	86% (13)	0.813
0.76–1.5 mm	87% (467)	86% (96)	0.120
1.5–2.5 mm	75% (261)	80% (85)	0.492
2.5–4.0 mm	70% (147)	64% (43)	0.871
>4.0 mm	49% (108)	36% (38)	0.149
Head/Neck			
<0.76 mm	92% (83)	< 100 (2)	0.660
0.76–1.5 mm	81% (164)	85% (48)	0.401
1.5–2.5 mm	81% (87)	71% (53)	0.832
2.5–4.0 mm	66% (51)	56% (33)	0.929
>4.0 mm	51% (54)	20% (16)	0.017

* Kaplan-Meier survival estimates.
(Courtesy of Slingluff CL Jr, Stidham KR, Ricci WM, et al: *Ann Surg* 219:120–130, 1994.)

distant metastases. Only 16% of ELND procedures are positive, and ELND does not necessarily prevent recurrent nodal disease in the dissected basin. The procedure offers no apparent survival advantage. Lymphoscintigraphy may be of value in the preoperative assessment of patients with ELND.

▶ This is a very large single-institution retrospective study. These authors concluded that ELND was of limited therapeutic value. The findings from this group as well as other randomized trials have led to the utilization of lymphoscintigraphy or vital dyes and sentinel node biopsy. The latter method has been particularly helpful in identifying patients who might benefit from therapeutic lymph node dissection.—T.J. Eberlein, M.D.

Hodgkin's Disease

With Modern Imaging Techniques, Is Staging Laparotomy Necessary in Pediatric Hodgkin's Disease? A Pediatric Oncology Group Study

Mendenhall NP, Cantor AB, Williams JL, Ternberg JL, Weiner MA, Kung FH, Marcus RB Jr, Ferree CR, Leventhal BG (Univ of Florida, Gainesville; Washington Univ School of Medicine, St Louis, Mo; Hackensack Med Ctr, NJ; et

al)
J Clin Oncol 11:2218–2225, 1993   140-95-12-44

Introduction.—The existence of effective treatments that do not require precise delineation of abdominal disease, the potential morbidity of laparotomy, and cost concerns have increased interest in reducing the use of staging laparotomy in Hodgkin's disease (table) patients. Whether imaging studies and clinical assessments can predict the information gained by staging laparotomy in children with Hodgkin's disease was determined.

Methods.—Two hundred sixteen consecutive children with Hodgkin's disease underwent laparotomy. The children were treated on 2 concurrent pediatric oncology group protocols. Imaging evaluation included CT of the chest, abdomen, and pelvis. Among the clinical factors examined were sedimentation rate, B symptoms, histologic findings, number and location of involved sites, mediastinal involvement, and age. The pretreatment CT scans of 88 children were reviewed for the presence and size of supradiaphragmatic and infradiaphragmatic lymph nodes, intrinsic splenic lesions, and splenic size. The investigators created models to predict the presence of abdominal disease, splenic or extensive splenic involvement, and upstaging at laparotomy.

Results.—The model for prediction of any abdominal disease—based on B symptoms, histologic findings, sedimentation rate, and the number and location of involved sites—was highly significant. However, it was of only limited value in predicting abdominal disease in individual patients, with a false negative rate of 26% and a false positive rate of 32%. False positive and false negative rates were similarly high for the significant models to predict splenic and extensive splenic involvement and upstaging at laparotomy (Fig 12–35).

Conclusion.—For most children with Hodgkin's disease, CT and clinical factors are unable to predict the findings of staging laparotomy. The models developed in this study can predict laparotomy findings in no more than 20% of patients.

Incidence of Stage Change by Laparotomy

Clinical Stage	No. of Patients	Pathologic Stage				Total Stage Changes	
		I/II	III₁*	III₂	IV	No.	%
I/II	181	133	36	9	3	48	27
III₁	9	2	3	4	—	6	67
III₂	9	—	2	7	—	2	22
IV	4	—	—	—	4	0	0

* Excludes 13 pathologic stage III, patients in whom clinical stage was not reported.
(Courtesy of Mendenhall NP, Cantor AB, Williams JL, et al: *J Clin Oncol* 11:2218-2225, 1993.)

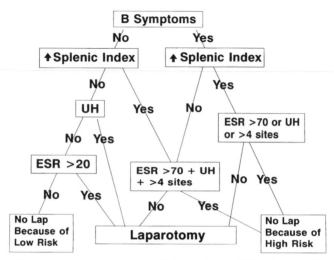

Fig 12–35.—Decision tree for laparotomy in Hodgkin's disease. *UH*, unfavorable histology (not lymphocyte-predominant or nodular sclerosis); *ESR*, erythrocyte sedimentation rate; *Lap*, laparotomy. (Courtesy of Mendenhall NP, Cantor AB, Williams JL, et al: *J Clin Oncol* 11:2218–2225, 1993.)

▶ With the advent of new CT and other noninvasive staging techniques, the need for a staging laparotomy has been called into question. This study of consecutive patients from the pediatric oncology group demonstrated that the ability to predict abdominal disease in any individual patient was very limited, thereby justifying a staging laparotomy until more effective noninvasive techniques can be developed.—T.J. Eberlein, M.D.

13 Plastic, Reconstructive, and Head and Neck Surgery

Introduction

The YEAR BOOK and I have laid out quite a plate for the reader in this section on plastic, reconstructive, and head and neck surgery. We have included 3 articles on breast reconstruction after mastectomy: the first, from M.D. Anderson Cancer Center on outcomes (Abstract 140-95-13–1), the second on trends over the past 10 to 15 years (Abstract 140-95-13–2), and a third paper that examines the complications in those reconstruction patients who also have adjuvant chemotherapy (Abstract 140-95-13–4). The reader will note that the trend is clearly toward the use of autogenous tissue (transverse rectus abdominis myocutaneous flap) rather than alloplastic materials (silicone implants) in postmastectomy breast reconstruction. This trend may have started well before the silicone crisis and may have its roots in the better aesthetic and functional results obtained. Judge for yourself.

The fourth paper (Abstract 140-95-13–3) is an example of the type of scientific investigation that is badly needed in the arena of clinical surgery, namely, outcomes studies. This study examined reduction mammaplasty to demonstrate the medical efficacy of the procedure. The single burn paper included (Abstract 140-95-13–5) examines the ongoing controversy regarding the use of homograft skin and immunosuppression.

Similar comments apply to the paper on long term follow-up of patients who have had flap reconstruction of median sternotomy wound dehiscence (Abstract 140-95-13–6). This paper should be read carefully, though, because of some problems in the study design. Two other papers (Abstracts 140-95-13–7 and 140-95-13–8) examine abdominal wall problems in postoperative surgery patients and are worth perusal. Goretex mesh continues to have problems with recurrence in the repair of abdominal wall hernias.

We have selected a wide range of papers in head and neck surgery to cover the topics of basic science, diagnoses, extirpation, reconstruction, and outcomes. The basic science studies continue to focus on efforts to determine tumor markers utilizing molecular biology and molecular genetic techniques. Clearly, these methods are experimental at present, and yet one has the distinct sense that we are on the brink of broad-based clinical applications of these techniques in the management of the head and neck cancer patient. I think you will find these papers quite readable and comprehensible, even with a novice's understanding of molecular biology (such as mine).

In the diagnostic section, the use of positron emission tomography (PET) scans on head and neck patients is discussed and some surprising results are reported. The second paper reexamines the topic of routine panendoscopy in head and neck patients and arrives at some sensible conclusions and methods for reducing the costs.

In the extirpative aspect, we allow the reader to examine several debatable topics regarding the head and neck. Included is a paper on carotid artery resection (Abstract 140-95-13–11), another on positive margins from an intergroup study (Abstract 140-95-13–13), and a third on the appropriate management of patients who have carcinoma of the thyroid that actively invades the airway (Abstract 140-95-13–15). The reader may reach a different conclusion from these investigations than do the authors. Included also is a paper on parotidectomy and melanoma (Abstract 140-95-13–12) that adopts a fresh examination of the efficacy of parotidectomy and node dissection in melanoma. The final paper in that section (Abstract 140-95-13–14) is a comparison of radiotherapy vs. microlaryngoscopy and excision in the treatment of T1 carcinomas of the larynx. The Pittsburgh group didn't just assess curage but weighed the costs as well.

Although a large number of papers on head and neck reconstruction passed over my desk, I made an effort to select those that had some element of assessment of outcomes rather than a "show and tell" format that is distressingly common in such papers. Included are 2 papers on reconstruction of the mandible with microvascular techniques. Both papers were included for separate reasons: One is an assessment of the rationale for aggressive pursuit of reconstruction at advanced disease and the other a measure of our success and use of the appropriate flaps to insure that success. Included also are papers on arteriovenous malformations, extensive skin cancer reconstruction, and a new approach to glossectomy reconstruction. A large series of free flaps (over 300) has also been selected to give the reader a perspective on 1 center's approach and results.

The section on head and neck surgery that I have dubbed "outcomes" is a collection of papers that assess and discuss functional status in head and neck cancer patients. We must be able to demonstrate in the future how we have beneficially affected quality of life and move beyond a discussion of cure rates and survival. The authors discuss the use of measurement tools that may facilitate this process. Other topics in this section include the elderly patient with head and neck cancer, organ preservation (besides the larynx) with utilization of induction chemotherapy plus radiotherapy; and another innovative technique, the use of photodynamic therapy in patients who have had field cancerization.

The best may have been saved for the last in a miscellaneous reconstruction category that includes some very exciting papers. The first abstract in this section (Abstract 140-95-13-30) concerns a small series of children with advanced and massive hemangiomas treated with interferon-α2a. The paper is immensely readable and gives the reader a background in the natural history of childhood hemangiomas. The second paper (Abstract 140-95-13-31), a report of the experience of the Mayo Clinic with infected peripheral vascular grafts, discusses salvage with the use of muscle flaps. The third (Abstract 140-95-13-32) is another highly innovative attempt to solve a difficult problem—pressure ulcers—with the use of drug therapy. Growth factors continue to dominate the fields of both experimental and clinical aspects of wound healing. The last 2 papers (Abstracts 140-95-13-33 and 140-95-13-34) fall into the category of "desperate appliances for desperate diseases" and include the use of latissimus muscle for a cardiomyoplasty and muscle reconstruction of sarcoma defects.

In summary, as one sage stated, some of these offerings on the readers' plate are for tasting and sampling only; others are to be more carefully contemplated and digested.

Edward A. Luce, M.D.

Breast

Bilateral Breast Reconstruction: Conventional Versus Free TRAM

Baldwin BJ, Schusterman MA, Miller MJ, Kroll SS, Wang B-g (MD Anderson Cancer Ctr, Houston)
Plast Reconstr Surg 93:1410–1416, 1994   140-95-13–1

Introduction.—The transverse rectus abdominis myocutaneous (TRAM) flap procedure is an effective form of breast reconstruction when used as a pedicled or free-tissue transfer. Transfer of a free TRAM flap now is routinely offered.

Study Plan.—The value of the free TRAM flap approach in bilateral breast reconstruction was examined in 46 patients, 18 of whom received free TRAM flaps and 28 of whom received conventional superior-pedicled TRAM flaps after bilateral mastectomies (Fig 13-1). Both bilateral pedicled and free flaps were usually placed in the ipsilateral breast pocket, using muscle-sparing flap elevation according to the surgeon's preference. The thoracodorsal vessels were the preferred recipient vessels. The 2 patient groups were similar in age, body weight, and stage of disease. A large majority of patients in each group underwent immediate reconstruction.

Results.—The conventional TRAM flap procedure required 6.6 hours on average and entailed blood loss of 313 c³. In contrast, free TRAM flap reconstruction took 9.6 hours and was attended by an average blood loss of 575 c³. The latter figures improved as more experience was

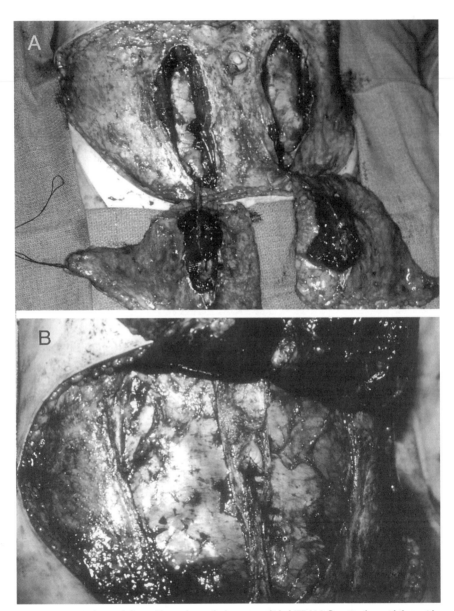

Fig 13–1.—**A,** donor defect with total muscle harvest pedicled TRAM flap. **B,** donor defect with muscle-splitting free TRAM flap. *Abbreviation: TRAM,* transverse rectus abdominis myocutaneous. (Courtesy of Baldwin BJ, Schusterman MA, Miller MJ, et al: *Plast Reconstr Surg* 93:1410–1416, 1994.)

gained, and the hospital stay was similar for the 2 patient groups. Seven conventional TRAM flaps but none of the free TRAM flaps were complicated by partial flap or fat necrosis. There were 3 flap losses in this group early in the series. Three patients in each operative group had seromas, and 1 given free TRAM flaps had a breast-pocket hematoma. The overall rate of complications was 50% in the patients having pedicled TRAM flap reconstruction and 33% with free flaps.

Conclusion.—Bilateral free TRAM flap reconstruction can prevent partial flap loss and fat necrosis, with the attendant delay in postoperative radiotherapy or chemotherapy. It is a more labor-intensive procedure than pedicle flap reconstruction, but may be useful for patients who have had abdominal surgery and others who are poor candidates for a pedicled flap procedure.

▶ The authors, from M.D. Anderson Cancer Center, in a series of publications on breast reconstruction have refined the process of breast reconstruction and examined the outcomes critically. An eloquent case is made in this paper for the use of free-tissue transfer of the TRAM flap for bilateral breast reconstruction, with the additional investment of operative time reaping dividends in abdominal wall integrity and decreased complications in the reconstruction site.—E.A. Luce, M.D.

Changing Trends in Postmastectomy Breast Reconstruction: A 13-Year Experience
Trabulsy PP, Anthony JP, Mathes SJ (San Francisco)
Plast Reconstr Surg 93:1418–1427, 1994   140-95-13–2

Introduction.—During the past 2 decades, there have been important developments in the techniques and materials used in ablative surgery for breast cancer and breast reconstruction. The trends in the timing and techniques of reconstruction over the past 15 years were reviewed and the efficacy analyzed.

Methods.—Data on mastectomy and reconstruction were derived from the hospital records, operative notes, and clinic charts of 381 women undergoing 455 postmastectomy breast reconstructions between 1979 and 1991. The data collected included mastectomy indications and techniques, tumor pathology, the timing and technique of the breast reconstruction, and results and complications of each procedure. The patients were divided into 3 groups: group I patients were treated in 1979 through 1983; those in group II were treated in 1984 through 1987; and those in group III were treated in 1988 through 1991. The data for each group were compared with those for the other groups to determine trends.

Results.—The groups did not differ in indications for mastectomy, but the use of radical mastectomy declined considerably during the study period. The chronological groups demonstrated a significant trend toward immediate, rather than delayed, reconstruction, from 6% in group I to 25% in group II and 28% in group III. Although in the majority of patients in all 3 groups nonautogenous reconstruction techniques were used, the use of autogenous flap reconstruction (both TRAM and free flaps) increased over time from 13% to 37%. Among those undergoing nonautogenous reconstruction, the use of implants alone decreased, the use of tissue expansion plus implant increased, and the use of a latissimus dorsi flap plus implant decreased over time. These trends tended to increase operative time, but the autogenous reconstruction involved fewer revisional procedures.

Discussion.—Although breast cancer pathology remained essentially unchanged, the extirpative and reconstructive treatments changed considerably, with fewer radical mastectomies, more immediate reconstruction, and more autogenous or tissue expander/implant techniques being used. These newly developed techniques allow more options for a customized approach to patients requiring postmastectomy breast reconstruction.

▶ This paper is an excellent summary of the evolution of breast reconstruction over the past 10 to 15 years and demonstrates the trend toward immediate breast reconstruction with autogenous material. Although the authors' numbers demonstrate a preference still for nonautogenous reconstruction, the much higher incidence of revision in the nonautogenous (expander plus implant) group is an eloquent argument for leaning toward the use of autogenous tissue. The authors, like many plastic surgeons, have reserved microsurgical techniques for breast reconstruction for the patient in whom pedicled tissue transfer might be more risky for a variety of reasons. Because microsurgery continues to become more sophisticated and efficient, if a further follow-up is published 5 years from now, the majority of reconstructions will probably be free (microvascular) transfer of autogenous tissue, probably still by means of the TRAM flap.—E.A. Luce, M.D.

Reduction Mammaplasty: A Way Helping Females With Neck, Shoulder and Back Pain Symptoms
Berg A, Stark B, Malec E (Karolinska Hosp, Stockholm, Sweden)
Eur J Plast Surg 17:84–86, 1994   140-95-13–3

Purpose.—Breast hypertrophy is a common cause of chronic pain in the neck, upper trunk, and shoulder area. Whether reduction mammaplasty improves the pain symptoms and functional disability associated with macromastia was determined.

Patients.—Of 113 women with hypertrophic breasts who underwent reduction mammaplasty in 1991, 93 completed a follow-up evaluation 1 year after operation. Seventy-five patients had a Strömbeck procedure and 18 had a Lejour's vertical mammaplasty. Seventy-nine patients com-

Change of Pain Symptoms Postoperatively (N = 79)			
Grade of improvement	Number of patients	Percentage	According to a ten point-scale
cured	37	46.8	0
> 50%	28	35.4	1–4
< 50%	11	13.9	5–9
unchanged	3	3.8	10

(Courtesy of Berg A, Stark B, Malee E: *Eur J Plast Surg* 17:84–86, 1994.)

plained of musculoskeletal pain, 40 patients had cosmetic complaints, and all patients had deep brassiere strap furrows. Ten patients had degenerative musculoskeletal or joint diseases before operation. Breast volume was measured before and after operation. Preoperative and postoperative pain in the head and neck, interscapular area, and shoulder girdle was rated on a 10-point scale.

Results.—Reduction mammaplasty significantly improved existing pain symptoms of the neck, shoulder, and upper trunk: 37 patients (47%) were cured, 28 (35%) were more than 50% improved, 11 (14%) still had more than 50% of their preoperative pain symptoms, and 3 (4%) were unchanged (table). In 8 patients, infections developed that required antibiotic therapy, and 4 patients needed revision procedures because of postoperative hemorrhage. Of 61 patients who had been unable to perform sporting activities before operation, 36 had started to do so after operation. Eighty-six patients reported that reduction mammaplasty had improved their self-esteem and sense of well being. At follow-up, 56 patients (60%) were very satisfied with the outcome, 30 (32%) were satisfied, and 7 (8%) were dissatisfied.

Conclusion.—Reduction mammaplasty should be considered as a primarily medical indication in women with musculoskeletal pain symptoms caused by the weight of their heavy breasts. The rate of postoperative complications after standard reduction mammaplasty is low, and excellent results can generally be expected.

▶ Plastic surgeons and general surgeons need more objective data to demonstrate the efficacy of procedures such as reduction mammaplasty. This paper is a major step in the right direction.—E.A. Luce, M.D.

Wound Complications in Patients Receiving Adjuvant Chemotherapy After Mastectomy and Immediate Breast Reconstruction for Breast Cancer

Furey PC, MacGillivray DC, Castiglione CL, Allen L (Univ of Connecticut, Farmington)

J Surg Oncol 55:194–197, 1994   140-95-13-4

Background.—In patients with breast cancer, immediate breast reconstruction after mastectomy can help to reduce psychological trauma. In addition, adjuvant chemotherapy can decrease the rate of breast cancer relapse in both node-positive and node-negative patients. Hence, many patients managed with mastectomy and immediate breast reconstruction also undergo treatment with adjuvant chemotherapy. The incidence and severity of perioperative wound complications was investigated in women undergoing mastectomy and immediate breast reconstruction with and without adjuvant chemotherapy.

Patients and Methods.—The medical records of 112 patients in whom immediate breast reconstruction after modified radical or simple mastectomy had been performed during a 5-year period were retrospectively reviewed. Information on wound incidence was available for 120 mastectomies. Complication rates were compared between 36 mastectomies treated with chemotherapy after surgery, and 84 mastectomies not treated with adjuvant therapy.

Results.—Overall, 25 wound complications were noted for the entire patient sample. Wound complications occurred in 10 of 36 mastectomies receiving adjuvant chemotherapy, and in 15 of 84 mastectomies not undergoing adjuvant treatment, yielding 27.8% and 17.9% incidence rates, respectively. However, these differences did not reach statistical significance. No delays in initiation of adjuvant therapy caused by wound complications secondary to immediate reconstruction were noted in any patient. No significant differences in wound type, severity, or method of treatment were noted between groups. Age, type of operation, tumor size, stage, number of lymph nodes harvested, prosthetic device, chemotherapy, and histopathology were not correlated with or predictive of complications as determined via logistic regression analysis.

Conclusion.—The frequency of wound complications was not increased in women undergoing mastectomy with immediate reconstruction and adjuvant chemotherapy. Thus, in patients undergoing this type of surgery, the administration of adjuvant chemotherapy need not be delayed.

▶ There was *some* difference between the 2 groups, but the numbers were small and significant differences may have been apparent with a larger series. Also, this group did not start the tissue expansion until *after* completion of cyclical chemotherapy, which did not even begin until 5 weeks after surgery. Also, these patients were reconstructed with expander implants only, not autologous tissue—a progressively (with time) moot point in the present legal climate that surrounds implants.—E.A. Luce, M.D.

Burns

Cyclosporin A Treatment Failed to Extend Skin Allograft Survival in Two Burn Patients

Eldad A, Benmeir P, Weinberg A, Neuman A, Chaouat M, Ben-Bassat H, Wexler MR (Israel Defense Forces Med Corps, Jerusalem; Hadassah Univ, Jerusalem)

Burns 20:262–264, 1994   140-95-13–5

Background.—Immunosuppressive drugs have occasionally been used to prolong the survival of skin allografts in patients with burns, but results have been mixed. Two pediatric patients were treated with cyclosporin A (CycA) and family-related skin allografts. Although 1 child survived, the results were not considered encouraging.

Patients, Methods, and Outcome.—The patients were an 11-year-old boy who sustained a high voltage electric burn and a 3-year-old boy who was severely burned while playing with matches. Both cases involved deep burns that covered at least 85% of the body surface area. Relatives donated 1:1.5 meshed fresh allografts, and CycA treatment was started before the operation. In both cases, the family-related allografts were rejected during CycA treatment after 14–18 days. The younger boy became septic after signs of rejection were noted in the allografts on day 17. He died the day of operation to replace the rejected allografts with frozen cadaver allografts. Antimortem blood cultures were positive for *Candida albicans*.

Discussion.—Both patients were monitored daily for blood levels of CycA, and findings were in the therapeutic range. The complication of Candida sepsis was rare at the study institution's burn unit, suggesting a possible link to immunosuppressive therapy. Cyclosporin A may lower immunocompetence and, thus, the chance of survival. In these 2 cases, allograft survival was not extended beyond the period that is usual without CycA treatment. Other factors may have contributed to rejection, however, including the use of fresh allografts and the lack of an HLA match between donors and recipients. Overall, CycA did not clearly provide a benefit to these patients with severe burns, and its use cannot be recommended without further investigation.

▶ Two swallows do not make a summer and 2 burn patients are not an indepth series, yet the authors report here that allograft survival was not extended with immunosuppression, and 1 patient burned over a 95% body surface area died.—E.A. Luce, M.D.

Trauma

Long-Term Results of Flap Reconstruction in Median Sternotomy Wound Infections

Ringelman PR, Vander Kolk CA, Cameron D, Baumgartner WA, Manson PN
(Johns Hopkins Univ, Baltimore, Md)

Plast Reconstr Surg 93:1208–1214, 1994   140-95-13–6

Background.—The early use of muscle and omental flaps in infected median sternotomy wounds can reduce the morbidity, length of hospital stay, and mortality. The long-term follow-up and functional outcome in such patients were evaluated.

Methods.—Over an 8-year period, 133 patients with mediastinal wound infection underwent debridement and muscle or omental flap closure. Seventy-six percent of the flaps were pectoralis major and 21% were rectus abdominis. The pectoralis major muscle was used primarily as a transposition flap. Eighty patients responded to a follow-up questionnaire, and 48 patients were given a physical examination. The average length of follow-up was 48 months.

Results.—The incidence of mediastinitis was 1.5%. The wounds healed in 99% of patients. The overall rate of confirmed sternal instability was 23%. After operation, pain and discomfort were reported by 51% of patients, and subjective postoperative weakness in the arm or shoulder was reported by 32.5%. Among the 14 patients who complained of arm and shoulder weakness and had a physical examination, 8 were found to have diminished strength and 6 had normal strength. Closer inspection revealed that, at most, a decrement of only 1 unit of strength occurred for the shoulder muscle tested. Thus, a total of 31% of patients had arm or shoulder weakness. The inability to perform preoperative activities was reported by 36% of patients. Among the patients eligible to return to work, 52% did not. Scars were good-to-excellent in 75% of patients. In 31% of patients, there were abdominal hernias and bulges. In 53% of patients with rectus abdominis flaps who had an examination, ventral hernia or fascial weakness was observed. The incidence of true hernia formation was 11%, and the incidence of fascial weakness/bulging was 42%. Shoulder strength dropped significantly in 1 patient after having bilateral pectoralis major transposition flaps.

Discussion.—Drawbacks can occur in this otherwise reliable, long-term closure of infected mediastinal wounds. The extent of sternal resection did not necessarily correlate with patients' complaints. The chest and axillary contour abnormalities might have been avoided by using the turnover flap method of pectoralis transfer more often.

▶ We need more long-term outcome studies of patients' quality of life after some of our heroic efforts, yet we must examine the study design carefully. In this instance, only about one third of the patients were available for examination, and only the most strident complainers might have agreed to participate to properly air their concerns. These results must be compared to those of a similar group of patients with uncomplicated coronary artery bypass grafts because of significant lifestyle changes that must be made (with dyspnea on exertion and chronic sternal pain) in this group as well. Clearly, few alternatives exist for closure in the infected sternum, and this paper perhaps arms the reconstructive surgeon for appropriate informed consent.—E.A. Luce, M.D.

Planned Ventral Hernia: Staged Management for Acute Abdominal Wall Defects
Fabian TC, Croce MA, Pritchard FE, Minard G, Hickerson WL, Howell RL, Schurr MJ, Kudsk KA (Univ of Tennessee, Memphis)
Ann Surg 219:643–653, 1994   140-95-13–7

Purpose.—Acute abdominal wall defects may result from necrotizing fascial infection and traumatic abdominal wall loss. Some newer approaches to patient management of these defects include open-abdomen techniques and scheduled relaparotomy for intra-abdominal infections. A number of different types of prostheses have been used for wound management, but there have been few direct clinical comparisons, nor any detailed studies of definitive reconstruction of these defects. A staged approach to the initial and definitive management of abdominal wall defects was described and evaluated.

Methods.—A 4-stage approach to management of acute abdominal wall defects was developed, beginning with placement of a prosthesis at the time of loss of abdominal wall integrity (Fig 13–2). Prostheses used

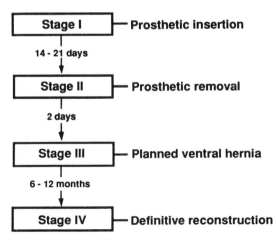

Fig 13–2.—Diagram of the four-staged management scheme for treating acute abdominal wall defects. (Courtesy of Fabian TC, Croce MA, Pritchard FE, et al: *Ann Surg* 219:643–653, 1994.)

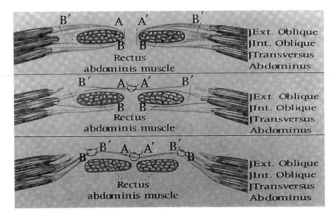

Fig 13–3.—Illustration of the modified components separation technique for abdominal wall reconstruction after mobilization of skin and subcutaneous fat from the muscular fascia out to the flank: 1) *top panel*—the external oblique fascia is incised just lateral to the anterior rectus sheath (**B'**) from epigastrium to inguinal region; 2) *middle panel*—the rectus abdominis muscle is separated from the posterior rectus sheath (**B**) and the internal oblique component of the anterior rectus sheath is divided (*dotted line*) from the epigastrium to the arcuate line; 3) *bottom panel*—the anterior rectus sheaths are approximated with monofilament suture in the midline (**A—A'**), and the medial border of the posterior rectus sheath is joined to the lateral border of the anterior rectus sheath (**B—B'**). (Courtesy of Fabian TC, Croce MA, Pritchard FE, et al: *Ann Surg* 219:643–653, 1994.)

included Prolene, Vicryl, Gore-tex, and plastic. In stage II, performed 2 or 3 weeks later when wound granulation had occurred, the prosthesis was removed. For patients with edema, attempts were made to gradually pleat and remove the mesh for 5 to 10 days to allow for delayed primary fascial closure. Gauze dressings were placed on the granulation defect and changed for a few days to decrease bacterial colonization and allow for hemostasis. Stage III followed in 2 or 3 days, with a planned ventral hernia by either split-thickness skin grafting or full-thickness skin and subcutaneous fat grafting. Finally—6 to 12 months after hospital discharge—the definitive reconstruction was performed. In patients with lesser amounts of abdominal wall resection or edematous patients in whom the abdominal wall could not be closed after stage II, a modification of the components separation method of reconstruction was used (Fig 13–3).

Results.—This approach was used in 88 patients over an 8.5-year period. The mortality rate was 26%, including 1 patient in whom a small bowel fistula developed as the result of Vicryl prosthesis erosion. Prolene was used in 51% of cases, Vicryl in 31%, and Gore-tex in 11%; the use of Vicryl increased with increasing experience. Of 39 patients with massive edema, half were able to undergo pleating and removal of the graft with fascial closure. The prostheses were in place for an average of 14 days. Eleven fistulas developed, 8 related to the management technique; all were controlled. Forty-eight percent of the patients have undergone definitive reconstruction an average of 9 months after the injury. Twelve of these 22 patients had prosthetic reconstruction. At a mean follow-up of 11 months, infections developed in 33% of patients with prosthetic repairs, and recurrent ventral hernias developed in another 33%. One infection requiring drainage developed in 9 patients who underwent reconstruction with the components separation method.

Conclusion.—This staged approach to the management of acute abdominal wall defects may be especially applicable to the patient with hypothermic, coagulopathic trauma who requires massive fluid resuscitation and in whom edema prohibits abdominal closure. As edema decreases, prostheses can be removed in about half of these cases for delayed primary fascial closure. The Vicryl mesh prosthesis is preferred because it is easier to remove than the Prolene prosthesis. For patients with moderate-sized midline defects, a modification of the components separation technique can be used. Mesh reconstructions can be used for larger defects, although with a significant rate of recurrent hernia.

▶ The authors have done a superb job of putting together the various components of an overall strategy for the management of these difficult problems. You may not agree with all their conclusions, but the reader will have to concur that the authors have taken a logical approach. Read particularly the discussants' additions at the end of the paper.—E.A. Luce, M.D.

Reherniation After Repair of the Abdominal Wall With Expanded Polytetrafluoroethylene

Simmermacher RKJ, Schakenraad JM, Bleichrodt RP (Sophia Hosp, Zwolle, The Netherlands; Univ of Groningen, The Netherlands; Twenteborg Hosp, Almelo, The Netherlands)
J Am Coll Surg 178:613–616, 1994   140-95-13–8

Introduction.—The repair of abdominal wall defects poses a difficult surgical challenge. Polypropylene (PP) mesh is most commonly used for these repairs, but a newer material, an expanded polytetrafluoroethylene (ePTFE) patch, has recently been introduced. Its clinical usefulness has been flawed, however, by the frequent development of herniations at the interface between fascia and patch. It was thought that these herniations occurred because of insufficient ingrowth of fibrocollagenous tissue with the ePTFE patch. This hypothesis was investigated by examining the anchorage of the ePTFE patch in rats.

Methods.—Full-thickness abdominal wall defects were created in 30 rats. The defects were repaired with an ePTFE soft tissue patch in 15 rats and with a PP patch in 15 rats. Eight weeks later, the patch was dissected free and examined for hernias and for adhesions between the patch and the omentum and intestines.

Results.—Nine of the 15 rats with ePTFE patches had herniations at the interface of the fascia and patch; none of the 15 rats in the PP group had herniations. All of the rats with PP patches had moderate omental

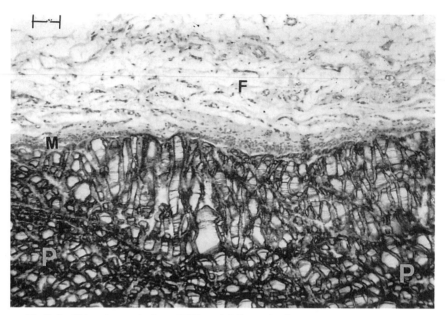

Fig 13-4.—Light micrograph of an ePTFE patch (**P**) 8 weeks after reconstruction of an abdominal wall defect in the rat. The ePTFE patch is separated from the adjacent fibrocollagenous tissue (**F**) by a thin layer of macrophages (**M**). There is no ingrowth of cells of the adjacent fibrocollagenous tissue into the patch. Toluidine and alkaline fuchsin staining. One cm bar is 100 μm. (Courtesy of Simmermacher RKJ, Schakenraad JM, Bleichrodt RP: *J Am Coll Surg* 178:613-616, 1994.)

and intestinal adhesions, whereas the rats with ePTFE patches had no or minimal omental or intestinal adhesions. Histologic examination of the dissected patches revealed that there was no ingrowth of fibrocollagenous tissue in the ePTFE patch (Fig 13-4), in contrast to the PP patch, which was fully incorporated in fibrocollagenous tissue continuous with the fibrous sheath of adjacent muscle.

Discussion.—These findings confirm the clinical evidence suggesting that the ePTFE soft tissue patch anchors poorly to adjacent fascia because there is no ingrowth of fibrocollagenous tissue into the patch. Although this lack of ingrowth increases the risk of reherniation, it also decreases the risk of visceral adhesions. The anchorage problem might be overcome if the surgeon used a double row of nonabsorbable sutures. It might also be overcome by modification of the ePTFE patch to create larger pores (at least 60 μm) to allow ingrowth of fibroblasts.

▶ The ePTFE (Gore-tex) patch is an attractive (although expensive) theoretical abdominal wall substitute. The nonreactivity of the material may actually be a detriment in the failure of scar tissue to adequately bridge the fascia patch interface. The authors suggest as a remedy a double layer of suture closure, but perhaps the solution needs to be more fundamental than simply another line of stitches.—E.A. Luce, M.D.

Head and Neck—Basic Science

p53 Gene Mutations as Markers of Tumor Spread in Synchronous Oral Cancers

Koch WM, Boyle JO, Mao L, Hakim J, Hruban RH, Sidransky D (Johns Hopkins Univ, Baltimore, Md)
Arch Otolaryngol Head Neck Surg 120:943–947, 1994   140-95-13–9

Background.—Molecular biological tools may soon be used for early detection of head and neck squamous cell carcinomas. These tools may also be useful for analyzing histopathologic margins and monitoring for recurrent disease. The ways in which genetic mutations may be used as specific markers for the study and management of head and neck squamous cell carcinomas were investigated.

Methods.—Synchronous primary squamous cell carcinomas of the head and neck from 1 patient were examined. Mutations in the p53 gene

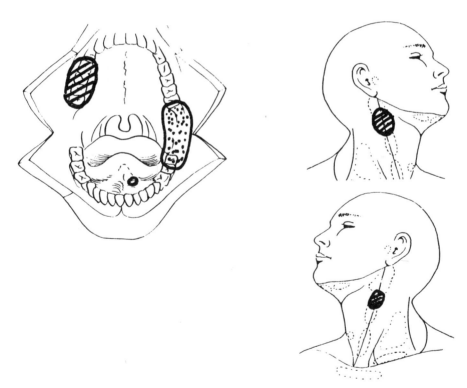

Fig 13–5.—Tumor map showing physical findings at initial presentation: right alveolar ridge lesion (*cross-hatching*), left retromolar trigone lesion (*stippling*), and floor of mouth leukoplakia (*open circle*). Bilateral clinically apparent neck masses are *cross-hatched* to indicate biological linkage to the right alveolar ridge. (Courtesy of Koch WM, Boyle JO, Mao L, et al: *Arch Otolaryngol Head Neck Surg* 120:943–947, 1994.)

were identified by DNA sequencing. Rare tumor cells were detected in surgical margins, lymph nodes, and swabs of the oral cavity by polymerase chain reaction and mutant-specific oligomer probes.

Findings.—Different missense mutations in the p53 gene were found in 2 synchronous primary invasive cancers. Metastases from both sides of the neck showed the mutated sequence from 1 primary tumor. Infiltrating cells from this biologically aggressive tumor were also found in a histologically normal surgical margin by a polymerase chain reaction–based assay and accurately predicted tumor recurrence (Fig 13–5).

Conclusion.—In 1 patient, p53 gene mutations were useful molecular markers distinguishing between tumors. The potential value of tumor cell detection in surgical margins and saliva by molecular methods merits additional research.

▶ This paper was included not as a comprehensive study (in fact, it is a case report) but rather as a clear demonstration of the use of molecular markers in head and neck cancer. The paper is easily readable and comprehensible to those outside the field of molecular biology. The techniques utilized in this instance to detect bilateral lymph node metastases from the right side of the 2 synchronous oral lesions, as well as the detection by molecular methods of a positive margin, might well represent a glimpse into their future application on a widespread basis.—E.A. Luce, M.D.

Tumor Angiogenesis as a Prognostic Factor in Oral Cavity Tumors
Williams JK, Carlson GW, Cohen C, Derose PB, Hunter S, Jurkiewicz MJ (Emory Univ, Atlanta, Ga)
Am J Surg 168:373–380, 1994   140-95-13–10

Background.—In patients with cancers of the oral cavity, lymph node metastasis is the single strongest predictor of survival. Tumor angiogenesis, which has been associated with metastasis in patients with breast cancer, may have prognostic value for other tumors as well. The possible correlation between angiogenesis—as shown by the percentage of factor VIII–related antigen immunostaining of endothelial cells—and the probability of the development of regional metastasis in clinically node-negative patients with squamous cell carcinomas of the oral cavity was investigated.

Methods and Findings.—Samples for analysis were obtained from 66 patients with clinically node-negative squamous cell carcinoma of the oral cavity. The percentage of tissue area stained for factor VIII was determined. The probability of metastasis was 2% for tumor staining of 10% or less and 93% for tumor staining of more than 10%. Patients with a tumor depth of 4 mm or less and 10% or less staining had a 2% recurrence rate. Patients with a tumor depth of more than 4 mm and staining of greater than 10% had a 100% recurrence rate (Fig 13–6).

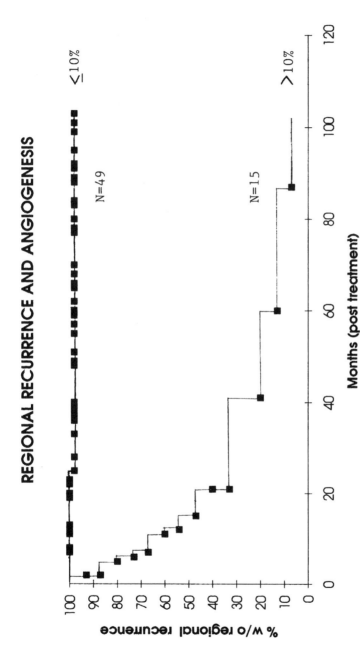

Fig 13-6.—Graph of regional recurrence and probability of patient being disease-free within a given percent staining group at time in months. At 30 months, the low-staining group will have a 98% probability of being disease-free, decreasing to 30% in the high-staining group. (Courtesy of Williams JK, Carlson GW, Cohen C, et al: *Am J Surg* 168:373–380, 1994.)

Conclusion.—Although tumor thickness suggested predictability, only angiogenesis significantly predicted recurrence in a multivariate analysis. Angiogenesis is strongly correlated with regional recurrence and may serve as an independent prognostic indicator.

▶ This is an eloquent study of the value of detection of tumor angiogenesis and a confirmation of work started by Judah Folkman a number of years ago.—E.A. Luce, M.D.

Head and Neck—Extirpative

Carotid Artery Resection for Cancer of the Head and Neck
Meleca RJ, Marks SC (Wayne State Univ, Detroit)
Arch Otolaryngol Head Neck Surg 120:974–978, 1994   140-95-13–11

Background.—Advanced squamous cell cancer of the head and neck may involve the carotid artery. Treatment options include carotid artery resection which is, in turn, associated with a high neurologic morbidity and mortality. Debate continues regarding the decision to ligate or replace the resected artery. The morbidity and mortality associated with ligation compared to reconstruction of the carotid artery after resection were examined.

Methods.—A retrospective record review of 1,784 patients who underwent surgery for head and neck cancer at the reporting institutions from January 1985 through June 1992 was conducted. Chi-square analysis was performed comparing the morbidity of those who underwent carotid resection and ligation with those who had replacement of the resected artery.

Results.—A total of 20 patients underwent carotid artery resection, with 12 undergoing ligation and 8 having interposition grafting. Neurologic complications occurred in 7 of the 12 patients (58%) with carotid artery ligation, whereas only 1 of the 8 patients (13%) with grafts had such complications (table). After surgery, 3 of 19 patients survived dis-

Morbidity and Mortality for Carotid Artery Resection		
	No. (%) of Patients	
	Ligation	Replacement
Morbidity	7/12 (58)	1/8 (13)*
Cerebrovascular accident	5/12 (42)	1/8 (13)*
Transient ischemic attack	2/12 (17)	0/8
Mortality	1/12 (8)	0/8

* P < .005.
(Courtesy of Meleca RJ, Marks SC: *Arch Otolaryngol Head Neck Surg* 120:974–978, 1994.)

ease-free for 1 year, and 1 survived 8 months disease-free. The median disease-free survival postoperatively was 6.3 months. Fourteen of 19 patients overall and 7 of 11 who survived for at least 5 months after surgery had local-regional control at the time of death or at their most recent follow-up.

Conclusion.—Nonsurgical therapy should be used because of the poor prognosis and high morbidity associated with surgery in patients with advanced squamous cell carcinoma of the head and neck involving the carotid artery. In individuals who have received radiation therapy and who have limited disease adherent to the carotid artery, resection can provide local-regional control and a possibility of prolonged disease-free survival. Interposition grafting should be used to minimize the risk of neurologic morbidity when carotid artery resection is performed.

▶ This paper does not convince this reviewer that carotid artery resection is a useful oncologic option. The 1-year disease-free survival rate is low (15% in this instance). Although locoregional control was reasonable, application of this option mandates for informed consent as much as possible with the patient and family. If carotid artery resection is selected though, this paper demonstrates a clear superiority of reconstitution by replacement over ligation alone.

Even though a vascular surgeon may be on notice, quite commonly the resection team elects to ligate because of stump pressures and angiographic results, or simply convenience. Stump pressure and angiograms correlate poorly with the occurrence of subsequent neurologic sequelae. Considerably more sophisticated techniques are available for determination of the availability of flow from the contralateral side. The biggest problem with this approach of carotid resection is the occurrence of tumor at the skull base because clearance of gross tumor and the availability of sufficient distal carotid stump for bypass may become mutually exclusive goals. Perhaps a better option is resection of a gross tumor from the artery, insertion of brachytherapy catheters, and coverage with a well-vascularized muscle flap.—E.A. Luce, M.D.

Evaluation of 107 Therapeutic and Elective Parotidectomies for Cutaneous Melanoma
O'Brien CJ, Petersen-Schafer K, Papadopoulos T, Malka V (Royal Prince Alfred Hosp, Sydney, Australia)
Am J Surg 168:400–403, 1994   140-95-13–12

Background.—Parotidectomy is often part of the treatment of head and neck melanoma because of the risk of metastasis to lymph nodes in the parotid gland. A prospective study of 107 patients treated by a single surgeon during a 6-year period examined the roles of elective and therapeutic parotidectomy and of adjuvant radiotherapy in cutaneous melanoma of the head and neck.

Patients and Methods.—The patient group included 80 men and 27 women with a median age of 57 years. The most common primary site was the face (57%), and the most frequently encountered type was nodular (36%). The median thickness of the melanoma was 2.6 mm. Twenty-five parotidectomies were therapeutic, performed for clinical metastatic disease in the parotid gland, and 82 were elective. Twelve elective procedures were in patients with clinical nodal disease in the upper neck from a primary site that could drain to the parotid gland. Only 7 of the parotidectomies were total (4) or subtotal (3). The facial nerve was sacrificed totally in 2 and partially in 8 of the therapeutic operations. Neck dissection was performed in all but 1 patient. Adjuvant radiotherapy came to be used more frequently when patients early in the series had recurrent disease when not given postoperative irradiation. Radiotherapy consisted of 5 fractions of 550 cGy during a 2.5-week period.

Results.—Pathologically positive lymph nodes were present in the parotid gland of 27 patients and in the neck of 15. Both parotid and neck metastases were found in 10 patients. The principal postoperative complication, facial nerve dysfunction, developed in 69% of those in whom the facial nerve was not sacrificed. Weakness of the lower lip because of mandibular nerve injury was the most common problem. Seventeen of 27 patients with positive parotid metastases received adjuvant radiotherapy. Parotid recurrences developed in 5 patients, 4 of whom were not irradiated, but the difference between the 2 groups was not significant. Melanoma-specific survival was 64% at 5 years and was significantly worse (40%) for patients with nodal involvement of the neck or parotid gland.

Conclusion.—Metastatic melanoma was found in only 2 clinically negative parotid glands and in the cervical lymph nodes of 3 other patients, raising questions about the need for elective parotidectomy and neck dissection. There appears to be no reason to remove parotid tissue deep to the plane of the facial nerve during elective procedures. Adjuvant radiotherapy was beneficial in cases of metastasis to the parotid gland.

▶ This paper makes 2 points. One is the low incidence of metastases in intermediate-thickness lesions and risk of facial nerve weakness. If this is so, informed consent for such patients would be to estimate about a 5% incidence of nodal disease vs. about a 1-in-3 chance of some permanent mandibular nerve weakness. The other point is the use of postoperative radiotherapy for better local and regional control.—E.A. Luce, M.D.

Is Surgical Resection Leaving Positive Margins of Benefit to the Patient with Locally Advanced Squamous Cell Carcinoma of the Head and Neck: A Comparative Study Using the Intergroup Study 0034 and the Radiation Therapy Oncology Group Head and Neck Database

Laramore GE, Scott CB, Schuller DE, Haselow RE, Ervin TJ, Wheeler R, Al-Sarraf M, Gahbauer RA, Jacobs JR, Schwade JG, Campbell BH (Univ of

Washington, Seattle; American College of Radiology, Philadelphia; Ohio State Univ, Columbus; et al)
Int J Radiat Oncol Biol Phys 27:1011–1016, 1993   140-95-13-13

Background.—An untested tenet of the management of individuals with advanced tumors of the head and neck has been that there is no role for surgery unless there is a high probability of achieving clear margins. Patients with squamous cell carcinomas of the head and neck were studied to determine whether they benefited from surgical resection that

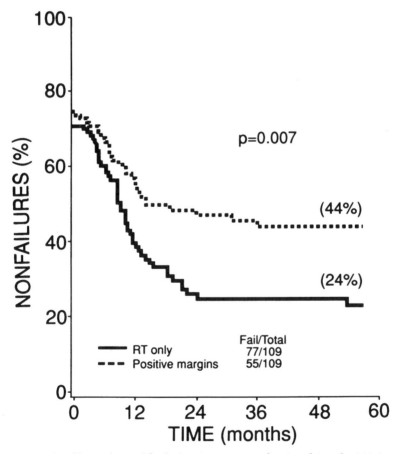

Fig 13–7.—Local/regional control for the 2 patient groups as a function of time after initiating therapy. The group treated with conventional radiotherapy alone is shown as the solid curve and the positive margin group is shown as the dotted curve. The difference between the two curves is statistically significant at the *P* = 0.007 level. (Courtesy of Laramore GE, Scott CB, Schuller DE, et al: *Int J Radiat Oncol Biol Phys* 27:1011-1016, 1993.)

left positive margins, followed by postoperative adjuvant therapy, compared with patients treated with radiotherapy alone.

Methods.—A group of 109 patients were excluded from a multigroup, cooperative clinical trial testing the efficacy of adjuvant chemotherapy for patients with resectable squamous cell carcinoma of the head and neck because they had positive surgical margins. These patients were followed prospectively for 2 end points: local-regional control and survival. Eight of these patients received no further treatment, 6 received postoperative chemotherapy alone, 71 received radiotherapy alone, and 24 received both radiotherapy and chemotherapy. The median dose of radiation given to those who received it was 60 Gy. This group was matched with a control group of head and neck cancer patients found through a computer database. The control patients received radiotherapy only, with a median dose of 66 Gy. The groups were matched for tumor site, tumor stage, nodal status, Karnofsky performance status, and closest age.

Results.—The positive margin group had a significantly higher rate of local-regional control (44% vs. 24%) at 4 years (Fig 13–7). The overall survival rates at 4 years were not significantly different (29% in the positive margin group vs. 25% in the radiotherapy only group).

Conclusion.—Although survival does not seem to be improved after incomplete excision and adjuvant therapy compared to radiation alone, significant improvements are found in local-regional control of the tumor. This finding may be applicable for palliative treatment. Caution is advised in changing resectability criteria before performing appropriate clinical trials.

▶ This intergroup study effectively dispels the old myth that patients who have positive margins and who will require radiotherapy are best treated with curative radiotherapy alone. Remember, though, that these are patients who were aggressively resected, yet had a persistent positive microscopic margin and were compared with a group of patients someone had decided would be best treated with radiation alone. Also, we know nothing from the paper about the stage of the disease. Regardless, the best option is not a choice between a positive margin plus radiotherapy vs. radiotherapy alone, but rather surgical resection with *negative* margins followed by postoperative radiotherapy, if needed.—E.A. Luce, M.D.

Microlaryngoscopic Surgery for T1 Glottic Lesions: A Cost-Effective Option

Myers EN, Wagner RL, Johnson JT (Univ of Pittsburgh, Pa; The Eye and Ear Inst of Pittsburgh, Pa)
Ann Otol Rhinol Laryngol 103:28–30, 1994   140-95-13–14

TABLE 1.—Costs of Treatment for Glottic Carcinoma

Type of Treatment	Total Costs*
Microlaryngoscopy plus excision with or without laser (1 procedure)	$6,478
Microlaryngoscopy plus excision with or without laser (2 procedures)	$12,956
Radiotherapy	$27,000
Hemilaryngectomy	$35,616
Total laryngectomy	$25,649
Laryngoscopy	$5,588

* Costs include hospital surgeon, radiology, radiation oncology, ancillary services, and both technical and professional components, where applicable (1992 figures).
(Courtesy of Myers EN, Wagner RL, Johnson JT: *Ann Otol Rhinol Laryngol* 103:28–30, 1994.)

Objective.—For the treatment of T1 glottic lesions, microlaryngoscopy (ML) with excision of the lesion with or without laser, vertical partial laryngeal surgery, and irradiation provides primary cure rates greater than 85%. In the present cost-conscious environment, there is a need to define treatment costs along with medical decision-making to provide cost-effective treatment.

Study Design.—The cost effectiveness of ML with or without laser was studied in a retrospective review of 50 patients with invasive and microinvasive squamous cell carcinoma who underwent treatment between 1978 and 1990. Cost analysis was performed for each treatment modality and hospitalization by averaging 10 hospital bills and related service bills and extrapolating 1992 health care costs into the treatment options

TABLE 2.—Costs for Theoretic Group of 100 Patients Undergoing Microlaryngoscopy With Excision for T1 Glottic Carcinoma

ML (100 patients) = ($6,478 × 2) × 100 patients = $1.3 million.
Eight patients would fail this regimen and need further treatment.
Two patients would have HL for salvage and 6 patients would undergo XRT. Therefore,
HL (2 failures) = $35,616 × 2 patients = $71,232
and
XRT (6 failures) = $27,000 × 6 patients = $162,000.
Finally, total costs for the entire ML patient group would be
C (total) = ML + HL + XRT or $1.5 million.

Abbreviations: ML, microlaryngoscopy; HL, hemilaryngectomy; XRT, radiotherapy; C, cost.
(Courtesy of Myers EN, Wagner RL, Johnson JT: *Ann Otol Rhinol Laryngol* 103:28–30, 1994.)

for T1 glottic carcinoma. Using previous reports, cost-effectiveness analysis was also performed for other treatment options for T1 glottic lesions, including hemilaryngectomy and radiotherapy.

Findings.—During an average follow-up of 48 months, 46 patients (92%) were cured by primary ML with excision, requiring an average of 2 procedures (range, 1–6 procedures). Four patients (8%) failed ML treatment, but all were successfully salvaged by hemilaryngectomy or irradiation. Similar cure rates of 95% have been reported after hemilaryngectomy or radiotherapy for T1 glottic lesions. The costs of treatment for T1 glottic cancer were $12,956 per patient for ML, $35,616 per patient with hemilaryngectomy, and $32,588 per patient with radiotherapy (Table 1). When these costs were extrapolated to a theoretic group of 100 patients, ML plus excision cost only $1.5 million (Table 2), providing savings of up to $2.4 million when compared with hemilaryngectomy ($3.6 million) or irradiation ($3.9 million).

Conclusion.—In T1 glottic carcinoma, ML plus excision provides similar cure rates as open conservation laryngeal surgery or radiotherapy, but with potential for savings. In selected patients, ML with excision is an effective, cost-conscious management option for early vocal cord cancer.

▶ Readers will begin to see more of these types of papers: a demonstration of efficacy *and* cost. Endoscopic excision accomplished with or without the laser was a clear winner over radiation therapy. Remember that these lesions were selected, namely, 50 cases over a 12-year period from an extremely busy head and neck service and were specifically midcord or anterior lesions (without involvement of the commissure), so perhaps the cure rates are not directly comparable. The point, though, that the authors also add and emphasize in the discussion is the dollars lost to the economic system (and patients) because of a prolonged period away from work for the 6–7 weeks of radiotherapy. If we do not start cost accounting for these factors, others will.—E.A. Luce, M.D.

Treatment of Patients With Carcinoma of the Thyroid Invading the Airway

Friedman M, Danielzadeh JA, Caldarelli DD (Rush Univ, Chicago; Univ of the Health Sciences/Chicago Med School, North Chicago, Ill)
Arch Otolaryngol Head Neck Surg 120:1377–1381, 1994   140-95-13-15

Introduction.—Because local invasion of the airway is the usual cause of death in patients dying of thyroid carcinoma, local control of invasive disease is essential. There is currently a lack of consensus regarding the surgical treatment of patients with laryngotracheal invasion by thyroid malignant neoplasms. A review of 34 patients who underwent a total of 48 procedures examined whether complete resection improved survival compared with incomplete resection.

Patients and Methods.—Patients reviewed for the study were treated between 1950 and 1987; had a tumor with invasion of the trachea, pharynx, larynx, or esophagus; and were followed for at least 5 years. Patients with anaplastic or medullary thyroid carcinoma were excluded. Fourteen patients (group 1) had complete tumor resection, 8 (group 2) had near-total resection with minimal tumor remaining, 10 (group 3) had resection with undetermined margins, and 2 (group 4) had gross unresectable tumor left behind. Local recurrence was confirmed by either open biopsy specimens or fine-needle aspiration; metastatic disease was not evaluated.

Results.—Most patients had either a papillary or mixed papillary pattern. Those in group 1, with complete tumor resection, had the most aggressive and/or the most advanced local disease. Nevertheless, only 27% of group 1 had local recurrence. Four of the 8 patients in group 2 died of local disease, 1 was disease-free after a total laryngectomy, and 3 have survived 3–10 years with locally recurrent disease and after additional surgical procedures. The local recurrence rate was 38% in group 3, but because the extent of their resection was uncertain, no conclusions can be drawn. Both patients in group 4 had unresectable tumors and died of persistent local disease. Survival was significantly better for group 1 vs. group 2 and group 4, and for group 3 vs. group 4. Only 1 patient in group 1 had a second operation.

Conclusion.—A review of articles for the past 30 years found recommendations ranging from limited resection to extensive surgery for patients with thyroid cancer locally invading the airway. This review found that leaving behind gross residual tumor increases morbidity and mortality and decreases survival. Thus, the goal should be tumor-free margins, except when adequate surgery poses an even greater risk.

▶ Differentiated thyroid carcinoma is often regarded as a "benign" neoplasm. But accumulating evidence indicates that once outside the gland (not necessarily nodal metastasis), the behavior may be entirely different. The discussion has raged for decades regarding management of airway involvement, namely, laryngeal/tracheal preservation.

These authors and their results come down squarely on the side of definitive resection and not reliance on ablation with ancillary means such as I-131. They caution the readers, though, that their series, like all series of this variant, are small and the analysis is retrospective. Unlike primary squamous cell carcinoma of the upper air/digestive tract, total laryngectomy may not be necessary. The tumor has invaded from the outside in, and a resection of cartilage and soft tissue with reconstruction can be accomplished.—E.A. Luce, M.D.

Head and Neck—Diagnoses

Positron Emission Tomography of Patients With Head and Neck Carcinoma Before and After High Dose Irradiation

Greven KM, Williams DW III, Keyes JW Jr, McGuirt WF, Watson NE Jr, Randall ME, Raben M, Geisinger KR, Cappellari JO (Bowman Gray School of Medicine, Winston-Salem, NC)
Cancer 74:1355–1359, 1994   140-95-13–16

Background.—Positron emission tomography (PET), a functional imaging technique, provides information about tissue perfusion and metabolism. By contrast, CT and MRI are mainly anatomical imaging techniques. Metabolic changes apparently associated with malignancy can be imaged by PET with 18F-2fluoro-2deoxyglucose (FDG). Also, PET may be able to predict outcomes after definitive radiotherapy and to distinguish viable tumor from normal tissue changes after radiotherapy. The patterns of FDG uptake in head and neck neoplasms before and after high-dose radiotherapy were investigated.

Methods and Findings.—Twenty-five patients were assessed prospectively with PET and standard clinical and radiographic techniques before and after radiotherapy (table). Twenty-four of 27 primary sites were identified on the initial PET scans. Primary sites were unknown in 2 patients. Eleven of 12 patients with clinically positive adenopathy before radiotherapy had increased FDG activity in cervical lymph nodes. In another 5 patients, regions of increased activity in the neck suggesting malignant adenopathy were identified on PET scans. One month after radiotherapy, all 22 patients studied had reduced FDG accumulation in the primary sites. Of the 16 with normal PET scans, 3 had documented persistent or recurrent disease. Persistent disease had been documented in all 6 patients with reduced but persistent FDG uptake. Cervical lymph

Pretreatment Positron Emission Tomography Scans of 25 Patients	
Primary sites	
Clinically positive	PET positive
27	24
Clinically negative	PET positive
2	2
Nodal sites	
Clinically positive	PET positive
12	11
Clinically negative	PET positive
25	5

(Courtesy of Greven KM, Williams DW III, Keyes JW Jr, et al: *Cancer* 74:1355–1359, 1994.)

node areas were also examined on the 1-month PET scans. In 15 patients, the scans were interpreted as normal. However, 2 of 3 patients undergoing a planned neck dissection had pathologically confirmed residual disease in the neck. Five of the 7 patients with abnormal FDG accumulation in the neck after radiotherapy underwent planned neck dissection. Pathologically positive tumor was found in all 5. Four months after radiotherapy, 11 patients had normal PET scans of the primary site. None had subsequent recurrences. Seven patients had abnormal FDG accumulation, 6 of whom had biopsy-confirmed recurrences.

Conclusion.—Irradiation apparently reduces FDG uptake into the tumor cell acutely, even though some tumor cells remain viable. Negative results on 1-month PET scans do not accurately indicate absence of disease. However, when findings on 1-month PET scans are positive for FDG uptake, the presence of persistent disease is likely.

▶ The specificity and sensitivity of PET are not, as the authors readily admit, sufficient to replace other modalities in the workup of the patient. What was particularly attractive about this paper, though, was the identification of radio-persistent tumor in a subset of patients that was considerably more reliable at 4 months than at 1 month. This is a difficult problem clinically because detection of submucosal persistent tumor may become quite advanced before becoming clinically evident. The other attractive aspect of PET is the *functional* nature of the imaging techniques rather than anatomical as in CT and MR scanning. I am certain we will hear more on PET in the next couple of years.—E.A. Luce, M.D.

Symptom-Directed Selective Endoscopy and Cost Containment for Evaluation of Head and Neck Cancer

Benninger MS, Enrique RR, Nichols RD (Henry Ford Hosp, Detroit)
Head Neck 15:532–536, 1993   140-95-13–17

Background.—Patients with squamous cell carcinoma of the head and neck commonly have synchronous and metachronous neoplasms of the upper aerodigestive tract. Routine screening for these lesions is commonly performed by panendoscopy; however, the diagnostic yield and cost effectiveness of this procedure have been questioned. The tumor identification rates and cost effectiveness of panendoscopy vs. symptom-directed selective endoscopy were assessed in a prospective study.

Methods.—One hundred consecutive patients with newly diagnosed, untreated squamous cell carcinoma were studied. Before any further evaluations were performed, all patients' symptoms were assessed to determine which specific studies might be selected to aid in identifying second primary neoplasms. Subsequently, all patients underwent chest radiography, barium esophagography, direct pharyngolaryngoscopy, esophagoscopy, and bronchoscopy with bronchial washings. The 2 approaches were compared for their rate of identification of primary neoplasms and their cost-effectiveness.

Results.—Six patients were found to have a total of 7 synchronous primary neoplasms; 1 of the patients had 3 separate tumors. Synchronous pharyngeal neoplasms were identified in 5 cases, 2 of which were asymptomatic, and oral cavity neoplasms in 2 cases. In 3 patients, all with symptoms of dysphagia and odynopagia, 2 primary cervical esophageal tumors and 1 synchronous esophageal tumor were found. Chest radiography detected 2 pulmonary metastases in patients whose bronchoscopies and bronchial washings had been negative. The use of selective, symptom-directed evaluations would have reduced the total cost by one third and minimized excessive diagnostic procedures and potential morbidity.

Conclusion.—Direct pharyngolaryngoscopy and chest radiographs appear to be indicated for all patients with squamous cell carcinoma of the neck for diagnosing synchronous primary neoplasms. However, esophagoscopy, esophagography, and bronchoscopy may be better reserved for patients with corresponding symptoms. Bronchial washings do not appear to be helpful in searching for additional primary tumors. With further study, indirect video pharyngolaryngoscopy may prove to be a useful alternative to direct operative pharyngolaryngoscopy.

▶ In the changing economic climate and with the emphasis increasingly placed on demonstrations of efficacy, this paper provides a model for such assessment. Based on clinical examination alone, the authors made a decision regarding the necessity for panendoscopy and then endoscoped all the patients. They discovered that routine bronchoscopy and esophagoscopy made little sense, although, for some inexplicable reason, they still recommended bronchoscopy until further data were obtained. Cost savings of approximately $100,000 for 100 patients were considerable as well. Nothing replaces a good clinical examination.—E.A. Luce, M.D.

Head and Neck—Reconstruction

Experience With Arteriovenous Malformations Treated With Flap Coverage
Yamamoto Y, Ohura T, Minakawa H, Sugihara T, Yoshida T, Nohira K, Shintomi Y (Hokkaido Univ, Sapporo, Japan; Soshundo Hosp, Sapporo, Japan)
Plast Reconstr Surg 94:476–482, 1994   140-95-13–18

Objective.—Fourteen patients with arteriovenous malformation (AVM) were treated by surgical resection of the malformation and free-tissue transfers or axial local flaps. This treatment protocol is based upon the hypothesis that well-vascularized tissue improves local hemodynamics and ischemia, offering long-term palliation.

Patients and Methods.—Patients ranged in age from 4 to 65 years. The congenital AVM was located on the face in 9 cases, the hand in 2, the knee in 2, and the foot in 1. Three patients had previously undergone a ligation or embolization procedure of the feeding arteries, and 3 had had previous partial excision of the AVM, all without success. Excision was performed as widely as possible after careful preoperative angiographic evaluation. Free flaps were used in 12 patients and axial local flaps in 2. The feeding vessels of the AVM were dissected and used as recipient vessels of the free-tissue transfer.

Results.—The flap transfer was successful in 13 of 14 patients. Partial necrosis of the flap developed in the remaining patient. With follow-up averaging 3 years 2 months, 12 of the patients had no clinical evidence of recurrence. Seven patients had angiographic follow-up; the AVM had completely disappeared in 2, was residual but stable in 3, and residual with increase in 2. The last 2 patients also had clinical evidence of recurrence. One had an intramaxillary recurrence at 1 year 3 months and the other had an intraorbital recurrence 3 years after surgery.

Conclusion.—The treatment of AVM has been a difficult and unresolved problem because of recurrence and persistence of the malformations. Surgical excision of the symptomatic area and replacement with well-vascularized tissue achieved palliation and results viewed as satisfactory in 86% of patients. The feeding arteries of the AVM were used for the recipient in all patients who required free flaps. A distant flap based on the different vascular system from the feeding vessels of the AVM should be used in the case of reconstruction with an axial local flap.

▶ The principal need here is long-term follow-up. The average follow-up was a little more than three years, and, of course, the AVMs may recur well after that date. The rationale is valid, though: to resect widely and to reconstruct with well-vascularized tissue.—E.A. Luce, M.D.

Management of Extensive Facial Basal Cell Carcinoma by Excision and Microvascular Tissue Transfer

Wilson GR, McLean NR, Beckingham IJ (Newcastle Gen Hosp, Newcastle upon Tyne, England)
Ann R Coll Surg Engl 75:405–410, 1993   140-95-13–19

Background.—Basal cell carcinoma is the most common skin malignancy in Australia. Frequency increases with age. Historically, advanced age has been considered a contraindication to major surgery in patients with basal cell carcinoma, but advances in surgical and anesthetic techniques now permit extensive elective procedures in the elderly.

Patients.—Six patients underwent a microvascular transfer of tissue procedure to provide skin and soft tissue coverage to large facial defects after excision of basal cell carcinoma. The patients were 4 men and 2 women aged 67–78 years. The site of the carcinoma was preauricular in 2 and the forehead, vertex of the scalp, occiput, and chin in 1 each.

Hierarchy of Wound
Closure Methods

Primary suture
Full-thickness skin graft
Split-thickness skin graft
Local flap
   Random pattern
   Axial pattern
   Fasciocutaneous
   Muscle
   Musculocutaneous
Distant flap
   Random pattern
   Axial pattern
   Fasciocutaneous
   Free microvascular transfer

(Courtesy of Wilson GR, Beckingham IJ, McLean NR: *Ann R Coll Surg Engl* 75:405–410, 1993.)

Three patients had had previous radiotherapy. Defect sizes ranged from 8 × 6 cm to 30 × 20 cm. Radial forearm flaps were used in 3 patients and latissimus dorsi flaps in the remaining 3. Follow-up ranged from 9 to 19 months. There were no complications.

Conclusion.—Management of large or recurrent basal cell carcinomas on the face can be difficult, especially when radiotherapy has been the primary treatment modality. Free-tissue transfer using microvascular surgery enables wide excision margins, ensuring tumor clearance. Closure problems do not compromise the procedure because the free flap can be designed after tumor excision and its size and composition can be individualized (table). Advanced age alone should not be a contraindication to this procedure.

▶ This series of 6 cases of elderly patients was designed to demonstrate the utility of free-tissue transfer. Actually, in some of these cases, reconstruction could have been accomplished with the use of regional flaps, which would have given an equal aesthetic result in shorter operative time. Yet, one should not be reluctant to utilize free-tissue transfer for reconstruction of large soft tissue defects created by the excision of skin cancer, particularly if the tissues are composite in nature. We need to ask 3 questions as we select an option in reconstruction: Is it the most simple? Most capable? Most consistent?—E.A. Luce, M.D.

A New Bilobed Design for the Sensate Radial Forearm Flap to Preserve Tongue Mobility Following Significant Glossectomy

Urken ML, Biller HF (Mount Sinai Med Ctr, New York)
Arch Otolaryngol Head Neck Surg 120:26–31, 1994   140-95-13–20

Objective.—The preservation of tongue mobility and the restoration of sensation are critical factors in oral rehabilitation. The radial forearm flap provides tissue that is thin, redundant, and pliable for reconstruction of the tongue. A new, bilobed design of the sensate radial forearm flap that permits separation of the mobile tongue from the reconstructed floor of the mouth and the gingiva was tested.

Technique.—The bilobed radial forearm free flap consists of 1 lobe used to restore the normal shape of the mobile tongue tip and a second lobe used to resurface the floor of the mouth and the gingiva. The depth of the division between these 2 lobes varies with the defect. For a longer separation between these lobes, a fascial subcutaneous bridge is preserved to insure adequate vascularity to both lobes. In defects that involve the tongue base and are deemed too large to close primarily, the length of the flap can be extended. Additional subcutaneous tissue is harvested to provide bulk where it is needed. This is accomplished by raising skin flaps on the forearm in a subdermal plane to minimize the size of the donor defect requiring coverage with a split-thickness skin graft. After the flap is inset, microvascular anastomoses are performed and the medial or lateral antebrachial cutaneous nerve is anastomosed to the lingual nerve. The lobe used to resurface the floor of the mouth and the gingiva should be fashioned with considerable redundancy to ensure that the mobile tongue is not tethered.

Outcome.—Ten patients who underwent significant glossectomy for squamous cell cancer have undergone tongue reconstruction using the bilobed radial forearm free flap. All patients had at least one half of the mobile tongue resected and a portion of the residual tongue had an intact motor supply. All 12 free flaps (2 patients who underwent segmental mandibulectomy had 2 flaps) were successfully transferred without partial or total necrosis. All patients had a mobile tongue tip and good articulation. Oral alimentation was restored in all but 1 patient. The earliest recovery of sensation in the reinnervated forearm skin was 6 weeks. There were 2 donor site complications.

Conclusion.—For reconstruction of the oral cavity after significant glossectomy, the new, bilobed radial forearm free flap provides thin, pliable, and redundant tissue to preserve tongue mobility while preventing tethering of the root of the tongue to the inner table of the mandible. Sensory re-education may improve functional sensation.

▶ For some reason, the belief has grown that glossectomy defects require bulk in reconstruction, such as a free or pedicled muscle/skin flap. Although that option may be useful in *total* glossectomy defects, what is needed in partial (greater than 50% in this series) defects is sufficient pliability to assure that the remaining native tongue can function properly. Would a similar approach be useful in the hemiglossectomy defects that are conventionally managed by closing the tongue upon itself?—E.A. Luce, M.D.

A Single Center's Experience With 308 Free Flaps for Repair of Head and Neck Cancer Defects

Schusterman MA, Miller MJ, Reece GP, Kroll SS, Marchi M, Goepfert H (MD Anderson Cancer Ctr, Houston)
Plast Reconstr Surg 93:472–478, 1994   140-95-13–21

Introduction.—Because of the aggressive character of head and neck cancers, radical—and usually disfiguring—surgery is frequently necessary. Simultaneous and reliable reconstructive surgery is important for restoring the patient's quality of life. The reliability of microvascular free-flap transfer in reconstructive surgery of the head and neck was investigated.

Methods.—A total of 308 free-flap procedures were performed from May 1988 through February 1992.

Results.—A total of 86% of flap procedures were performed at the time of the original surgery. Most of the patients were white male smokers who consumed alcohol. Most resections were the result of squamous cell carcinoma, most tumors were T3, T4, or recurrent, and most flaps were from the radial forearm. The average patient was followed for 14 months, and 206 were still alive at last follow-up. The complication rate was 36%, with a venous thrombosis rate of 7% and a flap loss rate of 6%. The flap salvage rate was 19%. Previous surgery and vein graft were significantly associated with flap loss.

Conclusion.—Microvascular surgery has improved the outcome of reconstructive surgery. Although the overall complication rate was 36%, only previous surgery and vein grafting increased the flap loss rate.

▶ This is probably the largest series of free-tissue transfer for head and neck extirpative defects, and the data are well presented. The authors compose an eloquent argument for the use of free-tissue transfer preferentially in ablative oral cavity and oropharyngeal defects, and their favorite seems to be the radial forearm.—E.A. Luce, M.D.

The Through-and-Through Oromandibular Defect: Rationale for Aggressive Reconstruction

Boyd JB, Morris S, Rosen IB, Gullane P, Rotstein L, Freeman JL (Univ of Toronto)
Plast Reconstr Surg 93:44–53, 1994   140-95-13–22

Introduction.—Surgical treatment of through-and-through oral cancer is challenging, as extensive microvascular reconstruction is required.

These patients are in the terminal stages of disease and are, therefore, often frail. Although the prognosis is poor, surgery may be justified to palliate their suffering, reduce hospitalization, and improve the quality of their remaining life. The iliac crest osteocutaneous flap allows composite microvascular tissue transfer in a single procedure. A retrospective evaluation was performed of 38 patients requiring reconstruction of bone, skin, and mucosa to assess the benefits of surgery in these patients.

Methods.—A study was made of the complete medical charts of 38 patients with through-and-through oral carcinoma who underwent a free vascularized tissue transfer to reconstruct the skin, mucosa, and a section of the mandible. The patients were followed for at least 1 year. In 34 of the 38 patients, reconstruction was performed at the time of tumor ablation and was accomplished with a radial forearm osteocutaneous flap, a free fibula with a radial cutaneous island, or the iliac crest osteocutaneous flap. In most of the patients, interosseous wires provided fixation, although some had Kirschner wires, miniplates, or reconstruction plates.

Results.—All 38 patients had stage T4 tumors; most had recurrent disease and had received preoperative radiation therapy. After reconstructive surgery, 92% had free-flap survival. There were no complications in 68% of the patients, although 1 postoperative death was attributed to respiratory obstruction. The mean hospital stay was 43 days. Most patients achieved normal or easily understood speech (65%) and could consume an oral diet (84%). Forty-nine percent drooled occasionally and 19% drooled continuously; the remaining 32% had normal oral continence. There was bony union in 73%. There were 12 patients still alive at the time of the evaluation. Of the patients who died, the average survival was 13 months.

Discussion.—A small number of patients with terminal stage disease were salvaged with ablative and reconstructive surgery. In the patients who died, symptoms were palliated. The single-stage procedures reduced the hospital stay and may reduce further hospitalizations. Ablative technique required radical bony excision, which could lead to debilitating deformity without bony reconstruction. The iliac crest provided sufficient soft tissue. A two-flap technique may be the best option for reconstructing massive, complex defects, especially the scapular osteocutaneous flap.

▶ What choice does a reconstructive surgeon have in these desparate instances? This series illustrates the thin, perhaps indistinguishable, line between reconstruction/rehabilitation and wound closure in far advanced cases of head and neck cancer. Some technical considerations are that perhaps the deep iliac donor site for microvascular transfer of bone and soft tissue is not the optimum choice for these frail and malnourished patients. Scapula is an attractive alternative but tends to prolong operative time because both teams (extirpative and reconstructive) cannot work simultaneously. Linked radial forearm (skin, soft tissue) and fibula (bone plus or minus skin) is a double free flap and has longer operative time. These are difficult decisions, but the point to be made is not reconstruction vs. no reconstruction, but rather palliation. Of course, the incidence of bony union (73%) could probably be enhanced with the use of plates instead of interosseous wires, a technique utilized in the earlier part of the series.—E.A. Luce, M.D.

Vascularized Bone Flaps in Oromandibular Reconstruction: A Comparative Anatomic Study of Bone Stock From Various Donor Sites to Assess Suitability for Enosseous Dental Implants
Moscoso JF, Keller J, Genden E, Weinberg H, Biller HF, Buchbinder D, Urken ML (Mount Sinai Med Ctr, New York)
Arch Otolaryngol Head Neck Surg 120:36–43, 1994   140-95-13–23

Background.—Oral cavity reconstruction has benefited greatly from the successful transfer of vascularized bone and sensate soft tissue as microvascular free flaps. Donor sites were identified from which vascularized bone could be harvested to accept osseointegrated implants of the minimum dimensions needed to ensure long-term implant stability.

Methods.—The most commonly used donor sites for vascularized bone in oromandibular reconstruction were studied in 28 cadavers. The ipsilateral fibula, iliac crest, radius, and lateral border of the scapula were harvested and sectioned at multiple predetermined sites. For each section, implantability was determined based on measurements of height, width, and cross-sectional area using computer planimetry.

Findings.—The most consistently implantable donor site was the iliac crest. Eighty-three percent of the sections satisfied the criteria for implantability. The corresponding percentages for the scapula, fibula, and radius were 78%, 67%, and 21%. At each donor site except the scapula, consistent regional differences in implantability were noted.

Conclusion.—These findings objectively confirm the clinical impression that the iliac crest is the most uniformly implantable source of vascularized bone for mandibular reconstruction. Unexpectedly, the lateral scapular border was the statistical equivalent of the iliac crest for overall implantability. The radius was the least reliable donor site, especially in female cadavers.

▶ Successful reconstruction of head and neck defects has moved from simply restitution of form to address of oropharyngeal functioning. Reconstruction of the mandible is an integral part of this approach. As the authors outline, the final margin of success in mandibular reconstruction is placement of endo-osseous implants.

Their work takes us further down the road toward understanding how to individualize reconstruction for specific patients. The iliac crest, within the framework of this study, is the preferable donor site for mandibular reconstruction, with a view towards eventual endo-osseous implants for denture fitting. Yet other considerations were ignored (as the authors remind us), including morbidity of the donor site (the iliac crest is a more difficult donor site dissection for vascularized bone than fibula in most hands) and the particular mandibular deficit. Many lateral mandibular defects do not need implants, and other donor sites than the iliac crest could be considered. Finally, this paper puts another nail in the coffin of the suitability (lack of same) of the radius as an *osseo*-cutaneous donor site.—E.A. Luce, M.D.

Head and Neck—Outcomes

Assessment of Quality of Life in Head and Neck Cancer Patients
Hassan SJ, Weymuller EA Jr (Univ of Washington, Seattle)
Head Neck 15:485–496, 1993   140-95-13–24

Background.—Over the past decade, concerns about the quality of life (QOL) as well as survival, have been increasing regarding patients with cancer. It has been agreed that the ideal QOL questionnaire should be short and easy to understand. The University of Washington (UW) QOL Head and Neck questionnaire, the Sickness Impact Profile (SIP), and the Karnofsky scales were examined.

Methods.—Seventy-five consecutive patients with head and neck cancer were selected to assess the UW QOL. The SIP and Karnofsky scales, already established evaluation tools, were used for comparison. Each assessment tool was administered several days before surgery, immediately after surgery, and 3 months after surgery.

Findings.—Ninety-seven percent of the patients found the UW QOL scale to be more acceptable than the SIP because it was more concise and easier to complete. When the SIP was used as a gold standard, the UW QOL scale had an average criterion validity of .849, and the average criterion validity of the Karnofsky scales was .826. The reliability coefficients for the UW QOL, Karnofsky scales, and SIP were more than .9, .8, and .87, respectively. In addition, the UW QOL was more effective at detecting change than the Karnofsky scales and the SIP.

Conclusion.—The validity and reliability of the UW QOL scale are comparable to those of the Karnofsky scales and the SIP. The UW QOL was more acceptable to patients and provided the best indicator of change in their QOL.

▶ Here is a crude and primitive but, nevertheless, first step in assessment of function in addition to simple survival. The questionnaire assesses only QOL issues in the head and neck; a more global picture would also require evaluation of overall functioning. These types of measurement tools will become more important as we demonstrate the effectiveness of our intervention by other means than the black-and-white of survival only.—E.A. Luce, M.D.

A Case-Control Study on Complications and Survival in Elderly Patients Undergoing Major Head and Neck Surgery

Kowalski LP, Alcantara PSM, Magrin J, Parise O Jr (AC Camargo Hosp, Sao Paulo, Brazil)
Am J Surg 168:485–490, 1994   140-95-13-25

Background.—With an increased life expectancy in Western nations, even 90-year-old individuals can anticipate living for another 6 years. Yet, older patients in good medical status are perceived to have a high surgical risk and are less likely than younger patients to receive standard treatment for cancer. A case-control study compared complications, mortality, and survival in a group of elderly patients and a comparable group of younger patients.

Patients and Methods.—Study subjects were drawn from patients admitted to the study institution from 1980 to 1990 for treatment of head and neck cancers. The older group included 115 consecutive patients aged 70 years or older who underwent radical surgery and 115 controls matched for cancer site, clinical stage, and choice of radical surgery. Controls ranged in age from 10 to 69 years (mean age, 54 years). The case group had more chronic heart and lung diseases and a larger proportion of females than the control group. Most tumors in both groups were located in the oral cavity, salivary glands, pharynx, or larynx.

Results.—Although disease extension was similar in subjects and controls, a highly significant number of cases were classified as operative risks III and IV. Standard surgical extension was not performed in 30% of the case subjects vs. 10% of the controls. The control group was more likely to have radical neck treatment, reconstructive procedures, and postoperative radiotherapy. Local and systemic complications occurred at a similar rate in the 2 groups. There were 5 postoperative deaths among subjects and 4 among controls. Risk of recurrence was slightly reduced in the case group. At the study closing date, 30% of the elderly subjects and 37% of younger controls were alive with recent follow-up information. Twenty-seven elderly patients and 9 controls had died of causes not related to cancer; cancer recurrence or treatment complications accounted for 34 case deaths and 39 control deaths. The 5-year actuarial survival rate was 43% for patients older than age 70 years vs. 56% for the younger controls.

Conclusion.—Treatment decisions regarding patients with head and neck cancer should be based upon clinical status rather than chronological age. This series of elderly patients undergoing radical surgery had rates of postoperative mortality and complications comparable to those of younger patients. Although older patients had 1.4 times the risk of death of younger patients, rates of cancer-related death were similar for the 2 groups.

▶ Once again we are reminded that in the management of head and neck cancer patients, elderly patients should be treated with standard protocols and will do as well in terms of morbidity, mortality, survival, and recurrence as their younger counterparts.—E.A. Luce, M.D.

Functional Status and Coping in Patients With Oral and Pharyngeal Cancer Before and After Surgery
Langius A, Björvell H, Lind MG (Karolinska Hosp, Stockholm, Sweden)
Head Neck 16:559–568, 1994   140-95-13-26

Introduction.—The treatment of oral and pharyngeal cancer, which usually consists of surgery and irradiation, often considerably affects the patient's quality of life. Reported problems include decreased eating ability, reduced social functioning, and disabilities in speech. A group of patients treated by surgery for oral or pharyngeal cancer were evaluated for functional status and coping ability. The usefulness of 2 questionnaires was also assessed.

Patients and Methods.—Forty-two of 71 eligible patients participated. Twenty-seven completed the assessment instruments 12 months after treatment and 15 were evaluated both before and after surgery. The Sickness Impact Profile (SIP) was used to measure functional status and the Sense of Coherence (SOC) scale was used to assess coping behaviors. Patients were classified according to the extent of their surgery: minor, moderate, or major. A healthy reference group was made up of a random sample of 75 women and 70 men; 6 comparison groups included patients with other disorders.

Results.—Scores on the SIP were higher overall for patients who had undergone surgery for oropharyngeal cancer than for the healthy reference group and for patients treated surgically for colorectal cancer and peripheral vascular disease. Patients with benign chronic pain had significantly higher SIP scores, however, both overall and on the physical and psychosocial dimensions of the scale. Functional limitations in the oropharyngeal cancer group were related to more extensive surgery and to less successful coping. The 15 patients studied prospectively perceived more dysfunction in the areas of ambulation and emotional behavior and communication 12 months after surgery; the area of work was perceived as better. Younger patients perceived more dysfunction, and women rated more functional impairments than men. Women also rated a weaker sense of coherence on the SOC scale than did men. There was a correlation between a stronger coping score and a lower functional impairment score.

Conclusion.—Both psychological and physical functioning are adversely affected by surgery for oral and pharyngeal cancer. Individual differences are considerable, however, and may depend on tumor size and location and on the patient's coping abilities. Patients should benefit from individualized rehabilitation programs that take into account their status as measured by the SIP and SOC scales.

▶ This is a landmark article not for the results—in fact the results are not important—but rather for the effort to develop quality-of-life measurements in head and neck cancer patients. Outcome studies that have focused on postoperative results have been concerned with either morbidity/mortality, survival, or quite discreet studies of rehabilitation of speech and deglutition. This study backs off several hundred yards and looks at aspects of coping and social/occupation functioning. The authors gained some experience with some qualitative life measurement tools that may be useful to other investigators.—E.A. Luce, M.D.

Laryngeal Preservation by Induction Chemotherapy Plus Radiotherapy in Locally Advanced Head and Neck Cancer: The M. D. Anderson Cancer Center Experience
Shirinian MH, Weber RS, Lippman SM, Dimery IW, Earley CL, Garden AS, Michaelson J, Morrison WH, Kramer A, Byers R, Peters L, Hong WK, Goepfert H (MD Anderson Cancer Ctr, Houston)
Head Neck 16:39–44, 1994   140-95-13–27

Introduction.—Total laryngectomy is generally performed in patients with locally advanced laryngeal and hypopharyngeal and some oropharyngeal cancers. Recent studies have suggested that cisplatin-based chemotherapy followed by radiation therapy may allow laryngeal preservation without reducing overall survival. This laryngeal preservation approach was evaluated in 2 consecutive prospective phase II studies in patients with locally advanced head and neck cancer.

Methods.—The studies included 64 patients with squamous cell carcinoma of the larynx, hypopharynx, or base of the tongue who would otherwise have required total laryngectomy. Both protocols used cisplatin-based induction chemotherapy: 31 patients received cisplatin–bleomycin–5-fluorouracil (PBF), and 33 received cisplatin–5-fluorouracil (PF). Both groups received definitive radiation therapy, with a total dose to the primary site of 76.6 Gy. Only patients with less than a partial response to chemotherapy and those with residual or recurrent cancer after chemotherapy plus radiation therapy underwent surgery.

Results.—Fifty-nine patients were evaluable for response to chemotherapy. The overall complete plus partial response rates were comparable for the 2 chemotherapy protocols: 73% for PBF and 79% for PF. There was no significant difference by tumor site, with response rates of 75% for laryngeal, 78% for hypopharyngeal, and 75% for oropharyngeal cancers. Forty-five patients with complete or partial responses received radiation therapy; 41 were evaluable for response. Complete response rates after this treatment were 88% for patients with laryngeal cancer, 83% for those with hypopharyngeal cancer, and 50% for those with oropharyngeal cancer. Eighteen patients required surgical salvage: 10 who did not respond to chemotherapy and 8 with persistent disease after chemoradiotherapy.

The most common hematologic toxicity of chemotherapy was neutropenia of less than 1,000 cells/mm³, which occurred in 16% of the PBF group and 44% of the PF group. Mucositis of grade 3 or greater occurred in 4% of the PBF group vs. 50% of the PF group. At follow-up of up to 54+ months, 44% of patients with laryngeal cancer, 28% of those with hypopharyngeal cancer, and 22% of those with oropharyngeal cancer were alive with laryngeal preservation. The overall 2-year survival rates in these 3 groups were 71%, 46%, and 38%, respectively.

Conclusion.—With cisplatin-based chemotherapy followed by radiation therapy, laryngeal preservation appears to be feasible in patients with locally advanced head and neck cancer. There is no compromise in survival, even for patients in whom surgery and radiation therapy are delayed because of chemotherapeutic failure. Further studies of laryngeal preservation approaches—including promising new chemotherapy regimens, different radiation therapy approaches, and elective neck dissection—are needed.

▶ The unit at M.D. Anderson Cancer Center has taken the next logical step after the publication of their 1991 V.A. trial of laryngeal preservation in advanced disease by combined chemoradiotherapy. These results confirm the VA cooperative trial and take the next step, namely, to begin to examine other primary sites. The reported 50% complete remission rate was obtained in oropharyngeal lesions that would have otherwise required laryngectomy as part of their surgical treatment. The numbers are low (6 patients) and the response is certainly lower than larynx-hypopharynx primaries. Yet, these are intriguing findings that demand further clinical trials of such an approach in other sites in the head and neck.—E.A. Luce, M.D.

Photodynamic Therapy of Malignant and Premalignant Lesions in Patients With 'Field Cancerization' of the Oral Cavity

Grant WE, Hopper C, Speight PM, Macrobert AJ, Bown SG (Royal Free Hosp, London)
J Laryngol Otol 107:1140–1145, 1993   140-95-13–28

Background.—The coexistence of premalignant lesions such as leukoplakia or erythroplakia with an existing primary tumor in the oral cavity, or the presence of a secondary tumor in the same anatomical site, indicates a high risk for malignancy in the entire mucosa. Surgical resection of such "field cancerization" is likely to be mutilating. Eleven patients with single or multiple primary cancers and associated areas of leukoplakia in the oral cavity underwent photodynamic therapy (PDT) as an alternative to surgery.

Patients and Methods.—Five patients had a primary cancer and 6 had multiple primary tumors, all with associated premalignant disease. All cases involved histologically proven early invasive squamous cell carcinomas diagnosed as stage I. Six patients had previously undergone surgical excision of oral tumors; no patient had received radiotherapy. Treatment consisted of photofrin at a dose of 2 mg/kg administered 48 hours before photoirradiation with 50–100 J/cm² of red laser light by surface illumination. Two patients with very extensive disease were treated on 2 separate occasions, and 10 patients required more than 1 spot to treat the target areas. The initial response was evaluated at 6–8 weeks.

Results.—Patients received PDT on an outpatient basis and tolerated the procedure satisfactorily. Treated areas healed fully in 3–5 weeks. At 6–8 weeks, 10 of the 11 patients had a complete response to PDT. The remaining patient had undergone 2 separate treatments because the entire surface of the tongue was involved. Although more than 75% of the treated area had healed, a patchy grey-white lesion persisted on the dorsum. With a mean follow-up of 11 months, no patient had evidence of recurrence of invasive squamous cell carcinoma at treated sites. Two patients subsequently required excision and radiotherapy for further metachronous primary carcinomas at other sites.

Conclusion.—Patients with early invasive and premalignant lesions in the oral cavity can benefit from PDT ablation. Unlike extensive surgery, the treatment does not result in unacceptable loss of function and cosmetic changes. In addition, PDT can be repeated without loss of normal tissue.

▶ Photodynamic therapy holds great promise for inclusion in the armamentarium of the head and neck surgeon; however, the exact role has yet to be defined. Limitations of the technique include the ability to treat only to a depth of a few millimeters and long-term photosynthesization of the patient. The patients treated in this series represented an extremely difficult problem, namely, widespread changes of the oral mucosa for which our only recourse in the past has been simply observation. We need more evidence in a larger series of patients, but this report is encouraging.—E.A. Luce, M.D.

Tracheostomal Stenosis After Total Laryngectomy: An Analysis of Predisposing Clinical Factors

Kuo M, Ho C-M, Wei WI, Lam K-H (Univ of Hong Kong)
Laryngoscope 104:59–63, 1994   140-95-13–29

Introduction.—Stenosis of the terminal tracheostome in patients who have undergone total laryngectomy is a complication that poses a cosmetic problem, precludes insertion of a voice prosthesis, and may lead to serious medical consequences. A retrospective study of 207 patients who underwent surgery for carcinoma of the larynx and hypopharynx analyzed potential contributing factors for stenosis of the terminal tracheostome.

Patients and Methods.—The patients had a median age of 63 years; 184 were men and 23 were women. All were treated by total laryngectomy and many also underwent radical neck dissection and/or immediate tracheoesophageal puncture. Laryngectomy was performed through a transverse skin incision, and the tracheostome was brought out through the middle of the lower flap. The median follow-up was 20 months, and all patients were reviewed at least 6 months postoperatively.

Results.—The overall incidence of tracheostomal stenosis was 13%; the mean period between operation and onset of stenosis was 3 months. Women were more likely to be affected than men (26% vs. 11%, a statistically significant difference). Factors associated with a higher incidence of tracheostomal stenosis included postoperative radiotherapy, pharyngeal reconstruction using the pectoralis major myocutaneous flap, tracheostomal infection, and immediate tracheoesophageal puncture. Multivariate analysis, however, found only female sex and tracheostomal infection to be independent determinants of the risk of tracheostomal stenosis.

Conclusion.—Reports of the incidence of tracheostomal stenosis after total laryngectomy have varied widely, from 4% to 42%. The technique of stomal reconstruction is thought to affect the development of stenosis. In this series of patients, the incidence of tracheostomal stenosis using 3- or 4-flap interdigitation was 13%. Factors significantly related to the development of stenosis were female sex and tracheostomal infection. The latter is an avoidable complication, and every effort should be made to minimize and treat it.

▶ The most important factor in determination of the occurrence of stomal stenosis after laryngectomy is the technique of initial stomal construction. Some method—most commonly, the use of interdigitating flaps—must be used to avoid the "straight-line" contracture consequent to a simple circle design. The authors also determined a higher incidence with immediate tracheopharyngeal puncture as well as pectoralis myocutaneous flap reconstruction. Perhaps the operative factor in both cases was some element of leakage that was not sufficiently clinically significant to be evident in this retrospective study, yet produced low-grade infection and later stenosis.—E.A. Luce, M.D.

Miscellaneous Reconstruction

Interferon-Alpha-2a for the Treatment of Complex Hemangiomas of Infancy and Childhood
Ricketts RR, Hatley RM, Corden BJ, Sabio H, Howell CG (Emory Univ, Atlanta, Ga; Med College of Georgia, Atlanta)
Ann Surg 219:605–614, 1994   140-95-13–30

Background.—Hemangiomas, the most frequent tumors of infants and children, most often grow rapidly until the infant is aged 6–8 months, at which time they stabilize and begin to involute in the second year of life. Complete resolution occurs in 90% of all children by age 10 years. Hemangiomas that do not follow this course may threaten vital organs and extremities and are associated with a 20% to 50% mortality rate. Typically, aggressive treatment has included high-dose steroids, arterial ligation, or surgical resection. Each of these treatments may have serious risks, or may be ineffective with, some individuals. The results of treating 4 infants and 1 child for complex hemangiomas with interferon-α-2a were examined.

Methods.—Interferon-α-2a was administered subcutaneously at a beginning dose of 1 million units/m² per day during a 1-week period. The dose was then advanced during a 1-week period to 3 million units/m² per day. Therapy was continued for 5–11 months, based on response of the lesion to treatment.

Results.—The 5 patients were aged 4 weeks to 28 months. There were 3 boys and 2 girls, 3 white and 2 black children. Two patients had received prior therapy, 1 with compression and 1 with prednisone plus blood product replacement therapy. Three patients had total or near total regression, 1 had partial regression, and 1 had stabilization for a mean of 7.4 months. Severe consumptive coagulopathy resolved immediately on initiation of therapy in 1 patient. All patients have grown and developed normally, and there have been no recurrences after a mean follow-up of 9.25 months. Minor, transient side effects occurred in 2 patients.

Conclusion.—The findings presented here are in agreement with studies presented elsewhere supporting the effectiveness of interferon-α-2a in treating complex hemangiomas. Interferon-α-2a should be considered as the first-line agent in the treatment of complex hemangiomas of infants and children.

▶ I would recommend this paper to the reader for 2 reasons: (1) the results obtained in this extremely difficult group of patients with innovative therapy with interferon-α-2a and (2) the paper provides an excellent summary of the clinical characteristics and behavior of hemangiomas and vascular malformations. As the discussants point out (the paper was presented at the Southern Surgical Association), the natural history of complex hemangiomas is so variable that separation or delineation of a therapeutic effect of a particular drug or intervention is quite difficult. Yet, these problems (loss of limb, life, or eyesight) merit such an approach.—E.A. Luce, M.D.

Muscle-Flap Coverage for Infected Peripheral Vascular Prostheses

Meland NB, Arnold PG, Pairolero PC, Lovich SF (Mayo Clinic and Found,

Rochester, Minn)
Plast Reconstr Surg 93:1005–1011, 1994   140-95-13–31

Background.—Reconstructive vascular operations with synthetic arterial substitutes are common. The loss of an extremity is a potential complication of infection in these protheses. Grade 3 infections, as classified by Szilagy et al., are infections surrounding and in contact with the graft, and they have been further classified into stages I, II, and III. Stage I includes infection of the graft material without secondary complications, stage II includes infection with minor secondary complications, and stage III includes infections complicated by massive recurrent bleeding, systemic sepsis, and thrombosis of the graft. The data were reviewed on a highly select group of patients with infected vascular grafts.

Methods.—The records of 20 patients with 24 grade 3 peripheral prosthetic graft infections were studied. The grafts were treated by debridement and muscle flap transposition. Seventeen grafts were stage I, 6 were stage II, and 1 was stage III. Twelve grafts were seen as a swollen, painful groin mass and leukocytosis, 6 as a draining cutaneous sinus, and 5 as a pseudoaneurysm. The infections were in the groin in 19 patients. Aortofemoral bypass grafting was performed in 14 patients, and femoral popliteal grafts were used in 6. The rectus femoris was the most commonly used muscle flap. The muscle was removed without overlying skin and was skin-grafted 48 hours after transposition and insetting.

Results.—Long-term graft coverage without recurrent infection was successful in 16 grafts. Eight grafts failed, and all failures were secondary to recurrent or persistent infections with thrombosis, hemorrhage, or sepsis. In graft failures, the mean recurrence time to infection was 5.6 months. The loss of an extremity occurred in 3 patients. The success rate of polytetrafluoroethylene grafts was 75%, and the success rate of Dacron grafts was 62.5%. In 7 of 9 patients, the sartorius muscle was used successfully. In 1 patient, the rectus abdominis muscle became necrotic immediately after transposition.

Discussion.—The standard treatment for infections in peripheral prosthetic vascular grafts has been removal of the graft and extra-anatomical bypass. These infections have also been treated successfully by debridement, continuous irrigation, and conservative local therapy with skin flaps, muscle flaps, and skin grafting. Muscle flaps have been shown to improve healing, lower bacterial counts, and bring in well-vascularized tissue to infected areas. The rectus femoris muscle is preferred for groin infections.

▶ These authors are careful to remind the reader that this approach of debridement, muscle flaps, and closed suction that yielded a salvage rate of two thirds of the grafts was accomplished in a selected group at a busy institution (the Mayo Clinic). In fact, these were *localized* infections and three fourths of them were stage I (infection without secondary complication of bleeding, thrombosis, or systemic sepsis). Less than one half of the stage II and III infections were salvaged, and perhaps another approach (excision and extra-anatomical bypass) would be preferable.

My criticisms of the series are as follows: (1) the mean debridements before muscle transfer was 3, not particularly expeditious; (2) the hospital stay was lengthy according to the protocol described of 14 days of closed suction and an additional week of parenteral antibiotics; and (3) the sartorius muscle was frequently used, and I have found that muscle skinny, thin, poorly vascularized, and just generally inadequate for these limb-threatening, and perhaps life-threatening, situations. The rectus femoris is a much better option.—E.A. Luce, M.D.

A Phase II Study to Evaluate Recombinant Platelet-Derived Growth Factor-BB in the Treatment of Stage 3 and 4 Pressure Ulcers

Mustoe TA, Cutler NR, Allman RM, Goode PS, Deuel TF, Prause JA, Bear M, Serdar CM, Pierce GF (Northwestern Univ, Chicago; California Clinical Trials, Beverly Hills; Univ of Alabama, Birmingham; et al)
Arch Surg 129:213–219, 1994   140-95-13–32

Background.—The B chain of platelet-derived growth factor (PDGF), a product of the v-*sis* oncogene, stimulates the proliferation of fibroblasts, smooth muscle cells, and possibly endothelial cells from wound capillaries. It also has chemotactic activity and activates neutrophils, macrophages, smooth muscle cells, and fibroblasts. Topically applied recombinant PDGF-BB (rPDGF-BB) has hastened the healing of surgical incisions in normal animals and those with impaired healing.

Study Design.—The efficacy of a daily topical application of rPDGF-BB was investigated in a prospective, double-blind, randomized study of 41 patients in a hospital or nursing home setting. The patients were predominantly elderly women who had clean pressure ulcers that had been adequately debrided. The ulcers were not a result of vascular disease. The patients were randomly assigned to daily topical treatment with 100 or 300 µg/mL of rPDGF-BB or a placebo. Saline gauze dressings were applied each day and the patients were turned frequently. The wound volume was measured by using alginate molds.

Results.—Both doses of rPDGF-BB reduced the volume of pressure ulcers, whereas only minimal change was seen in the placebo-treated patients. The time to 50% healing was shortest in the patients treated with 100 µg/mL of rPDGF-BB. After 28 days of treatment, the ulcers were much smaller in both active treatment groups, compared with placebo recipients. The treated lesions contained more activated fibroblasts and showed greater synthesis of procollagen type 1.

Conclusion.—Topical treatment with rPDGF-BB may be an effective means of hastening the healing of chronic pressure ulcers.

▶ Growth factors are the current "wonder drug" for wound healing, but this report is the first prospective, double-blind study to assess the efficacy of PDGF. The authors present a convincing case, but it would need confirmation with considerably larger studies than this model.—E.A. Luce, M.D.

The Use of Latissimus Dorsi Muscle Flap in Reconstructive Heart Surgery

Lalinde E, Sanz J, Bazán A, Ballesteros A, Mesa F, Elejabeitia J, Paloma V, Herreros J (Univ of Navarra, Pamplona, Spain)
Plast Reconstr Surg 94:490–495, 1994   140-95-13–33

Background.—The use of a skeletal muscle flap as a mechanical aid for the heart is being defined as dynamic cardiomyoplasty. This technique of ventricular assistance is indicated for the correction of left ventricular aneurysm and for cardiomyopathies in which heart transplantation is contraindicated. The initial experience with a clinical dynamic cardiomyoplasty program was reported.

Patients.—Four dynamic cardiomyoplasties were performed in 1991 and 1992. Two patients had New York Heart Association functional class IV ischemic cardiomyopathy with absolute contraindications for heart transplantation, and 2 had major left ventricle anteroapical aneurysm with no angiographic chance of coronary revascularization.

Technique.—The operation was performed after a 3-week training period in which the left latissimus dorsi muscle was conditioned by means of an external pulse-train generator. The cardiomyoplasty consisted of a left latissimus dorsi island flap rotated into the thorax. A sensing electrode was placed in the anterior wall of the right ventricle, and the left and right ventricles were wrapped in the latissimus dorsi muscle flap. At the end of the procedure, the electrodes were connected to the generator, which was placed under the fascia of the rectal muscle in the abdomen. The generator was activated 2 weeks after surgery, when the union between the flap and the heart was stable.

Results.—One of the patients with cardiomyopathy died of cerebral embolism 4 months after surgery. This patient was at functional class II at the time. The other 3 patients are alive at functional class I and performing normal activities. All patients had improved left ventricular function, as evaluated by echo-Doppler and scintigraphy studies. Significant increases were observed in ejection fraction and maximum minute blood flow rate.

Conclusion.—Preliminary experience shows that left ventricular function is significantly improved after dynamic cardiomyoplasty. Clinical improvement is correlated with increased ejection fraction and maximum minute flow rate of blood. Five more dynamic cardiomyoplasties have more recently been performed. There have been no further deaths, and significant improvements have been observed in all evaluation parameters.

▶ All four patients had quite significantly improved cardiac function with a dynamic cardiomyoplasty. The latissimus muscle is particularly advantageous for the reasons cited, namely, proximity, length of the vascular pedicle, and the size of the muscle. Yet, this technique is obviously still experimental, and clinicians must be certain that the patient is not a candidate (in instances of cardiomyopathy) for transplantation.—E.A. Luce, M.D.

Wound-Healing Complications After Soft-Tissue Sarcoma Surgery
Peat BG, Bell RS, Davis A, O'Sullivan B, Mahoney J, Manktelow RT, Bowen V, Catton C, Fornasier VL, Langer F (Univ of Toronto)
Plast Reconstr Surg 93:980–987, 1994   140-95-13–34

Introduction.—The success of reconstructive technique for limb salvage surgery in patients with soft tissue sarcoma is measured by the ability to achieve primary wound healing. Clinical evidence has suggested that wound healing is often complicated in patients treated with direct wound closure. An attempt to identify the factors that predict wound-healing complications and the impact of using vascularized tissue transfer in patients at risk for wound complications was undertaken.

Methods.—The clinical records of patients treated for soft tissue sarcoma over 5 years were reviewed. Surgical reconstruction followed surgical resection and preoperative irradiation if staging studies revealed tumor margins adjacent to neurovascular structures, or if the expected postoperative irradiation field would include the full limb circumference or radiation-sensitive structures. Of the 180 patients, direct wound closure was performed in 137. The remaining 43 patients were treated with soft tissue reconstruction because empirical evidence suggested anticipated wound closure complications.

Results.—Of the 137 patients treated with primary wound closure, 23 (17%) experienced major wound complications, whereas 2 of the 43 patients (11%) who had soft-tissue reconstruction had major wound complications. Univariate analysis identified cross-sectional resection diameter, preoperative irradiation, a history of diabetes or vascular disease, a history of smoking, and the width of the skin excision as factors that predicted wound complications. Multivariate analysis identified only the cross-sectional resection diameter and preoperative irradiation as factors predicting major wound complications.

Discussion.—The higher wound complication rate in patients with larger resection diameters is not surprising, because a larger width of deep tissue was generally excised. This reduced skin flap vascularization and created more wound closure tension (in the wounds closed directly) and a larger surgical dead space. Although preoperative irradiation significantly predicted wound complications, the advantages of this treatment outweigh the risks. Preoperative irradiation can allow more precise postoperative treatment planning by decreasing tumor size and density. Vascularized tissue transfer can fill the dead space and decrease the skin closure tension created by tumor resection, and by providing nonirradiated tissue, it can enhance wound repair.

▶ This study might raise more questions in the reader's mind than answers, partly because of the retrospective nature of the study and the lack of randomization between primary closure and tissue transfer. Yet, undeniably, the patients with large tissue volume resection *and* preoperative radiotherapy who had muscle flaps performed prospectively had only one third the wound complication rate of those with wounds closed primarily. This patient group was clearly at the most difficult end of the spectrum. Probably, the best case also that can be made for wound closure by tissue transfer in limb salvage situations is the necessity for prompt initiation of *postoperative* radiotherapy, because it requires a closed and healed wound.—E.A. Luce, M.D.

14 Vascular Surgery

Introduction

Multiple reports over the past year have provided new information that directly impacts on the day-to-day care of patients with peripheral vascular disease. Subsequent analyses of patients entered into the NASCET database reveal that patients with minor neurologic defects can safely undergo carotid endarterectomy shortly (< 30 days) after a stroke (Abstract 140-95-14–1) and that the presence of plaque ulceration appears to be a risk factor for stroke that is independent of the degree of carotid stenosis, even if patients undergo carotid endarterectomy (see Abstract 140-95-14–2). In addition, the use of regional anesthesia for carotid endarterectomy appears to reduce the cost of this procedure and potentially make it safer (Abstract 140-95-14–3).

Similarly, comparison of results of endovascular procedures to results of standard reconstructive vascular surgery have clarified the role of these less invasive procedures in patients with arterial occlusive disease. Randomized comparison of catheter-directed thrombolysis to standard surgical therapy in patients with limb ischemia (Abstracts 140-95-14–5 and 140-95-14–6) demonstrates that thrombolysis reduces the risk of therapy of acute limb ischemia but is less successful than surgery in the management of chronic limb ischemia. In addition, thrombolysis has been shown to be inferior to surgical thrombectomy in the management of occluded hemodialysis access grafts (Abstract 140-95-14–7). Furthermore, long-term results of treatment of arterial occlusive disease with atherectomy using the Rotablator (Abstract 140-95-14–8) have been shown to be so poor that this technique has little role in the management of patients with peripheral vascular disease.

Balloon angioplasty has also been shown to be cost effective compared to surgery only if it is done as an isolated procedure in patients with claudication, whereas the cost of balloon angioplasty with or without adjuvant surgical procedures in patients with critical ischemia is equivalent to that of surgery (Abstract 140-95-14–9). Finally, endoluminal aneurysm repair of aortic aneurysms has been reported to be a promising new technique, with early results being encouraging (Abstracts 140-95-14–10 and 140-95-14–11). However, many questions remain to be answered concerning the long-term outcome of endoluminal aneurysm repair, and these questions must be answered before general release of this procedure.

Surgical therapy remains the mainstay for the management of limb ischemia, and refinements of techniques of peripheral vascular reconstruction continue. Repeat leg bypass in properly selected patients can be successful, even after 2 or more bypass graft failures in the same leg (Abstract 140-95-14-14). Unconventional amputations can be used to salvage a functional limb, despite extensive forefoot ischemia (Abstract 140-95-14-15), and toe pressures can help predict the success of forefoot amputations (Abstract 140-95-14-16).

Magnetic resonance arteriography continues to develop and may soon replace contrast arteriography for imaging of the peripheral vascular tree (Abstract 140-95-14-17). Recognition of difficult problems, such as atheroembolism, and understanding the natural history of problems such as small popliteal aneurysms also are a key to good outcome in patients with peripheral vascular disease. Defining patients with high risk for deep venous thrombosis who will likely benefit from prophylaxis should also lead to improved outcomes. Surprisingly, in almost 20% of patients undergoing abdominal aortic aneurysm repair, deep venous thrombosis has been shown to develop, so prophylaxis for deep venous thrombosis should be routine in such procedures (Abstract 140-95-14-20). In addition, in up to the 4% of some high-risk trauma patients, pulmonary embolism will develop despite prophylaxis, and these patients may be best managed with a prophylaxis vena caval filter (Abstract 140-95-14-21).

James M. Seeger, M.D.

Early Endarterectomy for Severe Carotid Artery Stenosis After a Nondisabling Stroke: Results From the North American Symptomatic Carotid Endarterectomy Trial

Gasecki AP, Ferguson GG, Eliasziw M, Clagett GP, Fox AJ, Hachinski V, Barnett HJM (Univ of Western Ont, Canada; Univ of Texas, Dallas; Univ Hosp, London)

J Vasc Surg 20:288–295, 1994   140-95-14-1

Background.—There is continued debate over the timing of carotid endarterectomy (CE) in patients with recent nondisabling stroke. In the initial experience with CE, a delay of 4 to 6 weeks after acute stroke was a generally accepted policy; however, such a delay may put the patient with a less disabling stroke at risk of a major disabling stroke. Patients from the North American Symptomatic Carotid Endarterectomy Trial were reviewed to compare the prognostic implications of early and delayed CE.

Methods.—A subgroup of 100 surgical patients from the larger trial were reviewed. All had severe—i.e., 70% to 99%—stenosis of the carotid artery, as measured by angiography, and all were given a diagnosis of a nondisabling hemispheric stroke at entry to the trial. Forty-two patients underwent CE within 3 to 30 days after the stroke, and 58 had their operation delayed for 33 to 117 days. These early and delayed groups were compared for their risk of stroke after CE.

Results.—Although the baseline clinical characteristics of the 2 groups were similar, the delayed group had more lesions ipsilateral to the symptomatic side identified on preoperative CT scans. Stroke rates 30 days after CE were 4.8% in the early group and 5.2% in the delayed group, for a relative rate of .92. There were no deaths in the 30-day postoperative period. At 18 months after CE, the combined rates of stroke or death were 11.9% in the early group and 10.3% in the delayed group, for a relative rate of 1.15. In patients undergoing early CE, there was no association between an abnormal preoperative CT scan and subsequent risk of stroke.

Conclusion.—Early CE appears to be appropriate for patients with severe carotid artery stenosis who have had a nondisabling ischemic stroke. Morbidity and mortality rates are comparable with those of delayed CE. The practice of delaying operation for patients with symptomatic high-grade stenosis may expose them to some risk of recurrent stroke, which early operation may be able to avoid.

▶ It is becoming increasingly clear that delaying an indicated CE for 4–6 weeks after a minor, nondisabling stroke is unnecessary. This subanalysis of the NASCET data further supports this by demonstrating no difference in short- or long-term stroke risk in patients undergoing CE within 30 days of stroke, compared with those whose strokes had occurred more than 30 days before the procedure. In addition, this retrospective study also suggests that CT scanning is of little value in identifying patients at risk for recurrent postoperative stroke or intracranial hemorrhage.—J.M. Seeger, M.D.

Significance of Plaque Ulceration in Symptomatic Patients With High-Grade Carotid Stenosis
Eliasziw M, for the North American Symptomatic Carotid Endarterectomy Trial (John P Robarts Research Inst, London, Ont, Canada)
Stroke 25:304–308, 1994   140-95-14–2

Background.—Whether an ulcerated carotid plaque is a cause of cerebral ischemic symptoms remains uncertain. It also is not clear how important plaque ulceration is in symptomatic patients with severe carotid stenosis.

Methods.—The association between plaque ulceration and the risk of subsequent stroke was examined using the Cox proportional hazards regression method in 659 participants in the North American Symptomatic Carotid Endarterectomy Trial. The patients were symptomatic and had 70% to 99% carotid stenosis on angiography. Half the patients were randomized to having their plaques surgically removed, regardless of whether ulceration was present.

Results.—Both the type of treatment given (medical vs. operative) and the degree of ipsilateral carotid stenosis significantly influenced the outcome. In medically treated patients with ulcerated plaques, the risk of ipsilateral stroke within 2 years increased from 26% with 75% carotid stenosis to 73% with 95% stenosis. The risk of stroke remained constant at 21% in patients whose plaques were not ulcerated. In surgically treated patients with an ulcerated plaque, the risk of stroke increased only slightly at the highest degrees of carotid stenosis, and the overall risk of ipsilateral stroke occurring within 2 years was lowered by at least half when carotid endarterectomy was performed.

Conclusion.—In patients with symptomatic carotid stenosis who are managed medically, the presence of ulcerated plaque is associated with a substantially increased risk of stroke during 2 years of follow-up as the degree of stenosis increases. Carotid endarterectomy substantially lowers the risk of stroke, regardless of the degree of stenosis or the presence of plaque ulceration.

▶ Plaque ulceration is an identifier of increased stroke risk, which is independent of the degree of carotid stenosis, at least in symptomatic patients with 70%–99% stenosis. Even patients treated surgically who had an ulcerated plaque causing a 95% stenosis were at increased risk, compared with those without ulcerations. This suggests that the presence of plaque ulceration may identify a systemic process that independently increases the patient's risk of stroke.—J.M. Seeger, M.D.

The Influence of Anesthetic Technique on Perioperative Complications After Carotid Endarterectomy

Allen BT, Anderson CB, Rubin BG, Thompson RW, Flye MW, Young-Beyer P, Frisella P, Sicard GA (Washington Univ, St Louis, Mo)
J Vasc Surg 19:834–843, 1994   140-95-14-3

Background.—Despite the established benefits of carotid endarterectomy (CE) for high-grade carotid bifurcation stenoses compared with optimal medical treatment, perioperative morbidity and death—mainly from neurologic and cardiac complications—continue to be significant problems. An important factor in these complications is the anesthetic technique used during CE.

Methods.—Five hundred eighty-four consecutive patients undergoing 679 CEs were studied. Three hundred sixty-one had general anesthesia, and 318 had cervical block regional anesthesia. Perioperative complications, the use of a carotid artery shunt, duration of the operative procedure, and postoperative hospital course in the 2 groups were retrospectively compared.

Findings.—Overall, the perioperative stroke rate was 2.4% and the stroke death rate was 3.2%. These rates did not differ significantly between anesthetic groups or between patients who had symptomatic vs. asymptomatic disease. However, the use of cervical block anesthesia was associated with a significantly shorter operating time, fewer perioperative cardiopulmonary complications, and a briefer postoperative hospitalization than the use of general anesthesia. In addition, a carotid artery shunt was used in 19.2% of the patients receiving a cervical block anesthetic and 42.1% of those given a general anesthetic. In a multivariate analysis, age older than 75 years, operative time exceeding 3 hours, and the use of a carotid artery shunt were independent risk factors for perioperative cardiopulmonary complications. When a carotid artery shunt was not included in the multivariate analysis, general anesthesia became a significant risk factor for perioperative cardiopulmonary complications.

Conclusion.—Compared with the use of a general anesthetic, the use of cervical block anesthesia in patients undergoing CE is safer and requires fewer hospital resources. Cervical block anesthesia offers significant advantages over general anesthesia in overcoming the limitations of intraoperative cerebral monitoring and perioperative cardiac risk.

▶ The use of regional anesthesia for CE can make the procedure easier, more cost effective, and, possibly, safer. Previous randomized studies of regional anesthesia vs. general anesthesia in patients undergoing peripheral arterial reconstructive procedures failed to document a decrease in cardiopulmonary complications as was found in this retrospective, nonrandomized study of patients undergoing carotid surgery. Regardless, the reduced hospital stay and operative time associated with CE done using regional anesthesia demonstrates the value of this technique in these times when cost effectiveness is becoming paramount.—J.M. Seeger, M.D.

The Spectrum of Blunt Injury to the Carotid Artery: A Multicenter Perspective

Cogbill TH, Moore EE, Meissner M, Fischer RP, Hoyt DB, Morris JA, Shackford SR, Wallace JR, Ross SE, Ochsner MG, Sugerman HJ (Gundersen/Lutheran Med Ctr, La Crosse, Wis; Univ of Colorado, Denver; Univ of Washington, Seattle; et al)
J Trauma 37:473–479, 1994   140-95-14–4

Introduction.—Blunt trauma to the carotid artery frequently results in death or permanent neurologic impairment. Because this injury is rare, there are few comprehensive studies of its clinical presentation, treatment, and outcome. Patients from several medical centers were reviewed so that they could be stratified by type of arterial injury and guidelines for evaluation and management could be established.

Methods.—Inpatient hospital records from 11 institutions were retrospectively reviewed for carotid artery injuries from blunt trauma that occurred from January 1987 through December 1992. Available outpatient records were also examined for long-term follow-up. Neurologic function was classified as good, moderate impairment, or severe impairment.

Results.—Sixty blunt carotid artery injuries were identified in 49 patients during the 6-year study period. The median age of the group was 33 years; 63% of patients were male. Associated injuries were common and included craniocerebral trauma in 24 patients and facial fractures in 17. Twenty-four patients had a normal initial neurologic examination, but 14 showed significant neurologic deficits more than 12 hours after admission. The most common types of arterial injury were arterial dissection and arterial thrombosis. Angiography confirmed the diagnosis in 42 patients. All but 4 patients had CT of the head at admission; results were normal in 39%. Arterial dissection was managed nonsurgically in most patients, usually with anticoagulation; arterial thrombosis was managed with supportive care because of fixed deficits; arterial pseudoaneurysms were repaired surgically, and carotid-coronary fistulas were treated with balloon occlusion. All patients with carotid disruption died before treatment. Sixteen patients died, 13 as a direct result of the carotid artery injury. Among the 33 survivors, 22 had good functional neurologic outcome, 7 had moderate neurlogic deficits including monoplegia and hemiplegia, and 4 had to be institutionalized because of severe neurologic disability.

Conclusion.—Blunt injury to the carotid artery has diverse manifestations. Early diagnosis and stratification of injuries by type, location, and neurologic presentation are essential to the development of a successful treatment strategy. A high level of suspicion for carotid injury is required because neurologic symptoms may be delayed.

▶ Blunt injury to the carotid is uncommon; even this multicenter study from 11 busy trauma centers could identify only 60 injuries in 49 patients. A high index of suspicion based on the mechanism of injury should prompt investigation, perhaps initially using duplex ultrasound, especially in patients without neurologic deficits. More severe forms of injury, such as thrombosis or arterial disruption, have poor outcomes already established at the time of presentation, but pseudoaneurysms and patent internal carotid artery dissections can usually be successfully treated.—J.M. Seeger, M.D.

Results of a Prospective Randomized Trial Evaluating Surgery *Versus* Thrombolysis for Ischemia of the Lower Extremity: The STILE Trial
The STILE Investigators (Cleveland Clinic Found, Ohio)
Ann Surg 220:251–268, 1994   140-95-14–5

Introduction.—Catheter-directed thrombolysis has been used to manage patients with both acute and chronic arterial and graft occlusions. However, its therapeutic efficacy has been questioned. A prospective, randomized study assessed the relative effectiveness of catheter-directed thrombolysis and standard surgical intervention in patients with lower limb ischemia resulting from nonembolic arterial and bypass graft occlusion.

Methods.—Patients with worsening limb ischemia and nonembolic arterial or bypass graft occlusion identified by angiography were stratified for native artery occlusion or bypass graft occlusion and were randomly assigned to 1 of 3 treatment groups: surgical revascularization or catheter-directed thrombolysis with either recombinant tissue plasminogen activator (rt-PA) or urokinase. At 30 days after treatment, the composite clinical outcome was assessed, including the occurrence of ongoing or recurrent ischemia, death, major amputation, and major morbidity.

Results.—Patients in the thrombolysis group had a 61.7% adverse event rate, whereas 36.1% of the surgical patients had adverse events. In particular, thrombolysis patients had a significantly higher incidence of ongoing or recurrent ischemia (54% vs. 25.7%), life-threatening hemorrhage (5.6% vs. .7%), and vascular complications (9.7% vs. 3.5%) than did surgical patients. The rates of mortality and major amputation were comparable in the treatment groups. Thrombolysis with rt-PA or urokinase was equally effective, and the 2 had comparable bleeding complications. In the surgical group, patients with graft occlusions tended to have a higher amputation rate, and patients with native arterial occlusions tended to have a higher mortality rate, whereas in the thrombolysis group, outcome was similar in native arterial or graft occlusions. In addition, among patients with acute ischemia ($\leq$ 14 days), the surgical group had more major amputations, whereas among patients with chronic ischemia ($>$ 14 days), the surgical group had fewer major amputations and less ongoing/recurrent ischemia than the thrombolysis group. Because of this, surgery was associated with a lower death and amputation rate in patients with chronic ischemia, whereas thrombolysis was associated with a lower death and amputation rate in patients with acute ischemia.

Conclusion.—These findings suggest that patients with acute ischemia may be better managed with catheter-directed thrombolysis, and patients with chronic ischemia are optimally managed with surgical revascularization.

A Comparison of Thrombolytic Therapy With Operative Revascularization in the Initial Treatment of Acute Peripheral Arterial Ischemia

Ouriel K, Shortell CK, DeWeese JA, Green RM, Francis CW, Azodo MVU, Gutierrez OH, Manzione JV, Cox C, Marder VJ (Univ of Rochester, New York)
J Vasc Surg 19:1021–1030, 1994   140-95-14–6

Objective.—Intra-arterial thrombolytic therapy has come into widespread use for patients with peripheral arterial occlusive disease. However, there has been no randomized study to compare the efficacy of this treatment approach with that of operative revascularization procedures.

The 2 approaches were compared for the initial treatment of acute peripheral arterial occlusion in a prospective, randomized trial.

Methods.—All of the 114 patients in the trial had limb-threatening ischemia of less than 7 days' duration. They were randomized to undergo intra-arterial catheter-directed urokinase therapy or operative intervention. Any anatomical lesions discovered after thrombolysis were managed by balloon dilation or operation. Limb salvage and survival were the main study end points.

Results.—The occluding thrombus was dissolved by thrombolytic therapy in 70% of patients. The cumulative limb salvage rate at 1 year was about 82% in both groups. However, cumulative survival at the same time was significantly better in patients assigned to thrombolysis (84% vs. 58%). The mortality difference appeared to arise mainly from a 49% incidence of in-hospital cardiopulmonary complications in the operative treatment group, compared with just 16% in the thrombolysis group. The median duration of hospitalization was about 11 days in both groups, and costs were only somewhat higher in the thrombolysis group: median in-hospital costs were $15,700 vs. $12,300.

Conclusion.—For patients with acute peripheral arterial ischemia, intra-arterial thrombolytic therapy with urokinase appears to be a safe and effective alternative to operative revascularization. The incidence of in-hospital cardiopulmonary complications is lower with thrombolysis, with a corresponding increase in survival. The benefits of thrombolysis accrue with no appreciable increase in hospitalization time and only a modest increase in in-hospital costs. Lesions unmasked by thrombolysis should be managed aggressively. Further studies are needed to assess the value of thrombolysis in patients with subacute and chronic occlusions.

▶ These two randomized trials (Abstracts 140-95-14–5 and 140-95-14–6) significantly clarify the role of thrombolysis in patients with peripheral vascular disease. Although the risk of catheter-directed thrombolysis is not small (as demonstrated in Abstract 140-95-14–5), patients with acute ischemia (14 days duration or less) treated with thrombolysis have lower mortality, amputation, and complication rates than similar patients treated surgically. In contrast, patients with a longer duration of ischemia (> 14 days) do better after surgical therapy, and thrombolysis appears to have essentially no role in the management of these patients.—J.M. Seeger, M.D.

Thrombolysis Versus Thrombectomy for Occluded Hemodialysis Grafts
Schuman E, Quinn S, Standage B, Gross G (Good Samaritan Hosp, Portland, Ore)
Am J Surg 167:473–476, 1994   140-95-14–7

Background.—Graft thrombosis is the most common complication resulting from polytetrafluoroethylene (PTFE) grafts for hemodialysis. Surgical thrombectomy is the standard treatment for graft thrombosis; however, recently the use of fibrinolytic agents has shown varying rates of success. Thrombolysis was compared with standard surgical thrombectomy in an attempt to evaluate the safety and efficacy of both methods for declotting a dialysis graft.

Method.—Thirty-one patients with occluded PTFE grafts were randomly assigned to thrombolysis or surgical thrombectomy. After either treatment, the patients proceeded to dialysis. The procedure was considered successful if the patient was able to initiate dialysis that day.

Results.—Fifteen patients underwent thrombolysis and 16 had thrombectomy. The success rate for the thrombolysis group was 67%, compared to a 94% success rate in the thrombectomy group. No significant differences in primary and secondary patency rates were seen between the 2 groups, but the complication rates were higher and the time to completion longer in the thrombolysis patients. Charges for surgical treatment were $3,383 for thrombectomy, compared with $2,830 for thrombolysis.

Conclusion.—Although both thrombolysis and surgical thrombectomy can be used successfully, thrombectomy remains the optimal choice in the management of occluded dialysis grafts, showing a more rapid and successful initiation of dialysis and a lower rate of complications.

▶ As thrombolysis appears to be associated with more complications and surgical revision is much more effective in prolonging graft patency than angioplasty, thrombolysis appears to have a small role in the management of occluded hemodialysis grafts at present.—J.M. Seeger, M.D.

Peripheral Atherectomy With the Rotablator: A Multicenter Report
The Collaborative Rotablator Atherectomy Group (CRAG) (Univ of California, Los Angeles)
J Vasc Surg 19:509–515, 1994   140-95-14–8

Background.—The Food and Drug Administration has approved 4 atherectomy instruments for general use in treating peripheral arterial occlusive lesions. The efficacy and limitations of the Auth Rotablator, 1 of the devices recently approved, were investigated.

Methods.—Seventy-two patients from 3 medical centers underwent atherectomy with the Auth Rotablator between August 1987 and December 1990. Seventy-nine limbs and 107 arteries were treated, including 45 femoral, 31 tibial, 29 popliteal, and 2 iliac. The mean patient age was 69 years. Sixty-seven percent were men. Atherectomy was indicated by claudication in 43% and limb threat in 56%. The mean ankle-brachial index was .47, and the mean lesion length was 9 cm. Seventy arterial segments treated were less than 10 cm long and 37 were greater than 10 cm long. Arterial pulse examination, vascular laboratory Doppler measurement of ankle-brachial indices, and arteriography were performed in all patients before and after surgery and during a 15–41 month follow-up.

Results.—Initial angiographic success was achieved in 89% of the limbs and 77% of the arteries, including 50% of the iliac, 84% of the femoral, 83% of the popliteal, and 61% of the tibial arteries. Similarly, in-hospital clinical and hemodynamic success was attained in 77% of the limbs. Complications were hemoglobinuria in 13%, emboli in 10%, dissection in 6%, hematoma in 5%, perforation in 4%, and infection in 1%. Eleven percent had early thromboses and 2 device-related amputations were done. Most importantly, cumulative primary patency rates at 6, 12, and 24 months were only 47%, 31%, and 18.6%, respectively.

Conclusion.—Because of the frequent early thromboembolic complications and poor late patency rates associated with the Auth Rotablator, this device currently has limited application in peripheral atherectomy. Until these problems are solved, atherectomy is not generally recommended in the treatment of peripheral arterial occlusive lesions.

▶ Like many other endovascular techniques, atherectomy using the Rotablator has been promoted based on reports of acceptable results in patients followed for short periods after treatment. However, diffusely diseased peripheral arteries respond poorly to the extensive arterial wall injury that occurs during atherectomy, as documented by the approximately 80% failure rate by 2 years after therapy with the Rotablator. The cause of most long-term failures is intimal hyperplasia, and, until this process can be controlled, endovascular techniques such as atherectomy using the Rotablator will have limited value in patients with peripheral vascular disease.—J.M. Seeger, M.D.

Hospital Costs of Revascularization Procedures for Femoropopliteal Arterial Disease
Hunink MGM, Cullen KA, Donaldson M (Harvard Med School, Boston)
J Vasc Surg 19:632–641, 1994   140-95-14–9

Introduction.—A 1984 study reported that percutaneous transluminal angioplasty (PTA) was considerably more cost effective than bypass, suggesting that PTA may be the treatment of choice for peripheral vascular disease. However, the effectiveness of PTA procedures has been questioned and the cost of surgical revascularization has been decreasing, indicating the need for more recent data.

Methods.—Patients treated with femoropopliteal PTA or bypass between 1985 and 1991 were prospectively studied. Treatment choices were made on the basis of diagnostic evaluation. Hospital costs, excluding physician fees, related to PTA and bypass were compared for all admissions, then compared for admissions with and without unrelated additional procedures, and with and without related vascular procedures, including debridement or amputation. Multiple linear regression analyses examined the factors influencing costs.

Results.—The primary indication for admission was disabling claudication in the PTA group and critical ischemia in the bypass group. Additional major procedures were performed in 7% of each group. Patients in the PTA group required additional bypass and thrombolysis (34% and 16%, respectively) more commonly than did patients in the initial bypass group (3% and 7%, respectively). The mean hospital costs for all admissions were $16,341 for the PTA group and $17,076 for the bypass group. Excluding all additional procedures and comparing indications for admission, PTA costs were significantly lower than bypass costs for patients with claudication, whereas the cost differences were of only borderline significance for patients with critical ischemia. Hospital costs were significantly influenced by the primary procedure, additional unrelated procedures, additional related vascular procedures, and whether debridement or amputation was required.

Discussion.—These data indicate that PTA is not as cost effective compared with bypass as it was believed to be. Combining this evidence with questions about patient outcome after PTA suggests that the indications for PTA should be reevaluated.

▶ Decreased cost of therapy has been espoused as 1 of the major advantages of PTA. As shown in this study, this may be true for selected patients with claudication but not for patients with critical ischemia. In addition, as expected, PTA plus surgery is no less expensive than surgery alone. Interestingly, the cost of PTA appears to be increasing more rapidly than the cost of surgery.—J.M. Seeger, M.D.

Repair of Abdominal Aortic Aneurysm by Transfemoral Endovascular Graft Placement

Moore WS, Vescera CL (Univ of California Los Angeles Ctr for the Health Sciences)
Ann Surg 220:331–341, 1994   140-95-14-10

Background.—Direct repair of abdominal aortic aneurysm through excision and graft replacement has become standard practice. Yet, despite the high success rate of this procedure, approximately 15,000 patients die of ruptured abdominal aortic aneurysms yearly in the United States. This high incidence of rupture can be explained by the fact that surgery is sometimes withheld because of the patient's increased risk of operation compared with a relatively small aneurysm. A new device approved by the Food and Drug Administration for clinical investigation was described; it allows for the repair of abdominal aortic aneurysm by a transfemoral endovascular graft placement, thus permitting a more aggressive approach in the management of patients with smaller aneurysms or high-risk patients.

Method.—Sixty-nine patients with abdominal aortic aneurysms were screened, and 10 were found to have suitable anatomical and clinical characteristics for the endovascular graft system (EGS). Repair was carried out under general anesthesia. One femoral artery was surgically exposed and the EGS—consisting of an introducer sheath and a catheter-based delivery system containing a graft of appropriate size with fixation devices at each end—was inserted with fluoroscopic control through an open arteriotomy. Postoperative evaluation included documentation of the anatomical position of the graft as seen by the radiopaque self-expanding fixation devices at each graft extremity, and examination of a color-flow duplex scan indicating flow through the graft and showing evidence of perianastomotic reflux into the aneurysm. Finally, a CT scan was obtained to ensure the position of the graft, its function, and the presence or absence of contrast-enhanced blood within the aneurysm sac.

Results.—Eight of the 10 grafts were considered an immediate success and were entered into the follow-up protocol. Two graft deployments were considered failures and required conversion to an open repair. On follow-up, 7 of the 8 patients who underwent successful implantation are still alive. Four of the 8 patients had normal completion angiography at the time of surgery with no sign of perianastomotic reflux. Follow-up CT scans showed no evidence of contrast enhancement within the aneurysm sac, and color-flow duplex scan studies demonstrated normal graft flow without perianastomotic reflux. Six of the 8 patients have completely normally functioning grafts without any function of the thrombosed aneurysms. Two patients continue to show some evidence of perianastomotic reflux but no sign of aneurysm expansion.

Conclusion.—The results indicate that transfemoral endovascular graft placement appears to be safe and effective. Long-term follow-up studies of this procedure are now required.

Transluminal Placement of Endovascular Stent-Grafts for the Treatment of Descending Thoracic Aortic Aneurysms
Dake MD, Miller DC, Semba CP, Mitchell RS, Walker PJ, Liddell RP (Stanford Univ, Calif)
N Engl J Med 331:1729–1734, 1994   140-95-14–11

Purpose.—Thoracic aortic aneurysms are most often treated by surgical replacement with a prosthetic graft. However, this procedure is associated with considerable morbidity and mortality; 1 recent series of elective surgical repairs reported a mortality rate of 12%. Transluminally placed endovascular stent graft devices were studied as an alternative to surgical repair in patients with thoracic artery aneurysms.

Methods.—Thirteen patients with descending thoracic artery aneurysms were treated with transluminally placed stent grafts over a 2-year period. The patients were 11 men and 2 women (average age, 61 years). The series included patients with atherosclerotic, anastomotic, and post-traumatic true or false aneurysms, as well as patients with aortic dissection. The mean aneurysm diameter was 6 cm. A custom-designed endovascular stent graft, consisting of a self-expanding stainless-steel stent covered with a woven Dacron graft, was used in each patient.

Results.—The stent graft prostheses were successfully placed in all patients. Twelve patients had complete thrombosis of the thoracic aortic aneurysm surrounding the prosthesis, and the remaining patient had partial thrombosis. Small, residual patent proximal tracts into the aneurysmal sac were initially noted in 2 patients; in both cases, these tracts thrombosed within 2 months after the procedure. Four patients required 2 stent graft prostheses to bridge the aneurysm adequately. The average follow-up was 12 months, during which time there were no deaths and no cases of paraplegia, stroke, distal embolization, or infection. Surgical graft replacement was required 4 months later because of progressive dilation of the arch in 1 patient with extensive chronic aortic dissection.

Conclusion.—In appropriately selected patients, endovascular stent graft repair appears to be a feasible, safe, and effective approach to the management of thoracic aortic aneurysms. Careful long-term studies are needed to confirm these preliminary results. The effectiveness of this approach in patients with aortic dissection is more problematic, and its applicability to traumatic tears is unknown.

▶ Abstracts 140-95-14–10 and 140-95-14–11 document early clinical experience with transluminal stent graft repair of abdominal and thoracic aortic aneurysms. Initial results appear encouraging, but many questions regarding this procedure remain. Prospective trials comparing stent graft repair of abdominal aortic aneurysms to standard surgical repair are under way and, hopefully, these trials will provide such information before general use of this technique.—J.M. Seeger, M.D.

Natural History of Atherosclerotic Renal Artery Stenosis: A Prospective Study With Duplex Ultrasonography
Zierler RE, Bergelin RO, Isaacson JA, Strandness DE Jr (Univ of Washington, Seattle)
J Vasc Surg 19:250–258, 1994   140-95-14–12

Background.—Renal artery stenosis occurs in 30% to 40% of patients with peripheral arterial disease, and renal artery repair in selected patients with severe hypertension and/or renal insufficiency has been shown to be beneficial. However, the role of renal revascularization in patients without severe hypertension or kidney failure is debated. Duplex scanning, a noninvasive method, is ideally suited for screening and follow-up of renal artery disease. The natural history of renal artery stenosis was documented in patients in whom immediate renal revascularization was not required.

Methods.—Eighty-four patients with 1 or more abnormal renal arteries on duplex scanning were recruited from a group being screened for renal artery stenosis. Eighty patients with 139 renal artery/kidney sides were included in the follow-up protocol. The 44 women and 36 men (mean age, 66 years) were monitored for a mean of 12.7 months.

Findings.—Initially, 36 renal arteries were normal, 35 showed less than 60% stenosis, 63 showed 60% stenosis or more, and 5 were occluded. None of the initially normal renal arteries showed disease progression. In contrast, the mean cumulative incidence of progression from less than 60% to 60% or greater stenosis was 23% at 1 year and 42% at 2 years, and the cumulative incidence of progression from greater than 60% stenosis to occlusion was 5% at 1 year and 11% at 2 years. All renal arteries progressing to occlusion had 60% or greater stenosis initially, and the only clinical risk factor associated with disease progression was diastolic blood pressure.

Conclusion.—Progression of renal artery stenosis occurs at a rate of about 20% per year, and progression to occlusion is associated with a pronounced reduction in kidney length. However, it is unknown whether this natural history can be improved by earlier intervention for renal artery stenosis.

▶ The risk of subsequent renal artery occlusion in patients with a renal artery stenosis > 60%–80% is substantial. This appears to justify repair of asymptomatic renal artery lesions in conjunction with other aortic procedures if the renal artery repair can be done without increasing the overall risk of the procedure. However, the value of renal artery repair as a primary procedure in asymptomatic patients remains to be determined.—J.M. Seeger, M.D.

High-Attenuating Crescent in Abdominal Aortic Aneurysm Wall at CT: A Sign of Acute or Impending Rupture
Mehard WB, Heiken JP, Sicard GA (Mallinckrodt Inst of Radiology, St Louis, Mo; Washington Univ, St Louis, Mo)
Radiology 192:359–362, 1994   140-95-14–13

Background.—The CT signs of abdominal aortic aneurysm (AAA) rupture have been extensively studied, but only those criteria relating to size are able to recognize impending rupture. A high-attenuating crescent along the aortic margin in dissected AAA has been reported, which was ascribed to intramural hematoma without intimal rupture. A similar sign in AAAs on unenhanced CT scans of patients with back pain has been observed. The value of this finding as a sign of impending rupture was retrospectively evaluated.

Methods.—The study included 149 consecutive patients undergoing surgery for AAA who had undergone preoperative unenhanced CT. Seventy percent of the patients had aneurysm repair surgery within 1 month of the CT scan, and those with a high-attenuating crescent sign had repair within 2 weeks. The investigators correlated the finding of a peripheral high-attenuating crescent with the surgical findings of acute mural hematoma, acute rupture, or contained rupture. They also correlated the aneurysmal diameter with the presence or absence of pain at the time of CT scanning, a high-attenuating crescent, and aneurysmal complications.

Results.—Thirteen percent of the patients had a high-attenuating crescent sign on CT. Three of these 19 patients also had CT evidence of rupture; surgery, done the same day, documented the occurrence of frank rupture. Another 3 were found to have contained rupture, 3 to have acute intramural hematoma, and 1 to have had rupture in the interval between CT and surgery. The other 9 patients with a high-attenuating crescent sign were found to have uncomplicated aneurysms at surgery. Of the 130 patients with no high-attenuating crescent sign, 4 were eventually found to have frank ruptures and 2 to have small contained ruptures.

Thus, as an indicator of complicated aneurysm, the high-attenuating crescent sign had a sensitivity of 77%, a specificity of 93%, and a positive predictive value of 53%. Significant correlations were noted between the presence of this sign and large aneurysm size and pain at the time of CT scanning.

Conclusion.—The presence of a high-attenuating crescent sign on unenhanced CT in patients without evidence of frank aneurysm leakage should be considered a sign of impending AAA rupture. The peripheral high attenuation may result from acute hematoma within the aneurysmal wall or within adjacent mural thrombus, and this sign is particularly important in patients with pain.

▶ This is an interesting observation that may be of value in determining the urgency of repair in patients with equivocal symptoms and intact AAA. However, patients with symptomatic AAA are not truly without risk of rupture until the aneurysm is repaired.—J.M. Seeger, M.D.

Repeat Leg Bypass After Multiple Prior Bypass Failures
De Frang RD, Edwards JM, Moneta GL, Yeager RA, Taylor LM Jr, Porter JM
(Oregon Health Sciences Univ, Portland)
J Vasc Surg 19:268–277, 1994   140-95-14–14

Introduction.—Increasing numbers of patients are undergoing leg bypass for various arterial lesions, resulting in prolonged patency and excellent limb salvage rates. At the same time, most patients are being seen with severe lower extremity ischemia after multiple failed bypass procedures. An aggressive approach to limb salvage after graft failure is often recommended, but the role of repeat bypass after 2 or more failed attempts is unclear. Eighty-one patients were managed by a policy of repeated revascularization regardless of prior failures.

Patients.—The patients underwent a total of 85 revascularization procedures after failure of 2 or more prior infrainguinal bypasses in the same leg. The operation represented the third procedure in 72 cases, the fourth procedure in 6, and the fifth procedure in 7. The indication for the procedure was revision of a failing graft disclosed by routine surveillance in 26 cases and graft thrombosis in 59. Seventy-nine percent of procedures were autogenous and 21% were prosthetic reconstructions. The distal anastomosis was made to the infrapopliteal artery in 66 cases and the popliteal artery in 19.

Outcomes.—The operative mortality was 3.7%, and patients were followed for a mean of 17 months after their most recent operation. The 4-year primary patency rate for repeat bypass procedures by life table analysis was 80% and the limb salvage rate was 70%. These results did not differ for bypasses done with arm vein compared with other alternate vein sources or for procedures done after graft thrombosis compared with failing grafts. Fifteen percent of patients undergoing a detailed hematologic screening had an identifiable hypercoagulable disorder; all had anticardiolipin antibodies.

Conclusion.—Surprisingly good primary patency and limb salvage rates resulted in patients undergoing limb revascularization after 2 or more failed leg bypass procedures. Patient survival was also unexpectedly high at 4 years in this series. These results are believed to justify the aggressive policy of limb revascularization after multiple failed bypass procedures.

▶ These results demonstrate that in properly selected patients, good long-term results can be achieved, even after the failure of 2 or more arterial reconstructive procedures in the same leg. This is not surprising as bypass graft success is primarily determined by the quality of inflow and outflow arteries and whether venous conduit is available. However, hypercoagulability screening is important in these patients as 15%–20% will have hypercoagulable states.—J.M. Seeger, M.D.

Increased Limb Salvage by the Use of Unconventional Foot Amputations

Chang BB, Bock DEM, Jacobs RL, Darling RC III, Leather RP, Shah DM (Albany Med College, NY; VA Hosp, Albany, NY)
J Vasc Surg 19:341–349, 1994   140-95-14–15

Background.—When ischemic necrosis of the foot develops, salvaging the extremity necessitates revascularization followed by either debridement or partial amputation of the foot. An unconventional type of amputation may be necessary if necrosis extends beyond the toes and metatarsal heads.

Methods.—Infrainguinal revascularization was carried out on 2,105 ischemic extremities during a 15-year period. In 98 instances, extensive foot necrosis was managed by unconventional foot amputation. The techniques used included a modified Chopart amputation in 59 patients, a Lisfranc procedure in 14, a Pirogoff operation in 17, and the Syme amputation in 8. Patients ambulated in a "clamshell" prosthesis and foot spacer.

Results.—Early failure of the amputation was seen in 13 patients, 3 with bypass failure, 5 with inadequate foot perfusion despite a patent graft, 3 with diabetes and renal failure, and 2 with persistent infection. Late, functional limb salvage was achieved in 84%. The Lisfranc and the modified Chopart amputations most reliably resulted in limb salvage with long-term ambulatory function, and patients were able to get out of bed at night and ambulate short distances more easily with these amputations than with Pirogoff and Syme amputations.

Conclusion.—Major amputation is not always necessary when ischemic necrosis of the foot extends beyond the limits of conventional transmetatarsal amputation, as acceptable limb salvage and good functional results can be achieved with unconventional foot amputations.

▶ Lisfranc and Chopart amputations provide a functional limb which allows ambulation for short distances without a protheses. It should be strongly considered when necrosis extends beyond the level of a transmetatarsal amputation.—J.M. Seeger, M.D.

Wound Healing in Forefoot Amputations: The Predictive Value of Toe Pressure

Vitti MJ, Robinson DV, Hauer-Jensen M, Thompson BW, Ranval TJ, Barone G, Barnes RW, Eidt JF (Univ of Arkansas, Little Rock; John L. McClellan VA Med Ctr, Little Rock, Ark)
Ann Vasc Surg 8:99–106, 1994   140-95-14–16

Background.—A healing failure rate of 30% to 45% has been documented in patients undergoing forefoot amputation for the treatment of gangrene or severe infection. Preoperative toe pressure may predict the likelihood of wound healing in patients undergoing such procedures. Experience with this simple technique was reviewed.

Patients and Methods.—The medical records of 136 men who underwent forefoot amputation were reviewed. Data collected included age, smoking history, and the presence of diabetes mellitus, hypertension, hyperlipidemia, coronary artery disease, infection, preoperative arterial Doppler data, toe pressure, wound disposition, concomitant revascularization, and healing outcome.

Results.—The mean patient age was 64.8 years, with a range of 41–80 years. Most patients were diabetic. The mean toe pressure in healed patients was 71.8 mm Hg, significantly higher than the mean toe pressure of 45.1 mm Hg observed in the nonhealed group. In diabetic patients with a preoperative toe pressure of less than 38 mm Hg, primary amputation healing did not occur, whereas in revascularized diabetic patients, no healing occurred with a toe pressure of less than 40 mm Hg after bypass. In contrast, no failures occurred when the toe pressure was higher than 68 mm Hg or when there was an increase in toe pressure of 30 mm Hg or more after bypass. Among the nondiabetic patients, no threshold toe pressure values were noted. Age older than 60 years, diabetes mellitus, preoperative toe pressure, and revascularization were identified as significant independent predictors of forefoot amputation healing, based on logistic regression analysis.

Conclusion.—Preoperative toe pressure appears to be a valuable clinical tool for predicting the healing potential of an amputation procedure in any given forefoot.

▶ Toe pressures can be a valuable measure of the likelihood of healing of forefoot amputation sites with or without prior bypass. Broader utilization of this simple technique should decrease the incidence of failed amputation and its inherent risk and cost.—J.M. Seeger, M.D.

Peripheral Vascular Surgery With Magnetic Resonance Angiography as the Sole Preoperative Imaging Modality
Carpenter JP, Baum RA, Holland GA, Barker CF (Univ of Pennsylvania, Philadelphia)
J Vasc Surg 20:861–871, 1994   140-95-14–17

Background.—Magnetic resonance angiography (MRA), a developing technique, provides arteriograms without the risks associated with iodinated contrast and arterial puncture and without costly hospitalization. Previous reports have shown that peripheral vessel MRA enables accurate assessment of the aorta through pedal vessels. Whether vascular reconstructions could be planned and accomplished on the basis of MRA alone was investigated.

Methods.—Eighty consecutive candidates for bypass who had ischemic rest pain or tissue loss were assessed by preoperative outpatient MRA of the juxtarenal aorta through the foot. Magnetic resonance angiography findings were confirmed by intraoperative intra-arterial pressure measurements for proximal vessels and postbypass arteriography for the runoff.

Findings.—Except for 2 patients who could not tolerate MRA and needed contrast arteriography, all patients had reconstructive procedures based on MRA findings alone. In every patient, intraoperative findings of the suitability of inflow and outflow vessels confirmed the accuracy of the MR angiograms. None of the patients undergoing infrainguinal bypass had significant inflow occlusive disease, according to MRA. This was confirmed at surgery by pressure measurements of inflow vessels within 10 mm Hg of systemic pressure. The results of intraoperative completion arteriography and preoperative MRA were identical in all patients but 2, who showed minor discrepancies. All aortobifemoral reconstructions remained patent and all limbs were intact. At 21 months, infrainguinal reconstructions had an 84% limb salvage rate and a 78% primary graft patency rate. Each patient undergoing preoperative MRA alone had a cost savings of $1,288.

Conclusion.—Magnetic resonance angiography is a noninvasive, cost-effective outpatient imaging technique. If performed and interpreted properly, MRA is sufficient for planning peripheral bypass procedures, and its use may eventually supplant contrast arteriography in many patients.

▶ As MRA develops, this technique may some day replace contrast arteriography for arterial imaging in patients with peripheral vascular disease. However, at present, only selected centers can obtain results such as those presented in this article, and as the authors suggest, before MRA can be used as the sole imaging modality for decision-making in patients with peripheral vascular disease, it must be validated in each individual center against the gold standard of contrast arteriography.—J.M. Seeger, M.D.

Popliteal Artery Aneurysms: The Risk of Nonoperative Management
Lowell RC, Gloviczki P, Hallett JW Jr, Naessens JM, Maus TP, Cherry KJ Jr, Bower TC, Pairolero PC (Mayo Clinic and Found, Rochester, Minn)
Ann Vasc Surg 8:14–23, 1994   140-95-14–18

Background.—There is ongoing debate regarding the risk and management of popliteal artery aneurysms (PAAs), the most common type of peripheral artery aneurysm. In reported series, most patients are treated surgically to avoid catastrophic limb loss; only a few are treated conservatively. A series of 106 patients with PAAs were reviewed to assess the risk of nonoperative management.

Patients.—The patients were 103 men and 3 women (mean age, 70.5 years) who were seen from 1980 through 1985. The patients had a total of 161 PAAs and were followed for a mean of 7 years; follow-up was 92% complete. Seventy-seven percent of lesions were confirmed by ultrasound, 20% by physical examination only, and 4% by arteriography only. Fifty-two limbs had chronic symptoms, 15 had acute symptoms, and 94 were asymptomatic. Surgical repair was performed initially in 23 of the limbs with chronic symptoms, 10 limbs with acute symptoms, and 27 of the asymptomatic limbs. Amputation was done in 2 patients undergoing repair for chronic ischemia, 5 patients with acute ischemia, and 1 patient undergoing repair for an asymptomatic PAA.

Findings.—This left 67 asymptomatic limbs in which initial treatment was nonoperative. Symptoms eventually developed in 18% of limbs, and 92% of these limbs in which symptoms developed initially had at least 1 of 3 risk factors—size over 2 cm, thrombus, and poor run-off—compared with 38% of limbs that remained asymptomatic. Four percent (3 patients) went on to amputation, all after attempts at repair.

Conclusion.—Despite attempts at initial nonoperative management, symptomatic patients with PAAs continue to have high amputation rates. The risk factors mentioned above can predict the development of symptoms in patients seen with asymptomatic PAAs. Elective repair is warranted when any of these risk factors is present, even in an asymptomatic patient if a reasonable chance of long-term survival is present.

▶ Management of patients with small, asymptomatic PAAs remains controversial. The risk of symptom development in this series was only 18%, and eventual amputation occurred in 4.5%, not significantly different from the amputation risk of 4% in asymptomatic patients who underwent initial repair. Certainly those patients with large aneurysms containing thrombus should be repaired, even when no symptoms are present. However, conservative follow-up can be considered in patients with small, asymptomatic PAAs that do not contain thrombus, particularly when poor run-off may limit the success of repair.—J.M. Seeger, M.D.

An Institutional Experience With Arterial Atheroembolism

Baumann DS, McGraw D, Rubin BG, Allen BT, Anderson CB, Sicard GA (Washington Univ, St Louis, Mo)
Ann Vasc Surg 8:258–265, 1994   140-95-14–19

Objective.—The clinical manifestations of an atheroembolism vary significantly according to the level of the offending plaque. Atheroemboli can cause blue-toe lesions that are seemingly minor or they can cause serious problems such as limb loss, visceral ischemia, and death. Misdiagnosis can lead to delays in treatment and increased morbidity. One institution's experience with atheroembolism was reviewed.

Patients.—The authors' vascular surgery service treated 62 patients with atheroembolism from 1988 through 1991. All 62 patients had cutaneous manifestations of atheroembolic disease with no cardiac source of embolization. Thirty-one patients were women and 31 were men; their mean age was 63 years. Most had multiple risk factors for atherosclerosis, especially smoking and hypertension. The episode of atheroembolism was spontaneous in 62% of cases; however, 21% of patients had a recent, inciting invasive radiologic procedure, 16% were receiving antico-agulant drugs, and 1 patient had sustained abdominal trauma. A coinci-dental deterioration in renal function was noted in 29% of patients and intestinal infarction from atheroemboli in 6%.

Diagnosis and Treatment.—Ninety-seven percent of the patients un-derwent arteriography. The aorta and iliac arteries were implicated in 80% of cases, the femoral artery in 13%, and the popliteal and subclav-ian arteries in 3% each. Bypass grafting procedures were done after ex-clusion of the native diseased artery in 42 patients, extra-anatomical in 6. Endarterectomy was performed in 20 patients, 6 of whom received addi-tional bypass grafts. No corrective vascular procedure was performed in 5 patients.

Outcomes.—There was a 5% operative mortality rate after 30 days. Minor amputations were required in 31% of patients; major leg amputa-tions were needed in 2 patients. The overall limb salvage rate was 98%, i.e., 86 of 88 limbs. At a mean follow-up of 20 months, none of the pa-tients experienced further episodes of atheroembolism in the involved limb.

Conclusion.—A policy of urgent arteriography and surgical correction or bypass, with exclusion of the offending lesion, is recommended for patients with arterial atheroembolism. This aggressive surgical approach maximizes limb salvage with low operative mortality and excellent long-term relief of embolization. It is essential to differentiate cholesterol em-bolization from other embolic phenomena and from the other systemic diseases that it may mimic.

▶ Atheroembolism to the extremities, kidneys, or bowels is an uncommon and vexing problem. This report emphasizes that treatment is surgical and that visceral involvement is commonly associated with poor outcome. It also emphasizes again that anticoagulation plays a minor role in this disease, and, in fact, may be detrimental.—J.M. Seeger, M.D.

The Incidence of Deep Venous Thrombosis in Patients Undergoing Abdominal Aortic Aneurysm Resection

Olin JW, Graor RA, O'Hara P, Young JR (Cleveland Clinic Found, Ohio)
J Vasc Surg 18:1037–1041, 1993   140-95-14–20

Background.—Most recommendations concerning prophylaxis against postoperative deep venous thrombosis (DVT) are directed toward pa-tients undergoing general, orthopedic, and neurologic surgery. Little in-formation is available concerning prophylaxis in patients undergoing vas-cular surgery procedures. In part, this is because the incidence of DVT in such patients is poorly defined.

Methods.—A prospective venographic study enrolled 50 consecutive patients undergoing resection of an abdominal aortic aneurysm (42 men and 8 women; mean age, 70 years). None received prophylaxis against DVT before surgery. Venography was done bilaterally 5 days postoperatively.

Results.—Nine patients (18%) had venographic findings of acute DVT. None of the women were affected; the incidence in men was 21%. None of the patients had symptoms suggestive of DVT. Seven patients had thrombi in calf veins and 2 in more proximal venous segments. No patient had clinical evidence of pulmonary embolism.

Conclusion.—These findings warrant an effort to determine whether prophylaxis against DVT can lower the risk of thromboembolism developing after resection of an abdominal aortic aneurysm.

▶ It has been suggested that patients undergoing vascular surgery procedures may have a low incidence of DVT because of intraoperative anticoagulation. However, as this study shows, DVT is not an uncommon problem after abdominal aortic aneurysm repair, and prophylaxis should be routine, at least for patients undergoing aortic procedures.—J.M. Seeger, M.D.

Risk Factors Associated With Pulmonary Embolism Despite Routine Prophylaxis: Implications for Improved Protection

Winchell RJ, Hoyt DB, Walsh JC, Simons RK, Eastman AB (Univ of California, San Diego)
J Trauma 37:600–606, 1994   140-95-14–21

Background.—Although uncommon, pulmonary embolism (PE) can cause sudden death in patients with trauma who have otherwise survived their injuries. Even with current methods of prophylaxis and detection of patients at risk, PE is still a major cause of post-traumatic morbidity and mortality. Risk factors for PE were assessed in patients with trauma in whom this complication developed despite routine prophylaxis.

Methods.—The retrospective study included 9,721 patients with trauma discharged over an 8-year period. Thirty-six of the patients had clinically evident PE, an incidence of .4%. These complications occurred despite a policy of routine prophylaxis against deep venous thrombosis, including prophylactic vena caval filters placed in 29 patients. A detailed analysis was performed to identify injury-related risk factors for PE despite prophylaxis.

Results.—Eight of the 36 patients who had documented PE died, for a mortality rate of 22%. In no case did PE develop after an inferior vena caval filter was placed. On analysis of patterns of injury, 4 common combinations of significant risk factors were identified as high-risk patterns: head plus spinal cord injury (1.5% of patients), head plus long bone fracture (2.3%), severe pelvis plus long bone fracture (3.8%), and multiple long bone fracture (2.9%). Compared with the control group, the odds ratios of the high-risk groups for the development of PE ranged from 4.5 to 12.

Conclusion.—Improvement of outcome for trauma patients relies on consistent application of conventional care and consideration of other measures, such as prophylactic inferior vena caval filters, for patients at highest risk of PE. More research is needed to determine the efficacy and long-term complications of prophylactic filter placement in high risk patients. For now, it is suggested that patients whose estimated risk of PE is greater than 2% to 5%, despite prophylaxis, should be considered for prophylactic vena caval filter placement.

▶ Identification of trauma patients at high risk for PE despite deep venous thrombosis prophylaxis potentially will allow appropriate use of prophylactic vena caval filters. Studies such as this one provide a basis for rational use of such filters as well as a starting point for studies to identify the efficacy of such an approach.—J.M. Seeger, M.D.

Mesenteric Venous Thrombosis: Still a Lethal Disease in the 1990s

Rhee RY, Gloviczki P, Mendonca CT, Petterson TM, Serry RD, Sarr MG, Johnson CM, Bower TC, Hallett JW Jr, Cherry KJ Jr (Mayo Clinic and Found, Rochester, Minn)
J Vasc Surg 20:688–697, 1994   140-95-14–22

Purpose.—Mesenteric venous thrombosis (MVT) is a potentially lethal condition that is reported to account for 5% to 15% of all cases of acute mesenteric ischemia. The mortality rate is 15% to 40%, partly because of delayed diagnosis. With the increasing use of CT and ultrasonography, MVT may even be an incidental finding in patients without acute symptoms of bowel ischemia. Two decades of progress in the diagnosis, management, and outcome of MVT were reviewed in a series of 72 patients.

Patients.—The subjects were 45 men and 27 women (mean age, 57 years) treated for MVT at a tertiary referral center from 1972 to 1993. They accounted for 6% of all patients treated for mesenteric ischemia during this period. The condition was acute in 53 patients and chronic in 19. Secondary MVT was present in 79% of patients; the most frequent associated conditions were previous abdominal surgery and hypercoagulable states. When CT was performed, the results showed abnormalities in 100% of patients who had acute MVT and in 93% of those who had chronic MVT. In 5 of 7 patients, the diagnosis of acute MVT was made by angiography. The most frequent presenting signs and symptoms were abdominal pain, 83%; anorexia, 53%; and diarrhea, 43%. The symptoms were present for more than 48 hours in three fourths of the patients. An operation was performed in 64% of patients who had acute MVT. Thirty-one of these 34 patients required bowel resection; thrombectomy failed in 1 patient. Of the other 19 patients who had acute MVT, 7 received anticoagulation without surgery and 12 were observed. All 19 patients having chronic MVT were observed; 9 underwent anticoagulation. The diagnosis of acute MVT was delayed for a median of 48 hours throughout the study period.

Outcomes.—The recurrence rate of MVT was 36% and the 30-day mortality rate was 27%. Long-term survival was 36% for patients having acute MVT vs. 83% for those having chronic MVT. The most frequent complications in patients who had acute MVT were short bowel syndrome, 23%; wound infection, 21%; and sepsis, 17%. Among patients having acute MVT, survival was better in those who underwent anticoagulation, with and without surgery, than in those who were observed.

Conclusion.—This 22-year experience shows little improvement in survival for patients who have acute MVT. The most sensitive imaging procedure for MVT is CT scanning. For patients who have acute MVT, anticoagulation and surgery are associated with better survival. For those who have chronic MVT, the main determinant of survival is the underlying disease.

▶ Mesenteric venous thrombosis remains an important, but uncommon, cause of intestinal ischemia. The diagnosis is now easily confirmed using CT and/or mesenteric duplex scanning. Hypercoagulable states are common in patients with MVT, and anticoagulation plus surgery if peritonitis is suspected is the best treatment. Although associated medical conditions account for part of the high mortality rate associated with this disease, improved recognition and prompt treatment provide the best chance for improving short- and long-term survival in patients with MVT.—J.M. Seeger, M.D.

15 Noncardiac Thoracic Surgery

Introduction

This year's literature in general thoracic surgery continues to mark changes in the way we approach our patients with malignant disease. This Mosby-Year Book review will touch on several important areas for the surgeon practicing general thoracic surgery. Specifically, we will review some interesting approaches to the evaluation of patients with thoracic surgical therapy. In addition, we will look at an interesting report from the Brompton Hospital regarding the use of an old technique for treatment of bullous emphysema.

The resection of pulmonary metastases by the general thoracic surgeon is often 1 of the most difficult types of decisions to make. We review 6 articles in this year's Year Book that shed light on the appropriate indications and expected results in a variety of cell types of metastatic lung disease.

With the rising incidence of mesothelioma in the United States, it appeared appropriate to select for review 4 articles that deal with the pathophysiology of the disease, as well as interesting and unique therapeutic approaches that may help to clarify the standard treatment in disease.

We will take this opportunity to update surgeons practicing general thoracic surgery on recent reports of video-assisted thoracic surgical approaches to more substantial procedures such as lobectomy and pneumonectomy. We will look at an interesting report that seeks to compare the morbidity and mortality of video-assisted surgery vs. conventional techniques. Video-assisted surgery continues to advance, both in the level of complexity of the procedures performed as well as in new applications of this technique in the treatment of patients with benign and malignant diseases of the chest.

One of the areas where the standard treatment of non–small-cell lung cancer appears to be changing most radically is in the treatment of patients with stage III disease. The need for preresectional identification of mediastinal N2 adenopathy, advocated by those who would utilize neoadjuvant chemotherapy as well as surgery in the treatment of this disease, is contrasted to conventional surgical approaches. This year's literature review revealed 6 excellent articles combining large institutional experiences in the evaluation of surgical therapy, as well as multimodality therapy of state IIIA disease. The long-awaited prospective, randomized phase III trial confirming the efficacy of neoadjuvant chemotherapy in the setting of IIIA non–small-cell lung cancer from the group in Barcelona will also be carefully reviewed.

Phase II trials of multimodality therapy in stage IIIB disease are now beginning to find their way into the literature. This fact may signal the possibility of a surgical approach to patients with stage IIIB disease, particularly for those who are IIIB by virtue of a T4 primary tumor.

The need to perform radical tracheal surgery, often in palliative settings, is now being obviated by the proliferation of a variety of endotracheal stenting devices. We review 5 papers that look at a variety of stenting procedures using innovative new technology and combined technological approaches with both laser resection and mechanical stenting.

It is hoped that surgeons practicing general thoracic surgery will find this year's review helpful as they tailor their practice to accommodate advances in the preoperative assessment, staging, and therapy of patients with malignant disease with a variety of new technologies and therapeutic strategies. In addition, it is clear that further integration of video-assisted thoracic surgical techniques into the standard practice of the thoracic surgeon is occurring. To the extent that this review provides assistance to the surgeon practicing general thoracic surgery, in this regard, it will be counted as a success.

David J. Sugarbaker, M.D.

Assessment of Operative Risk in Patients Undergoing Lung Resection: Importance of Predicted Pulmonary Function

Kearney DJ, Lee TH, Reilly JJ, DeCamp MM, Sugarbaker DJ (Brigham and Women's Hosp, Boston; Beth Israel Hosp, Boston)
Chest 105:753–759, 1994   140-95-15-1

Introduction.—The most common cause of cancer death in the United States is lung cancer. The majority of the 168,000 estimated new patients this year will die within a year of diagnosis. Surgical resection remains the most viable curative option for patients with non–small-cell carcinoma. Although smoking is highly related to lung cancer, smoking also can result in chronic obstructive pulmonary disease and heart disease. Thus, the patient with a lung resection also may have significant cardiovascular disease and impairment of ventilation. In some recent studies, mortality has ranged from 2% to 11%. The decline in the risks for patients undergoing lung resection has resulted in a reappraisal of the predictive criteria for postoperative complications.

Methods.—The subjects were 331 patients who underwent lung surgery for cancer during a 2-year period. The preoperative data collection included history, functional status, blood gas analysis, spirometry, and oxygen saturation at rest and during a 6-minute walk. The postoperative forced expiratory volume in 1 second (FEV_1) was predicted from the preoperative pulmonary function testing data and information on the number of bronchopulmonary segments removed during surgery according to the following formula: predicted postoperative FEV_1 = preoperative FEV_1 × [1-(S × 5.26)/100] where S = the number of bronchopulmonary segments removed and 5.26 represents the percent of total lung function for each bronchopulmonary segment.

Results.—Complications were seen in 56 patients. Respiratory complications included 8 cases of pneumonia, 14 cases of atelectasis, 6 cases of respiratory failure, and the requirement of mechanical ventilation for more than 2 days after surgery in 4 patients. Cardiac complications included supraventricular tachycardia in 37 patients, ventricular arrhythmias in 4, the need for cardioversion in 1, and infarction in 2. Renal failure occurred in 4 patients and 3 died. The predictors of complications included age older than 60 years, male sex, a history of smoking, and the procedure performed. The postoperative complication rate was stratified according to the predicted postoperative FEV_1. Preoperative hypercarbia, oxygen desaturation during exercise, and a preoperative FEV_1 of less than 1L were not predictive of medical complications.

Conclusions.—The best indicator of any risk was the predicted postoperative FEV_1. Each 2-L decrease resulted in an odds ratio for complications of 1.46. When the other risk factors were controlled for in a multivariate analysis, the predicted postoperative FEV_1 was the only significant predictor of complications. This simple calculation may be of value in identifying patients at risk for postsurgical medical complications.

▶ This interesting review of thoracic surgery in high-risk patients highlights the need for careful preoperative assessment in patients who are deemed to be at high risk by conventional preoperative testing. Particularly, as the population in the United States ages, more patients will fall into a high-risk category purely on the basis of age. The importance of comorbidities in the area of cardiovascular disease and pulmonary disease are highlighted in this review. Of interest is the fact that preoperative hypercarbia, oxygen desaturation during exercise, and preoperative FEV_1 in the context of the amount of lung to be removed were not predictors of postoperative complications in this large group of patients. This study yielded a simple conclusion, i.e., the best predictor of any risk is the predicted postoperative FEV_1 in the context of the amount of lung to be removed. Each .2-liter decrease resulted in an odds ratio of 1.46. When all risk factors were controlled, the predicted postoperative FEV_1 was noted to be the best predictor of any postoperative complication. In the authors' experience, it is this simple calculation that has been most useful in predicting postoperative complications in the high-risk patient in whom less than an anatomic pulmonary resection is contemplated. Also of note in this report was the fact that parenchymal sparing procedures were used aggressively to afford these high-risk patients a chance at surgical cure.—D.J. Sugarbaker, M.D.

Surgical Treatment of Bullous Emphysema: Experience With the Brompton Technique

Shah SS, Goldstraw P (Royal Brompton Natl Heart and Lung Hosp, London)
Ann Thorac Surg 58:1452–1456, 1994   140-95-15–2

Background.—A technique first described by Monaldi for drainage of pulmonary cavities after tuberculosis has been modified and used to treat patients with bullous emphysematous lung disease. The technique and outcomes of 58 patients undergoing this procedure between 1983 and 1992 are examined.

Technique.—A 5- to 7-cm limited thoracotomy was performed, a segment of the underlying rib was resected, and the pleura was opened. The incision site was guided by CT findings, and corresponded to the area where the bulla came closest to the visceral pleura after decompression. After opening the bulla, 2 concentric Prolene pursestring sutures were placed around the opening, and any septa were perforated to permit free communication between adjacent loculi and bullae. The cavity was next insufflated with iodized talc, and a 32F Foley catheter was placed within the bulla. After inflating the balloon with 40 cc of air, the pursestring sutures were secured. An intrapleural chest drain was inserted, and the wounds were closed in routine fashion.

Results.—The median patient age was 57 years, and the median follow-up was 1.9 years. An operative mortality rate of 6.9% was noted. Symptomatic improvement, measured with the modified Medical Research Council of Great Britain dyspnea scale, was observed in 52 patients (mean preoperative value of 3.7–2.1 postoperatively). Symptom alleviation was accompanied by objective improvement in lung function, with a mean increase of 28% in forced expiratory volume in 1 second and a 12.3% improvement in total lung capacity. A decrease in the mean residual lung volume-total lung capacity ratio was observed (from 70% to 57% postoperatively). Significant predictors of poor prognosis included forced expiratory volume less than 500 mL in 1 second and carbon dioxide tension greater than 6.5 kPa. Two patients required further drainage of new bullae on the operated side, which was done percutaneously.

Conclusions.—This modified procedure is simple, safe, and effective for treatment of bullous emphysematous lung disease.

▶ The Monaldi technique for drainage of pulmonary cavities after tuberculosis infection is well reported in the literature. This approach has also been used in the surgical treatment of bullous emphysema. This review is particularly timely, given the renewed interest in the surgical therapy of emphysema in chronic obstructive pulmonary disease. The Monaldi technique has the advantage of minimizing the surgical procedure, including the morbidity and mortality of the approach, by shortening the operative incision. Reducing intrathoracic volume by collapsing and sclerosing the bullous lesion lets patients enjoy volume reduction, which in turn allows for expansion of the more-normal lung nearby and overall improvement in pulmonary function.

This report is a nice review of the Monaldi technique. The operative mortality rate of 6.8% with a 29% increase in forced expiratory volume at 1 second, however, would seem to be a slightly higher operative mortality than one would expect with an overall improvement of pulmonary function that seems to be in line with the resection of a single bullous lesion in the majority of patients with bullous emphysema.

If this technique is to be applied selectively, it would appear to be by patients who are at high risk for operative therapy. It should be tucked away in the armamentarium of surgeons performing general thoracic surgery.—D.J. Sugarbaker, M.D.

Surgical Resection of Pulmonary Metastases: Up to What Number?
Girard P, Baldeyrou P, Le Chevalier T, Lemoine G, Tremblay C, Spielmann M, Grunenwald D (Centre Médico-Chirurgical de la Porte de Choisy, Paris; Institut Gustave Roussy, Villejuif, France)
Am J Respir Crit Care Med 149:469–476, 1994   140-95-15-3

Background.—Specific conclusions regarding the surgical resection of a large number of pulmonary metastases (PM) have not yet been available. Thus, the risk-benefit ratio of this particular approach is open to debate. The medical records of a large patient cohort who underwent surgical resection of 8 or more PM were reviewed to determine whether such patients could benefit from surgery, and if so, to better define the selection criteria for this treatment option.

Patients and Findings.—Forty-four of 456 patients identified from this medical record review had undergone at least 1 resection for 8 or more PM between January 1, 1979 and December 31, 1990. Thirty-three had PM from osteogenic or soft tissue sarcoma. Overall 77 operations were performed in these 44 patients; 47 were bilateral and 9 were incomplete resections. After the first resection of 8 or more PM, the survival probabilities were 36% and 28% at 3 and 5 years, respectively. These findings did not differ significantly from those of the other 412 patients who underwent thoracic surgery for the resection of PM during the same period. All the long-term survivors, defined as 5 years or more, had osteogenic or soft tissue sarcoma. However, the probability of survival of these patients was not significantly different from that of the others. The only highly significant prognostic factor in patients undergoing resection for 8 or more PM was the quality of resection, whether it was complete or incomplete.

Conclusions.—At least in patients with osteogenic or soft tissue sarcoma, the prognostic value of the number of PM appears to be more dependent on associated resectability than on quantity. Thus, after careful preoperative patient selection, it is recommended that any PM that can be resected should be resected, regardless of the number.

▶ This study confirms the bias of many surgeons practicing general thoracic surgery as they treat patients with PM via metastasectomy. Dr. Noel Martini reported many years ago that those patients who could undergo complete "surgical resection" were those who would enjoy a survival advantage from a pulmonary metastasectomy. In this retrospective review a similar conclusion was reached. In addition, those patients with soft tissue sarcomas were noted most frequently to be the ones with multiple prime PM greater than 8 in number who underwent surgical resection.

Although this study emphasizes the importance of complete surgical resection during pulmonary metastasectomy, surgeons should be tempered in their enthusiasm for resecting more than 4 PM. Indeed, the ability to accomplish a complete surgical resection may be severely compromised as the number of PM increases. Nevertheless, this report does emphasize and clearly demonstrates the importance of complete surgical resection as the ultimate goal of the surgeon performing metastasectomy regardless of the number of lesions to be resected.—D.J. Sugarbaker, M.D.

Results of Pulmonary Resection of Metastatic Colorectal Cancer and Its Application

Yano T, Hara N, Ichinose Y, Yokoyama H, Miura T, Ohta M (National Kyushu Cancer Ctr, Fukuoka, Japan)
J Thorac Cardiovasc Surg 106:875–879, 1993   140-95-15–4

Background.—The 5-year survival rate for patients with colorectal cancer, after resection of pulmonary metastases, is between 9% and 42%. The differences appear to be due to the different indications for surgical resection. The 5-year survival rate and causes of death following resection of pulmonary metastases from colorectal cancer were examined.

Methods.—During an 8-year period, 27 patients had pulmonary resection of metastases from colorectal cancer. Records were reviewed for age, sex, colorectal cancer stage, number and diameter of pulmonary metastases, resection type, and survival after thoracotomy.

Results.—The 27 patients ranged in age from 27 to 81 years. The colon was the primary site in 13 patients and the rectum in the remaining patients. The primary tumor stage was Dukes' A in 2, B in 4, C in 16 and unknown in 5 patients. Unilateral pulmonary metastases were found in 14 and bilateral in 13 patients. Solitary metastases were found in 12 patients, whereas 5 had 2, 1 had 4, and 9 had 5 or more metastases. Surgical methods were wedge excision in 15 patients, segmentectomy in 3, lobectomy in 8, and pneumonectomy in 1 patient. The cumulative survival rate was 41% for all patients. For patients with solitary or 2 metastases, the survival rate was 54%, significantly higher than the survival rate for patients with more metastases. Factors about the metastases or surgical method had no influence on survival rate. The presence of controlled hepatic metastases did not have an adverse effect on survival. In 9 of the 13 patients who died a median of 24 months after thoracotomy, multiple pulmonary metastases developed causing death.

Conclusion.—In patients with primary colorectal cancer, the site should be fully explored and the number of pulmonary metastases considered when contemplating pulmonary resection.

▶ This review of pulmonary metastasectomy in patients with colorectal carcinoma points out the need to identify a subset of patients with metastatic colon cancer who develop pulmonary metastases only. In the author's experience, there is a subset of patients who develop pulmonary metastases with colorectal carcinoma who do not develop other visceral or bony metastases during the natural course of their disease. It is important to recognize this subset of patients by carefully examining their natural history before metastasectomy. In addition, it is suggested in the literature that these patients will have pulmonary metastases develop in the absence of elevation of serums, carcino-embryonic antigen (CEA). It is this subgroup in whom repeated pulmonary metastasectomy may be indicated by the lack of other visceral metastases during the course of disease. This study simply illustrates that the fewer metastases present at the time of resection, the better the overall expectant survival. The number of metastases in this setting appears to be a marker of the biological aggressiveness of the tumor.—D.J. Sugarbaker, M.D.

Surgical Treatment of Pulmonary Metastases From Soft Tissue Sarcomas: A Retrospective Study in The Netherlands

Van Geel AN, Van Coevorden F, Blankensteijn JD, Hoekstra HJ, Schuurman B, Bruggink EDM, Taat CW, Theunissen EBM (Dr Daniel den Hoed Cancer Ctr, Rotterdam, The Netherlands; Cancer Inst, Amsterdam; Academic Hosp, Groningen, The Netherlands; et al)
J Surg Oncol 56:172–177, 1994   140-95-15-5

Background.—Pulmonary metastases from soft tissue sarcomas no longer have a uniformly fatal outcome. Prolonged survival after surgical treatment has been achieved, and a 5-year postthoracotomy survival of 30% or more is possible. It is unclear which prognostic factors predict a favorable outcome. The National Cancer Institute in Bethesda, Maryland, offers the following section criteria: tumor doubling time of 20 days or more, no more than 4 metastatic nodules, and a disease-free interval of 12 months or less. However, these criteria are calculated for pulmonary metastasectomy of all types of cancer. Metastases to the lung only are characteristic of soft tissue sarcomas; in cases of soft tissue sarcoma these criteria are useful, but controversial. Reports of prognostic factors in metastatic surgery of soft tissue sarcoma are uncommon. A statistical analysis of prognostic factors was done in a retrospective study in the Netherlands to identify patients who might benefit from metastasectomy.

Methods.—The medical records were reviewed of 59 patients with soft tissue sarcoma who underwent complete resection of metastases in the lung. Three survival curves were calculated: the crude survival curve for death related to the disease, the overall survival curve for any death, and the disease-free survival cure for recurrence or death related to the disease.

Results.—The 3-year crude survival was 54%, overall survival was 52%, and disease-free survival was 49%. The 5-year crude survival was 45%, overall survival was 38%, and disease-free survival was 41%. Recurrence in the lung occurred in 40% of patients; in 5 patients the recurrence was in the opposite lung after unilateral thoracotomy, in 1 patient the recurrence was found after 10 years, and in 26 patients, the median time of the first sign of recurrence was 15 months. The only prognostic variable significantly related to disease-free survival was tumor grade.

Conclusions.—Surgery for lung metastases of soft tissue sarcoma should be standard treatment when complete resection is predicted. Analysis of prognostic factors related to survival is not conclusive. By adding chemotherapy to surgery, improved prognosis is probable.

Lung Metastasectomy in Patients With Soft Tissue Sarcoma
Robinson MH, Sheppard M, Moskovic E, Fisher C (Weston Park Hosp, Sheffield, England; Brompton Hosp, London; Royal Marsden Hosp, London)
Br J Radiol 67:129–135, 1994   140-95-15–6

Background.—High grade soft tissue sarcomas lead to metastases in 50% to 60% of patients, with the lung most often the site of first metastasis. Without treatment, this condition is inevitably fatal. Some reports have correlated survival after pulmonary metastasectomy with the duration of disease-free interval after treatment of the primary tumor. The outcomes of patients with soft tissue sarcoma undergoing this procedure were thus assessed and compared with those of patients not offered pulmonary metastasectomy.

Patients and Methods.—Lung metastases as the sole first site of disseminated disease was noted in 189 patients with soft tissue sarcoma between 1970 and 1990, of whom 44 underwent pulmonary metastasectomy. Medical records and radiologic and pathologic characteristics were reviewed in an effort to determine which patients benefit from surgery.

Results.—Patients undergoing surgery had a better overall 5-year survival at 70%, vs. 19% for those not receiving surgical treatment. The subsequent survival from the time lung metastases was detected was also improved in the 44 surgical patients, at 52% compared with 7.5% in the

145 not offered this procedure. Multivariate analysis showed that survival and control of lung disease after resection were not associated with number of metastases resected, completeness of excision, use of adjuvant chemotherapy, or presence of bilateral disease. The use of lung resection as treatment was identified as the most important factor, with a risk of .2 for death compared with those not undergoing surgery. Other factors associated with decreased risk of death were age less than 40 years and primary tumor in a lower limb site.

Conclusions.—Selected patients with soft tissue sarcoma after primary local cure should be considered for pulmonary metastasectomy, although randomized or prospective studies are needed to further elucidate the value of this procedure.

▶ These 2 reviews have nicely demonstrated the survival advantage afforded to patients with soft part sarcomas metastatic to the lung by pulmonary metastasectomy. In the first review by the group from the Netherlands, further evidence is placed in the literature for the aggressive use of pulmonary metastasectomy in patients with metastatic soft tissue sarcomas. Despite that fact that this is a retrospective study, it does appear to indicate the salvage potential in patients with pulmonary metastases from soft part sarcomas. Of interest was that the only prognostic variable in this group was the grade of the tumor, indicating again that the biological aggressiveness is the principal factor in determining survival in patients undergoing pulmonary metastasectomy. However, in concluding that pulmonary metastasectomy provides a survival advantage, this group has asked more from the retrospective phase II trial than it can deliver.

In the report by Robinson et al., an attempt is made to compare nonsurgical therapy of patients with pulmonary metastases to those patients undergoing surgical treatment. In the absence of a prospective, randomized, phase III trial, where the clear advantage of surgery could be demonstrated and definite conclusions drawn, this study does provide some evidence for the superiority of operative management in the treatment of patients with metastatic disease to the chest. Of interest was the fact that multivariate analysis showed that survival after resection was not associated with either the number of metastases resected or the completeness of resection, use of adjuvant therapy, or the presence of bilateral disease. In this particular study, only the use of lung resection as treatment was correlated with improved survival. These conclusions need to be considered in the context of previous reports in this review. We note the overwhelming support in the literature for the concept that complete resection is the gold standard and primary goal of the surgeon performing metastasectomy. This study should not be interpreted as endorsing a less than complete resection in patients undergoing metastasectomy.—D.J. Sugarbaker, M.D.

Pulmonary Resection of Metastatic Renal Cell Carcinoma

Cerfolio RJ, Allen MS, Deschamps C, Daly RC, Wallrichs SL, Trastek VF, Pairolero PC (Mayo Clinic and Found, Rochester, Minn)
Ann Thorac Surg 57:339–344, 1994   140-95-15-7

Background.—The factors associated with long-term survival in patients undergoing pulmonary resection for metastatic renal cell carcinoma (RCC) are not well defined. Review of experience with pulmonary resection for metastatic RCC addressed the prognostic features that influence extended survival.

Patients and Methods.—Ninety-six consecutive patients with a mean age of 63 years were included in this analysis. The time between nephrectomy and pulmonary resection was 0–18.4 years, with a median of 3.4 years. Solitary metastasis was noted in 48 patients, whereas 16 had 2, 18 had 3, and 14 had more than 3 metastases. Sixty-two patients underwent wedge excision, 3 had segmentectomy, 25 had lobectomy, 3 had bilobectomy, and 3 had pneumonectomy. Repeat thoracotomy was performed in 14 patients for recurrent metastases. Complete resection of limited extrapulmonary disease was also undertaken in 34 additional patients. The median follow-up was 3 years, with a range of 70 days to 19 years.

Results.—No operative deaths occurred. An overall 5-year survival rate of 35.9% was noted. Patients with solitary and multiple metastases had 5-year survival rates of 45.6% and 27%, respectively. Tumor-free intervals of more than 3.4 years were associated with improved survival, compared with intervals of 3.4 years or less. No differences between 5-year and overall survival were observed for patients undergoing repeat thoracotomy or complete resection of extrapulmonary disease.

Conclusions.—Pulmonary resection of metastatic RCC is safe and effective, with improved survival noted among patients with solitary metastasis.

▶ In this review of patients undergoing pulmonary metastasectomy for metastatic RCC, several important facts are highlighted. Once again, as was noted in patients with metastatic colon carcinoma, there is a subset of patients with metastatic RCC to the lung that appears to demonstrate pneumotropic tumors that have the propensity to metastasize only to lung parenchyma. The authors of this report have successfully identified this subset of patients, subjecting 14 of them to repeat thoracotomy and resection. It is important in this particular cell type to acquaint oneself with the natural history of the disease in a given patient. A repeat thoracotomy should be considered for recurrent disease in the lung in the absence of aggressive disease elsewhere. The overall 5-year predicted survivals in this report were encouraging particularly for the patients with solitary metastatic lesions. Again, the presence of a single metastatic lesion appears to be a mark of the biological activity of the tumor. It is also important to realize that as metastatic lesions manifest in the lung, they represent a spectrum of clones from the primary lesion, each of which may have different biological activity in terms of growth potential and cell kinetics.—D.J. Sugarbaker, M.D.

Pulmonary Resection for Metastatic Breast Cancer
McDonald ML, Deschamps C, Ilstrup DM, Allen MS, Trastek VF, Pairolero PC (Mayo Clinic and Mayo Found, Rochester, Minn)
Ann Thorac Surg 58:1599–1602, 1994   140-95-15–8

Introduction.—It is estimated that nearly 1 of 9 women will have breast cancer during her lifetime, making it the second leading cause of cancer-related death in women in the United States. A solitary pulmonary lesion can be seen on chest roentgenogram in approximately 3% of women with breast cancer, with more than 40% of those lesions being breast metastases. Although resection of these metastatic pulmonary lesions is thought to be helpful, the efficacy of the procedure has been demonstrated only with cancers originating in other sites. The efficacy of pulmonary resection for metastatic breast cancer was assessed.

Methods.—The records of 13,502 women treated for breast cancer during a 10-year period were reviewed. Pulmonary metastases were found in 60 of the patients; a median interval of 2.2 years elapsed between the time of primary breast surgery and the diagnosis of pulmonary metastases. Complete pulmonary resection was performed in 40 patients (consisting of wedge excision, lobectomy, and pneumonectomy). The remaining 20 patients had an incomplete or noncurative resection.

Results.—One patient died of complications after thoracotomy; 59 patients were assessable with a mean follow-up of 3.5 years. Thirty-two of 39 patients who underwent a complete resection had a recurrence of disease after a median disease-free interval of 1.6 years. Sites of recurrence included lung (15 patients), chest wall (4 patients), brain (3 patients), bone (2 patients), breast (2 patients), liver (1 patient), pericardium (1 patient), supraclavicular lymph node (1 patient), and disseminated (3 patients). Twenty-eight patients died of recurrent breast cancer. Seven patients remain disease-free and 4 are currently alive with disease. Of the 20 patients who underwent an incomplete (or noncurative) resection, 17 died of disseminated breast cancer and 3 remain alive with disease. For all patients, the 5- and 10-year survival rates were 37.8% and 8.1%, respectively. For the 40 patients who underwent a complete resection, 5- and 10-year survival rates were 35.6% and 13.4%, respectively, compared with a 5-year survival of 42.1% for patients who underwent an incomplete resection ($P > .05$).

Conclusion.—This study failed to demonstrate improved survival of patients after complete pulmonary resection for metastatic breast cancer. Of 13,502 patients, only 60 (.4%) had isolated pulmonary metastases. Therefore, a complete resection can be recommended for patients with a history of breast cancer who have a solitary pulmonary lesion to differentiate metastatic breast cancer from a new primary lung cancer.

▶ This review points to the fact that not all patients with metastatic carcinoma are candidates for pulmonary metastasectomy. In this well-done review, the authors have pointed out that patients undergoing complete resection of pulmonary metastases fared no better than patients undergoing incomplete palliative resection for metastatic breast disease. The lack of a survival advantage for patients undergoing complete resection would seem to discourage surgeons from performing routine metastasectomy in patients with documented metastatic breast carcinoma.

It should be stated, however, that in many clinical situations, particularly where the patient who has had breast cancer also has a smoking history, the presence of a solitary pulmonary nodule may actually represent a primary lung malignancy. At the time of resection it is often impossible for the pathologist to clearly elucidate whether the lesion represents a primary lung malignancy or metastatic breast carcinoma. Therefore, solitary lung lesions in patients with known breast cancer should be treated as primary lung malignancies in the majority of clinical settings unless it can be clearly demonstrated that they are of metastatic origin. Estrogen receptor (ER) and progesterone receptor (PR) positivity may or may not be helpful given the subset of patients with lung carcinoma who are ER positive as well as PR positive. The aggressive nature of breast carcinoma once it becomes metastatic would appear to preclude the use of pulmonary metastasectomy for the majority of cases.—D.J. Sugarbaker, M.D.

Intrapleural Treatment With Recombinant Gamma-Interferon in Early Stage Malignant Pleural Mesothelioma
Boutin C, Nussbaum E, Monnet I, Bignon J, Vanderschueren R, Guerin J-C, Menard O, Mignot P, Dabouis G, Douillard J-Y (Hôpital de la Conception, Marseille, France; Centre Hospitalier Intercommunal, Créteil, France; St Antonius Ziekenhuis, Nieuwegein, The Netherlands; et al)
Cancer 74:2460–2467, 1994   140-95-15–9

Background.—The response of diffuse malignant pleural mesothelioma to surgery, chemotherapy, and/or radiation therapy has been unsatisfactory. Although chemotherapy and radiation may be palliative, survival is not prolonged. Surgical therapy may be beneficial but is associated with high morbidity and mortality. Intracavitary immunotherapy, however, has shown promise. The cytokine gamma-interferon (γ-INF), in particular, may be effective against pleural mesothelioma because of its facilitation of cell differentiation, cytotoxic action on mesothelial cells, and stimulation of natural killer lymphocytes and macrophages. Preliminary results of a multicentric, prospective study documented 4 complete and 2 partial responses out of 22 affected patients. Response to therapy is reported for an additional 67 patients to confirm the preliminary results.

Methods.—Participants had stage I or II epithelial or mixed malignant mesothelioma. Those with fibrosarcomatous mesothelioma were not included because of the apparent inefficacy of γ-INF in 4 previous patients. Stage I was subdivided, based upon thoracoscopic findings, into stage IA, where the parietal or diaphragmatic pleura but not the visceral pleura was involved, and stage IB, where parietal, diaphragmatic, and visceral pleura were involved. In each patient human recombinant γ-INF was administered via either a 21 Fr chest tube, placed in the third or fourth intercostal space with the tip near the larger lesions, or an implantable port. Beginning 2 weeks after catheter or port placement 40, a million units of γ-INF were administered for 6 hours twice weekly for 8 weeks. The response to treatment was determined by CT 2 weeks after therapy, with thoracoscopy or thoracotomy and multiple biopsies performed if signs of improvement were seen.

Results.—Significant adverse effects noted in the 89 patients included fever in 100%, empyema in 8%, and asthenia in 3%. Clinical pathologic abnormalities were noted in 81% of patients, with elevated serum glutamic pyruvic transaminase and glutamic oxaloacetic transaminase, anemia, and neutropenia most common. Treatment was stopped in 13% of patients because of the severity of adverse reaction. There was no macroscopic or microscopic evidence of disease after therapy in 8 patients, and a greater than 50% decrease in tumor size in an additional 9, for a total response rate of 19.1%. The response rate varied with disease stage, with 44.8% of patients with stage I disease and only 6% of patients with stage II disease responding. Complete response occurred in 38.4% of patients in stage IA, 12% in stage IB, and 1.8% in stage II. The mean durations of remission were 17 months for complete responders and 19 months for partial responders.

Conclusions.—Immunotherapy using γ-INF may be a therapeutic alternative to surgery for patients with stage I epithelial or mixed malignant mesothelioma. Early diagnosis and treatment may significantly improve response to therapy, with few patients with stage II disease expected to respond to treatment. Further studies are necessary to explore response to other cytokines or cytokine mixtures and to combinations of cytokines with chemotherapy or surgery.

▶ This particular study demonstrates the profound effect of intrapleural γ-INF on early stage malignant pleural mesothelioma. Although the mechanism for the observed responses of early stage epithelial-type mesothelioma to installation of γ-INF is not clear, the demonstrated biological activity suggests that its use as an adjunctive agent may be of some value.

Of interest is the fact that in the United States, the detection of very early cases of malignant pleural mesothelioma is not the most common clinical presentation. We will follow these studies and will be interested to see the development of treatment strategies that use γ-INF in a multimodality schema. The authors of this review are specific about substaging these patients depending upon the visceral pleural involvement. It is not clear that this subtyping is of any clinical importance to those clinicians in the United States treating more advanced disease.—D.J. Sugarbaker, M.D.

Localized Malignant Mesothelioma: A Clinicopathologic and Flow Cytometric Study
Crotty TB, Myers JL, Katzenstein A-LA, Tazelaar HD, Swensen SJ, Churg A (Mayo Clinic and Found, Rochester, Minn; Crouse-Irving Mem Hosp, Syracuse, NY; Univ of British Columbia, Vancouver, Canada)
Am J Surg Pathol 18:357–363, 1994   140-95-15–10

Series.—Malignant pleural mesotheliomas occur only very rarely as a localized tumor mass. Six patients, 4 women and 2 men, 42 to 76 years of age, were seen with such tumors. Three of the 6 patients had a history of asbestos exposure.

Pathology.—Four mesotheliomas were sessile tumors having a broad pleural attachment, and 2 were pedunculated. Three of the tumors were purely epithelioid lesions. An ultrastructural study of 2 of these tumors revealed long, thin microvilli, well-developed desmosomes, and many tonofilaments. Immunohistochemical studies were positive for cytokeratin and negative for carcinoembryonic antigen in all instances. Only 1 of the 6 tumors stained focally for Leu-M1 in a peripheral membrane pattern. Flow cytometry demonstrated an aneuploid DNA content in 4 of the 5 lesions examined.

Outcome.—Local recurrences developed in 3 patients 4 to 18 months after excision of the primary tumor, and all 3 patients died of disease 1 to 2 years after diagnosis. The other 3 patients are well without disease, the first patient after 8 months, the second after 2 years, and the third after 8 years.

Conclusions.—A varient of malignant mesothelioma is a localized tumor that resembles classical diffuse mesotheliomas with respect to their histologic appearances and immunophenotypic characteristics. These tumors may behave aggressively, but complete excision may be curative in some instances.

▶ The rare clinical setting when mesothelioma presents as a primary mass often leads to the incorrect therapy of the disease based on an incomplete understanding of its tumor biology. This nice review of 6 cases performed at the Mayo Clinic demonstrates the need to have histologic confirmation of tumor type before the planned surgical procedure. It also highlights that there is a subset of patients with malignant mesothelioma that will present as a single mass as opposed to the diffuse studding of parietal and visceral pleura.

The author points out, however, the growing importance of thoracoscopy in fully assessing these patients to document before planned resection the extent of visceral involvement. It is the authors' experience that in many cases, although a dominant mass is noted on plain film and CT scan, direct inspection of the pleura will yield evidence of multifocal disease. Multifocality in this disease demands either aggressive pleurectomy or pleural pneumonectomy or pallidi of treatment. Resection of a local mass in the face of evidence of multifocal disease elsewhere in the pleura will provide only short-term palliation.—D.J. Sugarbaker, M.D.

A Phase II Trial of Pleurectomy/Decortication Followed by Intrapleural and Systemic Chemotherapy for Malignant Pleural Mesothelioma
Rusch V, Saltz L, Venkatraman E, Ginsberg R, McCormack P, Burt M, Markman M, Kelsen D (Mem Sloan-Kettering Cancer Ctr, New York)
J Clin Oncol 12:1156–1163, 1994   140-95-15–11

Introduction.—Surgical resection, radiation, and systemic chemotherapy have all had limited success in treating malignant pleural mesothelioma. Even multimodality regimens have achieved a median survival duration of only 1 year. The ideal treatment would control the local tumor and reduce the risk of distant disease. A new approach reported here combines surgical resection with immediate postoperative intrapleural chemotherapy followed by systemic chemotherapy.

Patients and Methods.—Eligible patients had biopsy-proven, resectable malignant pleural mesothelioma; none had extrathoracic disease or were previously treated. Surgical resection sought to remove all gross tumor while leaving the lung in place. Patients were hydrated with IV fluids at least 12 hours preoperatively in preparation for intrapleural chemotherapy (cisplatin 100 mg/m² and mitomycin 8 mg/m²), administered in the recovery room. Systemic chemotherapy, started 3 to 5 weeks postoperatively, consisted of IV infusions of cisplatin 50 mg/m² on days 1, 8, 15, 22, 36, 43, 50, and 57, and IV boluses of mitomycin 8 mg/m² on days 1 and 36. Patients were monitored every 3 months after completing systemic chemotherapy, for a period of at least 18 months or until death.

Results.—Twenty-seven of 36 patients who entered the study were potential candidates for the planned systemic chemotherapy. This group had a mean age of 62 years; 24 were men and 3 were women. Sixteen had a history of asbestos exposure. In 20 patients, a complete resection of all gross tumor was performed. Four of the 27 patients did not receive systemic chemotherapy. One died a month after surgical resection, 2 had renal insufficiency after intrapleural chemotherapy, and 1 had a poor performance status. The remaining 23 patients received a median of 80% and 87% of the planned total cisplatin and mitomycin doses, respectively. There were no grade 3 or 4 toxicities. Overall survival among the candidates for systemic therapy was 68% at 1 year and 40% at 2 years; median survival was 17 months. The most common form of relapse was locoregional disease, characterized by pleural-based tumor in the opposite hemithorax.

Conclusion.—Malignant pleural mesothelioma typically occurs in men who had an occupational exposure to asbestos from the 1940s through the 1960s. The short, aggressive multimodality regimen reported here has a potential for serious toxicity but yielded overall survival as good or better than that obtained with other combined treatments. Approaches designed to achieve local control are needed, because local recurrence remains a dominant problem.

▶ The treatment of malignant pleural mesothelioma in the United States has not been standardized. Indeed, the standard of care for pleural mesothelioma would appear to be in most centers only palliative, supportive therapy. Dr. Rusch and colleagues have in this report sought to evaluate the use of parietal pleurectomy and systemic chemotherapy in the treatment of this disease. The substantial morbidity incurred with this therapy and the guarded median survival of 17 months compares only slightly more favorably than supportive therapy alone. Nevertheless, this is an important paper that appears to evaluate in a single institution committed to this regimen the results of topical therapy combined with intravenous treatment in this disease. Unfortunately, the use of pleurectomy as a standard operative approach in this disease precludes any accurate surgical pathologic staging of these patients.

It appears clear that a staging system will need to be constructed based on complete resection of specimens with pathologic review of them and documentation of pathologic stage, if accurate prognosis is to be gained based on a surgical pathologic staging system.

It is clear that the lack of effective adjuvant treatment makes any surgical approach to these disease palliative in the majority of cases.

The lack of enthusiasm for subtotal resection in this disease and the encouraging results obtained with extrapleural pneumonectomy followed by adjuvant treatment have caused many clinicians to conclude that more aggressive treatment or no treatment are the appropriate courses of action.—D.J. Sugarbaker, M.D.

Thorascopy—Advances in Techniques

INTRODUCTION

The introduction of the microchip camera 5 years ago led to the reengineering of many thoracic surgical techniques. With the development of new instrumentation in video-assisted thoracic surgery, many surgical procedures have now begun to be reengineered. Whereas early reports concentrated on diagnostic procedures including simple pleuroscopy and poudrage, we are now beginning to see mature reports of prospective, randomized trials seeking to evaluate video-assisted techniques vs. accepted conventional surgical therapy. It is important to understand that we are seeing procedures in evolution being compared with standard procedures that were themselves the result of many years of surgical innovation. Therefore, reports showing equivalency between video-assisted thoracic surgery vs. conventional surgery should be seen as an early indicator of the potential of these new, minimally invasive techniques in the performance of routine thoracic surgical procedures. Certainly, it is clear that the avoidance of a standard posterolateral thoracotomy in the majority of cases will yield a decrease in morbidity and mortality for a large population of patients.

David J. Sugarbaker, M.D.

Postoperative Pain-Related Morbidity: Video-Assissted Thoracic Surgery Versus Thoracotomy

Landreneau RJ, Hazelrigg SR, Mack MJ, Dowling RD, Burke D, Gavlick J, Perrino MK, Ritter PS, Bowers CM, DeFino J, Nunchuck SK, Freeman J, Keenan RJ, Ferson PF (Univ of Pittsburgh, Pa; St Luke's Med Ctr, Milwaukee, Wisc; Humana Hospital, Dallas)

Ann Thorac Surg 56:1285–1289, 1993   140-95-15–12

Background.—Video-assisted thoracic surgery (VATS) may be associated with reduced postoperative morbidity, although objective comparisons between this approach and open thoracotomy techniques are limited. Early postoperative pain-related morbidity was evaluated in patients undergoing VATS pulmonary resection, and compared with that of patients treated with a limited lateral thoracotomy (LLT) approach.

Patients and Methods.—One hundred thirty-eight consecutive, nonrandomized patients with comparable demographic and preoperative physiologic parameters were included. Pulmonary resection of peripheral lung lesions 3 cm or less in diameter was accomplished using a VATS approach in 81 and an LLT approach in 57 patients. Wedge resection was done in 74 of the VATS and 19 of the LLT patients, whereas 7 patients had VATS lobectomy, and 38 patients had lobectomy performed through an LLT. Pain was quantitatively measured by postoperative narcotic requirements, the use of intercostal/epidural analgesia, and subjective pain index scoring. Shoulder and pulmonary function (forced expiratory volume in 1 second) were evaluated before surgery, on the third postoperative day, and at 3 weeks' follow-up.

Results.—Significantly less postoperative pain was noted in patients undergoing the VATS procedures. None of the patients in the VATS group required intercostal block/epidural analgesia, compared with 31 of the LLT group. The need for narcotics was also less among the VATS patients, which correlated with lower perception of pain index after surgery for these patients. At postoperative day 3, shoulder girdle strength was equally impaired, although function improved in the VATS patients at 3 weeks' follow-up. Patients undergoing wedge resection alone by LLT showed greater impairment in early pulmonary function compared with the VATS wedge resection group, although these differences were not observed at 3 weeks.

Conclusions.—Patients undergoing VATS pulmonary resection experience decreased pain, shoulder dysfunction, and early pulmonary impairment, compared with those treated with an LLT approach. The efficacy of the VATS approach in reducing the chronic postoperative morbidity of thoracic surgery remains to be determined. Additional studies are also needed to clarify the relative benefits of the VATS approach alone compared with LLT and epidural analgesia in decreasing the postoperative morbidity of major pulmonary resection.

▶ This study by Landreneau et al. was carefully conducted to attempt to evaluate prospectively the effect of VATS on early postoperative morbidity after thoracic surgery. It is interesting that, although patients undergoing VATS pulmonary resection experienced less pain, shoulder dysfunction, and early pulmonary impairment compared with those treated with a standard thoracotomy, this effect was transient and was not detectable in the extended postoperative period.

However, had this group of authors restricted their study to high-risk elderly and poor performance-status patients, this decrease in postoperative morbidity, pain, and shoulder dysfunction may have actually translated into reduced incidence of pneumonia, respiratory failure, and death. Whereas the reduction in postoperative morbidity via the VATS approach is intuitive for the majority of surgeons, we will require further studies of the extended postoperative period to determine the effect of the VATS approach on long-term morbidity related to these procedures.—D.J. Sugarbaker, M.D.

Initial Experience with Video-Assisted Thoracoscopic Lobectomy
Kirby TJ, Mack MJ, Landreneau RJ, Rice TW (The Cleveland Clinic Found, Ohio; Humana Hospital, Dallas; Univ of Pittsburgh, Pa)
Ann Thorac Surg 56:1248–1253, 1993   140-95-15–13

Objective.—The technical feasibility of video-assisted thoracic surgery (VATS) in early primary lung cancers was evaluated.

Patients.—Forty-four patients with primary bronchogenic carcinoma were accepted as potential candidates for VATS lobectomy. All patients had clinical stage I tumors on complete preoperative staging. All patients had normal arterial blood gases and adequate pulmonary reserve to undergo lobectomy, with forced expiratory volume in 1 second of more than 1.5 L.

Procedure.—Under single-lung anesthesia, VATS lobectomy was performed through 2 thoracoscopy ports and a non–rib-spreading 6- to 8-cm "access" thoracotomy. After dissection in the fissure and exposure of the interlobal artery, the arterial branches and venous drainage were divided using a vascular endostapler from which the knife blade was removed before firing. The vessels were then safely divided. The lobar bronchus was transected with a 30 Endo-GIA tissue stapler, and fissures were completed with multiple firings of a 3.5-mm endostapler and electrocautery. Special technical considerations for the right upper lobe included transection of the right upper lobe bronchus with anterior retraction of the distal bronchial stump to allow exposure of the arterial branches. For the right middle lobe, lobectomy was performed from an anterior approach by dividing the middle lobe vein and then the middle lobe bronchus. For the right lower lobe, it was necessary to separately transect the superior segmental artery and bronchus in the right lower lobe so as not to compromise the middle lobar artery and bronchus. For the left upper lobe, the often large anterior arterial branch was transected last after dividing the remaining arterial supply to the upper lobe, the superior pulmonary vein, and the upper lobe bronchus.

Outcome.—At the time of operation, 3 patients had N2 disease and did not have resection. Of the remaining 41 patients, 35 successfully underwent a VATS lobectomy during a mean operative time of 153 minutes. There were no major intraoperative complications that necessitated conversion to an open thoracotomy. All patients recovered uneventfully, with a mean hospital stay of 5.7 days.

Conclusion.—A VATS lobectomy is technically feasible and potentially safe. Although it offers many potential advantages over conventional surgery in terms of decreased postoperative pain, improved cosmesis, earlier hospital discharge, and faster return to work, major advances in thoracic imaging and instrumentation are necessary before this procedure will have potential for widespread acceptance. The majority of available instrumentation for VATS are designed for general surgical applications, so that much of the endoscopic equipment is inadequate or suboptimal for major chest operations. Furthermore, prospective, randomized trials are necessary to confirm these advantages.

Thoracoscopic Pulmonary Lobectomy: Early Operative Experience and Preliminary Clinical Results
Walker WS, Carnochan FM, Pugh GC (City Hospital, Edinburgh, Scotland)
J Thorac Cardiovasc Surg 106:1111–1117, 1993   140-95-15–14

Background.—Thoracoscopic video-assisted lobectomy techniques can be used to resect all the major pulmonary lobes. Preliminary experience with 11 pulmonary lobectomy procedures was evaluated.

Patients and Methods.—Eleven patients, including 7 men and 4 women, with a mean age of 66 years were evaluated. Peripheral pulmonary opacities were noted in 10 patients, including bronchogenic carcinomas in 8, an atypical carcinoid lesion in 1, and a pulmonary infarct in 1. Preoperative CT scanning was performed in these patients to rule out mediastinal lymphadenopathy. The remaining patient had a preoperative diagnosis of lobar bronchiectasis. Surgical access was provided through 3 stab incisions (1 cm) and 1 short submammary incision (7 cm), made without rib separation and used for specimen delivery. Four left upper, 2 left lower, 2 right upper, and 3 right lower lobes were resected.

Results.—All patients survived and were discharged from the hospital. Excision was complete for patients with neoplastic disease, and all bronchial stumps healed without complications. Postoperative bleeding was not a problem in any patient. Overall mean operative time and blood loss were 3.3 hours and 263 mL, respectively, in the first 6 patients. In the latter 5 patients, these figures were 2.3 hours and 100 mL, respectively, suggesting improvement with experience. Mean high-dependency unit time was 41 hours, and no patient required ventilatory assistance. A standard dissectional lobectomy with lobar lymph node clearance equal to that achieved at open thoracotomy was possible in each patient. Patients in this series had decreased postoperative pain, morphine consumption, and high-dependency unit stay, in comparison with a series of 33 who underwent open lobectomies.

Conclusions.—These findings support the development of video-assisted thoracoscopic pulmonary lobectomy for patients with small peripheral opacities or established benign disease.

▶ The use of thoracoscopic techniques in the performance of more advanced pulmonary procedures has been the subject of much debate in the thoracic surgical and general surgical community. Indeed, the feasibility of performing a complete anatomical lobectomy via a video-assisted technique has not been firmly established. In their multi-institutional report, Dr. Kirby et al. (Abstract 140-95-15–13) have nicely demonstrated the initial anatomical considerations in the performance of a variety of lobectomies in patients with T1, stage I non–small-cell carcinomas.

The emphasis on knowing the N2 status before thoracotomy, the careful selection of patients based on complete fissure presence of T1 lesions, and the absence of N1 lymph nodes make this report appear to be well considered and carefully constructed. Although the average hospital stay of 7.5 days lags considerably behind other centers performing conventional thoracic surgical procedures, this early report should be seen as an encouragement to surgeons seeking to develop alternative techniques in the performance of standard lobectomies via less morbid video-assisted techniques. The emphasis by Dr. Kirby et al. (Abstract 140-95-15–13) on the lack of thoracic surgical instrumentation is well placed. Indeed, at this time, the lack of instrumentation is the principal cause of the reluctance of many surgeons to move ahead with more complex thoracic surgical procedures to be performed via minimally invasive techniques.

The report by Dr. Walker et al. further confirms the feasibility of performing VATS lobectomies in selected centers with experience in thoracoscopic and video-assisted techniques. This well-illustrated article, like that of Dr. Kirby, uses 2 or 3 ports in addition to a utility thoracotomy of 8–10 cm, used without the aid of a rib spreader. Indeed it is this avoidance of rib spreading that is thought to obviate the majority of the pain and discomfort resulting conventional thoracic surgery.—D.J. Sugarbaker, M.D.

Video-Assisted Thoracoscopic Pneumonectomy

Walker WS, Carnochan FM, Mattar S (City Hosp, Edinburgh, Scotland)
Br J Surg 81:81–82, 1994   140-95-15–15

Introduction.—A 51-year-old woman was referred for surgical intervention for a 4-cm mass detected in the lingula and mediastinal glands of less than 5 mm diameter in which CT was used.

Surgical Technique.—The patient was positioned for a standard left thoracotomy. Access was gained using 3 stab incisions and one 6-cm submammary incision. A 10-mm laparoscope connected to a video camera with light source and monitor were introduced through the upper posterior incision. Pneumonectomy was required because the tumor crossed the oblique fissure and an obviously malignant lymph node that involved the basal stem artery was detected. The other incisions were used for laparoscopic dissection and insertion of stapling devices. After anterior and inferior lung retraction, sharp dissection was used to enter the sheath of the pulmonary artery. The pulmonary artery and superior and inferior pulmonary veins were clamped and divided before stapling. A conventional bronchial stapler was used to close the main bronchus. All peribronchial nodes were removed, and the lung was removed intact through the submammary incision without spreading the ribs. Small nodes on the aortic arch were removed. An intercostal drain was inserted through the lower posterior incision. Compared with patients having conventional thoracotomy, this patient required significantly less morphine for pain control, had significantly lower linear visual analogue pain scores, and a blood loss of 360 mL. Intercostal nerve blocks were not needed. The patient was discharged on day 5 and was well at the follow-up examination at 5 months.

Conclusion.—Pneumonectomy can be successfully achieved through video-assisted thoracic surgery. Node dissection around the main bronchus and lateral aortic arch was uncomplicated and suggests that extensive node clearance may be accomplished during video-assisted thoracic procedures.

▶ This report by Walker et al. from Edinburgh shows the feasibility in a single case of performing a video-assisted pneumonectomy. Strong caution should be emphasized to all surgeons contemplating this surgical approach. Incomplete lymph node dissection may be a significant drawback to thoracoscopic or video-assisted pneumonectomy. In addition, the possibility of massive bleeding from the main pulmonary artery should give most surgeons pause before performing this surgical procedure without adequate exposure. Indeed, incomplete assessment of patients at the time of proposed pneumonectomy may lead to inappropriate resection.

After those strong words of caution, however, it is interesting to note that surgeons are developing techniques using currently available instrumentation to perform video-assisted and thoracoscopic procedures of this magnitude.—D.J. Sugarbaker, M.D.

Thoracoscopic Drainage and Decortication as Definitive Treatment for Empyema Thoracis Following Penetrating Chest Injury

O'Brien J, Cohen M, Solit R, Solit R, Lindenbaum G, Finnegan J, Vernick J
(Thomas Jefferson Univ Hosp, Philadelphia; Crozer Chester Med Ctr, Upton, Pa)

J Trauma 36:536–540, 1994   140-95-15–16

Introduction.—Selected surgical settings, including thoracic surgery, have been revolutionized by the use of videoendoscopic techniques. The less-invasive nature makes the method very attractive as the causes of major morbidity are associated with incisions, rib spreading, and postoperative pain. The experience with thoracoscopic drainage and decortication as treatment for empyema thoracis after penetrating chest trauma is reported.

Methods.—Gunshots or stab wounds sent 8 patients to 2 hospitals for treatment. Initial treatment for a hemothorax or pneumothorax included a closed tube thoracostomy and antibiotics. All patients had an empyema develop and underwent 3-portal thoracoscopy while in the lateral decubitus position. Two chest tubes were placed after the procedure.

Results.—The median time from injury to diagnosis of the empyema was 16 days. The empyema resolved in all 8 patients. Chest tubes were removed 8.5 (range, = 2 to 25) days after surgery. The hospital stay averaged 19 (range, = 4 to 56) days. The time for surgery averaged 110 minutes with an average loss of blood of 200 mL in 7 of the 8 patients. One patient lost 2,800 mL of blood. Six of the 8 patients had cultures for *Staphylococcus* (n = 4), and 1 each with *Proteus* and *Streptococcus*. There were no further procedures for the empyema, but 2 patients had further thoracoscopic intervention for an air leak or a trapped lung.

Comment.—Thoracoscopic drainage and decortication is an alternative to thoracotomy for treatment of empyema thoracis after a penetrating chest injury. The procedure is safe and has a low morbidity.

▶ The use of thoracoscopic approaches in the treatment of benign disease of the chest would appear to be a suitable match of operative technique with underlying pathophysiology. The lack of a need for strict surgical resection including resection margins makes the application of thoracoscopic techniques to decortication a "natural." These authors, by delineating the appropriate use of thoracoscopic techniques in these series of cases, gives this well-written report its importance. The application of thoracoscopic and video-assisted techniques in the treatment of empyema in these authors' experience is best relegated to the setting of acute decortication.

In the setting of chronic decortication with a chronic peel restricting lung function, it is often difficult to establish the plains required for thoracoscopic surgery. On the contrary, however, in the setting of acute active infection or in the presence of previous hemothorax, video-assisted techniques provide an excellent alternative to standard thoracotomy for chest evacuation and reexpansion of lung parenchyma.

It is precisely in this setting where the thoracoscopic approach may provide a superior alternative to conventional thoracic surgical incisions. Again, the need for better instrumentation and visualization via advanced instrumentation may be identified by any surgeon who has experience with empyema thoracis and its treatment.—D.J. Sugarbaker, M.D.

Nd-YAG Laser Pleurodesis Via Thoracoscopy: Endoscopic Therapy in Spontaneous Pneumothorax Nd-YAG Laser Pleurodesis
Torre M, Grassi M, Nerli FP, Maioli M, Belloni PA (Niguarda Hosp, Milan, Italy)
Chest 106:338–341, 1994   140-95-15–17

Background.—The best treatment for spontaneous pneumothorax is still debated. In 1989, the use of a new endoscopic therapeutic approach with Nd-YAG laser phototherapy through thoracoscopy in the radical treatment of 14 patients was reported. The technique has been improved since then and applied to a larger series of patients.

Methods.—Eighty-five patients with spontaneous pneumothorax were treated between 1986 and 1993. The patients were 55 men and 30 women, aged 16 to 51 years. Treatment consisted of a new endoscopic procedure using an Nd-YAG laser beam via thoracoscopy to obtain permanent pleurodesis and to treat the lung lesion responsible for the air leak. The thoracoscope was introduced through a 1-cm incision in the anterior axillary line of the fourth intercostal space with the patients under general anesthesia.

Findings.—Small blebs were found and resected successfully with low-power Nd-YAG laser pulses in 68 patients. In 2 patients in whom lesions greater than 2 cm were found at thoracoscopy, the Nd-YAG laser did not seal the air leak, and thoracotomy was done. No air leaks were found at endoscopy in the remaining patients. After lung lesions were treated, the parietal pleura was abraded using laser energy. No adverse effects occurred. Eighty patients were treated successfully and had no recurrence at a maximum follow-up of 86 months. After 5 to 24 weeks, 3 other patients had recurrence of pneumothorax. Surgery was considered mandatory in 2 of them. In both patients, a small bleb was detected at thoracotomy in the lower lobe and resected. The entire upper lobe adhered strongly to the parietal pleura at the site of previous laser abrasion.

Conclusions.—Treatment with Nd-YAG laser via thoracoscopy is a viable option in patients with spontaneous pneumothorax. This treatment, with the eventual aid of an endoscopic stapler, should be consid-

ered the preferred therapy, with open thoracotomy reserved for complicated cases.

▶ Early in the development of thoracoscopic surgery, it appeared as though
lasers were going to be the first assistant of the thoracoscopic surgeon. The
ability to apply thermal energy to the lung and intrathoracic structures without the need for electric cautery appeared as an attractive alternative to conventional dissecting techniques.

However, as the evolution of thoracoscopy has continued, it appears that
lasers do not offer any particular benefit over stapling techniques. Indeed, it
appears that the delayed eschar formation and the production of a delayed
air leak may make the laser an unpredictable therapeutic tool. Nevertheless,
these results from Milan show that thoracoscopic surgery will lead to new
marriages of instrumentation as a variety of combinations of new technologies are brought to bear upon thoracic surgical disease. It appears that the
jury is still out on the use of YAG lasers in the intrathoracic treatment of pulmonary disease. Whereas the use of endobronchial lasers in the treatment of
endobronchial obstruction has been established and appears secure, the extension of laser technology into intrathoracic disease is not clear.—D.J.
Sugarbaker, M.D.

Thoracoscopic Implantation of Cancer With a Fatal Outcome
Fry WA, Siddiqui A, Pensler JM, Mostafavi H (Northwestern Univ, Evanston,
Ill)
Ann Thorac Surg 59:42–45, 1995   140-95-15–18

Background.—Thoracoscopy is used in numerous settings, including
evaluation of pleural disease, debridement of chronic empyema, and
performing pericardiectomies and biopsies of lung tissue and lymph
nodes. Controversy surrounds its use in resection of known or suspected
lung cancer. A case of chest wall tumor implantation occurred after
video-assisted thoracoscopic surgical excision of a small pulmonary adenocarcinoma.

Case Report.—Man, 74, had a 2-cm cavitary density in the left lower lung field
that was found on a screening chest roentgenogram. A CT scan showed a peripheral 2-cm cavitary lesion in the superior segment of the left lower lobe of the
lung. There was no evidence of intrathoracic lymphadenopathy or other lesion in
the lung. The patient underwent video-assisted thoracoscopic surgery; the lesion
was identified and easily removed. Evaluation of the specimen revealed well-differentiated adenocarcinoma. A completion left lower lobectomy was then performed. The patient was discharged and did well until 5 months later, when he
noticed a protuberance over his left lateral chest. Examination revealed a 4 cm
× 3-cm, firm, fixed, smooth, nontender mass over the left fifth rib at the midax-
illary line. Examination of the tissue obtained by biopsy revealed adenocarcinoma consistent with the original tumor. Chest wall resection was performed,

the cancer was removed, and reconstruction was performed. Two months later, the patient had chest wall pain, and 2 months after that, the pain became severe. Examination showed obvious chest wall tumor recurrence all around the reconstruction site. Four specimens were examined and 3 showed adenocarcinoma. No relief was obtained from attempts at symptom control and the patient died 10 months after the initial lung cancer resection and 5 months after the chest wall resection of the tumor implant.

Comment.—The evidence of implanting the tumor is both temporal and topographic. To date, there is only 1 other report of chest wall incisional metastasis after video-assisted thoracoscopic surgery. This problem may have more to do with the biological nature of tumors than with the size of incision. Modifications or precautions may be needed when dealing with endoscopic tumor retrieval. Similar fatal complications may become more frequent as minimal-access surgical procedures become more common.

▶ Therapeutic surgical treatment of malignant disease has resulted from an evolution of techniques during the past decades. Understanding of oncologic principles has been the foundation by which new procedures have been constructed. An understanding of the biology of disease let Halstead and others to propose resection of regional lymph nodes in the primary treatment of malignant tumors. Likewise, the avoidance of incision into tumors and the spillage of tumor cells into open wounds has been written about for the last half century.

It is therefore not surprising that if during the thoracoscopic removal of intrathoracic malignancies cells are allowed to implant in the wound, recurrence in the wound will result in a majority of patients. This occurrence should not be allowed to discourage or condemn the use of thoracoscopic approaches to intrathoracic malignancy. It should, however, be used to condemn sloppy surgical technique, which remains sloppy whether it is performed thoracoscopically or in an open setting. This report highlights the fact that all tumors removed from the chest should be bagged in commercially available tissue traps before their removal. This is particularly true when large tumors are being squeezed through small incisions in the chest.—D.J. Sugarbaker, M.D.

Surgery for Stage IIIa-N2 Non-Small Cell Lung Cancer
Mountain CF (Univ of Texas MD Anderson Cancer Ctr, Houston)
Cancer 73:2589–2598, 1994   140-95-15–19

Introduction.—The only definitive therapy for non–small-cell lung cancer is surgery. There is little argument about surgery for patients with stage I or II disease, yet the benefits for patients with stage IIIa-N2 cancer are unknown. The 5-year survival rates for patients with N2 disease range from 9% to 32%; however, patient selection makes comparison difficult. The use of surgery for selected N2 patients is discussed, focusing on patient selection criteria.

Methods.—The records from 2,883 patients who had surgery for lung cancer were reviewed. A subset of 307 patients with N2 disease were the focus of the study. In this group, the median time to death was 14 months, the median follow-up time was 30 months, with a follow-up time range of 133 months.

Results.—More nodal disease means a poorer prognosis. The 5-year survival rate was 62% in patients with no nodal disease, 43% in patients with intrapulmonary metastasis, and 31% in patients with ipsilateral mediastinal lymph node metastases. The extent of nodal involvement is underestimated if resection of all nodes is not performed. The number of positive nodes significantly influenced survival. Survival rates were 37%, 27%, and 17% for patients with 1, 2 to 4, or more than 4 positive nodes, respectively. Fifty-five percent of the patients had 1 positive node, 21% had 2 to 4 positive nodes, and 13% had more than 4 positive nodes. The location and level of the involved nodes were also significant determinants of survival. The poorest survival rates were in patients with both upper peritracheal and lower mediastinal levels of positive nodes. Histologic classification of tumor cells was not a significant determinant of survival, whereas T1 primary tumor status was a significant determinant.

Conclusion.—Patients with N2 disease may be candidates for surgery if their cardiopulmonary status allows them to undergo the surgery and the sacrifice of lung tissue, the mediastinal lymph node metastasis is limited to 1 level in either the upper peritracheal or lower mediastinal groups, and there is no evidence of extranodal disease. Surgery should be excluded in patients with positive thoracic inlet nodes.

Results of Surgical Resection in Patients With N2 Non–Small Cell Lung Cancer

Miller DL, McManus KG, Allen MS, Ilstrup DM, Deschamps C, Trastek VF, Daly RC, Pairolero PC (Mayo Clinic and Found, Rochester, Minn)
Ann Thorac Surg 57:1095–1100, 1994   140-95-15–20

Introduction.—When lung cancer has metastasized into the ipsilateral mediastinal lymph nodes, prognosis is adversely affected. If this N2 disease is found before thoracotomy, the risk of surgery can outweigh its benefit. Mediastinoscopy can be useful in the evaluation of lymph nodes, but when results of the procedure are positive, the 5-year survival is only 9%. Some patients who have a normal mediastinum are found to have N2 disease at surgery. A subgroup of these patients were reviewed.

Methods.—During a 4-year period, 167 patients with non–small-cell lung cancer and a normal mediastinum had N2 disease. The patients ranged in age from 31 to 86 years. Mediastinal nodes were grouped into 4 classes on the basis of their locations.

Findings.—Eighty percent of the patients had adenocarcinoma or squamous cell carcinoma. The most frequent location for lymph node station was the subcarinal area in 46% of patients. Forty percent of patients had 3 or more lymph node stations. There were 8 deaths at surgery for a mortality of 4.8%, and 21% had complications. The surviving patients were followed up for a median of 31 months. Recurrence occurred in two thirds of the patients. The 5-year survival rate was 23.7% in patients who had a complete resection. Ninety-five percent of patients who had an incomplete resection died within 3 years. Predictors of survival included the location of the mediastinal lymph node station, age, type of surgery, and adjuvant radiation therapy.

Conclusion.—In patients with N2 disease and negative findings in the mediastinum, a complete resection is recommended to result in a disease-free patient. Extensive dissection of the lymph nodes is required regardless of the location of the primary tumor. Survival is improved if adjuvant radiation therapy is given and chemotherapy protocols can be considered.

▶ The treatment of stage III lung cancer remains the focal point of controversy. Treatment advocates range from those who would propose nonoperative therapy with chemotherapy and radiation treatment alone to those who would advocate surgical resection only in patients demonstrating ipsilateral IIIA and II disease. Clearly the key to unraveling this controversy is the accurate preresection staging of all patients. The use of mediastinoscopy has been shown to be a very accurate, sensitive, and specific technique for detection in these patients before thoracotomy. These 2 reports demonstrate the difficulty in determining long-term survival in patients with ipsilateral N2 disease treatment through surgery alone.

In the report from the University of Texas, Dr. Mountain (Abstract 140-95-15–19) documents the poor survival in patients who have more than 1 positive node. The N2 nodal location in this study seems to suggest that for the majority of patients with N2 disease, surgical resection alone will leave them with a survival rate somewhere in the neighborhood of 20%. Indeed, the subsequent study by Miller et al. also demonstrates a dismal survival for the majority of patients with N2 disease. Of note is the fact that the 5-year survival of the 147 patients who underwent "a complete resection" was only 23%. This is in contrast to 19 of the 20 patients who underwent incomplete resection and who were dead within 3 years. However, when we look at all patients taken to surgery who underwent an attempt at surgical resection, the survival is substantially less than the 23%, which was the result in the completely resected group only.

This study confirms the dismal survival of patients with N2 disease who undergo thoracotomy and subsequent resection. Surgeons who approach patients with N2 disease, whether it is known or unknown at the time of planned thoracotomy, and who obviate the need to do mediastinoscopy based on the supposed technical resectability of the intrathoracic disease, will relegate patients to this dismal overall survival. If there is more effective therapy for this group of patients, then the onus will be on the surgeon to detect more N2 disease in a larger number of patients before planned thoracotomy.—D.J. Sugarbaker, M.D.

Surgical Management of Non-Small-Cell Lung Cancer With Ipsilateral Mediastinal Node Metastasis (N2 Disease)

Goldstraw P, Mannam GC, Kaplan DK, Michail P, Shields TW (Royal Brompton and Natl Heart and Lung Hosp, London)
J Thorac Cardiovasc Surg 107:19–28, 1994   140-95-15–21

Objective.—There is ongoing debate regarding the best management of non–small-cell lung cancer (NSCLC) associated with ipsilateral mediastinal node metastases, i.e., N2 disease. Conflicting results have led to divergent attitudes regarding the surgical treatment of these patients, the preoperative selection criteria, and the role of mediastinoscopy. The effectiveness of surgery in patients with N2 NSCLC and the relevant prognostic factors were investigated in a retrospective study.

Patients.—A total of 876 patients with NSCLC were referred to a surgical unit during a 10-year period. The clinical, radiologic, or bronchoscopic findings excluded surgery in 146 of these. One hundred fifty-one patients were judged to have inoperable lesions on the basis of the cervical mediastinoscopy or anterior mediastinotomy finding of mediastinal invasion or metastasis. The remaining 578 patients who underwent thoracotomy were believed not to have N2 disease, based on the findings of CT and/or mediastinal exploration. The exception was 1 patient found to have involvement of a single nodal station at mediastinoscopy.

Outcomes.—In 149 of the patients who underwent thoracotomy, routine mediastinal node dissection disclosed unsuspected N2 disease. Eighty-seven percent of those patients were able to undergo resection, whether by pneumonectomy, lobectomy, bilobectomy, or lesser resection. Complete resection was possible in 85% of cases; none received adjuvant therapy. Of the patients with unsuspected N2 disease, 72 had squamous cell carcinoma, 54 had adenocarcinoma, 14 had large-cell carcinoma, and 9 had mixed-type carcinoma.

There were 8 in-hospital deaths after thoracotomy. At a median follow-up of 27 months, actuarial 5-year survival for patients undergoing complete resection was 20%. Survival was significantly better in patients with squamous cell carcinoma and those with involvement of a single nodal station. However, long-term survival was unaffected by either the extent of resection or the involvement of any particular nodal station.

Conclusions.—More than one fourth of patients with NSCLC may have unsuspected mediastinal node involvement at the time of thoracotomy, even with rigorous preoperative investigation. Complete resection is justified in these patients—who have already experienced the morbidity and mortality of thoracotomy—as long as complete resection is possible. In well-selected patients with "unsuspected N2 disease," complete resection may be associated with reasonable long-term survival.

▶ This report by Goldstraw et al. is informative in that it highlights the large number of patients with ipsilateral mediastinal node mestastases that are not detected before resectional surgery. Indeed, in this group of 876 patients with NSCLC, routine mediastinal lymph node dissection disclosed unsuspected N2 disease in 149 patients. All patients had been carefully screened with computerized tomography and indicated mediastinoscopy. Indeed, complete resection was only possible in 85% of these cases. Therefore, it appears that one fourth of the patients with non–small-cell lung cancer in this series may be found to have unsuspected mediastinal node involvement at the time of thoracotomy. Surgical resection, as we saw in the previous 2 reports, will lead to a dismal 5-year survival in this subset. Indeed, if one could provide a substantial improvement in survival for this subset of patients, then the use of routine mediastinoscopy would likely be of additional benefit. In this study, the authors believe that complete resection is justified in patients in whom unsuspected N2 disease has been demonstrated because they have already incurred the morbidity of the thoracotomy. The use of mediastinoscopy in all of these patients would have reliably detected N2 disease in the majority of this group of unsuspected patients with N2 disease.—D.J. Sugarbaker, M.D.

Survival Related to Nodal Status After Sleeve Resection for Lung Cancer
Mehran RJ, Deslauriers J, Piraux M, Beaulieu M, Guimont C, Brisson J (Laval Univ, Ste Foy, Quebec, Canada)
J Thorac Cardiovasc Surg 107:576–583, 1994   140-95-15–22

Background.—Sleeve lobectomy, a lung-saving procedure indicated for central tumors, is the alternative for pneumonectomy. However, the relationship between survival and nodal status is controversial. In most series, the presence of N1 disease adversely affects the prognosis with few or no long-term survivors. A comparative analysis was done based on nodal status.

Methods.—From 1972 to 1992, 142 patients underwent sleeve resection at 1 center. The patient age ranged from 11 to 78 years. Surgery was indicated by a central tumor in 79%, a peripheral tumor in 13%, and compromised pulmonary function in 8% of patients. Histologic type was squamous in 72.5%, nonsquamous in 24.6%, and carcinoid in 2.8%.

Findings.—Resection was complete in 87% of the patients. Operative mortality was 2.1%. Survival rates at 5 and 10 years were 46% and 33%, respectively. The 73 patients with N0 status had 5- and 10-year survival rates of 57% and 46%, respectively. Corresponding rates in the 55 patients with N1 status were 46% and 27%, respectively. None of the 14 patients with N2 status survived 5 years (Fig 15–1, table). Twenty-three

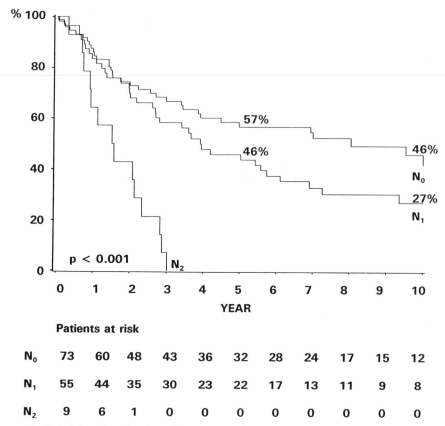

Fig 15–1.—Life-table analysis by nodal status showing the percentage of all patients remaining alive after sleeve resection of bronchogenic carcinoma. (Courtesy of Mehran RJ, Deslauriers J, Piraux M, et al: *J Thorac Cardiovasc Surg* 107:576–583, 1994.)

percent of the patients had local recurrences, but the prevalence did not differ significantly between those with N0 and N1 disease.

Conclusions.—Sleeve resection is an adequate treatment for patients with resectable lung cancer and N0 or N1 status. An N2 status makes the prognosis significantly worse and may be a contraindication to the use of this procedure.

▶ Further understanding of the effect of N2 disease is seen in this subset of patients who required sleeve resection for adequate control of their primary lesion. This group in Quebec is well known for their sleeve resection technique, and the influence of nodal status is seen to be profound in this subgroup of patients. Indeed, none of the 14 patients in this study with positive N2 nodes survived 5 years. Although not concluded by the authors of this report, it is this author's conclusion that mediastinoscopy should be performed in all patients in whom sleeve resection is contemplated. This opinion

Survival After Sleeve Resection for Lung Cancer

First author (yr)	Years of study	No. of patients	Five-year survival (%)	Ten-year survival (%)
Bennett (1978)	1958–1973	80	34	20
Faber (1984)	1962–1982	101	30	22
Frist (1987)	1962–1986	63	58	—
Watanabe (1990)	1975–1990	79	45	—
Van Schill (1991)	1960–1989	145	49	37

(Courtesy of Mehran RJ, Deslauriers J, Piraux M, et al: *J Thorac Cardiovasc Surg* 107:576–583, 1994.)

is due not only to the dismal outlook after surgical therapy alone as demonstrated in this report, but also to the possibility of improved survival that induction therapy may give if indeed this group of patients is selected prior to thoracotomy.—D.J. Sugarbaker, M.D.

Radical Systematic Mediastinal Lymphadenectomy in Non-Small Cell Lung Cancer: A Randomized Controlled Trial

Izbicki JR, Thetter O, Habekost M, Karg O, Passlick B, Kubuschok B, Busch C, Haeussinger K, Knoefel WT, Pantel K, Schweiberer L (Univ of Munich, Germany; Central Hosp Gauting, Germany)
Br J Surg 81:229–235, 1994   140-95-15-23

Introduction.—For any chance of a cure, classic lobectomy or pneumonectomy is the sole treatment for patients with non–small-cell lung cancer. It is claimed that pulmonary resection without mediastinal lymphadenectomy denies the patient a chance for a cure. It is also suggested that nodal sampling would avoid the increasing mortality and morbidity. Radical lymphadenectomy was compared with conventional lymph node dissection in patients with lung cancer.

Methods.—Patients with non–small-cell lung cancer were randomly assigned to 1 of the 2 surgical groups. Patients with distant metastases, contralateral or supraclavicular nodal involvement or N2 disease were excluded as were patients with severe cardiac, renal, or hepatic disease or poor pulmonary reserve. A total of 182 patients were studied. Patients were followed up at 6-month intervals.

Results.—The mean age of the patients was about 60 years. Systemic lymphadenectomy took an average of 20 minutes longer with no difference in blood loss or replacement. Six patients died in 30 days after surgery; 4 in the conventional group and 2 in the radical group. The most common complications were retained bronchial secretions and cardiac arrhythmias. Duration of stay in intensive care and the hospital was similar for both groups. Nearly 25% of each group had local recurrences. Distant metastases were found in 38% of patients who had conventional lymphadenectomy and 32% of patients who had radical lymphadenectomy. About 30% of each group died during the follow-up period. The mean time to death was 19 months in the patients undergoing conventional and 16 months in patients undergoing systematic lymphadenectomy.

Conclusion.—These data show that systematic lymphadenectomy is a safe procedure with acceptable mortality and morbidity rates. In terms of survival and local control of the tumor, there appears to be no significant advantage of the procedure over conventional methods.

▶ The importance of performing mediastinal node dissection in patients undergoing pulmonary resection for non–small-cell lung cancer has been emphasized by many authors. Indeed, the applied therapeutic advantage of performing radical lymph node dissection is in the balance of most manuscripts emanating from many large cancer centers in the United States. This is clear from the report by Dr. Goldstraw (Abstract 140-95-15–21) previously reviewed, that systematic lymph node dissection can accurately stage the mediastinum and lead to the diagnosis of unsuspected N2 disease in 25% of patients undergoing thoracotomy without previous mediastinoscopy. This report by Izbicki et al. from Munich is of particular interest in that it shows the results of a prospective, randomized control trial that was designed to compare radical lymphadenectomy with conventional lymph node dissection and sampling in a large group of patients with non–small-cell lung cancer. Although the radical lymphadenectomy took 22 minutes longer in the operating room, no overall difference in postoperative morbidity or mortality was noted. Even though the cohorts were similar in pathologic stage, there was no demonstrated survival advantage to systematic lymph node dissection. This study could have provided a better subset analysis of survival by stage, i.e., the effect of radical lymphadenectomy on advanced stages could have been better assessed. Nevertheless, it remains an important study and the first that has sought to prospectively randomize patients in the evaluation of the therapeutic efficacy of radical systematic mediastinal lymphadenectomy. The lack of therapeutic efficacy of radical lymphadenectomy in this report underlines the futility of surgery done in patients with N2 disease, the majority of whom will already have undetected systemic disease at the time of surgery.—D.J. Sugarbaker, M.D.

A Randomized Trial Comparing Preoperative Chemotherapy Plus Surgery With Surgery Alone in Patients With Non–Small-Cell Lung Cancer

Rosell R, Gómez-Codina J, Camps C, Maestre J, Padille J, Cantó A, Mate JL, Li S, Roig J, Olazábal A, Canela M, Ariza A, Skácel Z, Morera-Prat J, Abad A (Univ of Barcelona; Hosp La Fe, Valencia, Spain; Univ Hosp Germans Trias i Pujol, Barcelona)
N Engl J Med 330:153–158, 1994   140-95-15–24

Objective.—A randomized trial was planned to determine whether preoperative chemotherapy is a worthwhile addition to resection for non–small-cell lung cancer (NSCLC). Sixty patients with histologically confirmed stage IIIA NSCLC, all but 1 of them men, were included in the study.

Management.—Patients were randomly assigned to surgery only or to 3 courses of preoperative chemotherapy. All patients received mediastinal irradiation postoperatively in a cumulative dose of 50 Gy. Chemotherapy consisted of 6 mg of mitomycin per m², 3 g of ifosfamide per m², and 50 mg of cisplatin per m², all given IV at 3-week intervals. The 2 patient groups were comparable in most respects.

Results.—Sixty percent of the patients given chemotherapy had a partial or, in 2 cases, a complete radiographic response to treatment. The median disease-free survival time was 5 months for the surgical group and 20 months for patients given chemotherapy. The median overall survival times were 8 and 26 months, respectively. The surgical patients were followed up a median time of 19 months, and those given combined treatment for 2 years. Relapses developed during follow-up in 56% of patients given combined treatment and in 74% of those having surgery only.

Tumor Characteristics.—The prevalence of mutated K-*ras* oncogenes was more than twice as great in the surgical group. Those patients tended to have aneuploid tumor cells, whereas most of those given chemotherapy had tumors consisting of diploid cells.

Conclusion.—Preoperative chemotherapy prolongs the survival of patients having resection of NSCLC.

▶ This study represents a landmark report for the treatment of patients with IIIA NSCLC. The unequivocal long-term survival advantage enjoyed by patients undergoing treatment with induction chemotherapy in this study seems to confirm the therapeutic superiority of this approach. Indeed, the widely divergent survival and disease-free survival curves shown in this prospective, randomized, phase III trial will undoubtedly influence the treatment of a large number of patients in whom this disease is diagnosed. This study points out the importance of making the diagnosis of IIIA disease before thoracotomy. It is clear that once thoracotomy has been performed, the surgical momentum may carry the patient through surgical resection. The use of chemotherapy in the adjuvant setting has been previously studied. The Lung Cancer Study Group demonstrated no therapeutic efficacy of adjuvant chemotherapy in the treatment of patients with resected IIIA lung cancer. Therefore, the uniqueness of this report in demonstrating a substantial survival advantage in this subgroup seems to make the use of mediastinoscopy and the routine screening of appropriate patients imperative if this survival advantage is to be offered to as many patients with N2 disease as possible.

We have carefully reviewed the literature and defined the subsets of patients in whom unexpected, "occult" mediastinal node disease will be found in the mediastinum in up to 40% of cases (1). These particular clinical situations would be the ones in which routine mediastinoscopy might be used to identify the vast majority of patients with occult mediastinal disease before planned thoracotomy.

This landmark study will require prospective multi-institutional trials to confirm the therapeutic efficacy of this approach in patients with IIIA lung cancer. We are indebted to the authors of this trial for their demonstrated ability to randomize patients in this setting.—D.J. Sugarbaker, M.D.

Reference

1. Sugarbaker DJ, Strauss GM: Advances in Surgical Staging and Therapy of Non-Small Cell Lung Cancer. *Semin Oncol* 20:163–172, 1993.

Extended Operations After Induction Therapy for Stage IIIb (T4) Non–Small Cell Lung Cancer

Macchiarini P, Chapelier AR, Monnet I, Vannetzel J-M, Rebischung J-L, Cerrina J, Parquin F, Ladurie FLR, Lenot B, Dartevelle PG (Paris-Sud Univ, Le Plessis Robinson, France)
Ann Thorac Surg 57:966–973, 1994   140-95-15–25

Background.—Patients with stage IIIb non–small-cell lung cancer (NSCLC) invading adjacent organs (T4) and with or without involvement of supraclavicular or contralateral mediastinal or hilar (N3) nodes have a poor prognosis. This stage of disease is generally considered unresectable, and no long-term survivor of resection for N3 disease has been reported. There is evidence, however, that certain T4 tumors might be curable with surgery. Results in a consecutive series of 23 patients with stage IIIb (T4) NSCLC who underwent extended operation after induction chemotherapy, with or without radiation therapy, were evaluated.

Patients and Methods.—The patient group consisted of 21 men and 2 women with a median age of 54 years. There were 11 cases of squamous cell carcinoma, 9 of adenocarcinoma, and 3 of large-cell carcinoma. Six patients had histologically proved N2 disease. Excluded were patients with N3 disease, metastatic pleural effusion, and distant metastasis. Induction chemotherapy consisted of different phase II cisplatin-containing regimens. The number of courses and the use of radiation therapy depended on the type of protocol, not on the type of tumor response or tumor extension. Patients with an objective response or stabilization of disease after chemotherapy underwent thoracotomy. An attempt was made to remove the entire tumor area present at the time of initial staging.

Results.—Induction treatment resulted in 5 complete and 18 partial responses. Twelve patients received radiation therapy at a median dose of 40 Gy. Only 2 patients were unable to have all residual tumor at the primary site and involved structures resected. Procedures included 9 right tracheal and 11 intrapericardial pneumonectomies and 3 resections of apical tumors; 11 patients had radical mediastinal lymph node dissection. Six patients had major postoperative complications. The incidence of complications was significantly higher in patients who received radiation in addition to chemotherapy. Four patients died of early or delayed complications; 13 remain alive without evidence of disease at 12 to more than 39 months postoperatively. The projected 3-year survival rate was 54%.

Conclusion.—Early results of extended resection of stage IIIb (T4) NSCLC, after induction chemotherapy and with or without radiation, are encouraging. Patients selected for this combined treatment modality should have an adequate performance status and pulmonary function.

▶ The treatment of state IIIB lung cancer is the subject of this report by the group at Hôpital Marie-Lannelongue, France. Dr. Dartevelle's group is well known for their use of extended local resection in the treatment of patients with T4 lesions extending into mediastinal structures. They have now extended this experience to patients who have been treated with induction therapy with the presence of T4 disease as the source of their 3B stage designation. That they excluded patients with N3 disease is an important consideration in evaluating this report. In addition, patients with pleural effusions and distant metastases were not considered for resection. Nine patients were treated with a variety of platinum-based regimens, a distinct limitation of this report. Twelve patients received radiotherapy at a median dose of 40 Gy. Of note is the fact that these were the patients with substantial postoperative complications. Indeed, the incidence of complications was significantly higher in patients who received preoperative radiotherapy in addition to chemotherapy. This reluctance to use 2 modalities in the induction setting is shared by a variety of investigators. Nevertheless, the projected 3-year survival rate of 54% is very encouraging for this heretofore unresectable, untreatable group of patients. It appears clear that reports such as this lay the groundwork for further applications of the use of multimodality therapy in the treatment of patients with 3B NSCLC.—D.J. Sugarbaker, M.D.

Neoadjuvant Therapy: A Novel and Effective Treatment for Stage IIIb Non-Small Cell Lung Cancer

Rusch VW, Albain KS, Crowley JJ, Rice TW, Lonchyna V, McKenna R Jr, Stelzer K, Livingston RB, and the Southwest Oncology Group (Mem Sloan-Kettering Cancer Ctr, New York; Loyola Univ Chicago, Maywood, Ill; Cleveland Clinic, Ohio; et al)

Ann Thorac Surg 58:290–295, 1994   140-95-15–26

Background.—Neoadjuvant treatment is now accepted therapy for stage IIIa non–small-cell lung cancer. However, stage IIIb disease is usually considered incurable and treated nonoperatively. The feasibility of neoadjuvant treatment in patients with stage IIIb non–small-cell lung cancer was investigated in a prospective, multicenter trial.

Methods.—One hundred twenty-six patients were eligible for the study. All had pathologically documented T1-4 N2-3 disease. Treatment consisted of cisplatin, 50 mg/m², administered on days 1, 8, 29, and 36, plus VP-16, 50 mg/m², given on days 1–5 and 29–33, along with concurrent radiotherapy to a total dose of 4,500 cGy. If responses were stable, partial, or complete, surgical resection was done 3–5 weeks after the induction of medical treatment. Thirty-four men and 17 women, with a median age of 57 years, had stage IIIb tumors. Thirty-two patients, including 18 with T4 tumors and 14 with N3 disease, underwent resection of the primary tumor.

Findings.—Operative mortality was 5.2%. Operative time, blood loss, and length of hospitalization did not differ between the T4 and N3 patients. Overall 2-year survival was 39%. In all patients, the sites of relapse were primarily distant, even though patients with N3 disease did not initially have involved N3 nodes resected.

Conclusions.—The use of neoadjuvant therapy in patients with stage IIIb non–small-cell lung cancer is feasible. Such patients could be included in future trials designed to assess the role of surgical resection in the combined-modality therapy of stage III non–small-cell lung cancer.

▶ In this multi-institutional cooperative group trial, patients were prospectively evaluated and treated with induction chemotherapy and surgery for their 3B non–small-cell lung cancer. Patients were treated with a consistent regimen of platinum VP16 with concurrent radiotherapy. It is notable that the patients with T4 lesions appeared to enjoy improved survival over those patients who were IIIB by virtue of N3 contralateral disease. Indeed, those patients with residual and nodal disease in the mediastinum fared poorly in this study.

This study appears to endorse the concept that extended surgical resection for control of extensive tumors (T4) may be indicated in a selected subset of patients in whom induction chemotherapy or radiation therapy, or both, are utilized. The morbidity in this trial, conducted in a subset of institutions with experienced thoracic surgeons, demonstrates the need for careful patient selection in this subgroup. Nevertheless, the feasibility of this approach has been documented in this carefully conducted, phase II trial.—D.J. Sugarbaker, M.D.

Role of Radiotherapy in Combined Modality Treatment of Locally Advanced Non–Small-Cell Lung Cancer

Kubota K, Furuse K, Kawahara M, Kodama N, Yamamoto M, Ogawara M, Negoro S, Masuda N, Takada M, Matsui K, Takifuji N, Kudoh S, Kusunoki Y, Fukuoka M (Natl Kinki Central Hosp, Sakai, Japan; Osaka Prefectural Habikino Hosp, Japan)

J Clin Oncol 12:1547–1552, 1994   140-95-15–27

Objective.—For many years, radiotherapy (RT) has been a part of conventional therapy for patients with stage III non–small-cell lung cancer (NSCLC). However, there are few prospective data on the role of RT in these patients. Recent studies have shown excellent results with chemotherapy (CT) in patients with regionally advanced disease. A randomized trial comparing cisplatin-based CT with and without thoracic irradiation was conducted.

Methods.—The study included 92 patients with locally advanced NSCLC. The patients were randomly assigned to 1 of 3 arms of cisplatin-based CT: vindesine plus cisplatin; mitomycin plus vindesine plus cisplatin; or etoposide plus cisplatin, alternating with vindesine plus mitomycin. Patients who had stage III disease after 2 cycles of chemotherapy were randomly assigned to receive RT or no RT. The RT group received 50-60 Gy of thoracic irradiation in 5-6 weeks, 2 Gy/day in conventional fractions.

Results.—Sixty-three patients with stage III disease at reevaluation were randomly assigned to receive RT or not. The CT/RT and CT-only groups were similar in regard to age, sex, performance status, histologic findings, disease stage, and induction CT regimens. Median survival duration was 461 and 447 days, respectively. One-year survival was 58% in the CT/RT group vs. 66% in the CT-only group. Two-year survival was 36% vs. 9% and 3-year survival, 29% vs. 3%. There was 1 death from pneumonitis in the CT/RT group, but there were no CT-related deaths.

Conclusions.—The combination of cisplatin-based CT and chest irradiation in patients with locally advanced NSCLC results in significantly better long-term survival than chemotherapy alone. Irradiation is an essential component of combined-modality therapy for patients with bulky disease in the chest and should be included in further studies of treatment for locally advanced NSCLC. More studies to identify more active agents for CT and the optimal methods of combining CT and RT are needed.

▶ The use of RT in combination with CT in the treatment of unresectable IIIA and IIIB disease has been previously evaluated in the landmark study by Dillman et al (1). The survival advantage enjoyed by patients being treated with a combination of CT and RT was documented in that early study. Nevertheless, this study provides excellent affirmation of that finding by demonstrating the efficacy of CT and RT in the treatment of patients with unresectable stage IIIA or IIIB NSCLC. The authors have carefully studied prospectively this group of patients and have noted that those who were randomized to receive RT after systemic CT had a survival of 2 years (36%) vs. 9% 3 year survival of 29% versus 3%. Interestingly, all of these studies of the nonoperative treatment or operative treatment of patients with IIIA or IIIB NSCLC settle out at approximately 20%–25% extended survival. Certainly, this does raise the question of the efficacy of adding surgery to the treatment of this disease in its advanced stage. However, in both the study reported by Dr. Dillman (1) and in this study, local relapse was still a substantial problem in both groups. However, the local control was significantly improved in the patients receiving radiation therapy. Nevertheless, more than 30% of patients failed locally even in the radiation therapy arm. The majority of studies using surgery in the treatment of IIIA NSCLC would have local relapse rates under 20%.

This study points out the importance of combining radiation therapy with chemotherapy in the treatment of patients with unresectable stage III NSCLC.—D.J. Sugarbaker, M.D.

Reference

1. Dillman RO, Seagren SL, Propert KL, et al: A randomized trial of induction chemotherapy plus high-dose radiation versus radiation alone in stage III non-small-cell lung cancer. N Engl J Med 323:940–945, 1990.

Combined Radiosurgical Treatment of Pancoast Tumor
Maggi G, Casadio C, Pischedda F, Giobbe R, Cianci R, Ruffini E, Molinatti M, Mancuso M (Univ of Torino, Italy)
Ann Thorac Surg 57:198–202, 1994   140-95-15–28

Introduction.—Pancoast tumor, a superior sulcus tumor of the lung, is a distinct class of T3 bronchogenic carcinoma. Although considered fatal in the early 20th century, satisfactory results are obtained with radiotherapy followed by surgery. One of the largest cohorts of patients with Pancoast tumor and the responses to a combination of radiotherapy and surgery are reported.

Methods.—The subjects were 60 patients undergoing the combination of treatments. The mean age was 57 years and there were only 2 women. Rib and nerve root involvement was documented. The preoperative radiation dose was 30 Gy in 50 of the patients. Surgery was radical in 60% of the patients. Survival rates were plotted by surgical degree (radical or palliative resection).

Results.—Three patients died during the postoperative period. The complication rate was 21%. Seven patients had pain recur postoperatively. The overall 3- and 5-year survival rates were 34% and 17%, respectively. Survival in the palliative group was shorter than that of the radical group.

Conclusion.—The combination of radiation therapy and surgery is an appropriate option in managing patients with Pancoast tumor. Survival rates in patients who had radical surgery were similar to the rates for other T3 lung cancers. A poor outcome can be anticipated in the case of residual tumor. However, in most of the patients, good pain control was achieved.

▶ This study of the results of combined preoperative radiation and surgery in treatment of Pancoast tumors is important in that it points out the need for routine mediastinoscopy in this subgroup of patients. The survival of this cohort of patients of 34% and 17% at 3 and 5 years respectively, illustrates the dismal overall outlook for patients presenting with Pancoast lesions. Incomplete resection was also associated with a poor overall survival. The use of palliative surgical resection when the margins cannot be achieved intraoperatively remains in doubt.

The appropriate workup for a patient presenting with a Pancoast lesion should begin with a mediastinoscopy, and if positive mediastinal nodes are demonstrated, the palliative treatment should be considered particularly in the absence of a specific clinical research protocol for the use of induction therapy in this subgroup. The presence of a Pancoast tumor remains an absolute indication for mediastinoscopy regardless of the CT findings in the mediastinum because of the high rate of occult mediastinal nodes and poor survival in this subgroup with positive mediastinal nodes.—D.J. Sugarbaker, M.D.

Endobronchial Stents

INTRODUCTION

The use of endobronchial stents has become much more widespread in the last several years. This has been due to a larger group of thoracic surgeons who are now performing lung transplantation, sleeve resections, and tracheal resections. Indeed, the proliferation of lung transplant programs has allowed many surgeons to gain experience with airway surgery. The lung transplantation setting affords the most challenging application of bronchoplasty techniques. Experience gained in this setting has allowed the routine performance of tracheal surgery to become much more widespread. However, there are certain situations in which endobronchial obstruction in an unresectable situation is best treated by endobronchial stenting. As a rule, patients with extrinsic compression of the bronchus are better candidates for stenting, and patients with endoluminal tumors are better candidates for laser ablation. What follows are 5 reports of a variety of stenting techniques using new, expandable stents as well as the old standard silicone prostheses.

David J. Sugarbaker, M.D.

Balloon Dilatation and Self-Expanding Metal Wallstent Insertion: For Management of Bronchostenosis Following Lung Transplantation
Carré P, Rousseau H, Lombart L, Didier A, Dahan M, Fournial G, Léophonte P, and the Toulouse Lung Transplantation Group (Rangueil Hosp, Toulouse, France)
Chest 105:343–348, 1994   140-95-15–29

Background.—Airway obstruction after lung transplantation is a major complication. Cryoablation, laser treatment, and dilatation with a rigid bronchoscope provide immediate relief of symptoms, but the clinical improvement is usually short-lived. Balloon dilatation (BD) and insertion of self-expanding metal Wallstents (WS) were used in the treatment of lung transplant recipients with bronchial complications.

Patients.—During a 2-year study period, 10 lung transplant recipients were treated for 12 bronchial anastomotic complications localized primarily in the graft mainstem bronchus. Eight stenoses were treated with BD as the first-line treatment and a WS was inserted in the other 4 stenoses. All procedures were carried out under fluoroscopic guidance and without general anesthesia.

Outcome.—Both procedures were well tolerated and provided immediate relief of symptoms. The WS expanded with time, increasing the diameter of the bronchus to near-normal. Balloon dilatation also increased the diameter of the bronchus, but to a lesser extent. Early restenosis occurred in 4 of the 8 dilated stenoses, and all 4 cases were then treated with WS insertion. In 2 cases, the stenosis was located so that the lower end of the stent overlapped the upper lobe bronchus orifice. An Nd YAG laser was used to eliminate the filaments of the stent crossing the lobar orifice to prevent subsequent obstruction. After a mean follow-up of 15.3 months, 3 patients died of causes unrelated to the airway complications.

Conclusions.—Balloon dilatation and self-expanding metal stents can resolve most of the airway complications that occur after lung transplantation.

Bronchoscopic Diathermy Resection and Stent Insertion: A Cost Effective Treatment for Tracheobronchial Obstruction
Petrou M, Kaplan D, Goldstraw P (Royal Brompton National Heart and Lung Hosp, London)
Thorax 48:1156–1159, 1993   140-95-15-30

Introduction.—Resection remains the best treatment for patients with tracheobronchial obstruction from malignant or benign disease, but only in a minority of patients. In other patients, a cost-effective means of palliation is needed. The use of diathermy resection to relieve airway obstruction was studied.

Methods.—Tracheobronchial obstruction was present in 29 patients referred during a 7-year period. The patients' subjective opinions and objective tests of lung function were obtained before and after treatment. With the patient under general anesthesia, a rigid bronchoscope was inserted. The diathermy loop was inserted through the bronchoscope, the obstruction resected, and tissue samples removed. Nine patients were emergency cases.

Results.—Fifteen of the patients had prior treatment, and 5 patients required multiple treatment sessions. Ten patients received a stent. No intraoperative complication occurred. The average length of stay in the hospital was 5 days. Immediate symptomatic relief was seen in 28 of the 29 patients. In 8 patients in whom pretreatment lung function tests were available, forced expiratory volume in 1 second (FEV_1) improved 53% and forced vital capacity (FVC) improved 21%.

Conclusion.—In patients with airway obstruction, the use of bronchoscopic diathermy resection is a safe and effective method of palliation. It can be used in non-neoplastic as well as benign or malignant neoplastic tumors. It is also a useful emergency procedure.

Indications for an Expandable Metallic Stent for Tracheobronchial Stenosis

Nomori H, Kobayashi R, Kodera K, Morinaga S, Ogawa K (Saiseikai Central Hosp; Keio Univ, Tokyo)
Ann Thorac Surg 56:1324–1328, 1993   140-95-15–31

Background.—The expandable metallic stent (EMS) has been used to treat stenosis after tracheobronchial reconstruction, as well as cicatricial or inflammatory stenosis of the trachea. Indications and contraindications for use of the EMS were evaluated in a review of 9 patients treated for tracheobronchial stenosis.

Patients and Findings.—An EMS was used in 8 patients with malignant stenosis (6 with extrinsic compression and 2 with intraluminal tumor invasion), and 1 patient with nonmalignant stenosis. In the patient with nonmalignant stenosis, postreconstruction bronchomalacia and granulation tissue were affecting different parts of the tracheobronchial tree. The EMS was placed without difficulty in all patients. Migration of the EMS did not occur, and no EMS-related infections were noted. Successful dilation of the tracheobronchial stenosis was achieved in patients with extrinsic tumor compression and malacia. Conversely, the EMS proved ineffective for stenosis caused by intraluminal tumor invasion or granulation tissue, because tumor or granulation tissue growth tended to occur between the wires of the stent. An EMS covered with Dacron mesh was subsequently used to prevent further tumor growth in 1 patient with intraluminal tumor invasion. The stenotic area was satisfactorily opened without respiratory complications or infection. Autopsies were performed in 5 of 7 patients with malignant stenosis who died of disease progression. Microscopic examination revealed local erosion and mild inflammation at the EMS placement site, although no inflammation was noted beyond the tracheobronchial cartilage in any patient.

Conclusions.—The EMS can be used to treat tracheobronchial stenosis caused by extrinsic tumor compression with effective results. Although a mesh-covered EMS may be useful in patients with tracheobronchial stenosis caused by tumor invasion or granulation tissue, the risk of bacterial infection with use of the mesh-covered device has not yet been clarified.

Silicone Stents in the Management of Inoperable Tracheobronchial Stenoses: Indications and Limitations

Bolliger CT, Probst R, Tschopp K, Solèr M, Perruchoud AP (Univ Hospital, Basel, Switzerland)
Chest 104:1653–1659, 1993   140-95-15-32

Introduction.—Airway obstructions due to inoperable malignant stenoses are routinely treated with the Nd YAG laser. Should the airway be obstructed because of extrinsic compression, laser therapy must give way to mechanical dilation or placement of a stent. Stents may be made of either metal or silicone, with the removable silicone style being the most widely used. The technical aspects of the stents were tested as well as the long-term patency.

Methods.—A total of 31 patients with extrinsic compression of the central airways served as subjects. Dumon silicone stents were inserted using a rigid bronchoscope while the patient was under general anesthesia. Positioning of the stent was confirmed 24 hours later using radiography. Lung function tests, dyspnea, Karnofsky performance scale and the World Health Organization (WHO) activity index were evaluated pre- and post-treatment in all patients except those requiring an emergency procedure. In those patients, only post-treatment data were collected. The patency of the stent was evaluated monthly by the surgeon or general practitioner. Radiotherapy was begun no later than 2 weeks after stent placement to prevent a recurrence of the tumor around the stent opening.

Results.—Stents were placed easily in all patients. Five stents in 3 patients migrated and required emergency removal. Tolerance of the stent was excellent in 27 of the remaining 28 patients. One proximal stent was removed, and a lethal hemoptysis occurred hours after laser therapy and stent removal. No other complications were present. There was immediate and long-lasting improvement in lung function tests, Karnofsky scale, and WHO activity index in 28 of 31 patients. The role of radiotherapy was evaluated in a group of 10 patients with stage IIIB squamous cell carcinoma. Five patients received radiotherapy and 5 did not. The stents in 4 of 5 patients not receiving therapy were occluded by tumor recurrence within 2 months. Median survival was 4 months. No stents were occluded in the group receiving therapy. Median survival in this group was 6 months.

Conclusion.—The stents used in this study were easily placed and removed, were well tolerated and effective at relieving respiratory symptoms. Treatment of patients with extrinsic compression of central airways should include stent insertion, laser resection followed by radiotherapy for the prevention of tumor recurrence, and improved survival.

Temporary and Permanent Restoration of Airway Continuity With the Tracheal T-Tube

Gaissert HA, Grillo HC, Mathisen DJ, Wain JC (Harvard Med School, Boston)

J Thorac Cardiovasc Surg 107:600–606, 1994   140-95-15–33

Purpose.—In patients with critical stenosis of the upper airway that cannot be corrected by surgery, temporary or permanent tracheostomy is often necessary. The tracheal T-tube offers several advantages over a regular tracheostomy tube—including physiologic direction of air flow, preservation of laryngeal phonation, and better patient acceptance. An experience with the use of T-tubes, including some key factor in success or failure, was reviewed.

Patients.—A T-tube, or similar tube, was placed in 140 patients during a 23-year period. Seven patients received a TY-tube and 4 received a modified extended T-tube. The mean patient age was 43.8 years, with a range of 7 months to 95 years. Eighty-six patients had postintubation stenosis, 13 had burns, 12 had airway malignancies, and 29 had various other diagnoses. Thirty-one patients received temporary stenting with a rubber tube; 14 of them later had operative reconstruction. Another 49 patients had definitive, permanent tube insertion. The modified tube, placed in 4 patients with left main bronchial stenosis, provided effective long-term palliation in 3 cases. The tube was placed because of postoperative airway obstruction in 32 patients.

Outcome.—Twelve patients had T-tube placement above the vocal cords for subglottic stenosis; this was effective in 10 cases. Twenty percent of patients were unable to tolerate the T-tube, either because of obstruction of the upper limb or aspiration. Airway obstruction led to the need for tube removal in 5 of 10 patients younger than 10 years. Of 112 patients receiving long-term intubation, 49 had their tube in place for more than 1 year, and 12 for more than 5 years. When obstructive problems occurred, they were usually within 2 months of tube placement.

Discussion.—The tracheal T-tube is preferred for the management of patients with chronic airway obstruction that is not amenable to surgical reconstruction. It provides reliable restoration of airway patency, with excellent long-term results. Conditions associated with stent obstruction include subglottic or laryngeal edema, unreconstructable subglottic stenosis, and pediatric airway disease.

▶ In the authors' experience, the use of the laser to resect endobronchial tumor may be followed by the use of brachytherapy with the placement of afterloading catheters and endobronchial radiation treatment. As is pointed out by the group from the Royal Brompton Hospital, bronchoscopic diathermy may be substituted for laser ablation in a subset of patients with an expected palliative result that is acceptable.

In addition to the use of laser or diathermy, BD is often an effective way of restoring endoluminal patency before the placement of an expanding metal

WS. As noted in the report by Carré et al. (Abstract 140-95-15–29), this may be carried out safely and the stenotic process in a majority of patients successfully arrested. Indeed, the performance of BD without the use of general anesthesia has become routine at the Brigham and Women's Hospital as well. The balloon is much less traumatic on the airway, and the resultant, reactive stenosis is less in comparison to conventional rigid bronchoscopic dilatation of stenoses. The EMS is finding a variety of applications, as noted in the report from Nomori et al. (Abstract 140-95-15–31). However, its use when the tracheal broncho stenosis is caused by an extrinsic tumor is best demonstrated in this report. The long-term risks of bacterial infection or tumor ingrowth have not been satisfactorily determined in these studies. In the 2 studies from Switzerland and Boston, the use of silicone stents in the management of inoperative tracheal bronchial stenoses is noted. These stents were noted to be easily placed and removed when indicated and were well tolerated and effective in relieving respiratory symptoms and providing effective palliation in a selected group of patients. Situations in which stents may become acutely obstructed are important to identify. They include subglottic edema, unreconstructable subglottic stenoses, and progressive pediatric airway diseases.

The field of general thoracic surgery continues to move ahead, stimulated by advances in lung transplantation, lung reduction surgery, and thoracoscopic technique. We look forward in the next edition of the YEAR BOOK OF SURGERY to providing another year-end review of the exciting advances in this burgeoning field of surgery.—D.J. Sugarbaker, M.D.

Subject Index*

A

Abdomen
  closure
    in severe trauma with visceral edema,
      93: 90
    towel clip of skin, 93: 92
  inability to close because of visceral
    edema, 93: 85
  intra-abdominal infection
    critical, planned reoperation and
      open management, 93: 114
    relaparotomy in, planned, 93: 115
    study, of surgical infection society,
      management techniques and
      outcome, 94: 107
  intra-abdominal pressure increase, effect
    on blood flow, 93: 92
  surgery
    bile duct injury during, medicolegal
      analysis of, 95: 319
    decreasing carbohydrate oxidation
      and increasing fat oxidation in,
      growth hormone for, in total
      parenteral nutrition, 94: 201
    enteral feeding after, immediate,
      weight loss decrease and wound
      healing improvement due to (in
      rat), 93: 191
    wound dehiscence in, 93: 180
  trauma
    autotransfusion of potentially
      culture-positive blood in, 93: 98
    blunt, ultrasound results in, 95: 102
    closure in visceral edema, 93: 90
    massive, delayed gastrointestinal
      reconstruction after, 94: 89
    penetrating, antibiotic duration in,
      93: 100
    penetrating, aztreonam clindamycin
      superior to gentamicin clindamycin
      for, 95: 111
    penetrating, cephalosporin in,
      93: 100
    penetrating, laparoscopy to evaluate,
      93: 89
    penetrating and blunt, comprehensive
      algorithm for, 93: 107
    penetrating and blunt, septic
      morbidity after, enteral vs.
      parenteral feeding in, 93: 101
    severe, abdominal wall reconstruction
      after, tissue expanders for, 93: 96
  wall
    defects, acute, planned ventral hernia
      for, 95: 429

reconstruction after severe trauma,
  tissue expanders for, 93: 96
repair, reherniation after, with
  polytetrafluoroethylene, 95: 431
Abdominoperineal
  resection, for early rectal cancer,
    95: 375
Ablation
  of Barrett's esophagus epithelium,
    squamous mucosa restoration after,
    94: 242
Abscess
  "undrained," of multiple organ failure,
    and gastrointestinal tract, 94: 103
Academic
  health consortium, surgical resource
    consumption in, 95: 9
  medicine, and Health Security Act,
    94: 10
  role models, women surgeons as, 94: 12
  surgical group practice, and health
    reform, 95: 19
Achalasia
  esophagomyotomy in, thoracoscopic,
    93: 215
  esophagus, surgery of, long-term results,
    95: 285
  pneumatic dilatation for, causing
    esophageal perforation, surgical
    repair, 94: 253
Acidosis
  in critical injury, 93: 93
Acute illness
  of medical patients, mortality and
    hypomagnesemia, 94: 52
Adenocarcinoma
  adrenal, case review, 95: 196
  in Barrett's esophagus with high-grade
    dysplasia, 93: 214
  cardia, Barrett's metaplasia as source of,
    95: 282
  colorectal polyps containing,
    endoscopic polypectomy or
    colectomy, 93: 306
  esophageal, and Barrett's esophagus,
    93: 215
  invasive, and colorectal polyps, lymph
    node metastases risk in, 93: 303
  lung, ras gene mutations as prognostic
    marker, 93: 428
  rectal
    preoperative radiotherapy and surgery
      for, 93: 312
    surgical adjuvant, radiotherapy,
      5-fluorouracil and semustine in,
      93: 315

---

* All entries refer to the year and page number(s) for data appearing in this and the
previous edition of the YEAR BOOK.

537

glutamine, enteral diet supplement,
decreasing bacterial translocation in
burns (in mice), 95: 218
Albumin
leak after lower torso ischemia
reperfusion, complement activation
blockade preventing, 94: 41
Alcohol
nasopharyngeal carcinoma and, and
smoking, 93: 413
Alcoholic cirrhosis (*see* Transplantation,
liver, for cirrhosis,
alcoholic)
Allele
deletion on chromosome 17p in
advanced colorectal cancer,
95: 357
loss, of chromosome 18q, and
colorectal cancer prognosis,
95: 363
novel, in familial breast cancer, 95: 355
Allo-MHC peptides
inducing peripheral T cell anergy,
thymic recognition of, 95: 173
Allograft
skin, in burns, cyclosporin A failure to
extend allograft survival, 95: 427
Ambulatory
surgical patients, preadmission testing,
efficacy of, 93: 12
American Board of Surgery
in-training/surgical basic science
examination, telling about graduate
surgical education, 94: 1
success in examinations of, and surgery
resident performance, 94: 2
Amino acid
small bowel luminal, transport of,
starvation inducing (in rabbit),
95: 207
transport
regulated by growth hormone,
93: 205
by small intestine in total parenteral
nutrition, 94: 186
uptake by small intestine, growth
hormone enhancing, 95: 208
Aminoglycoside
in burns, with first-dose
pharmacokinetics, 94: 64
liposome delivery in burns, 93: 68
Amputation
foot, unconventional, for limb salvage
increase, 95: 482
forefoot, wound healing in, toe pressure
in, 95: 483
in peripheral vascular disease, 93: 372

of soft tissue sarcoma of extremity in
adults, 93: 346
vs. limb-sparing operations in soft tissue
sarcoma of extremity, 93: 344
Amrinone
improving myocardial performance and
oxygen delivery (in dog), 93: 45
thermogenic effect of, 95: 40
tumor necrosis factor production in
endotoxin shock and, 93: 44
Anabolic
therapy with growth hormone
accelerating protein gain in surgical
patients with nutritional
rehabilitation, 94: 203
Anal
canal carcinoma, recurrent squamous
cell, predictors of initial treatment
failure and salvage therapy results,
95: 388
ileal pouch anastomosis, failure patterns,
93: 251
Analgesia
in chest wall trauma, epidural vs.
intrapleural catheters for, 95: 110
Analgesic
requirements, patient-controlled vs.
standard, in cholecystectomy,
93: 15
Anastomosis
coloanal
with radiotherapy in resectable rectal
cancer, 94: 372
in rectal cancer (*see* Rectum, cancer,
coloanal anastomosis in)
coloanal and colorectal, after rectal
carcinoma resection, 93: 320
coloendoanal, for low rectal cancer,
95: 382
colon
bursting strength after corticosteroids,
95: 263
healing, epidermal growth factor, and
receptor genes of (in rat), 93: 188
ileal pouch-anal, failure patterns,
93: 251
infrainguinal anastomotic arterial graft
infection, graft preservation in,
93: 125
intestinal, transfusion impairing healing
of (in rat), 93: 55
side-to-side, to bypass small bowel,
93: 248
Anatomic dissection
public attitudes toward, 95: 28
Anemia
cisplatin-associated, erythropoietin trial
in, 93: 25

of gastric serosal blood perfusion, to
predict esophagogastrostomy
impaired healing, 95: 275
vs. oximetry, to predict wound healing
after extremity soft tissue sarcoma
excision, 95: 260

Fluconazole
for infection, disseminated, in critically
ill surgical patients candiduria as
early markers of, 94: 49

Fluid
breast cyst, multiple proliferative growth
factors in, 94: 219
resuscitation not restoring microvascular
blood flow in burns, 93: 75
wound, chronic, cell proliferation
inhibition by, 94: 214

Fluorescent
dextrans, transport across ilium after
skin burns (in rat), 95: 73

5-Fluorouracil
in breast cancer and mortality, 93: 262
in colonic healing (in rat), 93: 189
metabolism, hepatic, dietary protein
depletion in, 94: 208
in rectal adenocarcinoma, with
semustine and radiotherapy,
93: 315

Folinic acid
in colonic healing (in rat), 93: 189

Food
deprivation, hemorrhage in, glucose
infusion pretreatment preventing
fatal outcome after (in rat), 94: 171
intake, parenteral nutrition and brain
glycogen (in rat), 95: 229

Foot
amputation, unconventional, for limb
salvage increase, 95: 482
burns, grafts for, early ambulation and
discharge in, 94: 421

Forearm
flap, sensate radial bilobed, for tongue
mobility preservation after
glossectomy, 95: 449

Forefoot
amputation, wound healing in, toe
pressure in, 95: 483

Foregut
abnormalities, functional, in Barrett's
esophagus, 94: 240
symptoms, physiologic assessment in
surgical practice, 94: 251

Formula
enteral, specialized vs. standard, in
trauma, 95: 237

Fracture

face, reconstruction, fate and plates and
screws after, 93: 405
femoral shaft, incidence, management
and outcome, 95: 94
mandibular, rigid fixation, and
immediate function, 93: 406

Fundoplication
360-degree, dysphagia after, 93: 212
360 degree or partial, lower esophageal
sphincter characteristics and
esophageal acid exposure after,
93: 210
Nissen (see Nissen fundoplication)
total, in myotomized esophagus,
94: 254
wrap, vagus nerves isolated from,
95: 291

G

Gallbladder, 95: 305
mucin accelerating cholesterol
monohydrate crystal growth in
model bile (in cow), 94: 273
sludge, 93: 238

Gallstone
dropped, retrieval during laparoscopic
cholecystectomy, 95: 314

Gas
blood, changes during helium
pneumoperitoneum for
laparoscopic cholecystectomy,
95: 320
exchange improvement in respiratory
distress syndrome with
perfluorocarbon and mechanical
ventilation (in rabbit), 94: 31

Gastrectomy
in gastric carcinoma, pathology and
prognosis in, 93: 338
partial
for benign conditions, long-term
prognosis, 93: 219
with gastroduodenostomy, vs.
vagotomy for corporeal gastric
ulcer, 95: 301
R_1 subtotal vs. R_3 total, for antral
cancer, 95: 403
smoking-related death after, 93: 219

Gastric, 93: 218, 94: 255
acid production, effect of duodenal
switch procedure in, 93: 225
bypass, long-limb, in superobesity,
93: 222
cancer, 93: 333, 94: 376, 95: 399
advanced, immunochemosurgery of,
93: 333

X

Author Index

A

Abad A, 523
Abello PA, 60
Abner A, 345
Abraham E, 118, 120
Abu-Elmagd K, 169
Adachi J, 278
Ahrén B, 181
Albain KS, 526
Albala D, 193
Albear P, 26
Alcantara PSM, 454
Alexander JW, 64, 223
Alexander S, 157
Alexander SR, 155
Allen BT, 470, 486
Allen K, 33
Allen L, 426
Allen MS, 500, 501, 516
Allen PE, 312
Allman RM, 462
Al-Sarraf M, 438
Amery A, 300
Anderson CB, 470, 486
Anderson DC, 84
Andree C, 255
Andreola S, 382
Annas C, 119
Anthony JP, 423
Anvari M, 288
Aoki H, 54, 136
Ariza A, 523
Arnold PG, 460
Ashmore JD Jr, 297
Atkinson K, 114
Auger FA, 247
Avins AL, 124
Avrunin JS, 43
Azodo MVU, 473

B

Baba K, 281
Baba S, 373
Babayan VK, 214
Baize M, 318
Baker AR, 312
Baldauf C, 148
Baldeyrou P, 495
Baldini MT, 382
Baldwin BJ, 421
Ballesteros A, 463
Bandarenko N, 353
Barbareschi M, 350
Barclay JR, 32
Barker CF, 484
Barlan M, 149
Barnes RW, 483
Barnett HJM, 468
Barone G, 483
Barrow RE, 69

Bartelink H, 342
Baum RA, 484
Baumann DS, 486
Baumgartner WA, 428
Baxter JN, 320
Bazán A, 463
Bear M, 462
Beaulieu M, 519
Becker DA, 238
Beckingham IJ, 447
Behrman KH, 34
Bell RS, 464
Belli F, 382
Bellomi M, 382
Belloni PA, 513
Ben-Bassat H, 427
Benedetti E, 158
Benmeir P, 427
Benninger MS, 445
Berg A, 424
Berg RD, 220
Bergelin RO, 479
Bergenfelz A, 181
Berlakovich GA, 149
Bernard D, 162
Berry D, 353
Berthiaume F, 73
Bessey PQ, 207
Bethge N, 273
Beverly JL, 228, 229
Bevilacqua P, 350
Bignon J, 502
Biller HF, 449, 452
Billing A, 132
Bismuth H, 148
Bistrian BR, 214
Bittl M, 52
Bixler EO, 238
Björvell H, 455
Blackburn JH, 245
Blakeney P, 91
Blakslee JM, 203
Blankensteijn JD, 497
Blascovich J, 33
Blatchford GJ, 263
Bleichrodt RP, 137, 431
Bloedow DC, 45
Bock DEM, 482
Bode BP, 205
Boesken WH, 160
Bokey EL, 372
Bolliger CT, 533
Bolté E, 193
Bone RC, 45
Bongard F, 130
Bonten MJM, 234
Boracchi P, 350
Borger J, 342
Böttger TC, 410
Boucher BA, 111
Bouchier-Hayes D, 314
Boutin C, 502
Bowen V, 464
Bower TC, 485, 489

Bowers CM, 507
Bowling TE, 226
Bown SG, 457
Boyd JB, 450
Boyle JO, 433
Braccini G, 102
Bramwell V, 397
Braun WE, 163
Breeden MP, 252
Bremner CG, 282
Brennan MF, 232, 260, 395
Bresson-Hadni S, 148
Briegel J, 52
Brisson J, 519
Britten-Jones R, 288
Brochard L, 42
Brock WB, 180
Brodovsky H, 384
Broemeling L, 69
Bross DS, 23
Brown DR, 134
Brown RL, 252
Brown RO, 237
Brown RS, 8
Bruggink EDM, 497
Brun JM, 182
Brun-Buisson C, 42
Brunson ME, 168
Buchbinder D, 452
Büchler M, 52
Buchman AL, 227
Buchman TG, 60
Buchmiller TL, 262
Bueno-Cavanillas A, 44
Buesa J, 397
Bulajic P, 279
Bulkley GB, 60
Burdiles P, 282
Burgers M, 397
Burke D, 507
Burke GJ, 178
Burns RP, 180
Burt M, 505
Busch C, 522
Butterfield SL, 99
Byers R, 456

C

Caffo O, 350
Caldarelli DD, 442
Caleffi M, 351
Calhoun MC, 217
Camargo CA Jr, 152
Cameron D, 428
Cameron R, 411
Campbell BH, 438
Camps C, 523
Canela M, 523
Cantó A, 523
Cantor AB, 416
Cappellari JO, 444
Carey PD, 14